MARINO'S
The *Little* ICU Book

THIRD EDITION

MARINO'S
The *Little* ICU Book

THIRD EDITION

Samuel M. Galvagno Jr, DO, PhD, MS, MBA, FCCM
Professor and Chair
Department of Anesthesiology
University of Arizona College of Medicine-Phoenix
Phoenix, Arizona

Ronald F. Sing, DO, FACS, FCCM
Professor of Surgery
Department of Surgery
Wake Forest University School of Medicine
Atrium Health - Carolinas Medical Center
Charlotte, North Carolina

Based in part on the works of:

Paul L. Marino, MD, PhD, FCCM
Clinical Associate Professor
Weill Cornell Medical College
New York, New York

Illustrations by Patricia Gast

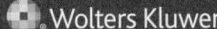

Philadelphia • Baltimore • New York • London
Buenos Aires • Hong Kong • Sydney • Tokyo

Acquisitions Editor: Keith Donnellan
Development Editor: Ashley Fischer
Marketing Manager: Kirsten Watrud
Senior Production Specialist: Bridgett Dougherty
Manager, Graphic Arts & Design: Stephen Druding
Illustrator: Patricia Gast
Manufacturing Coordinator: Lisa Bowling
Prepress Vendor: Absolute Service, Inc.

Third Edition

Copyright © 2026 Wolters Kluwer.

All rights reserved. This book is protected by copyright. No part of this book may be reproduced or transmitted in any form or by any means, including as photocopies or scanned-in or other electronic copies, or utilized by any information storage and retrieval system without written permission from the copyright owner, except for brief quotations embodied in critical articles and reviews. Materials appearing in this book prepared by individuals as part of their official duties as U.S. government employees are not covered by the above-mentioned copyright. To request permission, please contact Wolters Kluwer at Two Commerce Square, 2001 Market Street, Philadelphia, PA 19103, via email at permissions@lww.com, or via our website at shop.lww.com (products and services).

9 8 7 6 5 4 3 2 1

Printed in Mexico

Library of Congress Cataloging-in-Publication Data

Library of Congress Control Number: 2025944146

This work is provided "as is," and the publisher disclaims any and all warranties, express or implied, including any warranties as to accuracy, comprehensiveness, or currency of the content of this work.

This work is no substitute for individual patient assessment based on healthcare professionals' examination of each patient and consideration of, among other things, age, weight, gender, current or prior medical conditions, medication history, laboratory data, and other factors unique to the patient. The publisher does not provide medical advice or guidance, and this work is merely a reference tool. Healthcare professionals, and not the publisher, are solely responsible for the use of this work including all medical judgments and for any resulting diagnosis and treatments.

Given continuous, rapid advances in medical science and health information, independent professional verification of medical diagnoses, indications, appropriate pharmaceutical selections and dosages, and treatment options should be made and healthcare professionals should consult a variety of sources. When prescribing medication, healthcare professionals are advised to consult the product information sheet (the manufacturer's package insert) accompanying each drug to verify, among other things, conditions of use, warnings, and side effects and identify any changes in dosage schedule or contraindications, particularly if the medication to be administered is new, infrequently used, or has a narrow therapeutic range. To the maximum extent permitted under applicable law, no responsibility is assumed by the publisher for any injury and/or damage to persons or property, as a matter of products liability, negligence law or otherwise, or from any reference to or use by any person of this work.

shop.lww.com

To Karol, whose love grounds me, and to my daughters Aryanna and Gianna, who light my world with joy and purpose.

-SAMUEL M. GALVAGNO JR

I am deeply grateful to my wife, Victoria, whose unwavering love, patience, and encouragement make this work possible. To my children, you are the chapters I will always cherish the most.

-RONALD F. SING

Acknowledgments

Few in number, but sincere in sentiment, these acknowledgments reflect deep gratitude. First, we are immeasurably thankful for the trust Dr. Marino has placed in us to continue and build upon a remarkable book. We are eternally grateful for his mentorship, wisdom, and knowledge, and we accept this responsibility with humility and purpose. We also thank Patrica Gast, whose artistry and design talents—exemplified in the many prior versions of Dr. Marino's work—bring clarity and cohesion to this edition of *Marino's The Little ICU Book*. Finally, we extend our gratitude to Ashley Fischer, Harold Medina, and Keith Donnellan, whose expertise, insight, and editorial precision were instrumental in shaping this book.

Foreword

Almost 40 years have passed since I first conceived the idea for *The ICU Book*; that is, to create a basic textbook that focuses on fundamental concepts and practices that can be used in any ICU, regardless of the specialty designation of the unit. This was followed (years later) by the introduction of *The Little ICU Book*, to present the salient content of the larger textbook in a more succinct, and easily retrievable, format. Prior editions of these texts (seven in total) have been the product of a single author (myself), but this edition of *Marino's The Little ICU Book* marks a transition in authorship, as I have passed the mantle to two very distinguished critical care specialists: Drs. Samuel M. Galvagno and Ronald F. Sing. Both are former residents of mine whom I personally selected for this transition, and a few words about each is warranted.

Sam Galvagno is a critical care anesthesiologist who spent several years at the R Adams Cowley Shock Trauma Center at the University of Maryland where he gained multiple certifications in anesthesiology, critical care medicine, emergency medicine, neurocritical care, and critical care ultrasonography. Sam is currently Chairman of the Department of Anesthesiology at the University of Arizona College of Medicine and is also a colonel in the United States Air Force. Ron Sing is a trauma surgeon who has an added certification in surgical critical care and has served as Director of the Acute Care Surgery Fellowship at Carolinas Medical Center in Charlotte, NC. Ron has more than 230 major publications in peer-reviewed medical journals (contributed over a period of 30 years) and is currently Professor of Surgery at Wake Forest University School of Medicine. As intimated in these brief descriptions, both of these physicians have extensive experience in the care of critically ill patients, and both have achieved leadership positions in their respective fields.

A final word about the content of this book. While most of the chapter titles in the "little book" mirror those in the "big book" (i.e., the fifth edition of *Marino's The ICU Book*),

Sam and Ron have been given complete discretion to select and present the material in each chapter that they feel is most appropriate. They have also added chapters on Airway Management (Chapter 2), Extracorporeal Membrane Oxygenation (Chapter 30), and Traumatic Brain Injury (Chapter 45), which enhances the comprehensive quality of this endeavor. To conclude, I have no doubt that Sam Galvagno and Ron Sing will continue the tradition of *Marino's The Little ICU Book* as a densely packed and indispensable bedside resource for the care of critically ill patients.

Paul L. Marino, MD, PhD, FCCM

Preface

The third edition of *The Little ICU Book* (now known as *Marino's The Little ICU Book*) is the companion volume to Dr. Paul Marino's well-established critical care textbook, *Marino's The ICU Book*, now in its fifth edition. Over the years, The ICU Book has served as a trusted reference for intensivists, residents, fellows, medical students, and importantly, multidisciplinary teams of nurses, advanced practice providers, and many other medical professionals working in critical care environments worldwide. As critical care medicine has grown in complexity and scope, so too has the demand for more accessible, targeted resources that distill essential information while maintaining the depth and rigor that define the field.

This companion book was conceived with that need in mind.

Drawing on the foundation built by five editions of *Marino's The ICU Book*, and two editions of *Marino's The Little ICU Book*, we have curated and refined core content to address the daily practical challenges faced in the ICU. The aim of this book is to provide a text that enables one to quickly access essential knowledge, decision-making strategies, and evidence-based practices most relevant to frontline ICU providers. Our book is not intended to replace *The ICU Book*, but to complement it—serving as a concise, clinically oriented, "quick look up" guide for rapid consultation, bedside teaching, and ongoing learning.

As lifelong learners who embarked on our own journeys as intensive care physicians under the tutelage of Dr. Marino, we are deeply honored to continue Dr. Marino's efforts to provide a resource for the care of critically ill adults in any ICU. We remain indebted to Dr. Marino and the critical care community whose commitment, curiosity, and courage inspire this edition.

Samuel M. Galvagno Jr, DO, PhD, MS, MBA, FCCM
Ronald F. Sing, DO, FACS, FCCM

Contents

Acknowledgments vi
Foreword vii
Preface ix

SECTION I. COMMON PRACTICES

CHAPTER 1	Central Venous Access	1
CHAPTER 2	Airway Management	23
CHAPTER 3	Stress Ulcer Prophylaxis	45
CHAPTER 4	Prophylaxis for VTE	52
CHAPTER 5	Analgesia and Sedation	64
CHAPTER 6	Evaluation of Fever in the ICU	91

SECTION II. CRITICAL CARE MONITORING

CHAPTER 7	Bedside Echocardiography	109
CHAPTER 8	Oximetry and Capnography	124
CHAPTER 9	The Pulmonary Artery Catheter	136

SECTION III. RESUSCITATION FLUIDS

CHAPTER 10	Colloid and Crystalloid Fluids	153
CHAPTER 11	Fluid Management	176
CHAPTER 12	Anemia and Erythrocyte Transfusions	186
CHAPTER 13	Platelets and Plasma	210
CHAPTER 14	Coagulopathy Management	231

SECTION IV. SHOCK SYNDROMES

CHAPTER 15	Approaches to Clinical Shock	247
CHAPTER 16	Hemorrhagic Shock	260
CHAPTER 17	Cardiogenic Shock	275
CHAPTER 18	Inflammatory Shock	295

SECTION V. CARDIAC DISORDERS

CHAPTER 19	Acute Heart Failure(s)	311
CHAPTER 20	Dysrhythmias	328
CHAPTER 21	Acute Coronary Syndromes	352
CHAPTER 22	Cardiac Arrest	371

SECTION VI. RESPIRATORY DISORDERS

CHAPTER 23	Pulmonary Embolism	387
CHAPTER 24	Severe Asthma and COPD in the ICU	400
CHAPTER 25	Acute Respiratory Distress Syndrome	418

SECTION VII. RESPIRATORY MANAGEMENT

CHAPTER 26	Noninvasive Ventilation	431
CHAPTER 27	Conventional Mechanical Ventilation	443
CHAPTER 28	Ventilator-Associated Pneumonia	454
CHAPTER 29	Liberation from Mechanical Ventilation	474
CHAPTER 30	Extracorporeal Membrane Oxygenation	486

SECTION VIII. ACID-BASE DISORDERS

CHAPTER 31	Acid-Base Analysis	505
CHAPTER 32	Lactic Acidosis and Ketoacidosis	518

SECTION IX. RENAL & ELECTROLYTE DISORDERS

CHAPTER 33	Acute Kidney Injury	535
CHAPTER 34	Sodium and Chloride	556
CHAPTER 35	Potassium	575
CHAPTER 36	Magnesium	589
CHAPTER 37	Calcium and Phosphorus	598

SECTION X. THE ABDOMEN AND PELVIS

CHAPTER 38	Liver Failure	613
CHAPTER 39	Acute Pancreatitis	629
CHAPTER 40	Abdominal Infections	641
CHAPTER 41	Urinary Tract Infections	655

SECTION XI. NERVOUS SYSTEM DISORDERS

CHAPTER 42	Disorders of Consciousness	667
CHAPTER 43	Disorders of Movement	689
CHAPTER 44	Acute Stroke in the ICU	709
CHAPTER 45	Traumatic Brain Injury	727

Contents **xiii**

SECTION XII. NUTRITION AND METABOLISM

CHAPTER 46	**Nutritional Requirements**	741
CHAPTER 47	**Enteral Nutrition**	757
CHAPTER 48	**Parenteral Nutrition**	776
CHAPTER 49	**Adrenal and Thyroid Dysfunction**	790

SECTION XIII. OVERDOSES AND POISONS

CHAPTER 50	**Pharmaceutical Drug Overdoses**	807
CHAPTER 51	**Nonpharmaceutical Poisons**	825

SECTION XIV. APPENDICES

1	**Units, Conversions, and Ventilator Tidal Volumes**	843
2	**Clinical Calculators**	846

Index 851

SECTION I
COMMON PRACTICES

Chapter 1
Central Venous Access

There are four fundamental purposes for venous access, all of which are commonly required in ICU patients: fluid infusions (for both maintenance and resuscitation), intravenous medication administration, parenteral nutrition, and phlebotomy for laboratory testing. In addition, central venous access can allow for additional cardiorespiratory monitoring such as central venous pressure measurements and central venous oxygen saturation monitoring. Pulmonary artery catheters (see Chapter 9: The Pulmonary Artery Catheter) can measure right heart pressures, pulmonary artery pressures, cardiac outputs, and mixed venous oxygen saturations.

CATHETER SIZE

The size of vascular catheters is expressed in terms of their outside diameter. Size can be expressed in a metric-based *French* size or a wire-based *gauge* size.

- The French size is a series of whole numbers that increases in increments of 0.33 millimeters (e.g., 1 Fr = 0.33 mm, 2 Fr = 0.66 mm).
- The gauge size (originally developed for solid wires) has no definable relationship to other units of measurement and requires a table of reference.

PERIPHERAL INTRAVENOUS ACCESS

Peripheral intravenous (PIV) access is the most rapid and simplest method to gain venous access. The majority of fluids and IV medications can be infused via 22- or 20-gauge PIV.

Larger sizes have greater phlebitis risk. Generally, large bore PIV (16 gauge or larger) is preferred for rapid volume resuscitation due to access simplicity and rapid flow through shorter and larger bore PIV catheters as defined by Poiseuille's Law which illustrates that bore radius is a major contributing factor to flow rate (1). See Figure 1.1.

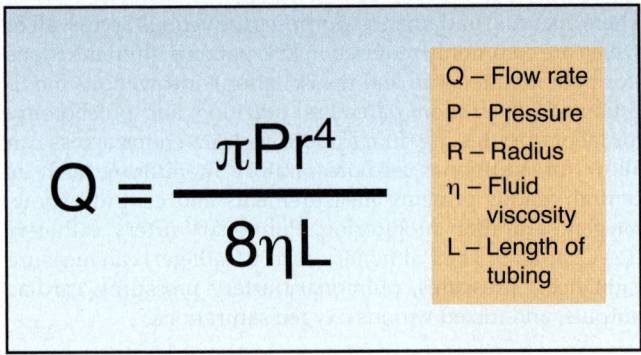

FIGURE 1.1. Poiseuille's Law.

For example, doubling the diameter of the catheter will increase flow rate by 16-fold. Catheter length and increased viscosity (e.g., blood products) also affect flow rates. Thus, blood product resuscitation for hemorrhage is typically through "large bore" (16 gauge or larger) (2). See Table 1.1.

In hypovolemic patients, however, large bore access may be challenging with collapsed and spasmed veins. The insertion of a 20-gauge PIV can be rapidly upsized to an 8.5 Fr rapid infusion catheter (RIC) over a 0.025-inch guidewire. A skin stab is required down the inserted wire to allow insertion of this large catheter. Comparison of common PIV catheters to RIC is shown in Figure 1.2. RIC catheter kit is shown in Figure 1.3.

TABLE 1.1 Flow Rates through Peripheral and Central Catheters

Gauge or French Size	Length	Gravity Flow Rate (mL/min)
20g	1.25 in (32 mm)	60
18g	1.25 in (32 mm)	105
16g	1.25 in (32 mm)	215
7 Fr Triple Lumen Catheter Distal Port (brown) 16g	200 mm	69
9 Fr Introducer Sheath	100 mm	150 Up to 300 mL/min with pressure bag
8.5 Fr Rapid Infusion Catheter	2.5 in (64 mm)	600

Adapted from Kalra A. Flow rates through peripheral and central catheters. In: *Pediatric Anesthesia Digital Handbook*. Boston, MA: Tufts Medical Center. Updated November 26, 2023.

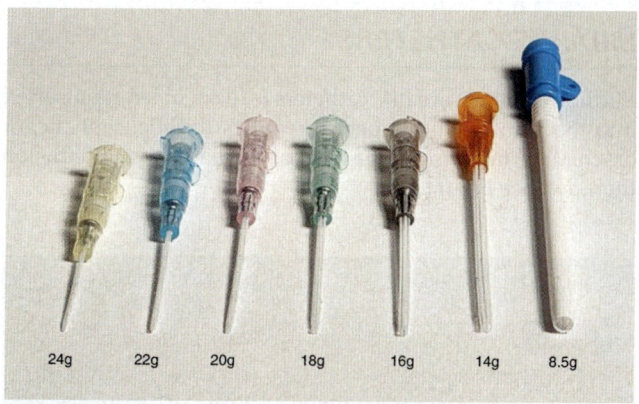

FIGURE 1.2. Peripheral intravenous (PIV) catheters.

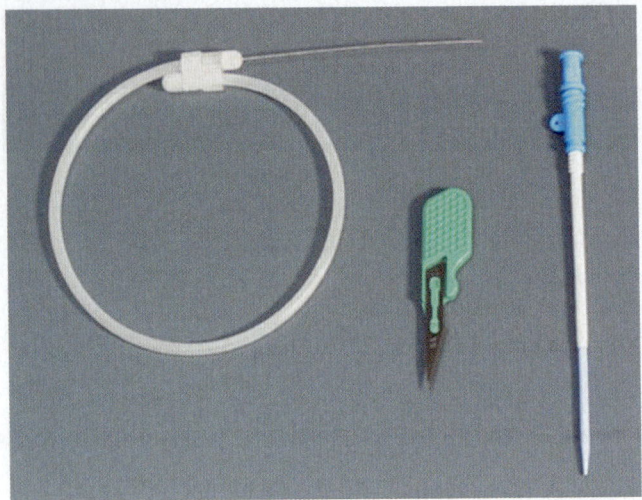

FIGURE 1.3. Rapid infusion catheter (RIC) set.

MIDLINE CATHETERS

Midline catheters are PIV catheters 8-10 cm in length inserted into the veins of the upper extremities (basilic, cephalic, or brachial) terminating at the level of the axillary vein (infusion therapy). See Figure 1.4.

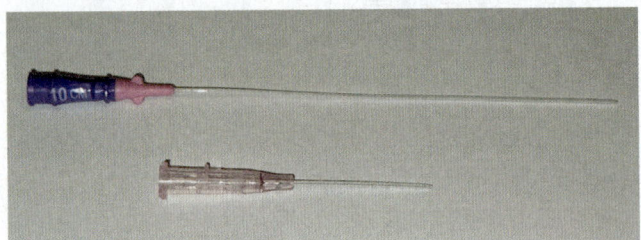

FIGURE 1.4. Midline catheters. 10 cm 20g midline catheter (top). 30 mm peripheral IV catheter (bottom).

Typically inserted by specialized vascular access teams, commonly with ultrasound guidance in patients with difficult peripheral access. Midlines have fewer bloodstream infections and less catheter occlusions than peripherally inserted central catheters (PICC lines) (3).

CENTRAL VENOUS ACCESS

Central venous access can be obtained via the insertion of flexible catheters into the internal jugular, subclavian, or femoral veins, and advanced into the superior vena cava or the inferior vena cava.

Central Venous Catheters

Modern central venous catheters (CVCs) have multiple infusion channels, like the popular triple-lumen catheter shown in Figure 1.5. This catheter has an outside diameter of 2.3 mm (Fr size 7) and is available in lengths of 16 cm (6 inches), 20 cm (8 inches), and 30 cm (12 inches). (Dimensions may vary by manufacturer).

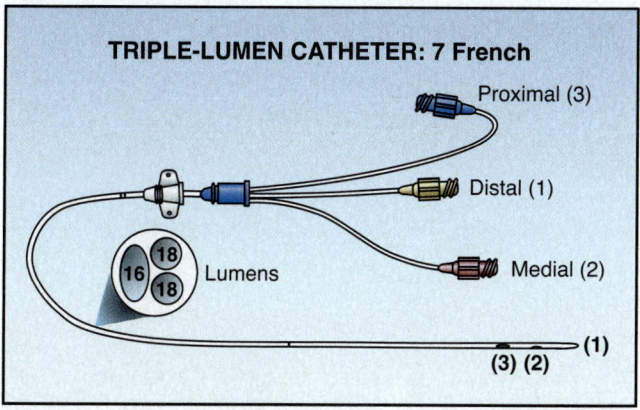

FIGURE 1.5. Triple-lumen central venous catheter, showing the gauge size of each lumen and the position of the outflow ports at the distal end of the catheter.

Introducer Sheaths

Introducer sheaths (4 Fr and larger) are used as a conduit for the insertion of other catheters and devices, e.g., pulmonary artery catheters, ECMO cannula insertion, temporary transvenous pacemakers, etc. The larger introducer sheaths (8 Fr plus) can be used in isolation as a large bore IV access for rapid volume resuscitation and transfusion, especially in hypotensive patients when PIV may be difficult. These catheters have a side port for infusion and a valve to allow insertion and extraction of catheters/devices without leaking blood. An example of an introducer sheath is shown in Figure 1.6. The obturator should be inserted whenever the insertion port is not in use. Rapid

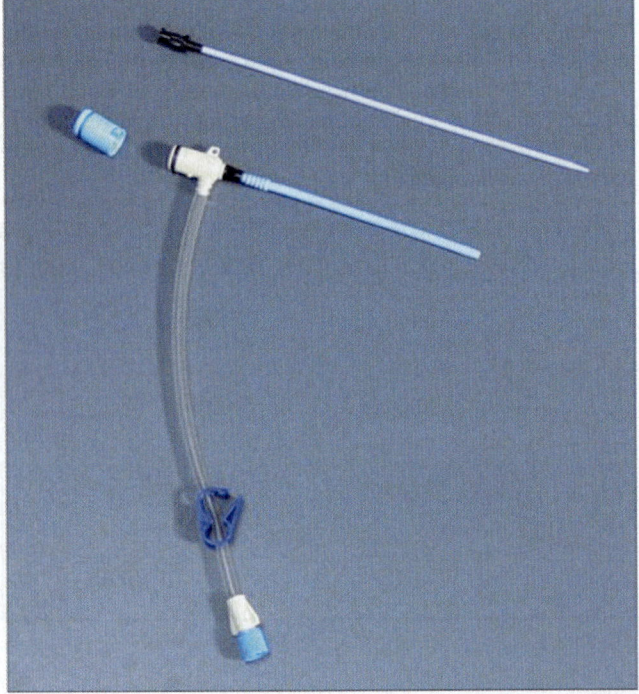

FIGURE 1.6. 9 Fr introducer sheath with dilator and obturator cap.

infusions without the obturator can cause entrainment of air into the circulation and resultant air embolism.

Antimicrobial Coating

CVCs are available with two types of antimicrobial coating:

1. Chlorhexidine and silver sulfadiazine (available from Arrow International)
2. Minocycline and rifampin (available from Cook Critical Care)

Each of these coatings can reduce the risk of catheter-related bloodstream infections (4). According to published guidelines (5), antimicrobial-coated catheters should be considered if the expected duration of catheterization is >5 days *and* if the incidence of catheter-related infections in an ICU is unacceptably high.

PICC Lines

Peripherally inserted central catheter (PICC) are long catheters that are inserted into arm veins just above the antecubital fossa and advanced into the superior vena cava. PICCs are available with multiple infusion channels, like CVCs, but they are narrower than CVCs (typically 5 Fr or 1.65 mm in

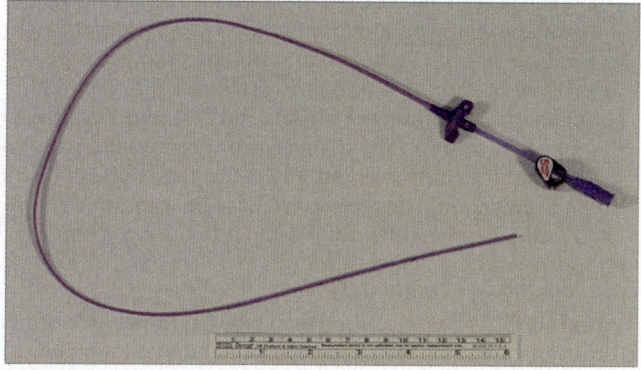

FIGURE 1.7. Peripherally inserted central catheter (PICC).

diameter) and are considerably longer than CVCs. PICCS are available in lengths of 50 cm (19.5 inches) and 70 cm (27.5 inches). As a result of the smaller diameter and longer length of PICCs, flow through PICCs is considerably slower than flow through CVCs. See Figure 1.7.

CANNULATION SITES

The following is a brief description of central venous cannulation at four different access sites:

1. Internal jugular veins
2. Subclavian veins
3. Femoral veins
4. PICC lines accessing via the veins emerging from the upper arm

Internal Jugular Vein

- The internal jugular vein (IJV) is located under the sternocleidomastoid muscle (SCM) and runs obliquely down the neck along a line drawn from the pinna of the ear to the sternoclavicular joint. In the lower neck region, the vein is often located just anterior and lateral to the carotid artery, but anatomic relationships can vary (6).
- At the base of the neck, the IJV joins the subclavian vein to form the innominate vein, and the convergence of the right and left innominate veins forms the superior vena cava.
- The right side of the neck is preferred for cannulation of the IJV because the vessels run a straight course to the right atrium. The distance from cannulation site to the right atrium is about 15 cm, so the shortest CVCs (~15 cm) should be used for right-sided cannulations (to avoid advancing the catheter tip into the right atrium).

Locating and Cannulating the Vein

Typical access is accomplished using the Seldinger technique. Ultrasound imaging has been recommended as a standard practice for locating and cannulating the IJV (7). Ultrasound guidance is associated with a higher success rate, fewer cannulation attempts, a shorter time to cannulation, and a reduced risk of carotid artery puncture (7-9). There are three approaches to the IJV relating to its position behind the SCM:

1. *Anterior:* The anterior approach is by the anterior border of the SCM.
2. *Medial:* The medial approach is at the apex of the splitting of the clavicular and sternal heads of the SCM.
3. *Lateral:* The lateral approach is via the posterior aspect of the SCM, typically where the external jugular vein crosses the SCM.

Whichever approach is taken, it is important not to cannulate the IJV through the SCM. See Figure 1.8.

To obtain a cross-sectional image of the IJV and carotid artery, place the ultrasound probe transversely across the SCM

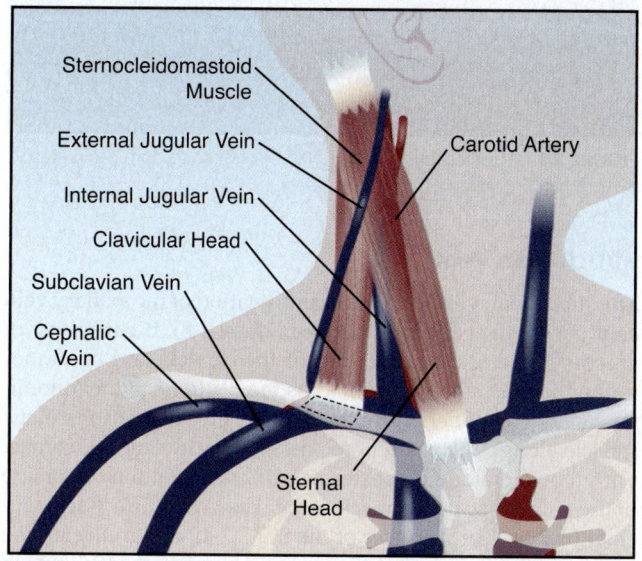

FIGURE 1.8. The large veins entering the thorax.

based on the approach selected. Typically, the IJV and carotid artery are easy to identify. Hypovolemic patients, however, can make this challenging. Compressing downward toward the vessels the neck with the ultrasound probe will collapse the IJV aiding in differentiating from the carotid artery. The access needle is visualized entering the IJV. See Figure 1.9.

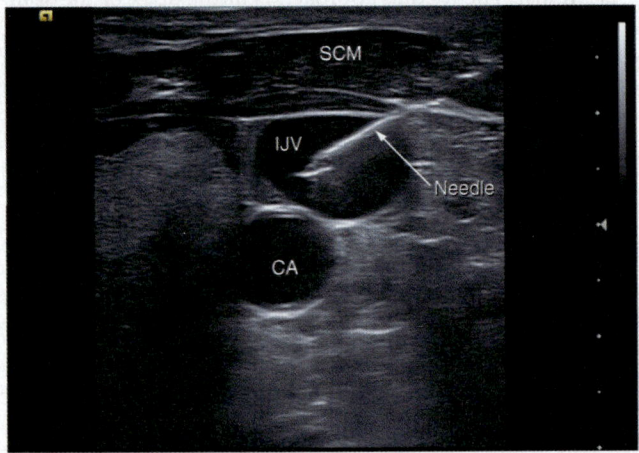

FIGURE 1.9. Access needle visualization. SCM: Sternocleidomastoid Muscle; IJV: Internal Jugular Vein; CA: Carotid Artery.

Subclavian Vein

The subclavian vein (SCV) is a continuation of the axillary vein as it passes over the first rib (see Figure 1.8). It runs most of its course along the underside of the clavicle and continues to the thoracic inlet, where it joins the IJV to form the innominate vein. The underside of the SCV sits on the anterior scalene muscle along with the phrenic nerve, which comes in contact with the vein along its posteroinferior side. On the underside of the anterior scalene muscle is the subclavian artery and brachial plexus. The diameter of the SCV (7-12 mm in the supine position) does not vary with respiration (unlike the IJV), which is attributed to strong fascial attachments that fix the vein to surrounding structures and hold it open (10). This is also the basis for the claim that volume depletion does not collapse the SCV (11), which is unproven.

Locating the Vein

The SCV is difficult to visualize with ultrasound imaging because the overlying clavicle blocks transmission of ultrasound waves. As a result, the use of surface landmarks continues to be the standard method of cannulating the SCV. The SCV can be located by identifying the clavicular head of the SCM (see Figure 1.8): The vein lies just underneath the clavicle at this point and can be cannulated from above or below the clavicle. This portion of the clavicle can be marked with a small rectangle, as shown in Figure 1.8, to guide insertion of the probe needle.

Femoral Vein

The femoral vein (FV) is a continuation of the long saphenous vein in the groin, where it is located in the femoral triangle along with the femoral artery and nerve, as shown in Figure 1.10. At the level of the inguinal crease, the vein lies just medial to the artery and is only a few centimeters from the skin. The FV is easier to cannulate when the leg is placed in abduction.

Locating the Vein

- The FV is easier to cannulate when the leg is placed in abduction.
- Locating the FV begins by palpating the femoral artery pulse, which is typically located just below and medial to the midpoint of the inguinal crease.
- If available, an ultrasound probe should be placed at the point where the femoral artery pulse is palpable to obtain cross-sectional images of the underlying vessels. The vein is then identified by its compressibility. If ultrasound imaging is not available, first palpate the femoral artery pulse and insert the probe needle (with the bevel at 12 o'clock) 1-2 cm medial to the pulse.

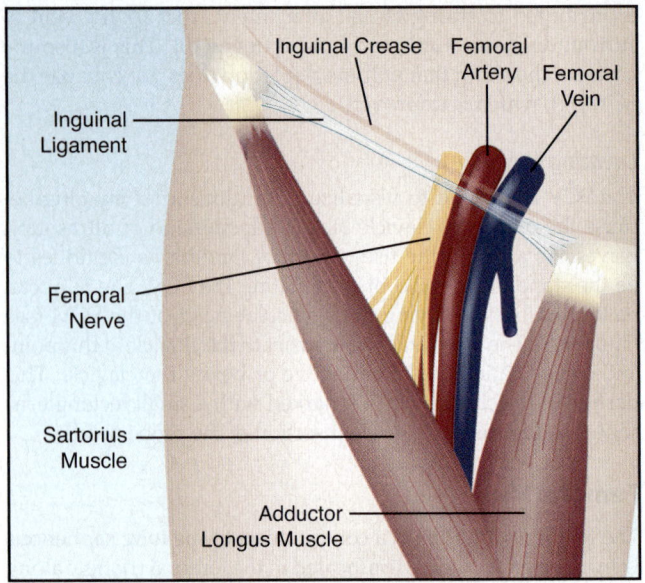

FIGURE 1.10. Anatomy of the femoral triangle.

PICC Lines

PICC lines are inserted into the basilic or cephalic vein in the arm and advanced into the superior vena cava. Like midlines, they are typically inserted by specialized vascular access teams. The basilic vein, which runs up the medial aspect of the arm, is preferred for PICC placement because it has a larger diameter than the cephalic vein, and it runs a straighter course up the arm. The benefits of PICCs over CVCs include enhanced patient comfort and mobility, and eliminating certain risks associated with CVC placement (e.g., pneumothorax).

COMPLICATIONS

Pneumothorax

The greatest risk for pneumothorax is SCV catheterization with a reported incidence of ≤5% (9,11); however, this complication is reported in 1.3% of IJV cannulations when surface landmarks are used to guide cannulation (8).

Portable chest x-rays are insensitive for the detection of pleural air, particularly in the supine position, where air collects anterior to the lung (12). Ultrasonography is a much more sensitive method of detecting pleural air when compared with portable chest radiography (13). If immediately available, bedside ultrasonography is the method of choice for the detection of pleural air in ICU patients. Rapid clinical deterioration can occur is critically ill patients, and the development of a tension pneumothorax can lead to cardiac arrest. This is a clinical diagnosis and should be rapidly treated (decompressed) with immediate needle decompression followed by tube thoracostomy. See Figure 1.11.

Cardiac Dysrhythmia

Ventricular dysrhythmias can occur during central line insertions using the Seldinger technique due to the insertion guidewire "tickling" the right ventricle. Ventricular premature complexes and ventricular tachycardia are easily remedied by withdrawing the guidewire until it is out of the ventricle. Rarely ventricular fibrillation may occur and require defibrillation.

Bleeding

Mediastinal hematomas, retroperitoneal hematomas, and hemothorax can occur during insertion, typically from overzealous insertion of dilators (overcoming the guidewire) or advancement of a dilator without a guidewire to advance the dilator. Wound hematomas are uncommon, with the risks being multiple attempts, coagulopathy, or anticoagulation.

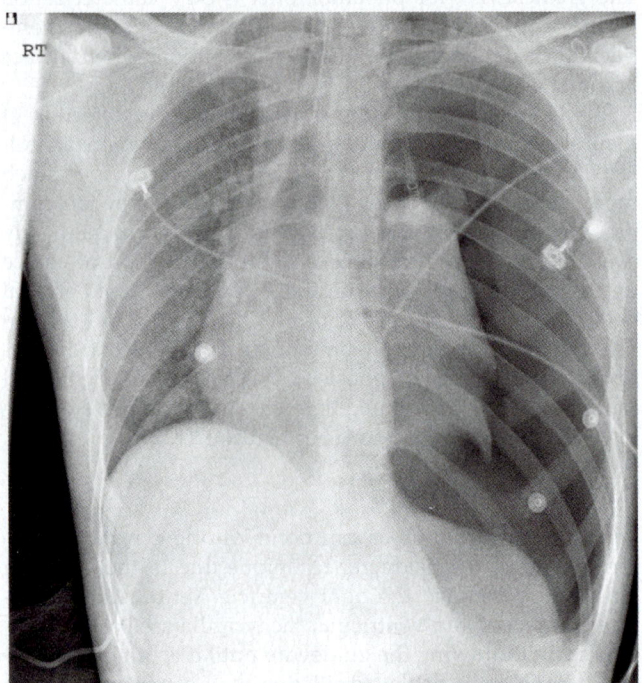

FIGURE 1.11. Tension pneumothorax showing mediastinal shift away from the pneumothorax side.

Arterial Injury

Arterial punctures are frequently inconsequential; however, puncture and/or cannulation can lead to hemorrhage and/or thrombosis. Carotid artery puncture is the most feared complication of IJV cannulation. The reported incidence is 0.5-11% when surface landmarks are used (8-9,14), and 1% when ultrasound imaging is employed (8).

Venous Air Embolism

Air entry into the central veins is a potentially lethal complication of central venous cannulation (15-16). When a vascular catheter is advanced into the thorax, the negative intrathoracic pressure generated during spontaneous breathing can draw air into the venous circulation if the catheter hub is open to the atmosphere. Both the volume and rate of air entry determine the consequences of venous air embolism. The consequences can be fatal when air entry reaches 200-300 mL (3-5 mL/kg) over a few seconds (15). See Figure 1.12 (17).

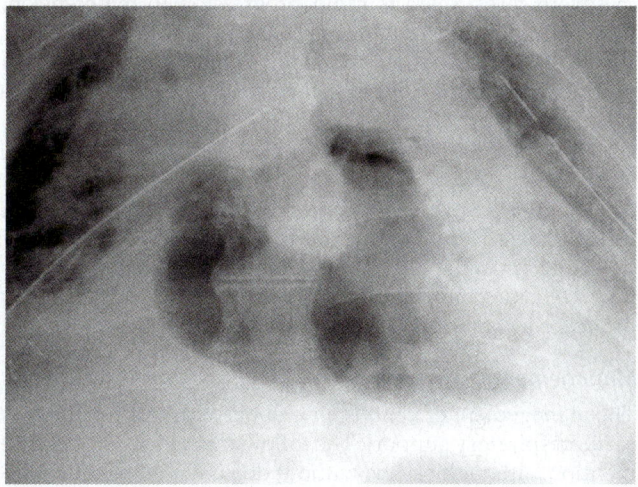

FIGURE 1.12. Venous air embolism. (Reprinted with permission from Novitsky YW, Mostafa G, Sing RF, et al. Fatal cardiac air embolism. Injury 2006;37[1]:78-80.)

Complications

The adverse consequences of venous air embolism include acute right heart failure (from an air lock in the right ventricle), leaky-capillary pulmonary edema, and acute embolic stroke (from air bubbles that pass through a patent foramen ovale) (15).

Positive-pressure ventilation is a deterrent to venous air embolism and can eliminate the problem if the intrathoracic pressure remains positive throughout the respiratory cycle. In spontaneously breathing patients, head-down body tilt (Trendelenburg position) can reduce the risk of air entry during IJV and SCV cannulation. Using appropriate precautions, the risk of symptomatic venous air embolism is <1% (16).

Venous air embolism can be clinically silent (16). In symptomatic cases, the earliest manifestation is sudden onset of dyspnea, which may be accompanied by a distressing cough. In severe cases, there is rapid progression to hypotension, oliguria, and depressed consciousness (from cardiogenic shock). The mixing of air and blood in the right ventricle can produce a drum-like, *mill wheel murmur* just prior to cardiovascular collapse (15).

Diagnosis

The diagnosis is usually a clinical diagnosis. If time permits, transthoracic Doppler ultrasound is a sensitive method of detecting air in the heart (15). (Doppler ultrasound converts flow velocities into sounds, and air in the cardiac chambers produces a characteristic high-pitched sound.)

Management

The management of venous air embolism primarily involves cardiorespiratory support. The following maneuvers deserve mention, although each is without documented benefit (15):

- If air entrainment is suspected through an indwelling catheter, you can attach a syringe to the hub of the catheter and attempt to aspirate air from the bloodstream.
- Pure oxygen breathing can reduce the volume of air in the pulmonary circulation promoting the egress of nitrogen from the pulmonary capillaries.
- Placing the patient in the left lateral decubitus position is a traditional maneuver aimed at relieving an air lock at the outflow of the right ventricle.

- Chest compressions can help to force air out of the pulmonary outflow tract and into the pulmonary circulation.

Insertion Site Thrombosis

Catheter-related thrombosis is more common than suspected but is clinically silent in most cases. Symptomatic catheter-related deep venous thrombosis incidence is 0.5% SCV, 0.9% IJV, and 1.4% FV (18). The most common complication of PICCs is catheter-induced thrombosis of the axillary and SCVs. Occlusive thrombosis with swelling of the upper arm is reported in 2-11% of patients with indwelling PICCs (19-20); the highest incidence occurs in patients with a history of venous thrombosis (19) and in cancer patients (21).

TABLE 1.2	The Central Line Bundle
Components	Recommendations
Hand Hygiene	Use an alcohol-based handrub or a soap and water handwash before and after inserting or manipulating catheters.
Barrier Precautions	Use maximal barrier precautions, including cap, mask, sterile gloves, sterile gown, and sterile full body drape, for catheter insertion or guidewire exchange.
Skin Antisepsis	Apply a chlorhexidine-based solution to the catheter insertion site and allow 2 minutes to air-dry.
Cannulation Site	When possible, avoid femoral vein cannulation.
Catheter Removal	Remove catheter promptly when it is no longer needed.

Adapted from O'Grady NP, Alexander M, Burns LA, et al. Guidelines for the prevention of intravascular catheter-related infections. Clin Infect Dis 2011;52:e162-93 and Gupta P, Thomas M, Patel A, et al. Bundle approach used to achieve zero central line-associated bloodstream infections in an adult coronary intensive care unit. BMJ Open Qual 2021;10:e001200.

Catheter-Associated Bloodstream Infection (CLABSI)

CLABSIs result in increased length of stay, healthcare costs, and mortality (18). The rate for PICCs occurs at a rate of 1 infection per 1,000 catheter days, which is similar to the rate of infection from CVCs (22). CLABSI prevention measures are two-fold: insertion-related and maintenance (23-24). The infection prevention measures recommended for central venous cannulation are shown in Table 1.2 (5,25).

Catheter Location

Because malposition of catheters occurs in 5-25% of CVC and PICC insertions (9,22), post-procedural chest x-rays are obtained routinely to evaluate catheter location and to exclude pneumothorax.

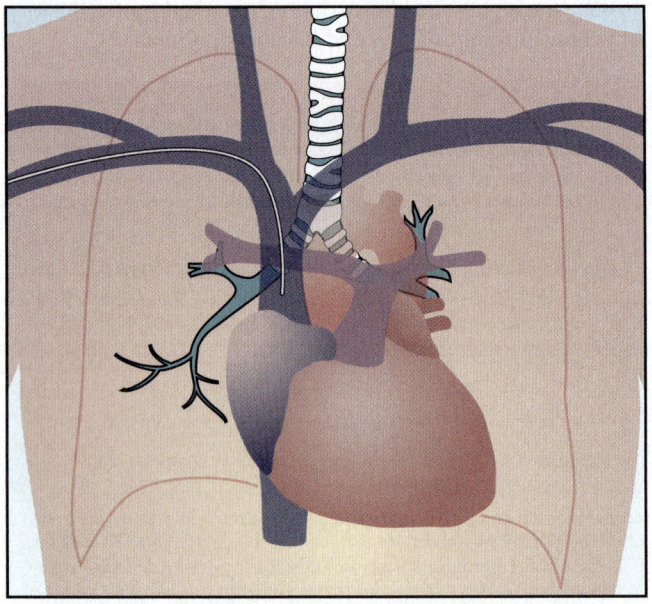

FIGURE 1.13. Properly placed upper torso central venous catheter (CVC) or peripherally inserted central catheter.

Proper Placement

A properly placed upper torso CVC or PICC should be in the superior vena cava (SVC), with the catheter tip 1-2 cm above the right atrium. The tracheal carina (i.e., the bifurcation of the trachea to form the right and left mainstem bronchi) is located just above the junction between the SVC and the right atrium, which makes it a useful landmark for evaluating catheter tip location (26). See Figure 1.13.

Left-sided CVCs, especially from the left SCV, enter the SVC at an almost 90-degree angle. It is important that the catheter tip be oriented in a vertical position, so it does not abut against the SVC wall and erode, leading to perforation. The catheter tip for femoral lines should lie within the inferior vena cava. The appropriate position for insertion via the upper torso CVC is shown in Figure 1.14. Note that the tip of the catheter is just below the tracheal carina.

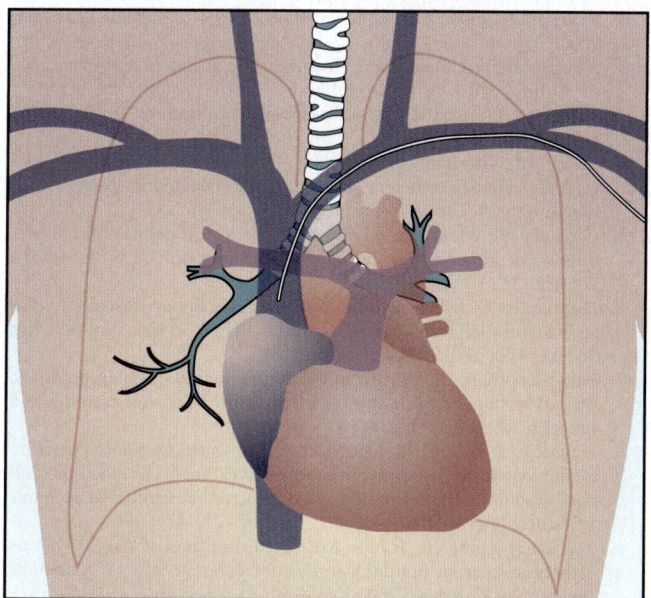

FIGURE 1.14. Position for insertion via the upper torso central venous catheter (CVC).

Catheter Tip in Right Atrium

A catheter tip that extends below the tracheal carina on a portable chest x-ray is likely to be in the right atrium. This creates a risk of right atrial perforation and cardiac tamponade (27), so retraction of catheters is generally advised when the tip is located below the carina. However, right atrial placement of CVCs is a common occurrence, with an incidence of 25% in one study (28), while right atrial perforation is a rare complication of CVC placement (27), so the need to reposition catheters advanced into the right atrium is questionable.

References

1. Reddick AD, Ronald J, Morrison WG. Intravenous fluid resuscitation: was Poiseuille right? Emerg Med J 2011;28:201-2.
2. National Association of Emergency Medical Technicians. *PHTLS: Prehospital Trauma Life Support*. 9th ed: Jones & Bartlett Learning; 2006.
3. Swaminathan L, Flanders S, Horowitz J, et al. Safety and Outcomes of midline catheters vs peripherally inserted central catheters for patients with short-term indications: a multicenter study. JAMA Intern Med 2022;182:50-8.
4. Casey AL, Mermel LA, Nightingale P, Elliott TS. Antimicrobial central venous catheters in adults: a systematic review and meta-analysis. Lancet Infect Dis 2008;8:763-76.
5. O'Grady NP, Alexander M, Burns LA, et al. Guidelines for the prevention of intravascular catheter-related infections. Clin Infect Dis 2011;52:e162-93.
6. Hernandez D, Diaz F, Rufino M, et al. Subclavian vascular access stenosis in dialysis patients: natural history and risk factors. J Am Soc Nephrol 1998;9:1507-10.
7. Feller-Kopman D. Ultrasound-guided internal jugular access: a proposed standardized approach and implications for training and practice. Chest 2007;132:302-9.
8. Hayashi H, Amano M. Does ultrasound imaging before puncture facilitate internal jugular vein cannulation? Prospective randomized comparison with landmark-guided puncture in ventilated patients. J Cardiothorac Vasc Anesth 2002;16:572-5.
9. Ruesch S, Walder B, Tramer MR. Complications of central venous catheters: internal jugular versus subclavian access—a systematic review. Crit Care Med 2002;30:454-60.

10. Fortune JB, Feustel P. Effect of patient position on size and location of the subclavian vein for percutaneous puncture. Arch Surg 2003;138:996-1000; discussion 1.
11. Fragou M, Gravvanis A, Dimitriou V, et al. Real-time ultrasound-guided subclavian vein cannulation versus the landmark method in critical care patients: a prospective randomized study. Crit Care Med 2011;39:1607-12.
12. Tocino IM, Miller MH, Fairfax WR. Distribution of pneumothorax in the supine and semirecumbent critically ill adult. AJR Am J Roentgenol 1985;144:901-5.
13. Collins GR, Clarke LE. Delayed pneumothorax: a complication of central venous catheterization. Surg Rounds 1994;17:589-94.
14. Reuber M, Dunkley LA, Turton EP, et al. Stroke after internal jugular venous cannulation. Acta Neurol Scand 2002;105:235-9.
15. Mirski MA, Lele AV, Fitzsimmons L, Toung TJ. Diagnosis and treatment of vascular air embolism. Anesthesiology 2007;106:164-77.
16. Vesely TM. Air embolism during insertion of central venous catheters. J Vasc Interv Radiol 2001;12:1291-5.
17. Novitsky YW, Mostafa G, Sing RF, et al. Fatal cardiac air embolism. Injury 2006;37:78-80.
18. Parienti JJ, Mongardon N, Megarbane B, et al. Intravascular complications of central venous catheterization by insertion site. N Engl J Med 2015;373:1220-9.
19. Evans RS, Sharp JH, Linford LH, et al. Risk of symptomatic dvt associated with peripherally inserted central catheters. Chest 2010; 138:803-10.
20. Hughes ME. PICC-related thrombosis: pathophysiology, incidence, morbidity and the effect of ultrasound-guided placement technique on occurrence in cancer patients. J Assoc Vasc Access 2011; 16:8-18.
21. Marin A, Bull L, Kinzie M, Andresen M. Central catheter-associated deep vein thrombosis in cancer: clinical course, prophylaxis, treatment. BMJ Support Palliat Care 2021;11:371-80.
22. Ng PK, Ault MJ, Ellrodt AG, Maldonado L. Peripherally inserted central catheters in general medicine. Mayo Clin Proc 1997;72: 225-33.
23. Bell T, O'Grady NP. Prevention of central line-associated bloodstream infections. Infect Dis Clin North Am 2017;31:551-9.
24. Haddadin Y, Annamaraju P, Regunath H. Central Line Associated Blood Stream Infections. In: StatPearls. Treasure Island (FL): StatPearls Publishing; 2022.
25. Gupta P, Thomas M, Patel A, et al. Bundle approach used to achieve zero central line-associated bloodstream infections in an adult coronary intensive care unit. BMJ Open Qual 2021;10:e001200.

26. Stonelake PA, Bodenham AR. The carina as a radiological landmark for central venous catheter tip position. Br J Anaesth 2006;96:335-40.
27. Booth SA, Norton B, Mulvey DA. Central venous catheterization and fatal cardiac tamponade. Br J Anaesth 2001;87:298-302.
28. Vezzani A, Brusasco C, Palermo S, et al. Ultrasound localization of central vein catheter and detection of postprocedural pneumothorax: an alternative to chest radiography. Crit Care Med 2010;38:533-8.

Airway Management

Chapter 2

Airway management is one of the most frequently performed procedures in the ICU (1-2); however, one in four major airway events (i.e., death, anoxic brain injury, surgical airway, hypoxemia) are more likely to occur in the ICU compared to the operating room (2), and more than half of all airway events in the ICU are considered preventable (3). Hence, prompt, safe, and definitive management of the airway is a fundamental priority for ICU patients. A comprehensive discussion of specific airway techniques is beyond the scope of this chapter; the reader is referred to several excellent textbooks that describe these techniques in detail (4-6). This chapter focuses on endotracheal intubation—the most commonly employed technique for securing a definitive airway in the ICU.

ASSESSMENT OF THE DIFFICULT AIRWAY

Definition

A difficult airway exists when a conventionally trained anesthesiologist, or other healthcare provider skilled at airway management, encounters difficulty with facemask ventilation of the upper airway, difficulty with tracheal intubation, or both (7). Others include failure to place a supraglottic airway (SGA) as part of the definition (8). Up to 20% or more airways in the ICU may be considered *difficult* using these definitions (9).

Assessment

A variety of bedside tests have been described to identify patients at risk for having a difficult airway. No single test is sensitive and specific, and the clinical utility of using these tests has been questioned (10). An assessment of multiple patient factors is recommended, preferentially in a stepwise approach (Figure 2.1) (6,11).

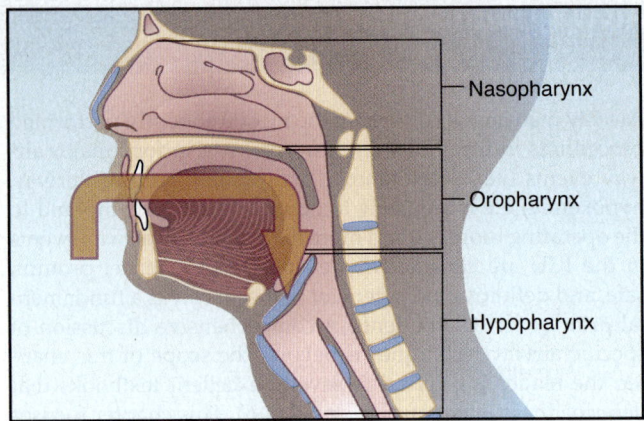

FIGURE 2.1. Bedside airway assessment. The examiner begins externally, examining the teeth, followed by an intraoral exam, and then additional external landmarks (see Table 2.1).

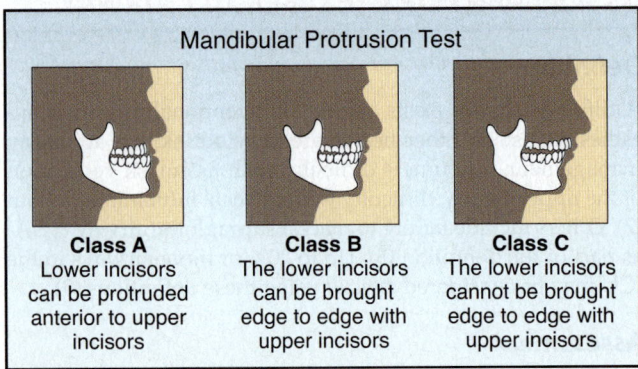

FIGURE 2.2. Mandibular protrusion test. The patient is asked to bite the upper lip. Inability to bite the upper lip (i.e., assuming a prognathic position) is associated with decreased jaw mobility.

Factors associated with difficult laryngoscopy are listed in Table 2.1. (See also Figures 2.2-2.4.)

TABLE 2.1 A 10-step Technique for the Assessment of Potentially Difficult Endotracheal Intubation

Step	Parameter	Significance
1	Length of upper incisors	May prevent axis of laryngoscope from entering mouth caudally
2	Presence of "buck teeth"	Prevents caudad entry of laryngoscope
3	Ability to assume prognathic position (upper lip bite test; Figure 2.2)	Inability to bite the upper lip suggests temporomandibular limitation or mandibular immobility
4	Mouth opening (5 cm or ~3 finger widths)	Prevents insertion of laryngoscope
5	Tongue size / Mallampati classification (Figure 2.3)	Large tongue / correlation with poor laryngoscopic views
6	Height and width of palate	Estimates lateral volume of the oropharynx; if narrow, laryngoscope will not fit
7	Thyromental distance (6 cm; Figure 2.4)	Smaller thyromental distance corresponds with potentially more anterior airway
8	Mandibular compliance	Less compliance associated with narrower airway
9	Neck length	Shorter neck associated with more difficult intubation
10	Cervical range of motion	Neck immobility prevents proper alignment of pharyngeal, laryngeal, and oral axes

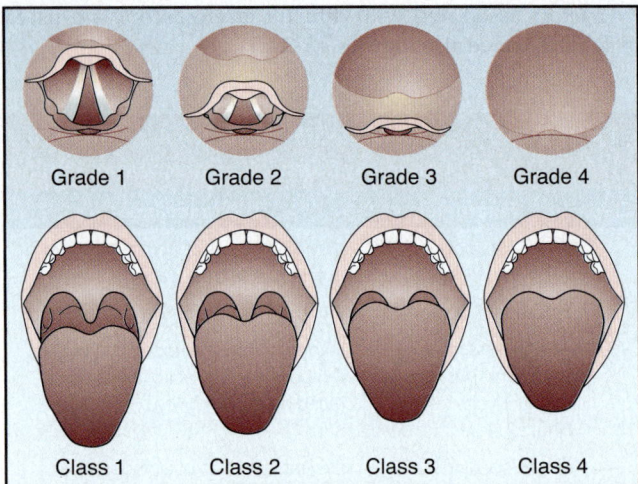

FIGURE 2.3. The Mallampati classification. Examination of the tongue and pharynx (class) corresponds to laryngoscopic view (Cormack-Lehane view). (Adapted from Mallampati SR, Mallampati SR, Gatt SP, et al. A clinical sign to predict difficult tracheal intubation: a prospective study. Can Anaesth Soc J 1985;32[4]:429-34 and Cormack RS, Lehane J. Difficult tracheal intubation in obstetrics. Anaesthesia 1984;39:1105.)

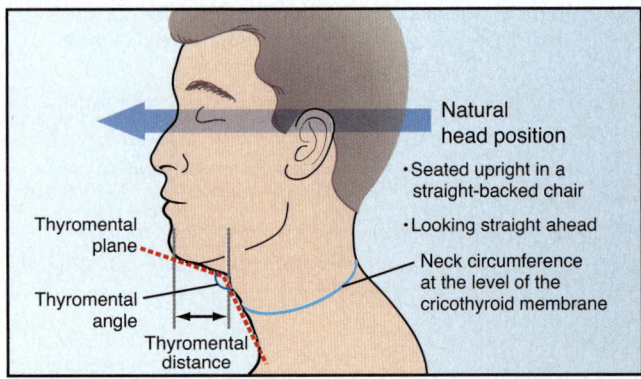

FIGURE 2.4. Thyromental distance. The distance is measured from the inside of the mentum to the thyroid notch. A distance less than 6 cm may suggest a difficult airway.

Multiple factors (Table 2.2) have been independently associated with difficult or impossible mask ventilation (12).

TABLE 2.2　Factors Associated with Difficult or Impossible Mask Ventilation

Age >55
BMI >26 kg/m^2
Presence of a beard
Lack of teeth (edentulous)
History of snoring
Poor mandibular protrusion

From Kheterpal S, Han R, Tremper KK, et al. Incidence and predictors of difficult and impossible mask ventilation. Anesthesiology 2006;105(5):885-91.

Ultrasound

Upper airway ultrasound is another point-of-care option for identifying anatomical features that may be associated with difficult intubation. Anatomical parameters indicating a potentially difficult airway include:

- Inability to visualize the hyoid bone;
- Hyomental distance <1 cm; or
- Pretracheal tissue >28 cm (anterior neck thickness [14])

Ultrasound can also be helpful for identifying the location of the cricothyroid membrane prior to cricothyrotomy (13-14).

PREPARATION FOR ENDOTRACHEAL INTUBATION

Critically ill patients who require endotracheal intubation are at higher risk for adverse events including hypoxemia, hypotension, and cardiac arrest. Notwithstanding anatomical factors, critically ill patients may also have a *physiologically* difficult airway due to physiological derangements that increase the risk of complications (15). In this section, preparatory measures are described to minimize or prevent adverse events during endotracheal intubation.

Preoxygenation

Critically ill patients frequently have decreased lung compliance, compression of airways, impaired ventilation-perfusion matching, and reduction of lung volumes and lung capacities, including functional residual capacity. These pathophysiological features are exacerbated in obese patients (16). Thus, critically ill patients are at high risk for hypoxemia and measures to increase the fraction of alveolar oxygen (FAO_2) should be taken prior to the administration of induction include pre-oxygenation to remove nitrogen (denitrogenation). Preoxygenation can be performed using a variety of techniques, each with advantages and disadvantages (Table 2.3).

Positioning

Head and body positioning prior to endotracheal intubation is essential to maximize first-pass success rates and to prevent further decreases in functional residual capacity and

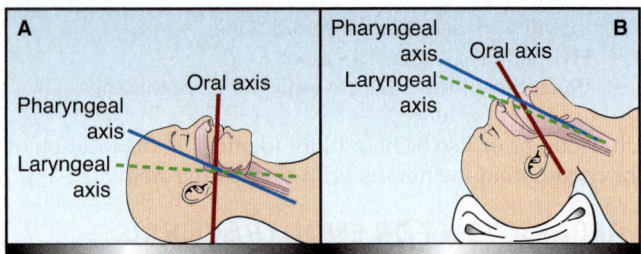

FIGURE 2.5. The sniffing position. In (A), the axes are not optimally aligned. In (B), using a combination of flexion of the neck and extension of the head, the sniffing position is achieved, aligning all three axes, and facilitating the optimal laryngoscopic view. (Redrawn from Mace SE. Challenges and advances in intubation: airway evaluation and controversies with intubation. Emerg Med Clin North Am 2008;26[4]:977-1000.)

TABLE 2.3 Techniques to Ensure Adequate Pre-oxygenation / Denitrogenation Prior to Endotracheal Intubation

Technique	Advantages	Disadvantages
Bag-valve mask (BVM) with 100% FiO_2, 15 lpm	• Standard of care in the operating room and other environments, whenever possible • Best method for denitrogenation/increasing FAO_2	• Requires a tight seal • Not tolerated by agitated/delirious patients
BVM with nasal cannula (10-15 lpm)	• Provides additional FiO_2 • Apneic oxygenation during intubation attempt (nasal cannula is left on) • Nasal dryness/epistaxis rare	• BVM seal violated (if used with BVM) • Requires two O_2 sources (not an issue in most ICUs)
Noninvasive ventilation (CPAP/BiPAP at 10-15 cm H_2O, 100% FiO_2)	• Best "safe apnea" time compared to face mask or non-rebreathing mask	• Requires additional equipment (mask, machine) • Contraindicated in patients at risk for aspiration
High flow nasal cannula (50-60 lpm, 100% FiO_2)	• Easy to apply • Humidification allows higher flows • Can be used in conjunction with BVM • Higher PaO_2 attained compared with simple facemask • May provide apneic oxygenation during attempts	• Requires additional equipment (nasal prongs, machine) • BVM seal violated (if used with BVM) • Minimal positive airway pressure delivered • Requires two O_2 sources (not an issue in most ICUs)

hypoxemia. The *sniffing* position (Figure 2.5) is recommended for patients without cervical spine injuries or immobility because this position aligns the pharyngeal, laryngeal, and oral axes to provide the optimal laryngeal view.

In obese patients, the use of blankets or a ramp device can help improve first-pass success rates while also prolonging the safe apnea time (Figure 2.6) (17).

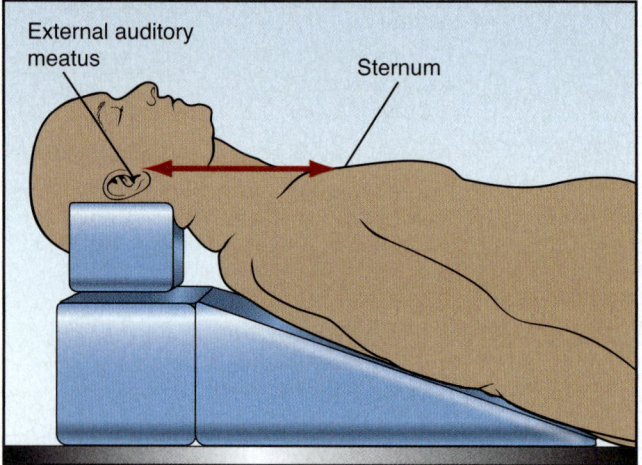

FIGURE 2.6. The ramp position. The external auditory meatus is aligned with the sternum/sternal notch. This position is particularly useful for obese patients.

When the sniffing or ramp position cannot be implemented, use of the reverse Trendelenburg position has been shown to both prolong safe apnea time and assist with a more rapid recovery from hypoxemia (18).

Equipment

A list of recommended equipment for endotracheal intubation is provided in Table 2.4.

TABLE 2.4 Equipment List for Endotracheal Intubation in the ICU

- Oxygen mask/nasal cannula/bag-valve mask (BVM)
- Oxygen source
- Suction catheter and suction source
- Oral and nasal airways
- Tongue depressor
- Laryngoscope handles and blades
- Endotracheal tubes
- Intubation stylet
- Videolaryngoscope (with associated stylet)
- Gum elastic bougie
- Magill's forceps
- End-tidal CO_2 (colorimetric) detector or in-line monitoring
- Stethoscope
- 10 mL syringe for cuffed tube inflation
- Tape
- Induction drugs
- Local anesthetics (if performing an awake intubation)
- Fiberoptic scope (for potentially difficult airways)
- #10 or #11 blade scalpel
- Free-flowing intravenous or intraosseous access
- Vasopressors (syringes and intravenous bags)
- Blood products (for actively hemorrhaging patients)

RAPID SEQUENCE INDUCTION AND INTUBATION

Rapid sequence induction and intubation (RSII) is the technique frequently used to establish a definitive airway in critically ill patients (19). RSII is predicated on the assumption that critically ill patients have a full stomach and will be at risk for aspiration if excessive BVM ventilation is provided.

Preparation

RSII involves a highly organized sequence of events starting with preoxygenation for at least three minutes followed by administration of induction agents, adjuncts, and neuromuscular blockers (NMBs).

Mask Ventilation

Although avoidance of BVM ventilation has been the traditional recommendation in RSII, many practitioners find that gentle mask ventilation (inspiratory pressure <20 cm H_2O) is acceptable during the induction sequence. Gentle mask ventilation may help prevent hypoxemia in obese, pregnant, pediatric, and critically ill patients, and allows testing for the adequacy of mask ventilation if intubation attempts fail.

Preoxygenation with Nasal Cannula

A nasal cannula or high-flow nasal cannula can be applied before intubation as described previously.

Gastric Decompression

For patients with severe gastric distention, some have proposed placing a gastric tube for decompression prior to RSII to remove undigested food particles (20). Use of gastric tubes must be carefully weighed against the risks of inducing emesis, trauma to the aerodigestive track, increases in intra-cranial pressure (in neurosurgical patients or traumatic brain injury patients) and delays in airway management to perform the procedure.

Gastric Ultrasound

Bedside ultrasound can be utilized to assess aspiration risk by quantitating the amount of gastric volume. A volume greater than 200-300 mL suggests the presence of severe distension with increased risk for aspiration (Figure 2.7) (20-21).

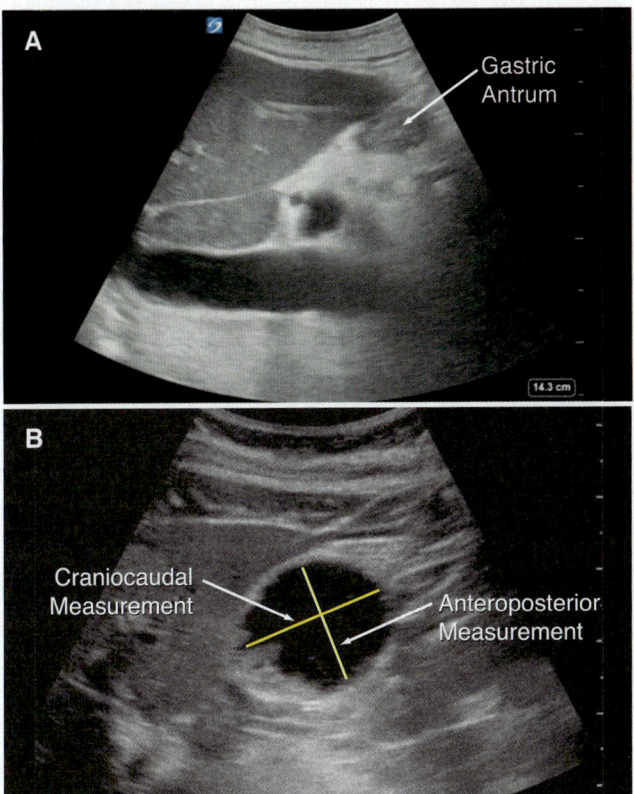

FIGURE 2.7. Gastric ultrasound. (A) The gastric antrum is visualized. The antrum appears flat, indicating low gastric volume. (B) The antrum is clear and distended, indicating the presence of fluid. With the measurement of craniocaudal and anteroposterior dimensions, the gastric volume can be estimated with the following equation: volume (mL) = 27 + (14.6 × CSA) − (1.28 × age). CSA (cross-sectional area) = ¼ × 3.14 × (anteroposterior × craniocaudal length in cm). Ideally, the patient should be examined in a longitudinal plane with a curvilinear probe (1-8 MHz) with the patient positioned head up at less than 45° and examined in both the supine and right lateral decubitus position.

TABLE 2.5 Induction Agents Used for Rapid Sequence Induction and Intubation (RSII)

Induction Agent	Dose for RSII	Onset	Duration of Action	Comment
Propofol	1-3 mg/kg	10-30 s	8-10 min	Dose usually reduced, sometimes by as much as 1/10 the recommended induction dose; causes decreased systemic vascular resistance and hypotension
Ketamine	1-2 mg/kg IV 2-4 mg/kg IM	30-60 s	5-20 min	Acceptable for use in patients with increased ICP; direct myocardial depressant but has indirect stimulatory effects (best avoided in patients with coronary artery disease)
Etomidate	0.2-0.3 mg/kg	30-45 s	10-20 min	A single dose causes adrenocortical suppression; controversial in septic shock
Remifentanil	1 µg/kg	30-60 s	<10 min	250 times more potent than morphine; may cause hypotension; not a reliable amnestic; does not accumulate; metabolized by non-specific esterases
Midazolam	0.3-0.6 mg/kg	2-3 min	20-30 min	When combined with opioids, can cause marked hypotension and respiratory depression

Induction

Before NMBs are administered, an induction agent is administered. Induction agents used in the ICU are reviewed in Table 2.5.

Neuromuscular Blockade

Succinylcholine (1-1.5 mg/kg) or rocuronium (0.8-1.2 mg/kg) is administered for neuromuscular blockade to abolish airway reflexes that may cause laryngospasm. Succinylcholine can be administered intramuscularly if an intravenous line is not established, but an increased dose of 3-4 mg/kg is recommended for this route. In most patients, both succinylcholine and rocuronium (at a dose of 1.2 mg/kg) provide optimal intubating conditions by 60 seconds (22).

Priming Doses

Priming doses of nondepolarizing agents are usually not considered for critically ill patients since these agents must be administered at least three minutes before the loading dose of muscle relaxant is administered, and in elderly or debilitated patients, pretreatment with a small dose of muscle relaxant may predispose to aspiration.

Succinylcholine

Succinylcholine is contraindicated in patients with burns, open globe injuries, neuromuscular disorders, hyperkalemia, pseudocholinesterase deficiency, severe crush injuries, or chronic paralysis.

Rocuronium

Rocuronium, a nondepolarizing agent, is an alternative when succinylcholine is contraindicated, but this agent cannot be administered intramuscularly, and the duration of action is much longer (typically up to 45 minutes) than succinylcholine (6-10 minutes). Rocuronium can be immediately reversed by sugammadex at a dose of 16 mg/kg, a selective NMB binding agent, but rapid NMB reversal is not usually an option in the ICU.

Adjuncts

Pharmacological adjuvants, such as opioids, may be considered during RSII, but owing to time pressure, these agents are frequently omitted. If administered, fentanyl (2 µg/kg), alfentanil (20-30 µg/kg) or remifentanil (1 µg/kg) may help attenuate hemodynamic responses to intubation, but opioids alone do not provide adequate amnesia and are usually not recommended as sole induction agents for RSII due to the potential for patient recall.

Midazolam

Midazolam is a short acting benzodiazepine with excellent amnestic properties that may also be given intramuscularly, but this agent may take 2-3 minutes to work.

Lidocaine

Following preoxygenation, intravenous lidocaine may be considered (1.5-2 mg/kg) for the theoretical benefit of preventing rises in intracranial pressure (ICP), although evidence to support the use of lidocaine is tangential and largely extrapolated from nontrauma populations (23). Lidocaine may precipitate hypotension—an undesirable side effect in critically ill patients.

Endotracheal Intubation – Cricoid Pressure, Video Laryngoscopy, Suction

The reader is referred to several excellent references regarding techniques for endotracheal intubation (4-6). Three technical aspects that are pertinent for endotracheal intubation in the ICU are discussed next: cricoid pressure, use of video laryngoscopes, and suction-assisted laryngoscopy.

Cricoid Pressure

Cricoid pressure (i.e., the "Sellick" maneuver) involves the application of backward and upward pressure to the cricoid cartilage with the goal of occluding the esophagus to prevent aspiration of gastric contents into the lungs. A significant amount of pressure is required to perform the technique. While the patient is awake, a 10 N or 1 kg pressure is applied until induction agents have been delivered. After the patient is induced and paralyzed, approximately 30 N or 3 kg is applied in a posterior direction to the cricoid ring. This technique has been associated rarely with complications including airway compromise, cricoid fracture, esophageal rupture, and potential exacerbation of cervical spine injuries (24). Furthermore, in a large multicenter randomized trial, cricoid pressure was not found to be any better than a sham procedure for the prevention of pulmonary aspiration (25). If cricoid pressure is used, pressure should be released if the laryngoscopic view is poor.

Video Laryngoscopy

Video laryngoscopy has evolved as a technology that enhances situational awareness for all ICU team members by allowing the entire team to visualize the airway during endotracheal intubation. Video laryngoscopy is readily available worldwide and can be used during all stages of intubation including initial laryngoscopy and awake intubation. In a large multicenter randomized trial conducted in 17 emergency departments and ICUs, video laryngoscopy resulted in a higher first-pass success rate compared to conventional laryngoscopy (26). In another meta-analysis, video laryngoscopy was associated with a reduced risk of difficult intubation and a higher first-pass success rate in adult ICU patients (27).

Suction Assisted Laryngoscopy (Ducanto Technique)

Blood and emesis can significantly impede laryngoscopic visualization during either direct or video laryngoscopy. Suction-assisted laryngoscopic and airway decontamination (SALAD), also known as the Ducanto technique, involves the use of preemptive rigid suctioning prior to and during introduction of a laryngoscope blade (28). The technique involves the following steps:

1. Following appropriate positioning of the patient, a rigid suction catheter is introduced with the right hand and swept from side-to-side prior to advancing the laryngoscope blade.
2. The suction catheter is gripped like a laryngoscope and used to displace the tongue prior to laryngoscopy.
3. The suction catheter is then withdrawn and reinserted into the left side of the mouth with the suction catheter tip advanced until positioned near the upper esophagus.
4. The suction catheter is then "parked" in this position to allow for continuous suctioning of the hypopharynx while endotracheal intubation is completed.
5. Following successful placement of the endotracheal tube, a soft suction catheter is used to suction the endotracheal tube to remove any residual contaminants.

Supraglottic Airway Devices

A variety of supraglottic airway (SGA) devices are available for use when attempts at endotracheal intubation or BVM ventilation fail. Commonly used SGAs are listed in Table 2.6. SGAs, like endotracheal intubation, require considerable training and all must be eventually replaced with a definitive airway.

Awake Fiberoptic Intubation

When the use of neuromuscular blocking drugs has the potential to cause immediate airway collapse (i.e., mediastinal mass or airway mass) or a high probability of airway loss (i.e., tracheal stenosis, known difficult airway), awake oral fiberoptic intubation may be considered. The term *awake* is a misnomer; the patient maintains spontaneous ventilation throughout the procedure under sedation with amnestic agents. This method may also be advantageous for patients with an unstable cervical spine injury as the potential to exacerbate the injury with laryngoscopy may be avoided. Steps for this technique, using topicalization with local anesthetics, are listed in Table 2.7. Alternatively, the topicalization techniques

TABLE 2.6 Commonly Used Supraglottic Airway Devices (SGAs)

Device	Considerations	Potential Advantages
Laryngeal Mask Airway (LMA)	• Oldest (invented in 1983) and most commonly used SGA device • Multiple variants including devices to facilitate gastric suction	• Inexpensive • Prevalent in most operating rooms and emergency departments
King LTS-D™	• Laryngeal tube designed to intubate the esophagus • Two cuffs: 1) distal esophageal 2) proximal oropharyngeal • Some versions have gastric decompression ports • Depth markings give an indication of the distance to the vocal cords when properly inflated	• Adult sizes based on height
i-gel™	• Non-inflatable SGA • Three adult sizes; color coded for weight • Black line indicates proper position at the incisors • Gastric channel and intubation conduit in newer versions	• Less tissue compression, no syringe required • Epiglottic blocker to prevent epiglottis from obstructing the airway after placement
Air-Q™	• Laryngeal airway with removable connector to allow intubation with standard endotracheal tube • Integrated bite block	• No syringe required • Accommodates standard endotracheal tubes (for conversion to definitive airway) • Aperture deflates slightly during BVM deflation (theoretical benefit of less blood vessel compression)

described in the table can also be used with a videolaryngoscope (i.e., "awake" video laryngoscopy).

TABLE 2.7 Steps Required for Awake Fiberoptic Intubation (Topicalization Method)

I. Preparation/ Sedation	a. Glycopyrrolate 0.2-0.4 mg IV (to help reduce secretions) b. Midazolam 0.5 mg IV, titrated to effect (avoid concomitant use of opioids) c. Dexmedetomidine • Time permitting: 10 minute loading infusion 0.5-1.0 μg/kg • Continuous infusion: 0.2-0.7 μg/kg/min • Effects noticeable in 5-10 minutes
II. Equipment	a. Fiberoptic scope b. Multiple endotracheal tube sizes c. Lubricant d. Long suction tubing for the fiberoptic scope e. Gauze pads
III. Topicalization/ Technique	a. Apply nasal cannula/nasal cannula with capnography capability b. Maintain spontaneous ventilation at all times c. Glossopharyngeal nerve topicalization: • Place 2-3 mL 5% lidocaine ointment on a tongue depressor and apply to the back of the tongue (this anesthetizes the glossopharyngeal nerve) d. Superior laryngeal nerve topicalization: 1. Using cotton balls or 4×4 cm gauze, soak with 4% or 1% lidocaine 2. Using either a Magill forceps or right angle tonsil holder, grab the cotton ball or 4×4 gauze and introduce gently into the posterior oropharynx, past the base of the tongue 3. Hold in place for 60-90 seconds 4. Repeat for each side e. Recurrent laryngeal nerve topicalization: 1. Place an oral airway to prevent biting down on the fiberoptic scope (with proper topicalization, this should be tolerated without gagging) 2. Inject 1-2 mL of 1% lidocaine through the injection port on the fiberoptic scope directly onto the vocal cords 3. Place the endotracheal tube and confirm placement with capnography/fiberoptic visualization

The Surgical Airway

A patient committed to RSII and who subsequently cannot be ventilated or intubated requires a surgical airway. Options include a surgical cricothyrotomy (also referred to as *cricothyroidotomy*) or tracheostomy; cricothyrotomy is the technique of choice given a lower incidence of bleeding and greater ease for successful performance.

Cricothyrotomy Procedure

Key steps in cricothyrotomy procedure are as follows:

1. In cases where a difficult airway is anticipated, it is best to palpate and mark the cricothyroid membrane prior to RSII.
2. Once the decision is made to proceed with cricothyroidotomy, the neck is rapidly prepared with chlorhexidine or iodine and the thyroid notch, thyroid cartilage, cricothyroid membrane, cricoid cartilage, and trachea are identified by palpation.
3. The thyroid cartilage is stabilized with the nondominant hand while a 2.0 to 2.5 cm vertical incision is made over the cricothyroid membrane with a #10 or #11 surgical blade.
4. A hemostat or tracheal spreader (or reverse end of the scalpel handle) is introduced into the incision and rotated 90° to widen the aperture.
5. Either a cuffed endotracheal tube (5.0 or 6.0) or tracheostomy tube is inserted through the incision. Alternatively, a gum elastic endotracheal tube introducer (i.e., "bougie") can be inserted into the opening and an endotracheal tube or tracheostomy tube may be passed over the device into the airway.
6. Following inflation of the cuff, the placement of the tube is confirmed by lung auscultation, chest rise, and capnography.

References

1. Pfuntner A, Wier LM, Stocks C. Most frequent procedures performed in U.S. hospitals, 2011. 2013 Oct. In: Healthcare Cost and Utilization Project (HCUP) Statistical Briefs [Internet]. Rockville (MD): Agency for Healthcare Research and Quality (US); 2006 Feb-. Statistical Brief #165. https://www.ncbi.nlm.nih.gov/books/NBK174682/
2. Admass BA, Endalew NS, Tawye HY, et al. Evidence-based airway management protocol for a critical ill patient in medical intensive care unit: systematic review. Ann Med Surg (Lond) 2022; 80:104284.
3. Needham DM, Thompson DA, Holzmueller CG, et al. A system factors analysis of airway events from the Intensive Care Unit Safety Reporting System (ICUSRS). Crit Care Med 2004;32(11):2227-33.
4. Brown CA, Saldes JC, Mick NW, et al., eds. *The Walls Manual of Emergency Airway Management*. 6th ed. Wolters Kluwer; 2023.
5. Gropper MA, Eriksson LI, Fleisher LA, et al., eds. *Miller's Anesthesia*. 9th ed. Philadelphia, PA: Elsevier; 2019.
6. Hagberg CA, ed. *Hagberg and Benumof's Airway Management*. 5th ed. Elsevier; 2022.
7. Apfelbaum JL, Hagberg CA, Caplan RA, et al. for the American Society of Anesthesiologists Task Force on Management of the Difficult Airway. Practice guidelines for management of the difficult airway: an updated report by the American Society of Anesthesiologists Task Force on Management of the Difficult Airway. Anesthesiology 2013;118(2):251-70.
8. Law JA, Broemling N, Cooper RM, et al. for the Canadian Airway Focus Group. The difficult airway with recommendations for management—part 1—difficult tracheal intubation encountered in an unconscious/induced patient. Can J Anaesth 2013;60(11): 1089-118.
9. Heuer JF, Barwing TA, Barwing J, et al. Incidence of difficult intubation in intensive care patients: analysis of contributing factors. Anaesth Intensive Care 2012;40(1):120-7.
10. Roth D, Pace NL, Lee A, et al. Bedside tests for predicting difficult airways: an abridged Cochrane diagnostic test accuracy systematic review. Anaesthesia 2019;74(7):915-28.
11. Philip S, Nizar FF. Prediction of difficult laryngoscopy in patients undergoing endotracheal intubation: a comparative study of various airway assessment tests. Astrocyte 2016;3:90-5.
12. Kheterpal S, Han R, Tremper KK, et al. Incidence and predictors of difficult and impossible mask ventilation. Anesthesiology 2006;105(5):885-91.

13. Osman A, Sum KM. Role of upper airway ultrasound in airway management. J Intensive Care 2016;4:52.
14. Keum JSS, Ikuine T, Ladd S, et al. *Techniques in Adult Cricothyroid Membrane Emergency Ultrasound Localization*. Keum Biomedical Sciences Inc.; 2021.
15. Mosier JM, Joshi R, Hypes C, et al. The physiologically difficult airway. West J Emerg Med 2015;16(7):1109-17.
16. Seyni-Boureima R, Zhang Z, Antoine MMLK, Antoine-Frank CD. A review on the anesthetic management of obese patients undergoing surgery. BMC Anesthesiol 2022;22(1):98.
17. Kristensen MS. Airway management and morbid obesity. Eur J Anaesthesiol 2010;27(11):923-7.
18. Hassan EA, Baraka AAE. The effect of reverse Trendelenburg position versus semi-recumbent position on respiratory parameters of obese critically ill patients: a randomised controlled trial. J Clin Nurs 2021;30(7-8):995-1002.
19. El-Orbany M, Connolly LA. Rapid sequence induction and intubation: current controversy. Anesth Analg 2010;110(5):1318-25.
20. Salem MR, Khorasani A, Saatee S, et al. Gastric tubes and airway management in patients at risk of aspiration: history, current concepts, and proposal of an algorithm. Anesth Analg 2014;118(3):569-79.
21. Van de Putte P, Perlas A. Ultrasound assessment of gastric content and volume. BJA: British Journal of Anaesthesia 2014;113(1):12-22.
22. Tran DTT, Newton EK, Mount VAH, et al. Rocuronium vs. succinylcholine for rapid sequence intubation: a Cochrane systematic review. Anaesthesia 2017;72(6):765-77.
23. Robinson N, Clancy M. In patients with head injury undergoing rapid sequence intubation, does pretreatment with intravenous lignocaine/lidocaine lead to an improved neurological outcome? A review of the literature. Emerg Med J 2001;18(6):453-7.
24. Salem MR, Khorasani A, Zeidan A, Crystal GJ. Cricoid pressure controversies: narrative review. Anesthesiology 2017;126(4):738-52.
25. Birenbaum A, Hajage D, Roche S, et al. Effect of cricoid pressure compared with a sham procedure in the rapid sequence induction of anesthesia: the IRIS Randomized Clinical Trial. JAMA Surg 2019;154(1):9-17.
26. Prekker ME, Driver BE, Trent SA, et al. Video versus Direct Laryngoscopy for Tracheal Intubation of Critically Ill Adults. N Engl J Med 2023;389(5):418-29.

27. Vargas M, Servillo G, Buonanno P, et al. Video vs. direct laryngoscopy for adult surgical and intensive care unit patients requiring tracheal intubation: a systematic review and meta-analysis of randomized controlled trials. Eur Rev Med Pharmacol Sci 2021;25(24):7734-49.
28. Root CW, Mitchell OJL, Brown R, et al. Suction Assisted Laryngoscopy and Airway Decontamination (SALAD): a technique for improved emergency airway management. Resusc Plus 2020; 1-2:100005.

Stress Ulcer Prophylaxis — Chapter 3

STRESS-RELATED MUCOSAL INJURY

Mucosal erosions of the gastric mucosa are visible in 75-100% of patients within 24 h of ICU admission (1). These erosions (called *stress ulcers*) are usually confined to the gastric mucosa and are typically clinically silent. However, erosions can extend into the submucosa and produce clinical bleeding.

Clinically apparent bleeding from stress ulcers is reported in up to 15% of ICU patients (2), but clinically significant bleeding (i.e., requires blood transfusion) occurs in only less than 3% of patients but has been associated with a mortality of close to 50% (1,3-4).

Pathophysiology

Fundamentally, stress ulceration is mucosal ischemia resulting from hypoperfusion (shock), reperfusion, and inflammatory responses to critical illness (3,5). Specific acute disease states have been associated with acute gastrointestinal ulcerations with morphologies that differ from the classic stress ulcerations which are typically diffuse. Despite differing pathophysiology, prophylaxis remains the same.

Cushing's Ulcer

In acute elevated intracranial pressure, vagal overstimulation (6) leads to the hypersecretion of gastrin and pepsin, resulting in elevated acid production, which causes deep ulcers and even perforation (6-7). This is unlike stress ulcers which are not associated with elevated gastric acid production.

Curling's Ulcer

This ulcer occurs in patients with greater than 20% total body surface area burns and occurs in both the stomach and duodenum (7-8).

Risk Factors

Multiple risk factors for stress ulceration in critically ill patients have been described (Table 3.1) over the past several decades (1,3-5,9-10).

TABLE 3.1 Risk Factors for Stress Ulcer Bleeding	
Independent Risk Factors[1]	**Other Risk Factors[2]**
Mechanical Ventilation >48 h	Shock — Severity of Illness
Coagulopathy	Sepsis — Major Trauma
• Platelet Count <50,000/mm³	Male — Age >50 years
• INR >1.5	Corticosteroid Therapy
• PTT <2X control	Acute Kidney Injury
	Chronic Hepatic Disease

[1]From Reference 9.
[2]From References 1, 3-5, 10.

Note that the only two independent risk factors (i.e., require no other risk factors to promote bleeding) are mechanical ventilation for longer than 48 h and coagulopathy (defined as platelet count <50,000/mm³, INR >1.5, or PTT >2X control) (9). Simply stated, if your patient is in an ICU on mechanical ventilation and/or coagulopathic, stress ulcer prophylaxis is indicated. If a patient is critical enough to require mechanical ventilatory support, they are at risk.

Pharmacologic Prophylaxis

Despite the understanding that mucosal stress ulceration is typically not associated with increased acid and pepsin excretion, their role in ulcerogenesis is due to the mucosal compromise from ischemia and inflammation. Therefore, control of pH remains the principal approach to stress ulcer prophylaxis. The goal is a pH >4 in gastric secretions, but this is rarely monitored.

Antacids

Although the drug costs of using antacids for stress ulcer prophylaxis (SUP) are minimal, they require frequent pH monitoring (every 2 to 4 h), making this modality resource intensive (4). Furthermore, head-to-head trials of antacids versus histamine H_2 blockers have demonstrated higher bleeding rates with antacids (10).

Histamine H_2 Receptor Antagonists (H_2RA)

1. Famotidine is the most often used H_2RA for stress ulcer prophylaxis. It can be given intravenously using the dosing regimens shown in Table 3.2.
2. H_2RA are less effective in reducing gastric acidity with continued use, but this does not reduce their effectiveness in preventing stress ulcer bleeding (11).
3. Dose reduction is therefore required in renal dysfunction (creatinine clearance <50 mL/min). This can be accomplished by increasing the dosing interval (to 24 h for ranitidine, and 36-48 h for famotidine) (12).

TABLE 3.2 Drugs Used for Stress Ulcer Prophylaxis

Drug	Routes	Dosage
H_2 Blocker:		
Famotidine	PO, NG, IV	20 mg every 12 h[†]
Proton Pump Inhibitors:		
Pantoprazole	PO, NG, IV	40 mg daily
Esomeprazole	PO, NG, IV	40 mg daily
Omeprazole	PO, NG	40 mg daily
Lansoprazole	PO, NG	30 mg daily
Cytoprotectant:		
Sucralfate	PO, NG	1 gram every 6 h (dissolved in 10 mL saline for NG administration)

PO = oral; NG = nasogastric; IV = intravenous.
[†]Dose reduction of 50% is recommended for creatinine clearance <50 mL/min.

Proton Pump Inhibitors

1. Proton pump inhibitors (PPIs) are replacing H_2RA for stress ulcer prophylaxis because they produce a more complete inhibition of gastric acid secretion, and there is no response attenuation with continued use (13).
2. Despite their pharmacologic advantages, there is no data to support *PPIs as more effective than H_2RA for preventing stress ulcer bleeding* (14-15).
3. The prophylactic dosing regimens for current PPIs are shown in Table 3.2. Pantoprazole and esomeprazole drug can be given intravenously, which is the recommended route for stress ulcer prophylaxis (13).
4. Adverse effects of PPIs are primarily related to the reduced gastric acidity (see next section). One drug interaction deserves mention: PPIs impede the activation of clopidogrel (a popular antiplatelet agent) in the liver (16). Although the significance of this interaction is unclear, current opinion favors avoiding PPIs, if possible, during antiplatelet therapy with clopidogrel.

Cytoprotection

Sucralfate. The cytoprotective agent, sucralfate, provides an alternative to gastric acid suppression for stress ulcer prophylaxis. An aluminum salt of sucrose sulfate, sucralfate has multiple physiologic effects (17):

1. Adheres to damaged areas of the gastric mucosa acting as a protective barrier shielding damaged mucosa from the damaging effects of pepsin and gastric acidity.
2. Absorbs pepsin, decreasing its concentration.
3. Increases mucus production by increasing prostaglandin production.
4. Increases prostaglandin-dependent and independent bicarbonate production.
5. Binds growth factors to the damaged mucosa facilitating healing/repair.

See Table 3.2 for dosing and administration.

Sucralfate has multiple drug interactions in the bowel lumen (Table 3.3), which can reduce their bioavailability (15,17). When these drugs are given enterally, sucralfate doses should be separated by at least 2 h.

TABLE 3.3 Sucralfate Drug Interactions

Drug Interactions that can Decrease Serum Concentrations	Interactions that can Decrease Absorption or Delay Onset of Actions
• Digoxin	• Naproxen
• Levothyroxine	• Potassium Phosphate
• Furosemide	• Levoketoconazole
• Quinolones	• Baloxavir
• Oral phosphate supplements	
• Warfarin	

From Reference 15.

Sucralfate does not elevate plasma aluminum levels, even with prolonged use (18).

Enteral Feedings

Enteral feeding has trophic effects including increased mesenteric blood flow on gastrointestinal mucosa, so it is theoretically beneficial regarding preventing stress ulcer development and bleeding. (For additional details and benefits of enteral nutrition see Table 47.1 in Chapter 47: Enteral Nutrition.) To date, however, there are no prospective evaluations of this hypothesis. Currently the data remains controversial, with even increased stress ulcer hemorrhage in the face of SUP (19). The Society of Critical Care Medicine and American Society of Health-System Pharmacists guideline recommends SUP continued with enteral nutrition if the patient possesses continued risk factors (5).

Stop!

When the risk factors for stress ulceration have resolved, SUP should be discontinued, preferably prior to transfer out of the ICU.

References

1. Bardou M, Quenot JP, Barkun A. Stress-related mucosal disease in the critically ill patient. Nat Rev Gastroenterol Hepatol 2015;12(2):98-107.
2. Krag M, Perner A, Wetterslev J, et al. Stress ulcer prophylaxis versus placebo or no prophylaxis in critically ill patients. A systematic review of randomised clinical trials with meta-analysis and trial sequential analysis. Intensive Care Med 2014;40:11-22.
3. Buendgens L, Koch A, Tacke F. Prevention of stress-related ulcer bleeding at the intensive care unit: risks and benefits of stress ulcer prophylaxis. World J Crit Care Med 2016;5:57-64.
4. Nathens AB, Maier RV. Prophylaxis and management of stress ulceration. In: Holzheimer RG, Mannick JA, eds. *Surgical Treatment: Evidence-based and Problem-oriented*. Munich: Zuckschwerdt Verlag; 2001.
5. MacLaren R, Dionne JC, Granholm A, et al. Society of Critical Care Medicine and American Society of Health-system Pharmacists Guideline for the Prevention of Stress-related Gastrointestinal Bleeding in Critically Ill Adults. Crit Care Med 2024;52:e421-e30.
6. Kumaria A, Kirkman MA, Scott RA, et al. A reappraisal of the pathophysiology of cushing ulcer: a narrative review. J Neurosurg Anesthesiol 2024;36:211-7.
7. Silen W, Merhav A, Simson JN. The pathophysiology of stress ulcer disease. World J Surg 1981;5:165-74.
8. Choi YH, Lee JH, Shin JJ, Cho YS. A revised risk analysis of stress ulcers in burn patients receiving ulcer prophylaxis. Clin Exp Emerg Med 2015;2:250-5.
9. Cook DJ, Fuller HD, Guyatt GH, et al. Risk factors for gastrointestinal bleeding in critically ill patients. Canadian Critical Care Trials Group. N Engl J Med 1994;330:377-81.
10. Mohebbi L, Hesch K. Stress ulcer prophylaxis in the intensive care unit. Proc (Bayl Univ Med Cent) 2009;22:373-6.
11. Huang J, Cao Y, Liao C, et al. Effect of histamine-2-receptor antagonists versus sucralfate on stress ulcer prophylaxis in mechanically ventilated patients: a meta-analysis of 10 randomized controlled trials. Crit Care 2010;14:R194.

12. Self TH, Gilless JP, Hudson JQ. Minimizing risk of mental status changes with H_2 blockers: dosage adjustment in kidney dysfunction. Consultant 2014;54:922-4.
13. Pang SH, Graham DY. A clinical guide to using intravenous proton-pump inhibitors in reflux and peptic ulcers. Therap Adv Gastroenterol 2010;3:11-22.
14. Lin PC, Chang CH, Hsu PI, et al. The efficacy and safety of proton pump inhibitors vs histamine-2 receptor antagonists for stress ulcer bleeding prophylaxis among critical care patients: a meta-analysis. Crit Care Med 2010;38:1197-205.
15. Song MJ, Kim S, Boo D, et al. Comparison of proton pump inhibitors and histamine 2 receptor antagonists for stress ulcer prophylaxis in the intensive care unit. Sci Rep 2021;11:18467.
16. Egred M. Clopidogrel and proton-pump inhibitor interaction: viewpoint and practical clinical approach. Br J Cardiol 2011;18:84-7.
17. Kudaravalli P, Patel P, John S. Sucralfate. In: StatPearls. Treasure Island (FL): StatPearls Publishing; 2025.
18. Tryba M, Kurz-Muller K, Donner B. Plasma aluminum concentrations in long-term mechanically ventilated patients receiving stress ulcer prophylaxis with sucralfate. Crit Care Med 1994;22:1769-73.
19. Ye Z, Reintam Blaser A, Lytvyn L, et al. Gastrointestinal bleeding prophylaxis for critically ill patients: a clinical practice guideline. BMJ 2020;368:l6722.

Chapter 4: Prophylaxis for VTE

Deep venous thrombosis (DVT) and pulmonary embolism (PE) constitute venous thromboembolism (VTE). Annually, VTE affects up to 900,000 people, with up to 100,000 deaths, leaving many others with long-term complications (1). This chapter presents the current practices for the prevention, diagnosis, and treatment of venous thrombosis and pulmonary embolism. The major focus of this chapter is prevention, because VTE is considered the leading cause of preventable deaths in hospitalized patients (1).

RISK FACTORS

Rudolf Virchow, a 19th century physician postulated 3 factors predisposing to the development of VTE. Virchow's observations remain relevant today. See Table 4.1.

TABLE 4.1 Virchow's Triad
1. Hypercoagulable State
2. Venous Stasis
3. Endothelial Injury

Multiple scoring systems are available to define the level of VTE "risk," yet even in patients receiving anticoagulant prophylaxis, risk assessment models perform poorly (2).

Hypercoagulable State

Severe illness leads to a systemic inflammatory response. The association of inflammation and thrombosis is well-known–inflammation activates cellular and humoral responses (i.e., cytokines, complement pathway, etc.) that have direct effects on initiating coagulation pathways (3-5).

Venous Stasis

Immobility in the ICU is multi-factorial, e.g., mechanical ventilation, sedation, shock, neuromuscular blockade. During slow blood flow, levels of coagulation factors are locally high promoting platelet aggregation and thrombosis (6). Venous stasis is associated with a 17-fold increase in VTE (7). Clearly, the VTE risk due to the immobility of critically ill patients, is compounded by the hypercoagulability of critical illness.

Endothelial Injury

A healthy endothelium provides an antithrombotic surface that when damaged converts towards pro-coagulation (8). Although thrombosis may be obvious at the site of injury, this injury incites coagulation cascades and can lead to systemic coagulopathy. Major surgery with general anesthesia is an example, as it is recognized as a cause of VTE in hospitalized patients. This risk can persist for several weeks, even post-discharge (9). Even the presence of a central venous catheter is a known risk for VTE (2,9-10).

Fundamentally, critically ill patients have all 3 factors on admission to the ICU and are therefore "high-risk" and should receive anticoagulant prophylaxis unless contraindicated (10-11).

VTE PROPHYLAXIS

Anticoagulant prophylaxis for VTE is a standard measure for all ICU patients (except those that are fully anticoagulated) and is started on the day of admission. Appropriate preventive measures can vary in different high-risk conditions, as indicated in Table 4.2 (12-19).

Unfractionated Heparin

Standard or *unfractionated* heparin is a heterogeneous mix of mucopolysaccharide molecules that vary in size and anticoagulant activity.

TABLE 4.2 Thromboprophylaxis with Parenteral Agents

Agent	Prophylactic Dosing Regimen
Unfractionated Heparin	Standard: 5,000 units SC every 8-12 h Obesity: 7,500 units every 8 h for BMI ≥40 kg/m^2 Renal: No dose adjustment
Enoxaparin (Lovenox)	Standard: 40 mg SC once daily, or 30 mg SC every 12 h Obesity: 40 mg SC every 12 h for BMI ≥40 kg/m^2 Renal: If Cr CL <30 mL/min, reduce dose to 30 mg SC once daily, or use UFH.
Dalteparin (Fragmin)	Standard: 2,500-5,000 units SC once daily Obesity: Not adequately studied Renal: No dose adjustment
Fondaparinux (Arixtra)	Standard: 2.5 mg SC once daily Obesity: No recommendations Renal: If Cr CL = 35-50 mL/min, reduce dose to 1.5 mg SC once daily. Do not use if Cr CL <30 mL/min.

SC = subcutaneous; Cr CL = creatinine clearance; UFH = unfractionated heparin.
From References 12-19.

Actions

- Heparin is an indirect-acting drug that must bind to a cofactor (antithrombin III or AT) to produce an anticoagulant effect. The heparin-AT complex inactivates multiple coagulation factors, and inactivation of factor IIa (antithrombin effect) is 10 times more sensitive than the other anticoagulant reactions (20).
- Heparin also binds to a specific protein on platelets to form an antigenic complex that induces the formation of IgG antibodies. These antibodies can cross-react with the platelet binding site and activate platelets, which promotes thrombosis and a consumptive thrombocytopenia.

Prophylactic Dosing

The potent antithrombin activity of the heparin-AT complex allows low doses of heparin to inhibit thrombogenesis without producing systemic anticoagulation.

- The standard regimen of *low-dose unfractionated heparin* (LDUH) is 5,000 units by subcutaneous injection every 12 h. There is a more frequent dosing regimen (5,000 units every 8 h), but there is no evidence of superiority over twice daily dosing (15,21).
- Studies in ICU patients (22) and postoperative patients (23) have shown a 50-60% reduction in the incidence of leg vein thrombosis with LDUH.
- The standard LDUH regimen may be less effective in obese patients because of the increased volume of drug distribution in obesity. The recommended dosing for LDUH in obesity is included in Table 4.2 (19,24). A systematic review and meta-analysis of weight-adjusted dosing compared with fixed-dose prophylaxis did not show a lower risk of VTE in obese patients (25).

Complications

- The risk of major bleeding with LDUH is <1% (15), and anticoagulation monitoring is not necessary.
- Heparin-induced thrombocytopenia has been reported in 0.5-1% of patients receiving LDUH (26).

Low-Molecular-Weight Heparin

Low-molecular-weight heparin (LMWH) is produced by enzymatic cleavage of heparin molecules, which produces smaller molecules of more uniform size. This results in more potent and predictable anticoagulation than occurs with unfractionated heparin. LMWH must still bind to anti-thrombin III, and the major anticoagulant reaction is inactivation of factor Xa.

Advantages

LMWH has the following advantages over unfractionated heparin:

- A more predictable dose-response relationship, and no routine monitoring of anticoagulant activity (7).
- Reduced DVT rate without increased bleeding risk (11).
- A much lower risk of heparin-induced thrombocytopenia (0.1-0.5% for LMWH vs. 0.5-1.0% for LDUH) (26).

Disadvantages

The major disadvantage of LMWH is its renal clearance, which creates the need for dosage adjustments in patients with renal failure. However, the tendency to accumulate in renal failure varies with individual LMWH preparations.

Prophylactic Dosing

The LMWH preparations studied most extensively for thromboprophylaxis are enoxaparin (Lovenox®) and dalteparin (Fragmin®). Prophylactic dosing regimens for these agents are summarized in Table 4.2.

Enoxaparin

The standard enoxaparin dose for thromboprophylaxis is 40 mg by subcutaneous injection once daily (12). In conditions with a very high risk of VTE (e.g., major trauma, hip and knee surgery), the dose is 30 mg twice daily (12). Dosing adjustments for renal failure (12) and morbid obesity (27) are shown in Table 4.2.

Dalteparin

Dalteparin has two advantages over enoxaparin:

1. It is given only once daily (28), and
2. It has been used safely without dose reduction in renal failure (14).

The appropriate dose of dalteparin in morbid obesity is not known.

Mechanical Aids

External compression of the lower extremities can promote venous outflow from the legs and reduce the risk of VTE. This approach is typically used in place of pharmacologic VTE prophylaxis in patients who are actively bleeding or have a high risk of bleeding but may also be used in combination with anticoagulant prophylaxis. There are two methods of external leg compression.

Graded Compression Stockings
- Graded compression stockings (GCS) are designed to create 18 mm Hg external pressure at the ankles and 8 mm Hg external pressure in the thigh (29). The resulting 10 mm Hg pressure gradient acts as a driving force for venous outflow from the legs.
- These stockings have been shown to reduce the incidence of VTE when used alone after major surgery (30), but they are not recommended as the sole method of thromboprophylaxis in ICU patients (31).

Intermittent Pneumatic Compression

Intermittent pneumatic compression (IPC) is achieved with inflatable bladders that are wrapped around the lower extremities and connected to a pneumatic pump (Figure 4.1).

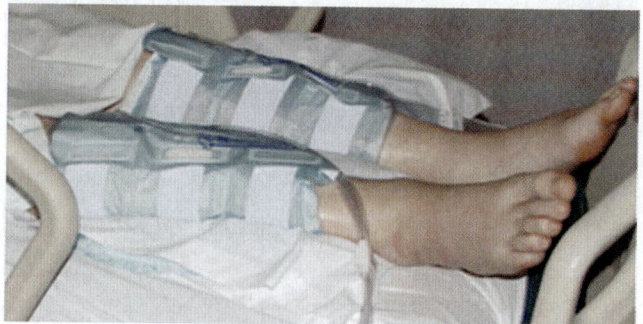

FIGURE 4.1. Intermittent pneumatic compression.

There are multiple variations that cover just the foot to covering the entire lower extremity. Repeated inflation and deflation of the bladders creates a pumping action that augments venous outflow from the legs. Another variation, "sequential compression devices" (SCD) inflate successively from distal to proximal to promote flow, although there is a paucity of data to demonstrate a benefit of any variation (32).

Vena Cava Filters

Vena cava filters prevent venous thrombotic emboli from reaching the lungs (pulmonary emboli). They are by definition prophylactic as they do not treat PE or DVT. Figure 4.2 demonstrates a venous thrombus trapped in a vena cava filter.

The use of vena cava filters as primary VTE prophylaxis, even with contraindication to anticoagulant prophylaxis cannot be routinely recommended (33). Specific high-risk

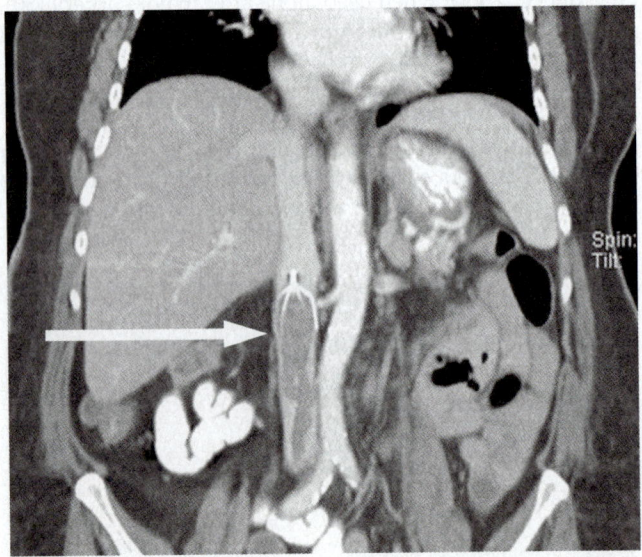

FIGURE 4.2. CT scan image showing venous thrombus trapped in vena cava filter (*arrow*).

patients may be considered after multi-disciplinary discussion on a case-by-case basis.

Percutaneous Interventional Procedures

Percutaneous interventional procedures are common in the intensive care setting with most being low-risk and do not require interruption of VTE prophylaxis (e.g., central venous catheters and chest tubes). Guidelines for management of anticoagulant prophylaxis from the Society of Interventional Radiology are shown in Table 4.3 (34).

TABLE 4.3	Management Recommendations for Anticoagulant Prophylaxis from the Society of Interventional Radiology	
Low-Dose UFH	• Low Risk	• Do not withhold
	• High Risk	• Procedure may be performed 6 h after last dose
LMWH	• Low Risk	• Do not withhold
	• High Risk	• Withhold 24 h before procedure

UFH = unfractionated heparin; LMWH = low molecular weight heparin.

From Patel IJ, Rahim S, Davidson JC, et al. Society of Interventional Radiology Consensus Guidelines for the Periprocedural Management of Thrombotic and Bleeding Risk in Patients Undergoing Percutaneous Image-Guided Interventions-Part II: Recommendations: endorsed by the Canadian Association for Interventional Radiology and the Cardiovascular and Interventional Radiological Society of Europe. J Vasc Interv Radiol 2019;30:1168-84.e1.

Neuraxial Analgesia

Anticoagulant prophylaxis can promote hematoma formation during the insertion and removal of intrathecal and epidural catheters with catastrophic outcomes (e.g., paralysis). To limit this risk, the insertion and removal of intrathecal and epidural catheters should be performed at a time when anticoagulant effects are minimal. The American Society of Regional Anesthesia and Pain Medicine evidence-based guideline is shown in Table 4.4 (35).

TABLE 4.4 Management of Pharmacologic VTE Prophylaxis with Neuraxial (Epidural) Catheters, from the American Society of Regional Anesthesia and Pain Medicine Evidence-Based Guidelines (Fourth Edition)

LMWH	• 12-h interval for between LMWH administration and placement or removal of an epidural catheter • Subsequent administration of LMWH should be delayed for 4 h after catheter removal
Low-Dose UFH	• 6-h interval between Low-Dose UFH administration and placement or removal of an epidural catheter • Subsequent administration of Low-Dose UFH should be delayed for 4 h after catheter removal

UFH = unfractionated heparin; LMWH = low molecular weight heparin.

From Horlocker TT, Vandermeulen E, Kopp SL, et al. Regional anesthesia in the patient receiving antithrombotic or thrombolytic therapy: American Society of Regional Anesthesia and Pain Medicine Evidence-Based Guidelines (Fourth Edition). Reg Anesth Pain Med 2018;43:263-309.

References

1. Centers for Disease Control and Prevention. Data and statistics on venous thromboembolism. Atlanta, GA 2024. https://www.cdc.gov/bloodclots/data-research/facts-stats/index.html
2. Al-Dorzi HM, Arishi H, Al-Hameed FM, et al. Performance of risk assessment models for VTE in patients who are critically ill receiving pharmacologic thromboprophylaxis: a post hoc analysis of the pneumatic compression for preventing VTE trial. Chest 2025; 167(2):598-610.
3. Chakraborty RK, Burns B. Systemic Inflammatory Response Syndrome. In: StatPearls. Treasure Island (FL): StatPearls Publishing; 2024.
4. Costantini TW, Kornblith LZ, Pritts T, Coimbra R. The intersection of coagulation activation and inflammation after injury: what you need to know. J Trauma Acute Care Surg 2024;96:347-56.
5. Stark K, Massberg S. Interplay between inflammation and thrombosis in cardiovascular pathology. Nat Rev Cardiol 2021;18:666-82.
6. Lichota A, Szewczyk EM, Gwozdzinski K. Factors affecting the formation and treatment of thrombosis by natural and synthetic compounds. Int J Mol Sci 2020;21.

7. Heit JA. The epidemiology of venous thromboembolism in the community. Arterioscler Thromb Vasc Biol 2008;28:370-2.
8. Kushner A, West WP, Khan Suheb MZ, Pillarisetty LS. Virchow Triad. In: StatPearls. Treasure Island (FL): StatPearls Publishing; 2024.
9. Nicholson M, Chan N, Bhagirath V, Ginsberg J. Prevention of venous thromboembolism in 2020 and beyond. J Clin Med 2020;9:2467.
10. Viarasilpa T, Panyavachiraporn N, Marashi SM, et al. Prediction of symptomatic venous thromboembolism in critically ill patients: the ICU-venous thromboembolism score. Crit Care Med 2020;48:e470-9.
11. Helms J, Middeldorp S, Spyropoulos AC. Thromboprophylaxis in critical care. Intensive Care Med 2023;49:75-8.
12. Enoxaparin. In: *AHFS Drug Information 2012*. American Society of Health-System Pharmacists; 2012:1491-501.
13. Ageno W, Riva N, Noris P, et al. Safety and efficacy of low-dose fondaparinux (1.5 mg) for the prevention of venous thromboembolism in acutely ill medical patients with renal impairment: the FONDAIR study. J Thromb Haemost 2012;10:2291-7.
14. Douketis J, Cook D, Meade M, et al. Prophylaxis against deep vein thrombosis in critically ill patients with severe renal insufficiency with the low-molecular-weight heparin dalteparin: an assessment of safety and pharmacodynamics: the DIRECT study. Arch Intern Med 2008;168:1805-12.
15. King CS, Holley AB, Jackson JL, et al. Twice vs three times daily heparin dosing for thromboembolism prophylaxis in the general medical population: a metaanalysis. Chest 2007;131:507-16.
16. Miano TA, Cuker A, Christie JD, et al. Comparative effectiveness of enoxaparin vs dalteparin for thromboprophylaxis after traumatic injury. Chest 2018;153:133-42.
17. Nutescu EA, Spinler SA, Wittkowsky A, Dager WE. Low-molecular-weight heparins in renal impairment and obesity: available evidence and clinical practice recommendations across medical and surgical settings. Ann Pharmacother 2009;43:1064-83.
18. Turpie AG, Lensing AW, Fuji T, Boyle DA. Pharmacokinetic and clinical data supporting the use of fondaparinux 1.5 mg once daily in the prevention of venous thromboembolism in renally impaired patients. Blood Coagul Fibrinolysis 2009;20:114-21.
19. Wang TF, Milligan PE, Wong CA, et al. Efficacy and safety of high-dose thromboprophylaxis in morbidly obese inpatients. Thromb Haemost 2014;111:88-93.
20. Garcia DA, Baglin TP, Weitz JI, Samama MM. *Parenteral anticoagulants: Antithrombotic Therapy and Prevention of Thrombosis*, 9th ed: American College of Chest Physicians Evidence-Based Clinical Practice Guidelines. Chest 2012;141:e24S-e43S.
21. Sorgi MW, Roach E, Bauer SR, et al. Effectiveness and safety of twice daily versus thrice daily subcutaneous unfractionated heparin for

venous thromboembolism prophylaxis at a tertiary medical center. J Pharm Pract 2022;35:190-6.
22. Cade JF. High risk of the critically ill for venous thromboembolism. Crit Care Med 1982;10:448-50.
23. Collins R, Scrimgeour A, Yusuf S, Peto R. Reduction in fatal pulmonary embolism and venous thrombosis by perioperative administration of subcutaneous heparin. Overview of results of randomized trials in general, orthopedic, and urologic surgery. N Engl J Med 1988;318:1162-73.
24. Medico CJ, Walsh P. Pharmacotherapy in the critically ill obese patient. Crit Care Clin 2010;26:679-88.
25. Ceccato D, Di Vincenzo A, Pagano C, et al. Weight-adjusted versus fixed dose heparin thromboprophylaxis in hospitalized obese patients: a systematic review and meta-analysis. Eur J Intern Med 2021;88:73-80.
26. Arepally GM, Padmanabhan A. Heparin-induced thrombocytopenia: a focus on thrombosis. Arterioscler Thromb Vasc Biol 2021;41:141-52.
27. Martin AM, Polistena P, Mahmud A, et al. Optimal enoxaparin dosing strategies for venous thromboembolism prophylaxis and treatment of high body weight patients. Thromb Res 2021;207:116-22.
28. Dalteparin. In: *AHFS Drug Information 2012*. American Society of Health-System Pharmacists; 2012:1482-91.
29. Goldhaber SZ, Morpurgo M. Diagnosis, treatment, and prevention of pulmonary embolism. Report of the WHO/International Society and Federation of Cardiology Task Force. JAMA 1992;268:1727-33.
30. Sachdeva A, Dalton M, Lees T. Graduated compression stockings for prevention of deep vein thrombosis. Cochrane Database Syst Rev 2018;11:CD001484.
31. Guyatt GH, Akl EA, Crowther M, et al. for the American College of Chest Physicians Antithrombotic Therapy and Prevention of Thrombosis Panel. *Executive summary: antithrombotic therapy and prevention of thrombosis*, 9th ed: American College of Chest Physicians Evidence-Based Clinical Practice Guidelines. Chest 2012;141:7S-47S.
32. Pavon JM, Williams JW Jr, Adam SS, et al. Effectiveness of intermittent pneumatic compression devices for venous thromboembolism prophylaxis in high-risk surgical and medical patients. In: *VA Evidence-based Synthesis Program Reports*. Washington, DC: Department of Veterans Affairs; 2015.
33. Shenoy R, Cunningham KW, Ross SW, et al. "Death Knell" for prophylactic vena cava filters? A 20-year experience with a venous thromboembolism guideline. Am Surg 2019;85:806-12.
34. Patel IJ, Rahim S, Davidson JC, et al. Society of Interventional Radiology Consensus Guidelines for the Periprocedural Management of Thrombotic and Bleeding Risk in Patients Undergoing Percutaneous Image-Guided Interventions-Part II: Recommendations:

endorsed by the Canadian Association for Interventional Radiology and the Cardiovascular and Interventional Radiological Society of Europe. J Vasc Interv Radiol 2019;30:1168-84.e1.

35. Horlocker TT, Vandermeuelen E, Kopp SL, et al. Regional anesthesia in the patient receiving antithrombotic or thrombolytic therapy: American Society of Regional Anesthesia and Pain Medicine Evidence-Based Guidelines (Fourth Edition). Reg Anesth Pain Med 2018;43:263-309.

Analgesia and Sedation
Chapter 5

In surveys of patients who have been discharged from the ICU, anxiety and unalleviated pain are the dominant recollections of the ICU stay (1). Hence, the principal function for clinicians in the ICU is not to save lives—which is impossible on a consistent basis—but *to relieve pain and suffering*. This chapter describes the pharmacological approach to pain and stress relief in the ICU, with a focus on intravenous drug regimens and recommendations from expert commentaries and consensus guidelines (2-6). Nonpharmacological measures are not discussed here but may be reviewed in a clinical practice guideline that is referenced in this chapter (3).

ASSESSMENT OF PAIN IN THE ICU

Unrelieved pain is the most frequently cited stressor in the ICU (7), and the frequency of painful experiences is equivalent in surgical and medical ICUs (8). Pain is defined as an unpleasant sensory experience (9). In ICU patients, the sensation of pain is often magnified (i.e., *hypernociception*) and even a minor event such as the act of turning a patient can be a painful experience. Failure to recognize the exaggerated pain sensation in ICU patients is a source of inadequate pain control.

Assessment Instruments

Pain is a subjective sensation, so a patient's self-assessment is the most accurate measure of pain intensity. *Changes in heart rate or blood pressure are not reliable indicators of pain* (2,8). In patients capable of self-assessment, the *Numeric Ranking Scale* (NRS) is recommended to quantify pain intensity (3). The NRS is a horizontal scale with 10 equally spaced markings, numbered 1 (no pain) to 10 (maximum pain). When patients are not capable of self-assessment (i.e., deep sedation), the Behavioral Pain Scale (Table 5.1) can be used.

TABLE 5.1	The Behavioral Pain Scale	
Item	Description	Score
Facial Expression	• Relaxed	1
	• Partially tightened	2
	• Fully tightened	3
	• Grimacing	4
Upper Limbs	• No movement	1
	• Partially bent	2
	• Fully bent, fingers flexed	3
	• Permanently retracted	4
Compliance with Ventilation	• Tolerating ventilator	1
	• Coughing, but tolerating ventilator	2
	• Fighting ventilator	3
	• Unable to control ventilation	4
	Total Score	

Score	Interpretation
3	No Pain
≥6	Unacceptable pain
12	Maximal pain

From Payen JF, Bru O, Bosson JL, et al. Assessing pain in critically ill sedated patients by using a behavioral pain scale. Crit Care Med 2001;29(12):2258-63.

ANALGESIA WITH OPIOIDS

Terminology

An *opiate* is a natural derivative of opium, a compound extracted from the poppy plan, *Papaver somniferum*. An *opioid* is a naturally occurring or synthetic derivative of opium that acts by stimulating a family of opioid receptors (i.e., mu, delta, kappa). A *narcotic* is an outdated term for an opioid but has also been adopted by law enforcement agencies to refer to an opioid that is obtained illegally and used for non-medicinal purposes. The term *opioid* is preferred because this term is clear, unambiguous, and includes both natural and synthetic opiates used in the ICU (10). In addition to analgesic effects, opioids produce mild sedation but without amnestic effects (11).

Dosing

The recommended intravenous dosing for fentanyl, hydromorphone, and morphine are shown in Table 5.2.

TABLE 5.2 Equivalent Dosage of Opioids Used in the ICU[†]

Drug	Equivalent Opioid Dosage (mg)			
	IV	Oral	IV: Oral Dosing Ratio	Equianalgesic Dose Ratio Compared to Morphine
Morphine	10	30	1:3	—
Fentanyl	0.1 (100 µg)	—	—	IV: 10:1 Oral: 300:1
Hydromorphone	1.5	7.5	1:5	IV: 7:1 Oral: 4:1
Oxycodone	—	20	—	Oral: 1.5:1
Methadone	1	1	1:1	Oral: 1-20 mg/day 4:1 21-40 mg/day 8:1 41-60 mg/day 10:1 >61-80 mg/day 12:1
Remifentanil	0.05-0.1 (50-100 µg)[†]	—	—	IV: 10:1[†]

[†]According to some references, remifentanil is reported to up to 250 times more potent than equianalgesic doses of morphine.

From References 5, 14, and 15.

It is important to emphasize that opioid dose requirements can vary widely in individual patients, and therefore, the effective dose of an opioid is determined by each patient's response, and not by the recommended dosing of the drug. Additionally, when patients are admitted to the ICU with a history of prior or current opioid use, or when patients experience adverse effects or the inability to tolerate a certain opioid formulation, opioid conversion is often required (12). Opioid conversion often involves a reduction of new opioid dosing by 50% or more due to incomplete cross-tolerance (i.e., the presence of different opioid receptor subtypes) (12-15).

Drugs

The opioids used most frequently in the ICU are fentanyl, hydromorphone (Dilaudid), and morphine. These opioids are metabolized in the liver and the metabolites are excreted in the urine.

Morphine

Morphine was historically used frequently for pain control in the ICU, but in recent years, several disadvantages have curbed its popularity:

1. Morphine has active metabolites, including morphine 3-glucuronide, that accumulate in renal failure. This metabolite can produce agitation with myoclonus and seizures (16). Another metabolite, morphine-6-glucuronide, has more potent analgesic properties than the parent drug (17). To avoid side effects related to the accumulation of metabolites, the maintenance dose of morphine should be reduced by 50% in patients with renal failure (18).
2. Morphine promotes the release of histamine, which produces systemic vasodilation and hypotension, but not bronchoconstriction (19). Morphine-related hypotension is more often seen in patients with a hyperadrenergic state and increased peripheral arterial tone (2).

Fentanyl

Fentanyl is a synthetic opioid that has replaced morphine as the most popular opioid used in the ICU (7). Advantages of fentanyl over morphine include the following:

1. Fentanyl is 600 times more lipid soluble than morphine and thus has a more rapid onset of action. This

lipophilicity is also a disadvantage as fentanyl can accumulate in the brain and fatty tissues following prolonged use or high dose infusions.
2. Fentanyl does not promote histamine release. Thus, the risk for hypotension is less, compared to morphine (19).
3. Fentanyl has no active metabolites, though the parent drug can accumulate in renal failure, and some recommend avoiding fentanyl in patients with end-stage renal disease (4).

Hydromorphone

Hydromorphone (Dilaudid) is a semi-synthetic derivative of morphine that may produce more effective analgesia than morphine (20). It seems to be favored for the treatment of cancer-related pain but has no proven advantages over fentanyl for analgesia. Although considered safer for use in patients with renal impairment, hydromorphone also has potentially neurotoxic metabolites (i.e., hydromorphone-3-glucuronide) that can accumulate in renal failure (21-23). Therefore, a dosing decrease of 50% is recommended when the creatinine clearance falls below 60 mL/min (21-23).

Remifentanil

Remifentanil is an ultra-short-acting synthetic opioid that is occasionally used in ICUs for brief periods of intense analgesia (13). Remifentanil has been reported to be at least equivalent to fentanyl and up to 250 times more potent than morphine (5,13). The recommended dose begins with a loading dose of 1.5 µg/kg and follows with a continuous infusion at 0.5-15 µg/kg/h (2). Remifentanil is not hepatically metabolized but undergoes rapid hydrolysis by non-specific tissue and plasma esterases, which gives it a rapid onset (<1 min) and short duration of action (i.e., elimination half-life of 10-20 min). Hence, drug metabolism does not take place in the liver or kidneys, so dose adjustments are not necessary in renal or hepatic failure.

Patient-Controlled Analgesia

For patients who are awake and capable of drug self-administration, *patient-controlled analgesia* (PCA) can be an effective method for pain control. *Mechanical ventilation is not a contraindication for the PCA method if the patient is awake and capable of activating self-administration.* The PCA method uses an electronic infusion pump that can be activated by the patient. When pain is sensed, the patient presses a button connected to the pump to receive a small intravenous bolus of drug. After each bolus, the pump is disabled for a mandatory time period called the *lockout interval* to prevent overdosing. Opioid dosing regimens for PCA are listed in Table 5.3.

TABLE 5.3	Commonly Used Intravenous Opioids		
	Morphine	Hydromorphone	Fentanyl
Onset	5-10 min	5-15 min	1-2 min
Bolus Dosing	2-4 mg q 1-2 h	0.2-0.6 mg q 1-2 h	0.35-0.5 µg/kg q 0.5-1 h
Infusion Rate	2-30 mg/h	0.5-3 mg/h	0.7-10 µg/kg/h
PCA Demand (bolus) Lockout Interval	0.5-3 mg 10-20 min	0.1-0.5 mg 5-15 min	15-75 µg 3-10 min
Lipid Solubility	x	0.2x	600x
Active Metabolites	Yes	Yes	No
Histamine Release	Yes	No	No
Dose Adjustment for Renal Failure	↓ 50%	↓ 50%	—

From References 2 and 4.

Adverse Effects of Opioids

Respiratory Depression

Opioids produce a centrally mediated, dose-dependent decrease in respiratory rate and tidal volume (with resulting hypercapnia), but *respiratory depression and hypoxemia are uncommon when opioids are given in the usual doses* (24). Patients with sleep apnea syndrome or chronic hypercapnia are particularly prone to respiratory depression from opioids.

Cardiovascular Effects

Opioid analgesia is often accompanied by decreases in blood pressure and heart rate, which are the result of decreased sympathetic activity and increased parasympathetic activity. These effects are usually mild and well-tolerated (24-25). Decreases in blood pressure can be more pronounced in patients with hypovolemia or heart failure, where there is an increased baseline sympathetic tone, or when opioids are given in combination with benzodiazepines (25). Opioid-induced hypotension is rarely a threat to tissue perfusion, and the blood pressure usually improves with intravenous fluids or a bolus doses of vasopressors.

Gastrointestinal Effects

Opioids are well known for their ability to depress bowel motility via activation of opioid receptors in the GI tract. This is a source of troublesome constipation, and not reliably reversed with the administration of methylnaltrexone, a peripheral opioid receptor antagonist (26). In critically ill patients, impaired GI motility can promote reflux of enteral tube feedings into the oropharynx, creating a risk for aspiration pneumonitis. Opioids can promote vomiting via stimulation of the chemoreceptor trigger zone in the lower brainstem (24). All opioids are equivalent in their ability to promote vomiting, but vomiting induced by one opioid occasionally resolves when another opioid is used.

ANALGESIA WITH NON-OPIOIDS

Concerns regarding opioid dependency and adverse effects have prompted recommendations to reduce opioid consumption in ICU patients whenever possible. Several alternative analgesics are available and listed with dosing recommendations in Table 5.4.

TABLE 5.4 Intravenous Non-Opioid Analgesia

Drug	Dosing Regimens and Comments
Acetaminophen	Dosing: 1 g IV every 6 h. Daily dose should not exceed 4 g. Comment: Has no anti-inflammatory activity.
Ketorolac	Dosing: 30 mg IV every 6 h. Reduce dose by 50% for patients with renal failure, age ≥65 yrs, or body weight <50 kg. Comment: Serious complications (e.g., renal impairment) are uncommon with short-term use.
Ketamine	Dosing: 60-120 µg/h in combination with an opioid. Comment: Psychomimetic effects are not prominent at the doses used for opioid-sparing analgesia.

From Analgesia and Sedation in the ICU. In: Marino PL. *Marino's The ICU Book*. 5th ed. Wolters Kluwer; 2025:86-104. Table 6.3.

Acetaminophen (Paracetamol)

Acetaminophen (North America) and paracetamol (Europe and other nations) are two generic names for a chemical substance known as *para-acetylaminophenol* (there is no difference between the two agents and acetaminophen is used here). Acetaminophen (Tylenol) was approved for intravenous use in 2010 and is indicated for the short-term treatment of pain and fever in postoperative patients who are unable to receive the drug via oral or rectal routes.

Dosing Regimen

The recommended dose is 1 g IV every 6 h, with a maximum allowable dose of 4 g daily (to prevent acetaminophen hepatotoxicity) (27). The major disadvantage of acetaminophen, in addition to the risk of hepatotoxicity, is the lack of an anti-inflammatory effect. IV acetaminophen is not superior for acute and postoperative pain when compared to oral or rectal acetaminophen when administered in equal doses (28). Therefore, IV acetaminophen, which is more costly than oral or rectal preparations, should be reserved for use when oral or rectal administration is not safe or possible.

Ketorolac

Ketorolac is a nonsteroidal anti-inflammatory drug (NSAID) that produces analgesia without respiratory depression. The drug can be used alone for mild pain but is more often used in combination with an opioid analgesic for moderate-to-severe pain. Ketorolac co-administration can reduce the opioid dose by 25-50% (29).

Dosing Regimen

Ketorolac can be given by IV or intramuscular (IM) injection, but IM injections of ketorolac can produce hematomas, so the IV route is preferred. The recommended dosing regimen for moderate-to-severe pain is 30 mg IV every 6 h (30). A 50% dose reduction (15 mg every 6 h) is recommended for patients with renal impairment, advanced age, and for those with a body weight <50 kg (30).

Adverse Effects and Risks

The beneficial actions of ketorolac and other NSAIDs are attributed to inhibition of prostaglandin production, but this also creates a risk for gastric mucosal injury and impaired renal function. These adverse effects are typically associated with excessive dosing or prolonged exposure to NSAIDs, and they are uncommon with short-term ketorolac use in the recommended doses (30). The use of NSAIDs such as ketorolac in postoperative ICU patients has been tempered by the perceived increased risk of bleeding because NSAIDs block the formation of thromboxane A2, a platelet-activating eicosanoid. However, multiple studies have shown that NSAIDs are unlikely to be the cause of postoperative bleeding complications, though use is not advised immediately following surgical cases with a high risk for bleeding (e.g., massive blood loss, acute traumatic coagulopathy) (31-32).

Ketamine

Ketamine is an anesthetic agent with sedative and analgesic properties that was first synthesized and tested in the 1960s as an alternative to phencyclidine (PCP) (5,33-34). Ketamine is highly lipophilic, crossing the blood brain area quickly with a near-immediate onset of action when given as an IV bolus. The dissociative effect associated with ketamine places a patient in a cataleptic state; the patient may seem awake but cannot process or respond to sensory input (33-34). Other notable effects of ketamine include increases in blood pressure and heart rate (sympathomimetic effects), bronchodilation, nausea and vomiting, and hypersalivation (rare) (33-34). The sympathomimetic effects may be advantageous in patients with circulatory shock (33), while the bronchodilation is desirable in patients with asthma or bronchospasm (34). Ketamine has analgesic properties and has been shown to reduce opioid consumption (33-34).

Dosing Regimen

The dissociative effect of ketamine, an effect that some patients find intensely unpleasant, is typically observed when ketamine is given at a dose >0.5 mg/kg over 40 min (35). When used for sedation in the ICU, a wide variety of IV infusion dosing ranges have been described (0.06-2.0 mg/kg/h). Less dissociation has been reported when lower doses are used (33-34,36).

Drugs for Neuropathic Pain

Non-opioid analgesia is usually required for neuropathic pain (e.g., from diabetic neuropathy), and the recommended drugs for this type of pain are *gabapentin*, *pregabalin*, and *carbamazepine* (2). These drugs must be given enterally. Effective drug doses vary in individual patients, but typical doses are 600 mg every 8 h for gabapentin, 25 mg once daily (or 50-150 mg/day in 2-3 divided doses) for pregabalin and 100 mg every 6 h for carbamazepine.

ANXIETY IN THE ICU

Anxiety and related disorders (agitation and delirium) are observed in as many as 85% of patients in the ICU (37). These disorders can be defined as follows:

1. *Anxiety* is characterized by exaggerated feelings of fear or apprehension that are sustained by internal mechanisms more than external events.
2. *Agitation* is a state of anxiety that is accompanied by increased motor activity.
3. *Delirium* is an acute confusional state that may, or may not, have agitation as a component. Although delirium is often equated with agitation, there is a hypoactive form of delirium that is characterized by lethargy (delirium is described in more detail in Chapter 42: Disorders of Consciousness).

A common finding in these disorders is the *absence of a sense of well-being*.

Sedation

Sedation is the process of relieving anxiety and establishing a state of calm. This process includes general supportive measures (like frequent communication with patients and families) and drug therapy. Several drugs are available for sedation in ICU patients, including benzodiazepines (e.g., midazolam), propofol, dexmedetomidine, and haloperidol.

Monitoring Sedation

The use of sedation scales is instrumental in achieving effective sedation in the ICU. The most widely used sedation scale is the Richmond Agitation-Sedation Scale (RASS), which is shown in Table 5.5 (38).

The routine use of sedation scales is instrumental for achieving effective sedation in the ICU. The optimal RASS score is zero (alert and calm). The RASS allows clinicians to monitor serial changes in a patient's mental state while titrating sedative medications to an acceptable end point (i.e., a RASS score of −1 to −2, which represents light sedation).

BENZODIAZEPINES

Benzodiazepines have been the traditional sedative agents used in the ICU, but they are gradually losing ground to other sedatives because of drug accumulation with prolonged use, and an increased risk of ICU-related delirium (see Chapter 42: Disorders of Consciousness). There are two benzodiazepines that are favored for intravenous delivery: midazolam (Versed) and lorazepam (Ativan). Diazepam (Valium) is generally avoided because of the long half-life (90 h) and the presence of active metabolites which promote prolonged sedation, especially with renal impairment. The intravenous dosing regimens for midazolam and lorazepam are shown in Table 5.6 (3).

Advantages

The advantages of sedation with benzodiazepines include the following:

1. The rapid onset of action makes benzodiazepines well-suited for the acute management of anxiety and agitation.

TABLE 5.5 The Richmond Agitation-Sedation Scale

Score	Term	Description
+4	Combative	Overly combative or violent; immediate danger to staff
+3	Very agitated	Pulls on or removes tube(s), catheter(s), or aggressive behavior
+2	Agitated	Frequent non-purposeful movement or patient-ventilator asynchrony
+1	Restless	Anxious or apprehensive but movements not aggressive or vigorous
0	Alert & calm	
-1	Drowsy	Not fully alert, but awakens for >10 sec, with eye contact, to voice
-2	Light sedation	Any movement (but no eye contact) to voice
-3	Moderate sedation	Less compliance associated with narrower airway
-4	Deep sedation	No response to voice, but movement to physical stimulation
-5	Unarousable	No response to voice or physical stimulation

To determine the RASS, proceed as follows:

Step 1 Observation: Observe the patient without interaction. If patient is alert, assign the appropriate score (0 to +4). If patient is not alert, go to Step 2.

Step 2 Verbal Stimulation: Address the patient by name in a loud voice and ask the patient to look at you. Can repeat once if necessary. If patient responds to voice, assign the appropriate score (-1 to -3). If there is no response, go to Step 3.

Step 3 Physical Stimulation: Shake the patient's shoulder. If there is no response, rub the sternum vigorously. Assign the appropriate score (-4 to -5).

From Sessler CN, Gosnell MS, Grap MJ, et al. The Richmond Agitation-Sedation Scale: validity and reliability in adult intensive care units. Am J Resp Crit Care Med 2002;166:1338-44.

2. Benzodiazepines cause a dose-dependent anterograde amnesia that is distinct from the sedative effect (6,11). Short-term memory is less affected than long-term memory.
3. Benzodiazepines are the sedatives of choice for the management of alcohol and opioid withdrawal as well as status epilepticus (see Chapter 43: Disorders of Movement) (39).

TABLE 5.6	Sedation with Intravenous Benzodiazepines	
Feature	Midazolam	Lorazepam
Bolus Dose	0.01–0.05 mg/kg	0.02–0.04 mg/kg
Onset of Action	3–5 min	5–15 min
Duration	1–2 h	2–6 h
Continuous Infusion	0.02–0.1 mg/kg/h	0.01–0.1 mg/kg/h
Lipid Solubility	+++	++
Active Metabolites	Yes	Yes
Concerns	Active Metabolites	Propylene Glycol Toxicity

From Barr J, Fraser GL, Puntillo K, et al. Clinical practice guidelines for the management of pain, agitation, and delirium in adult patients in the intensive care unit. Crit Care Med 2013;41:263-306.

Disadvantages

The disadvantages of sedation with benzodiazepines are the following:

1. Benzodiazepines have a tendency to accumulate and produce excessive sedation and delayed awakening, which can delay weaning from mechanical ventilation and prolong the ICU stay. This is more of a problem with midazolam compared with lorazepam (discussed in the section that follows).
2. Clinical studies have shown a strong relationship between benzodiazepine use and delirium in ICU patients (3-4).

Preventive measures can be used to prevent oversedation and delirium. Sedation "holidays" (i.e., daily interruption of infusions), careful titration of agents to the appropriate sedation

(RASS) level, or avoidance of benzodiazepines for prolonged sedation are strategies than can minimize detrimental effects.

Drugs

Midazolam

Midazolam is a short-acting drug that is favored for procedural sedation. Sedative effects are apparent within 5 min and last for 1-2 h. Midazolam is highly lipid soluble and will accumulate in the central nervous system when infused continuously. To avoid prolonged sedation from drug accumulation, *midazolam infusions should be limited to ≤48 h* (3). An exception to this axiom is *refractory status epilepticus*, where midazolam infusions are usually started at a dose of 0.2 mg/kg/h and increased until seizures cease, to a maximum dose of 2.9 mg/kg/h (39-40). Midazolam is metabolized by the cytochrome P450 system in the liver, and drugs that interfere with this system (e.g., diltiazem, erythromycin) can potentiate sedative effects. Midazolam has a metabolite that is cleared by the kidneys, so renal impairment may lead to prolonged sedation (3-4).

Lorazepam

Lorazepam was once used more frequently in the ICU but has fallen out of favor due to a longer half-life than midazolam and concerns for propylene glycol toxicity. Propylene glycol is added to intravenous lorazepam to enhance drug solubility in plasma. Propylene glycol is converted to lactic acid in the liver, and excessive intake can produce a clinical syndrome characterized by a metabolic (lactic) acidosis, altered mentation, systemic inflammation, and renal failure (41). The risk for toxicity is highest when the lorazepam infusion rate exceeds the upper limit of the recommended rate (0.1 mg/kg/h), or is >10 mg/h, for longer than 48 h. Plasma levels of propylene glycol are not routinely available, and lactate levels are not reliable for predicting toxicity, but an elevated osmolal gap (i.e., >10 mOsm/kg H_2O) has shown a good correlation with propylene glycol accumulation (42).

Remimazolam

Remimazolam is a newer short acting benzodiazepine that has a fast onset of action (i.e., 3 min to peak sedation) and a short duration of action (i.e., time to full alertness typically occurs 10-15 min after the last dose) (43). Remimazolam holds promise as a potential benzodiazepine for use in the ICU due to its unique pharmacological properties, but additional large-scale ICU studies are required to confirm data regarding safety and efficacy in critically ill patients (44).

SEDATION WITH RAPID AROUSAL AGENTS

Propofol

Propofol (Diprivan) is a rapidly acting GABAergic sedative that was introduced for the induction of general anesthesia and has subsequently become a standard agent for sedation during mechanical ventilation. A profile of this drug is presented in Table 5.7.

TABLE 5.7	Sedation with Rapid Arousal Agents	
Feature	Propofol	Dexmedetomidine
Loading Dose	5 μg/kg/min over 5 min	1 μg/kg over 10 min
Onset of Action	1-2 min	5-10 min
Maintenance Infusion	5-50 μg/kg/min	0.2-0.7 μg/kg/h
Time to Arousal	10-15 min	6-10 min
Respiratory Depression	Yes	No
Adverse Effects	• Hypotension • Hyperlipidemia • Propofol Infusion Syndrome	• Hypotension • Bradycardia

Dosing recommendations from Reference 2.

Actions

Propofol has sedative, amnesic, and anticonvulsant effects, but is devoid of analgesic effects (45). Propofol is used in the ICU as a continuous infusion to provide sedation. The arousal time is dependent on the depth and length of sedation as depicted in Table 5.8.

TABLE 5.8	Factors that Influence Emergence from Propofol Sedation	
	Arousal Time	
Infusion Time	Light Sedation	Deep Sedation
24 h	13 min	25 h
72 h	34 min	59 h
7 days	3.3 h	71 h
14 days	3.4 h	74 h

From Barr J, Egan TD, Sandoval NF, et al. Propofol dosing regimens for ICU sedation based upon an integrated pharmacokinetic-pharmacodynamic model. Anesthesiology 2001;95:324-33.

Dosing

Dosing recommendations are listed in Table 5.7. Of note, higher doses are occasionally used (up to 100 µg/kg/min) but are associated with adverse effects, as discussed below. Propofol is suspended in a 10% lipid emulsion that has a caloric density of 1 kcal/mL, which should be accounted for as part of the daily caloric intake. Propofol dosing is based on *ideal rather than actual body weight*, and no dose adjustment is required for renal failure or hepatic insufficiency (45).

Adverse Effects

The most common side effects of propofol are respiratory depression and hypotension. Hypotension is attributed to decreased systemic vascular resistance (SVR) and may be more pronounced in conditions such as hypovolemia and heart failure (4). Other side effects include hypertriglyceridemia, necrotizing pancreatitis (rare), anaphylactoid reactions (rare), and a greenish hue in urine (caused by harmless phenolic metabolites) (45-46). Propofol was previously contraindicated in patients with allergies to eggs, egg products, or soybeans, but multiple studies have confirmed that use of propofol is safe in patients with these allergies and should only be avoided if prior allergic reactions were severe (4,25).

Propofol-Related Infusion Syndrome. Propofol-related infusion syndrome (PRIS) is a rare (<1%) but highly lethal (>30% mortality) complication associated with prolonged (i.e., >48 h) and/or high dose (i.e., >5 mg/kg/h or >80 µg/kg/min) infusions, though the syndrome has been reported to occur at lower infusion dose ranges (47-50). PRIS is characterized by an abrupt onset of systolic heart failure, lactic acidosis (may be a late sign), elevated creatinine phosphokinase (>5,000 IU/L), and acute renal failure, with rapid progression to multiple organ failure (47-48). There is no single clinical feature present in all cases, and lipemia is only present in 20-40% of patients with PRIS. Primary and secondary features are listed in Table 5.9 (47-49). *The diagnosis of PRIS should be strongly considered when one or more otherwise unexplained primary or secondary features are present in critically ill patients who receive high or prolonged doses of propofol* (47-49).

TABLE 5.9 Features of Propofol-Related Infusion Syndrome

Primary Features	Secondary Features
Metabolic acidosis	Acute kidney injury
ECG changes (i.e., Brugada-like changes; coved-type ST-segment elevation in V_1-V_3)	Hyperkalemia
	Lipidemia (only present in 20-40%)
	Cardiogenic shock
Rhabdomyolysis (creatinine phosphokinase >5,000 IU/L)	Elevated liver enzymes
	Elevated lactate
	Fever

From References 47-49.

Following immediate cessation of propofol in suspected cases, treatment is supportive. Hemodialysis and extracorporeal membrane oxygenation are often required (see

Chapters 30: Extracorporeal Membrane Oxygenation and 33: Acute Kidney Injury).

Dexmedetomidine

Dexmedetomidine (Precedex) is a central α_2 adrenergic agonist that has sedative, amnesic, and mild analgesic effects, and does not depress ventilation (51). A brief profile of the drug is presented in Table 5.7.

Advantages

Dexmedetomidine is associated with the following advantages:

1. Sedation with dexmedetomidine allows arousal to be maintained, despite deep levels of sedation. This obviates the need for periodic or daily sedation interruptions.
2. Dexmedetomidine has minimal effects on respiratory function and can be used in patients who require sedation but are not mechanically ventilated.
3. Dexmedetomidine has modest analgesic properties and opioid-sparing effects.
4. Delirium is less frequent with dexmedetomidine compared with propofol (52).

Disadvantages

1. When given as a rapid bolus, transient hypertension and bradycardia (baroreceptor effect) may occur as the result of initial *peripheral* α_2B receptor activation.
2. Dexmedetomidine produces dose-dependent decreases in heart rate, blood pressure, and circulating norepinephrine levels (sympatholytic effect), and this effect is particularly marked in conditions where heart rate and blood pressure are supported by increased sympathetic activity (e.g., heart failure with reduced ejection fraction) (5,51).
3. Dexmedetomidine can have a withdrawal syndrome characterized by signs of sympathetic overactivity (i.e.,

tachycardia, hypertension, and agitation). Dexmedetomidine withdrawal is reported in 30% of patients and is unrelated to the infusion rate or duration (53).
4. Doses higher than 1.5 µg/kg/h are not effective (54).

ANTIPSYCHOTIC AGENTS

Several antipsychotic agents are used for sedation and anxiolysis in hospitalized patients, including *atypical* antipsychotic agents such as ziprasidone (Geodon), quetiapine (Seroquel), risperidone (Risperdal), olanzapine (Zyprexa), and the *typical* antipsychotic agent, haloperidol (Haldol).

Haloperidol

Haloperidol is a dopamine receptor antagonist that promotes sedation without respiratory depression or cardiovascular compromise (although hypotension is a risk in hypovolemic patients) (55). The principal use of haloperidol has been for the treatment of agitation and delirium that are not the result of alcohol or drug withdrawal.

Dosing

Table 5.10 lists a suggested dosing regimen for haloperidol.

TABLE 5.10 Intravenous Haloperidol for Sedation

1. Begin with 5 mg of haloperidol as an intravenous bolus.
2. For severely agitated or disruptive patients, add midazolam (1 mg) for a more rapid onset of sedation.
3. Wait 15 min.
4. If no response, double the dose of haloperidol (10 mg IV).
5. If no response after the second dose, switch to another agent.
6. If the response is satisfactory, maintain sedation with periodic doses of haloperidol (at 25% of the effective dose) given at 6-h intervals.

From Analgesia and Sedation in the ICU. In: Marino PL. *Marino's The ICU Book*. 5th ed. Wolters Kluwer; 2025:86-104. Table 6.8.

Haloperidol should not be used if the corrected QT interval (QTc) on the ECG is >500 msec.

Adverse Effects

The following adverse effects are associated with haloperidol:

1. *Extrapyramidal syndrome* (EPS) reactions (e.g., rigidity, spasmodic movements) are dose-related side effects when haloperidol is given orally, but these reactions are uncommon when haloperidol is given intravenously (55).
2. Prolongation of the QT interval may occur with haloperidol, triggering a polymorphic ventricular tachycardia in 3-4% of patients (*torsades de pointes*, described in Chapter 20: Dysrhythmias). Most reported cases have occurred when the daily dose of haloperidol is > 35 mg and when the QTc is >500 msec (56).
3. Haloperidol can trigger the *neuroleptic malignant syndrome*, which is an idiosyncratic reaction that presents with hyperpyrexia, severe muscle rigidity, and rhabdomyolysis (see Chapter 6: Evaluation of Fever in the ICU).
4. Haloperidol has been associated with increased mortality or cardiopulmonary arrest in adults aged 65 years and older; caution should be exercised when prescribing this drug in older adults (57).

Other Antipsychotics

The use of atypical antipsychotics (e.g., ziprasidone, quetiapine, risperidone, olanzapine) has become more popular in ICUs for treating anxiety and delirium, even though the use of these drugs for the prevention and management of delirium is discouraged in international guidelines (3,58). Atypical antipsychotic drugs may be helpful for managing sedation when other sedatives are not tolerated or contraindicated. When choosing a particular agent, the receptor binding profile may helpful (Table 5.11).

TABLE 5.11	Receptor Binding Profiles for Commonly Used Atypical Antipsychotics					
Drug	**Receptor Site of Action**					
	D_1	D_2	D_3	$α_1$	Histamine 1	Serotonin 5-HT$_{2A}$
Risperidone	+++	++++	+	++++	++	++++
Olanzapine	++++	++	+	++	++++	++++
Quetiapine	+	+	0	++	++++	+
Ziprasidone	+	++++	?	++	++	++++
Receptors	**Function/Adverse Effects**					
D_1	• Mediates hallucinations, delusions • Adverse effects: EPS, elevated prolactin levels					
D_2	• Mediates hallucinations, delusions • Adverse effects: EPS					
D_3	• May enhance motivation and cognitive dysfunction • Adverse effects: EPS (lower risk compared to D_2)					
$α_1$	• Adverse effects: orthostatic hypotension, dizziness, drowsiness					
Histamine 1	• Adverse effects: sedation, weight gain, impaired cognition					
Serotonin 5-HT$_{2A}$	• Balances D_2 blockade and attenuates EPS, plays role in circadian rhythm and may mediate hallucinations					

From References 59 and 60.

For example, if less orthostatic hypotension is desired, a drug with less $α_1$ receptor antagonism could be chosen (e.g., olanzapine, ziprasidone). If more sedation is desired, an agent with greater histamine-1 receptor blocking activity could be used (e.g., quetiapine) (59-61).

PUTTING IT ALL TOGETHER

An algorithm for managing pain, agitation, delirium, and sedation (PADS) in the ICU is presented in Figure 5.1 (delirium

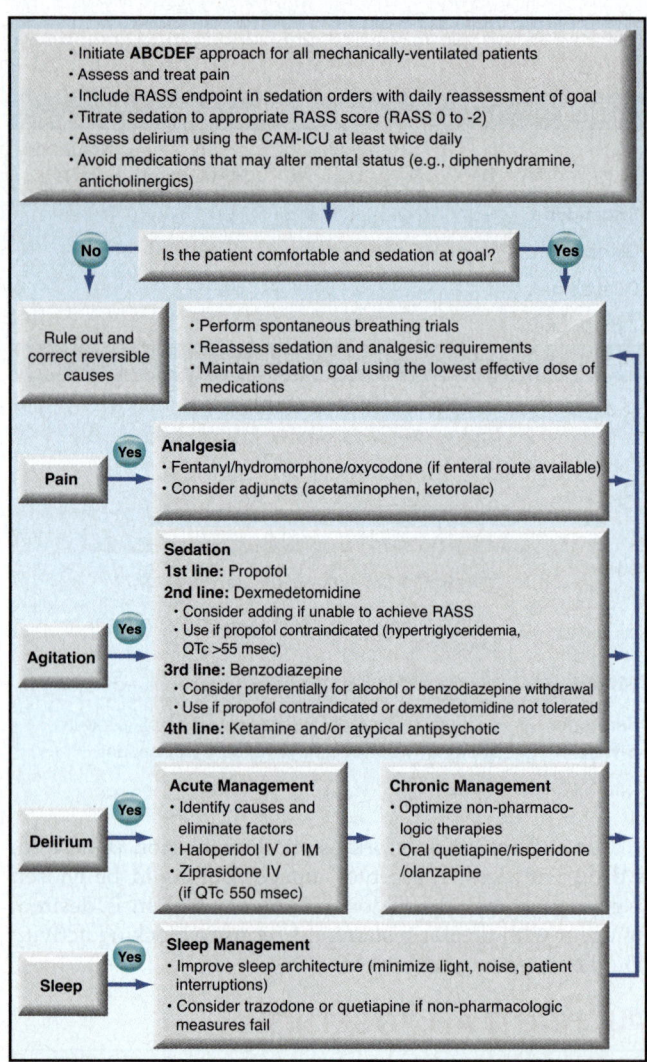

FIGURE 5.1. Pain, agitation, delirium, and sleep (PADS) algorithm. See Chapter 42 for additional details about delirium management.

is discussed more extensively in Chapter 42: Disorders of Consciousness).

References

1. Rotondi AJ, Chelluri L, Sirio C, et al. Patients' recollections of stressful experiences while receiving prolonged mechanical ventilation in an intensive care unit. Crit Care Med 2002;30:746-52.
2. Barr J, Fraser GL, Puntillo K, et al. Clinical practice guidelines for the management of pain, agitation, and delirium in adult patients in the intensive care unit. Crit Care Med 2013;41:263-306.
3. Devlin JW, Skrobik Y, Gélinas C, et al. Clinical practice guidelines for the prevention and management of pain, agitation/sedation, delirium, immobility, and sleep disruption in adult patients in the ICU. Crit Care Med 2018;48:e825-e873.
4. Devlin JW, Roberts RJ. Pharmacology of commonly used analgesics and sedatives in the ICU: benzodiazepines, propofol, and opioids. Crit Care Clin 2009;25:431-49.
5. Panzer O, Moitra V, Sladen RN. Pharmacology of sedative-analgesic agents: dexmedetomidine, remifentanil, ketamine, volatile anesthetics, and the role of peripheral mu antagonists. Crit Care Clin 2009;25:451-69.
6. Azevedo K, Johnson M, Wasserman M, Evans-Wall J. Drugs of abuse—opioids, sedatives, hypnotics. Crit Care Clin 2021;37:501-16.
7. Payen J-F, Chanques G, Mantz J, et al. for the DOLOREA Investigators. Current practices in sedation and analgesia for mechanically ventilated critically ill patients. Anesthesiology 2007;106:687-95.
8. Chanques G, Sebbane M, Barbotte E, et al. A prospective study of pain at rest: incidence and characteristics of an unrecognized symptom in surgical and trauma versus medical intensive care unit patients. Anesthesiology 2007;107:858-60.
9. Pain terms: a list with definitions and notes on usage, recommended by the IASP subcommittee on taxonomy. Pain 1979;6:249.
10. Scholten W. Make your words support your message. J Pain Palliat Care Pharmacother 2015;29(1):44-7.
11. Veselis RA, Reinsel RA, Feshchenko VA, et al. The comparative amnestic effects of midazolam, propofol, thiopental, and fentanyl at equisedative concentrations. Anesthesiology 1997;87:749-64.
12. Davis MP, McPherson ML, Reddy A, Case AA. Conversion ratios: why is it so challenging to construct opioid conversion tables? J Opioid Manag 2024;20(2):169-79.
13. Shafi A, Berry AJ, Sumnall H, et al. Synthetic opioids: a review and clinical update. Ther Adv Psychopharmacol 2022;12:20451253221139616.
14. Tan S, Lee E, Lee S, et al. Morphine equianalgesic dose chart in the emergency department. J Educ Teach Emerg Med 2022;7(3):L1-L20.

15. Payen JF, Bru O, Bosson JL, et al. Assessing pain in critically ill sedated patients by using a behavioral pain scale. Crit Care Med 2001;29(12):2258-63.
16. Smith MT. Neuroexcitatory effects of morphine and hydromorphone: evidence implicating the 3-glucuronide metabolites. Clin Exp Pharmacol Physiol 2000;27:524-8.
17. Pasternak GW. Pharmacological mechanisms of opioid analgesics. Clin Neuropharmacol 1993;16:1-18.
18. Aronoff GR, Berns JS, Brier ME, et al. *Drug Prescribing in Renal Failure: Dosing Guidelines for Adults.* 4th ed. American College of Physicians; 1999.
19. Rosow CE, Moss J, Philbin DM, Savarese JJ. Histamine release during morphine and fentanyl anesthesia. Anesthesiology 1982;56:93-6.
20. Felden L, Walter C, Harder S, et al. Comparative clinical effects of hydromorphone and morphine: a meta-analysis. Br J Anesth 2011; 107:319-28.
21. Coluzzi F, Caputi FF, Billeci D, et al. Safe use of opioids in chronic kidney disease and hemodialysis patients: tips and tricks for non-pain specialists. Ther Clin Risk Manag 2020;16:821-37.
22. Lee KA, Ganta N, Horton JR, Chai E. Evidence for neurotoxicity due to morphine or hydromorphone use in renal impairment: a systematic review. J Palliat Med 2016;19(11):1179-87.
23. Babul N, Darke AC, Hagen N. Hydromorphone metabolite accumulation in renal failure. J Pain Symptom Manage 1995;10(3):184-6.
24. Bowdle TA. Adverse effects of opioid agonists and agonist-antagonists in anaesthesia. Drug Safety 1998;19:173-89.
25. Darrouj J, Karma L, Arora R. Cardiovascular manifestations of sedatives and analgesics in the critical care unit. Am J Ther 2009;16(4): 339-53.
26. Patel PB, Brett SJ, O'Callaghan D, et al. Methylnaltrexone for the treatment of opioid-induced constipation and gastrointestinal stasis in intensive care patients. Results from the MOTION trial. Intensive Care Med 2020;46:747-55.
27. Yeh YC, Reddy P. Clinical and economic evidence for intravenous acetaminophen. Pharmacother 2012;32:559-79.
28. Ibrahim T, Gebril A, Nasr MK, et al. Unlocking the optimal analgesic potential: a systematic review and meta-analysis comparing intravenous, oral, and rectal paracetamol in equivalent doses. Cureus 2023;15(7):e41876.
29. Gillis JC, Brogden RN. Ketorolac. A reappraisal of its pharmacodynamic and pharmacokinetic properties and therapeutic use in pain management. Drugs 1997;53:139-88.
30. Ketorolac drug monograph. In: *AHFS Drug Information, 2022.* American Society of Health System Pharmacists; 2022:2060-71.
31. Bongiovanni T, Lancaster E, Ledesma Y, et al. Systematic review and meta-analysis of the association between non-steroidal anti-

inflammatory drugs and operative bleeding in the perioperative period. J Am Coll Surg 2021;232(5):765-790.e1.
32. Sheth KR, Bernthal NM, Ho HS, et al. Perioperative bleeding and non-steroidal anti-inflammatory drugs: an evidence-based literature review, and current clinical appraisal. Medicine (Baltimore) 2020;99(31):e20042.
33. Mazzeffi M, Johnson K, Paciullo C. Ketamine in adult cardiac surgery and the cardiac surgery Intensive Care Unit: an evidence-based clinical review. Ann Card Anaesth 2015;18(2):202-9.
34. Erstad BL, Patanwala AE. Ketamine for analgosedation in critically ill patients. J Crit Care 2016;35:145-9.
35. Krystal JH, Karper LP, Seibyl JP, et al. Subanesthetic effects of the noncompetitive NMDA antagonist, ketamine, in humans. Psychotomimetic, perceptual, cognitive, and neuroendocrine responses. Arch Gen Psychiatry 1994;51(3):199-214.
36. Patanwala AE, Martin JR, Erstad BL. Ketamine for analgosedation in the intensive care unit: a systematic review. J Intensive Care Med 2017;32(6):387-95.
37. Ely EW, Inouye SK, Bernard GR, et al. Delirium in mechanically ventilated patients: validity and reliability of the confusion assessment method for the intensive care unit (CAM-ICU). JAMA 2001;286:2703-10.
38. Sessler CN, Gosnell MS, Grap MJ, et al. The Richmond Agitation-Sedation Scale: validity and reliability in adult intensive care units. Am J Resp Crit Care Med 2002;166:1338-44.
39. Brophy GM, Bell R, Claassen J, et al. Guidelines for the evaluation and management of status epilepticus. Neurocrit Care 2012;17(1):3-23.
40. Rossetti AO. Refractory and super-refractory status epilepticus: therapeutic options and prognosis. Neurol Clin 2025;43(1):15-30.
41. Zar T, Graeber C, Perazella MA. Recognition, treatment, and prevention of propylene glycol toxicity. Semin Dial 2007;20:217-9.
42. Barnes BJ, Gerst C, Smith JR, et al. Osmolal gap as a surrogate marker for serum propylene glycol concentrations in patients receiving lorazepam for sedation. Pharmacotherapy 2006;26:23-33.
43. Teixeira MT, Goyal A. Remimazolam. Adv Anesth 2024;42(1):131-50.
44. Orjuela RB, Ripoll JG. Con: Remimazolam: the new miracle cure for critically ill patients. J Cardiothorac Vasc Anesth 2025;39(4):1082-6.
45. McKeage K, Perry CM. Propofol: a review of its use in intensive care sedation of adults. CNS Drugs 2003;17:235-72.
46. Barr J, Egan TD, Sandoval NF, et al. Propofol dosing regimens for ICU sedation based upon an integrated pharmacokinetic-pharmacodynamic model. Anesthesiology 2001;95:324-33.
47. Hemphill S, McMenamin L, Bellamy MC, Hopkins PM. Propofol infusion syndrome: a structured literature review and analysis of published case reports. Br J Anaesth 2019;122(4):448-59.

48. Anjankar SA. Propofol-related infusion syndrome: a clinical review. Cureus 2022;14:e30383.
49. Krajčová A, Waldauf P, Anděl M, Duška F. Propofol infusion syndrome: a structured review of experimental studies and 153 published case reports. Crit Care 2015;19:398.
50. Li WK, Chen XJC, Altshuler D, et al. The incidence of propofol infusion syndrome in critically-ill patients. J Crit Care 2022;71:154098.
51. Weerink MAS, Struys MMRF, Hannivoort LN, et al. Clinical pharmacokinetics and pharmacodynamics of dexmedetomidine. Clin Pharmacokinet 2017;56(8):893-913.
52. Lewis K, Alshamsi F, Carayannopoulos KL, et al. on behalf of the GUIDE group. Dexmedetomidine vs other sedatives in critically ill mechanically ventilated adults: a systematic review and meta-analysis of randomized trials. Intensive Care Med 2022;48:811-40.
53. Pathan S, Kaplan JB, Adamczyk K, et al. Evaluation of dexmedetomidine withdrawal in critically ill adults. J Crit Care 2021;62:19-24.
54. Venn M, Newman J, Grounds M. A phase II study to evaluate the efficacy of dexmedetomidine for sedation in the medical intensive care unit. Intensive Care Med 2003;29(2):201-7.
55. Beach SR, Gross AF, Hartney KE, et al. Intravenous haloperidol: a systematic review of side effects and recommendations for clinical use. Gen Hosp Psychiatry 2020;67:42-50.
56. Sharma ND, Rosman HS, Padhi ID, Tisdale JE. Torsade de pointes associated with intravenous haloperidol in critically ill patients. Am J Cardiol 1998;81:238-40.
57. Basciotta M, Zhou W, Ngo L, et al. Antipsychotics and the risk of mortality or cardiopulmonary arrest in hospitalized adults. J Am Geriatr Soc 2020;68(3):544-50.
58. Tomlinson EJ, Schnitker LM, Casey PA. Exploring antipsychotic use for delirium management in adults in hospital, sub-acute rehabilitation and aged care settings: a systematic literature review. Drugs Aging 2024;41(6):455-86.
59. Gareri P, De Fazio P, Stilo M, et al. Conventional and atypical antipsychotics in the elderly: a review. Clin Drug Investig 2003;23(5):287-322.
60. Bouman WP, Pinner G. Use of atypical antipsychotic drugs in old age psychiatry. Adv Psychiatr Treatment 2002;8(1):49-58.
61. Shafiekhani M, Mirjalili M, Vazin A. Psychotropic drug therapy in patients in the intensive care unit—usage, adverse effects, and drug interactions: a review. Ther Clin Risk Manag 2018;14:1799-812.

Evaluation of Fever in the ICU

Chapter 6

Fever is always a source of concern in a hospitalized patient, especially in the ICU. Unfortunately, the etiology can be obscure.

FEVER

Fever in the ICU is defined by the Society of Critical Care Medicine (SCCM) and the Infectious Diseases Society of America (IDSA) as a single body temperature ≥38.3° C (101° F) (1). In neutropenic patients, a lower threshold of 38.0° C (100.4° F) for >1 h is used (2). Outside of these definitions, there are no standardized grades of fever, although some authors define a high-grade (severe) fever as >39° C (102.4° F) and hyperthermia as a temperature >40° to 41° C (104° to 105.8° F) (3).

Core body temperatures obtained via thermistor-equipped catheters placed in the pulmonary artery, esophagus, or urinary bladder are more accurate than measurements obtained with rectal, oral, and tympanic temperature probes. If core measurements are not available, then rectal or oral temperatures are recommended (1), whereas axillary and temporal artery sites are not endorsed for temperature measurements. Thermistor-equipped catheters have the advantage of continuous monitoring.

INFLAMMATION VERSUS INFECTION

Fever is the result of inflammatory cytokines (called *endogenous pyrogens*) that act on the hypothalamus to elevate the body temperature. Any condition that triggers a systemic inflammatory response will produce a fever. Therefore, fever is an indication of inflammation, not necessarily an infection, and around 50% of ICU patients who develop a fever have no apparent infection (4-5). The severity of a fever does not correlate with the presence or severity of infection. High fevers can be the result of a noninfectious condition such as a drug fever (see later), while fever can be minimal or absent in life-threatening infections (2). The distinction between inflammation and infection is an important one, not only for the evaluation of fever, but also for curtailing the "knee jerk" response of using antibiotics to treat fever.

Inflammatory (Noninfectious) Etiologies

Noninfectious etiologies of fever in the ICU are widespread. Examples are shown in Table 6.1.

TABLE 6.1   Examples of Non-Infectious Sources of ICU Fever

- Aspiration Pneumonitis
- Venous Thromboembolism
- Acalculous Cholecystitis
- Febrile Transfusion Reaction
- Drug Fever
- Adrenal Insufficiency
- Pancreatitis
- Thyroid Storm
- Autoimmune Disease
- Malignancies

Aspiration Pneumonitis

Aspiration Pneumonitis does not require antibiotics in stable patients. In unstable patients, antibiotic coverage is warranted for community-acquired organisms. Antibiotic coverage for nosocomial infections is indicated for patients admitted within a healthcare facility for >72 h (6).

Venous Thromboembolism

Both deep venous thrombosis (DVT) and pulmonary embolism (PE) can result in fever. The incidence with PE is approximately 15% (7). Fever associated with DVT carries a worse outcome, but concurrent infection likely contributes (8).

Acalculous Cholecystitis

Acalculous Cholecystitis is caused by impaired gallbladder emptying as opposed to the typical cholecystitis caused by a gallstone obstructing the cystic duct. Risk factors include prolonged fasting and/or total parenteral nutrition, recent myocardial infarction, or major surgery (9). Prolonged distention can lead to necrosis and perforation, thus acalculous can be infected as well. Laboratories will demonstrate elevated liver function studies and a leukocytosis. Gallbladder distention and thickening of the gallbladder wall will be visible on ultrasonography. The placement of a percutaneous cholecystostomy tube is temporary in patients who are unstable.

Febrile Transfusion Reaction

Between 1% and 3% of transfusions result in febrile, non-hemolytic reactions occurring during the transfusion or up to six hours following it (10).

Anti-leukocyte antibodies in recipient blood react with antigens on donor leukocytes, triggering the release of endogenous pyrogens from phagocytes, causing the febrile response (11).

Drug Fever

Any drug can trigger a fever (as a hypersensitivity reaction). Even commonly used analgesics also used as antipyretics, i.e., acetaminophen and ibuprofen, have been reported as causing a drug fever (12-13). Common drug classes associated with drug fever are shown in Table 6.2 (14).

TABLE 6.2 Common Drug Classes Associated with Drug Fever

Antibiotics	*Anti-arrhythmics*
• Especially beta-lactams	• e.g., quinidine and procainamide
Anti-epileptics	• Diuretics
• Especially phenytoin	• Heparins

Derived from Achaiah NC, Bhutta BS, Ak AK. Fever in the Intensive Care Patient. [Updated 2023 Aug 17]. In: StatPearls [Internet]. Treasure Island (FL): StatPearls Publishing; 2025 Jan-.

Drug fever is poorly understood. Over 75% of drug fevers show no evidence of a hypersensitivity reaction (15). The median onset of the fever is 2 to 8 days (12) but can vary from a few hours to more than three weeks in most cases (12,14). In the case of neuroleptics and neuroleptic malignant syndrome, the onset can occur years later with chronic use (see below). Suspicion of drug fever usually occurs when there are no other likely sources of fever. When suspected, possible offending drugs should be discontinued. The fever should disappear in 2 to 3 days, but it can persist for up to 7 days (12,16).

Three drug-related hyperthermic presentations that are not considered "drug fevers" are worth further discussion.

1. *Malignant Hyperthermia (MH)* is an inherited disorder that produces muscle rigidity, hyperpyrexia, and rhabdomyolysis in response to halogenated inhalational anesthetics and the depolarizing neuromuscular relaxant, succinyl choline (17). MH may present immediately or in the early postoperative period. Succinyl choline is commonly used as a paralytic for endotracheal intubations in both the operating room and ICU. Rapid diagnosis and treatment with dantrolene sodium will decrease the mortality from ~30% to <5% (17). The clinical manifestations of MH are shown in Table 6.3 (17).

TABLE 6.3 Clinical Manifestations of Malignant Hyperthermia

Exposure to Volatile Anesthetics (e.g., Halothane and Sevoflurane) or Succinyl Choline	
Respiratory acidosis	End-tidal CO_2 >55 mm Hg; $PaCO_2$ >60 mm Hg
Cardiac	Sinus tachycardia, ventricular tachycardia, or ventricular fibrillation
Metabolic acidosis	Base deficit >8 mmol/L; pH <7.25
Muscle rigidity	
Rhabdomyolysis	Myoglobinuria, serum creatine kinase >20,000 U/L
Hyperthermia	Temperature >38.8° C

Derived from Rosenberg H, Davis M, James D, et al. Malignant hyperthermia. Orphanet J Rare Dis 2007;2:21.

2. *Neuroleptic Malignant Syndrome (NMS)* is a life-threatening syndrome associated with "neuroleptics" which are drugs that block or alter central nervous system dopamine (18,19). Neuroleptics encompass several groups of medications including (18):
   - Typical neuroleptics, e.g., haloperidol, thorazine, chlorpromazine
   - Atypical neuroleptics, e.g., olanzapine, risperidone, quetiapine
   - Antiemetics, e.g., droperidol, metoclopramide, promethazine
   - Dopaminergic agents (withdrawal), e.g., levodopa, amantadine, dopamine agonists

   Table 6.4 lists the criteria for diagnosing NMS (18).

TABLE 6.4 Criteria for Diagnosing Neuroleptic Malignant Syndrome*

Major Criteria (all required)	Other Criteria (at least 2 required)	
• Exposure to neuroleptic • Severe muscle rigidity • Fever	• Diaphoresis • Dysphagia • Tremor • Incontinence • Altered mental status	• Mutism • Tachycardia • Leukocytosis • Elevated or labile blood pressure • Elevated creatine phosphokinase

*Based on American Psychiatric Association. *The Diagnostic and Statistical Manual of Mental Disorders*. 5th ed. American Psychiatric Association Publishing; 2013.

From Simon LV, Hashmi MF, Callahan AL. Neuroleptic Malignant Syndrome. [Updated 2023 Apr 24]. In: StatPearls [Internet]. Treasure Island (FL): StatPearls Publishing; 2025 Jan-.

3. *Serotonin Syndrome (ST)* has symptoms ranging from mild to life-threatening, resulting from excess serotonin activity that can occur from therapeutic medication use, drug interactions, and overdose (20-21). Mechanisms of ST include the inhibition of serotonin uptake and metabolism, altered serotonin release, synthesis, and activation

of serotonin receptors involving a wide spectrum of drugs affecting serotonin. The most common interaction is the combination of selective serotonin reuptake inhibitor (SSRI) and a monoamine oxidase inhibitor (MAOI) (21). ST usually occurs within 24 h of a new serotonergic agent or dose change (20). Clinical manifestations of ST are shown in Table 6.5 (20-21).

TABLE 6.5 Clinical Manifestations of Serotonin Syndrome*	
• Tremor	• Hyperreflexia
• Mydriasis	• Fever (in severe cases >41° C)
• Diaphoresis	• Delirium
• Myoclonus	• Muscle rigidity

*Clinical manifestations can range from mild to severe.

Derived from Simon LV, Torrico TJ, Keenaghan M. Serotonin Syndrome. [Updated 2024 Mar 2]. In: StatPearls [Internet]. Treasure Island (FL): StatPearls Publishing; 2025 Jan-.

Less Common Etiologies

The following diagnoses are more typically comorbid conditions or reasons for ICU admission, but they can exacerbate or arise during an ICU stay.

- *Pancreatitis* is the most common etiologies for acute pancreatitis are gallstones and ethanol use. Drug-induced pancreatitis is responsible for 0.1-2% of pancreatitis diagnoses.
- *Adrenal Insufficiency* and critical illness-related corticosteroid insufficiency are discussed in Chapter 49: Adrenal and Thyroid Dysfunction.
- *Hyperthyroidism* and *Thyroid Storm* have both been reported after tracheostomy (22-23).
- *Rheumatologic* diseases comprise a large list of diseases such as systemic lupus erythematosus, scleroderma, rheumatoid arthritis, vasculitis, etc., that are all "inflammatory" processes that can be provoked in critical illness.

- Malignancies, through a variety of mechanisms such as tumor necrosis, cytokine production, and elevated pyrogens (interleukins) can cause fever (24).

Early Postoperative Fever

Fever in the first postoperative day following major surgery is common (15-40%), and in most cases, there is no apparent infection (5,25-27). These fevers usually resolve within 24-48 h, and most likely represent an inflammatory response to tissue injury sustained during the surgical procedure. Tissue injury occurring from surgery can induce interleukin-1, interleukin-5 production or other "damage-associated molecular patterns" known as "DAMPs" that cause release of pyrogens (28-29).

The traditional five "Ws" for postoperative fever deserve analysis. See Table 6.6 for their rationale.

TABLE 6.6		The Five "W's" of Postoperative Fever
1	**W**ind	Postoperative pain can contribute to poor pulmonary toilet (poor cough and low tidal volumes) leading to *atelectasis*.
2	**W**ater	Manipulation of the urinary tract, i.e., indwelling urinary catheters risk a catheter-associated urinary tract infection.
3	**W**ound	Any break in the skin is a risk of a surgical site infection, superficial or deep.
4	**W**alking	• Ambulation is critical to postoperative recovery. • Prolonged immobilization (anesthesia and confined to bed) along with the inflammatory response to surgery are risks for venous thromboembolism.
5	**W**onder Drugs	Numerous drugs are associated with fever.

1. *Wind*. There is a longstanding misconception that atelectasis is a common cause of fever in the early postoperative period, likely due to the concomitant nature

of fever and atelectasis. The incidence of atelectasis is no different in patients with postoperative fever than those without (27). A systematic review of eight studies concluded there was no evidence regarding an association of atelectasis and fever (30). However, persistent atelectasis is a pneumonia risk (31).

2. *Water.* An indwelling urinary catheter is a risk for urinary tract infection. See Chapter 41: Urinary Tract Infections for discussion of catheter-associated urinary tract infections and asymptomatic bacteriuria.
3. *Wound.* Clearly all surgical incisions are at risk of infection and require daily (minimum) examinations. This includes peripheral intravenous and phlebotomy sites.
4. *Walking.* See previous section, *Inflammatory (Non-Infectious) Etiologies.* Chapter 4: Prophylaxis for Venous Thromboembolism discusses venous thromboembolism and appropriate prophylaxis.
5. *Wonder Drugs.* Antibiotics are one of the most common causes of drug fever. However, the patient's entire medication history should be reviewed. See discussion of *Drug Fever* in the previous section.

Iatrogenic Fever

Faulty thermal regulators in water mattresses and aerosol humidifiers can cause fever by transference (32). Checking the temperature settings on heated mattresses and ventilators is a brief investigation, but explaining why such a simple cause of fever was missed might take much longer.

Most Common ICU Infections

Approximately 12% of ICU admissions with a length of stay >48 h will develop at least one nosocomial infection (33). Four infections account for about three-quarters of the infections encountered in the ICU (33-34).

1. Ventilator-associated pneumonias are described in Chapter 28: Ventilator-Associated Pneumonia.

2. Urinary tract infections are described in Chapter 41: Urinary Tract Infections.
3. Central line associated bloodstream infections (CLABSI).
4. Surgical site infections.

Central Line-Associated Bloodstream Infections (CLABSI)

Central venous access is a common necessity for many ICU patients. Unfortunately, over 30,000 annual CLABSIs in ICUs and hospital wards across the United States occur as a result (35).

CLABSI prevention strategies are shown in Chapter 1: Central Venous Access, Table 1.2. Examination of central line sites and along the tunnel should occur daily and if infection is suspected, the catheter should be removed. Physical signs may not be present, therefore at least two blood cultures should be obtained: one peripherally and one from the catheter.

Surgical Site Infections (SSI)

SSI typically appear after 5-7 days and can be superficial (involves skin and subcutaneous tissue), deep (extends to fascia, muscle, etc.), or organ/space (involving organ, or space such as joint, thorax abdomen, etc.). Management of deep SSIs includes a combination of drainage, debridement, and antibiotics. The pathogens involved in SSIs can differ, e.g., *Staph epidermidis* is the leading pathogen in SSIs following open heart surgery (36), while SSIs following bowel surgery typically involve gram-negative aerobic bacilli and anaerobes (2).

Necrotizing wound infections appear in the first few postoperative days and are produced by *Clostridium* species (most commonly *Clostridium perfringens*) or β-hemolytic streptococci (2,37). Usually, these infections manifest as a high-grade fever. Necrotic tissue frequently causes severe wound pain. Marked edema, fluid-filled bullae, and crepitance can evolve. Spread to deeper structures is rapid, leading to rhabdomyolysis and myoglobinuric renal failure. Treatment involves extensive debridement and intravenous penicillin. A rapid diagnosis is important to avoid the >60% mortality when treatment is delayed.

Other Notable ICU Infections

Sinusitis

Sinusitis is an underappreciated cause of fever in ICU patients with nasogastric tubes or nasotracheal tubes (which can block the ostia draining the paranasal sinuses). In one study of unexplained fever in mechanically ventilated patients (orotracheal tubes) with nasogastric tubes, 42% had culture-proven evidence of sinusitis (38). Clinical signs include purulent nasal drainage and/or malodor emanating from the nares and sometimes the oropharynx in intubated patients. The diagnosis is suggested by radiographic evidence of sinusitis (i.e., opacification or air-fluid levels in the involved sinuses), and is then confirmed by a positive culture of an aspirate (transnasal or trans-orally) obtained from the involved sinus (38-40). Aspiration of the involved sinus is necessary to document infection, because about 30% of patients with radiographic evidence of sinusitis have sterile sinus aspirates (39-40). CT scans are optimal for the detection of sinusitis, but portable sinus films (obtained at the bedside) can suffice (38). The maxillary sinuses (which are almost always involved) can be viewed with a single occipitomental view, called a "Waters view" (40).

Empiric antibiotics should cover the most common isolates in ICU-acquired sinusitis. The common isolates are gram-negative aerobic bacilli (60% of cases), followed by gram-positive aerobic cocci (particularly *Staph aureus* and *Staph epidermidis*) in 30% of cases, and yeasts (mostly *Candida albicans*) in 5-10% of cases (2).

The use of oro-enteral, oro-gastric access for drainage, or enteral feeding is preferred over nasal access for mechanically ventilated patients with endotracheal tubes.

Clostridium difficile *Infection*

An ICU-acquired fever that is associated with new-onset diarrhea should always prompt suspicion of *Clostridium difficile* enterocolitis. The diagnosis and management of this condition is described in Chapter 40: Abdominal Infections.

Invasive Candidiasis

About 15% of infections in ICU patients are attributed to *Candida* species (41), with emergence of increasingly multi-resistant species, i.e., *Candida glabrata* and *Candida auris*. Risk factors include indwelling central venous catheters, parenteral nutrition, abdominal surgery, corticosteroids, and recent exposure to broad spectrum antibiotics (42-43). Invasive candidiasis often goes undetected because blood cultures are sterile in >30% of cases (42). More sensitive methods of detection (e.g., DNA by polymerase chain reaction assays) have been developed. Candidiasis should be suspected in high-risk patients who have persistent fever after 3 days of broad-spectrum antibiotic therapy. The most recent IDSA guidelines (2016) recommend echinocandins (caspofungin, micafungin, anidulafungin) as first-line therapy, followed by fluconazole for suspected and culture-confirmed invasive candidiasis (44).

Pressure Ulcers

The prevalence of pressure ulcers in critically ill patients range from 14.3% to 26.6% (45-47). There are multiple contributing factors including, immobility, length of stay, hemodynamic instability, nutritional status, tissue hypoxia, etc., that contribute to the development of pressure ulcers, and ultimately infection if uncontrolled.

ASSESSMENT OF FEVER IN THE ICU

History and Physical Assessment

The significance of a detailed history and physical (H&P) to assess a new fever cannot be understated. Many unnecessary and costly diagnostic tests (e.g., CT scans) and inappropriate therapies can be avoided by understanding recent events and targeting diagnostics based on these events and physical exam findings. Each patient brings a unique compilation of medical history, medications, co-morbid conditions, recent events, and physical exam findings to help target appropriate studies.

Laboratories

C-reactive protein or *procalcitonin elevations* cannot be used to eliminate the presence of a bacterial infection (1).

Complete Blood Count
- *White blood cell count (WBC)* itself is not diagnostic of infection, whether low, normal, or elevated. An elevation (leukocytosis) is indicative of inflammation and can be helpful as part of a clinical response to therapy. A low count, especially neutropenia (see detailed discussion below) denotes immunocompromise. Eosinophilia has multiple implications to a fever work-up, including allergic reactions.
- *Platelet count* is commonly decreased in sepsis.
- *Amylase*, lipase, and liver function testing should be considered if the H&P or other clinical data (e.g., labs) suggests a pancreatic or hepatobiliary source, i.e., pancreatitis, acalculous cholecystitis.
- *Cultures* such as respiratory and urine should be based on suspicion. Blood cultures are indicated in patients without an obvious source of infection, especially in the presence of a central venous catheter (1). Two sets of blood cultures should be obtained from separate sites (1).

Imaging Studies

Chest radiography should be a routine study in the evaluation of an ICU fever (1). Further evaluation with ultrasound or CT scan may be considered to further delineate pathologic processes, i.e., effusions versus infiltrates seen on a chest radiograph.

Computed tomography, ultrasonography, magnetic resonance imaging and nuclear medicine studies should all be based on history, clinical signs, and symptoms.

Empiric Antimicrobial Therapy

Empiric antibiotic therapy is recommended for all ICU patients with fever, unless there is a high likelihood of a non-infectious source. Prompt initiation of therapy is considered essential, *particularly in patients with neutropenia* (absolute neutrophil count <500), where delays of only a few hours can have a negative impact on outcomes (48). Appropriate cultures should be obtained prior to antibiotic administration without causing a substantial delay (49).

Broad-spectrum antibiotics for empiric coverage should be guided by likely pathogens and local susceptibility patterns (50).

An *antifungal agent* should be considered when unexplained fever persists for longer than 3 days after the start of antibiotics, particularly in patients with risk factors for invasive candidiasis mentioned previously. The preferred agents are the echinocandins (*caspofungin, micafungin*, or *anidulafungin*) because of their broad spectrum of activity against azole-resistant *Candida* species (44,48).

ANTIPYRETIC THERAPY

The SCCM and IDSA guidelines (2016) recommend *against* the routine use of antipyretics to reduce fever (weak recommendation) (1). The balance of increased oxygen consumption and hypermetabolism needs to weigh against the protective role of fevers, including decreased bacterial growth and an increased immunologic response (cytokines, neutrophils, T cells, etc.) (14). In fact, a moderate fever (37.5° to 38.4° C) was associated with a decreased mortality (51). Certain populations, however, such as neurologically injured, recent cardiac arrest, even minimal elevations in temperature can have a negative impact on outcome and should be controlled. Interestingly, a fever of >40° C and no evidence of infection is associated with increased mortality (14).

Antipyretic Drugs

Prostaglandin E mediates the febrile response to endogenous pyrogens, and drugs that interfere with prostaglandin E synthesis are effective in reducing fever (52). These drugs include aspirin, acetaminophen, and nonsteroidal anti-inflammatory agents (NSAIDs). Only the latter two are used for fever suppression in the ICU.

External Cooling

Cooling Blankets

Although the febrile response mimics the physiological response to a cold environment, external cooling has been used effectively for short-term (48 h) fever suppression in patients with septic shock (53). External cooling (to maintain a body temp around 37° C or 98.6° F) may be preferred to antipyretic drugs because it provides more continuous temperature control and avoids the risk of adverse effects from antipyretic drugs.

References

1. O'Grady NP, Alexander E, Alhazzani W, et al. Society of Critical Care Medicine and the Infectious Diseases Society of America guidelines for evaluating new fever in adult patients in the ICU. Crit Care Med 2023;51:1570-86.
2. O'Grady NP, Barie PS, Bartlett JG, et al. Guidelines for evaluation of new fever in critically ill adult patients: 2008 update from the American College of Critical Care Medicine and the Infectious Diseases Society of America. Crit Care Med 2008;36:1330-49.
3. Balli S, Shumway KR, Sharan S. Physiology, Fever. In: StatPearls. Treasure Island (FL): StatPearls Publishing; 2025.
4. Commichau C, Scarmeas N, Mayer SA. Risk factors for fever in the neurologic intensive care unit. Neurology 2003;60:837-41.
5. Peres Bota D, Lopes Ferreira F, Melot C, Vincent JL. Body temperature alterations in the critically ill. Intensive Care Med 2004;30:811-6.
6. Agency for Healthcare Research and Quality. Aspiration Pneumonitis/Pneumonia Accessed March 12, 2015. https://www.ahrq.gov/sites/default/files/wysiwyg/antibiotic-use/best-practices/asp-pneumonitis-one-page.pdf

7. Stein PD, Afzal A, Henry JW, Villareal CG. Fever in acute pulmonary embolism. Chest 2000;117:39-42.
8. Barba R, Di Micco P, Blanco-Molina A, et al. Fever and deep venous thrombosis. Findings from the RIETE registry. J Thromb Thrombolysis 2011;32:288-92.
9. Jones MW, Ferguson T. Acalculous Cholecystitis. In: StatPearls. Treasure Island (FL): StatPearls Publishing; 2025.
10. Wang H, Ren D, Sun H, Liu J. Research progress on febrile nonhemolytic transfusion reaction: a narrative review. Ann Transl Med 2022;10:1401.
11. King KE, Bandarenko N, Campbell-Lee SA, Cooling LW, Cushing MM. *Blood Transfusion Therapy: A Physician's Handbook*. 9th ed: American Association of Blood Banks; 2008.
12. Someko H, Kataoka Y, Obara T. Drug fever: a narrative review. Ann Clin Epidemiol 2023;5:95-106.
13. Zylicz Z, Krajnik M. Paracetamol/acetaminophen-induced fever and malaise in a juvenile patient. J Pain Symptom Manage 2005; 29:429-30.
14. Achaiah NC, Bhutta BS, Ak AK. Fever in the Intensive Care Patient. In: StatPearls. Treasure Island (FL): StatPearls Publishing; 2025.
15. Mackowiak PA, LeMaistre CF. Drug fever: a critical appraisal of conventional concepts. An analysis of 51 episodes in two Dallas hospitals and 97 episodes reported in the English literature. Ann Intern Med 1987;106:728-33.
16. Cunha BA. Drug fever. The importance of recognition. Postgrad Med 1986;80:123-9.
17. Rosenberg H, Davis M, James D, et al. Malignant hyperthermia. Orphanet J Rare Dis 2007;2:21.
18. Simon LV, Hashmi MF, Callahan AL. Neuroleptic Malignant Syndrome. In: StatPearls. Treasure Island (FL): StatPearls Publishing; 2025.
19. Wijdicks EFM, Ropper AH. Neuroleptic malignant syndrome. N Engl J Med 2024;391:1130-8.
20. Simon LV, Torrico TJ, Keenaghan M. Serotonin Syndrome. In: StatPearls. Treasure Island (FL): StatPearls Publishing; 2025.
21. Volpi-Abadie J, Kaye AM, Kaye AD. Serotonin syndrome. Ochsner J 2013;13:533-40.
22. Kalpakam H, Dhooria S, Agarwal R, et al. A rare complication of bedside tracheotomy: thyroid crisis. Lung India 2019;36:77-9.
23. Pradeep P, Kazi MH. Thyroid storm: a dreaded complication of percutaneous tracheostomy. J Endocr Soc 2021;5(Suppl 1):A963-4.
24. Kallinich T, Gattorno M, Grattan CE, et al. Unexplained recurrent fever: when is autoinflammation the explanation? Allergy 2013;68: 285-96.
25. Engoren M. Lack of association between atelectasis and fever. Chest 1995;107:81-4.

26. Freischlag J, Busuttil RW. The value of postoperative fever evaluation. Surgery 1983;94:358-63.
27. Lim L, Lee J, Hwang SY, et al. Early postoperative fever and atelectasis in patients undergoing upper abdominal surgery. J Am Coll Surg 2023;237:606-13.
28. Crompton JG, Crompton PD, Matzinger P. Does atelectasis cause fever after surgery? Putting a damper on dogma. JAMA Surg 2019;154:375-6.
29. Roh JS, Sohn DH. Damage-associated molecular patterns in inflammatory diseases. Immune Netw 2018;18:e27.
30. Mavros MN, Velmahos GC, Falagas ME. Atelectasis as a cause of postoperative fever: where is the clinical evidence? Chest 2011;140:418-24.
31. Grott K, Chauhan S, Sanghavi DK, Dunlap JD. Atelectasis. In: StatPearls. Treasure Island (FL): StatPearls Publishing; 2025.
32. Gonzalez EB, Suarez L, Magee S. Nosocomial (water bed) fever. Arch Intern Med 1990;150:687.
33. European Centre for Disease Prevention and Control. Healthcare-associated infections acquired in intensive care units. ECDC. 2024. Accessed March 19, 2025. https://www.ecdc.europa.eu/sites/default/files/documents/healthcare-associated-infectionsin-tensive-care-units-annual-epidemiological-report-2020.pdf
34. Blot S, Ruppe E, Harbarth S, et al. Healthcare-associated infections in adult intensive care unit patients: changes in epidemiology, diagnosis, prevention and contributions of new technologies. Intensive Crit Care Nurs 2022;70:103227.
35. National Healthcare Safety Network. Bloodstream Infection Event (Central Line-Associated Bloodstream Infection and Non-central Line Associated Bloodstream Infection) Accessed March 5, 2025. https://www.cdc.gov/nhsn/pdfs/pscmanual/4psc_clabscurrent.pdf.
36. Gudbjartsson T, Jeppsson A, Sjogren J, et al. Sternal wound infections following open heart surgery—a review. Scand Cardiovasc J 2016;50:341-8.
37. Abdelmaseeh TA, Azmat CE, Oliver TI. Postoperative Fever. In: StatPearls. Treasure Island (FL): StatPearls Publishing; 2025.
38. van Zanten AR, Dixon JM, Nipshagen MD, et al. Hospital-acquired sinusitis is a common cause of fever of unknown origin in orotracheally intubated critically ill patients. Crit Care 2005;9:R583-90.
39. Balsalobre Filho LL, Vieira FM, Stefanini R, et al. Nosocomial sinusitis in an intensive care unit: a microbiological study. Braz J Otorhinolaryngol 2011;77:102-6.
40. Holzapfel L, Chevret S, Madinier G, et al. Influence of long-term oro- or nasotracheal intubation on nosocomial maxillary sinusitis and pneumonia: results of a prospective, randomized, clinical trial. Crit Care Med 1993;21:1132-8.

41. Vincent JL, Rello J, Marshall J, et al. International study of the prevalence and outcomes of infection in intensive care units. JAMA 2009;302:2323-9.
42. Calandra T, Roberts JA, Antonelli M, et al. Diagnosis and management of invasive candidiasis in the ICU: an updated approach to an old enemy. Crit Care 2016;20:125.
43. Logan C, Martin-Loeches I, Bicanic T. Invasive candidiasis in critical care: challenges and future directions. Intensive Care Med 2020;46:2001-14.
44. Pappas PG, Kauffman CA, Andes DR, et al. clinical practice guideline for the management of candidiasis: 2016 update by the Infectious Diseases Society of America. Clin Infect Dis 2016;62:e1-50.
45. Cox J, Edsberg LE, Koloms K, VanGilder CA. Pressure injuries in critical care patients in US hospitals: results of the International Pressure Ulcer Prevalence Survey. J Wound Ostomy Continence Nurs 2022;49:21-8.
46. Isfahani P, Alirezaei S, Samani S, et al. Prevalence of hospital-acquired pressure injuries in intensive care units of the Eastern Mediterranean region: a systematic review and meta-analysis. Patient Saf Surg 2024;18:4.
47. Labeau SO, Afonso E, Benbenishty J, et al. Prevalence, associated factors and outcomes of pressure injuries in adult intensive care unit patients: the DecubICUs study. Intensive Care Med 2021;47:160-9.
48. Freifeld AG, Bow EJ, Sepkowitz KA, et al. Clinical practice guideline for the use of antimicrobial agents in neutropenic patients with cancer: 2010 update by the Infectious Diseases Society of America. Clin Infect Dis 2011;52:e56-93.
49. Rhodes A, Evans LE, Alhazzani W, et al. Surviving sepsis campaign: international guidelines for management of sepsis and septic shock: 2016. Intensive Care Med 2017;43:304-77.
50. Khasawneh RA, Almomani BA, Al-Shatnawi SF, Al-Natour L. Clinical utility of prior positive cultures to optimize empiric antibiotic therapy selection: a cross-sectional analysis. New Microbes New Infect 2023;55:101182.
51. Lee BH, Inui D, Suh GY, et al. Association of body temperature and antipyretic treatments with mortality of critically ill patients with and without sepsis: multi-centered prospective observational study. Crit Care 2012;16:R33.
52. Plaisance KI, Mackowiak PA. Antipyretic therapy: physiologic rationale, diagnostic implications, and clinical consequences. Arch Intern Med 2000;160:449-56.
53. Schortgen F, Clabault K, Katsahian S, et al. Fever control using external cooling in septic shock: a randomized controlled trial. Am J Respir Crit Care Med 2012;185:1088-95.

SECTION II

CRITICAL CARE MONITORING

Chapter 7

Bedside Echocardiography

The use of point-of-care ultrasound (POCUS) has become prevalent in the ICU. The purpose of this chapter is to briefly review functional aspects of critical care echocardiography and other ultrasound techniques (i.e., lung ultrasound, transesophageal echocardiography). A review of ultrasound physics, image acquisition, and other calculations is beyond the scope of this text, as many excellent references are available to learn more about these technical aspects (1-4). The objective of this chapter is to review key echocardiographic findings that can be used to aid in the management of critically ill patients.

TRANSTHORACIC ECHOCARDIOGRAPHY

Types of Exams

Various transthoracic echocardiography (TTE) exams have been described for use in the critical care unit (5-8). Each of these exams may be used for assessment of hemodynamic status in various types of shock. The Rapid Ultrasound for Shock and Hypotension (RUSH) exam uses a three-step protocol for assessment of the "pump (cardiac status), tank (intravascular volume), and pipes (vascular assessment)" (Table 7.1) (8).

TTE examination protocols can be used to assess specific anatomical structures and physiological function.

Left Ventricular Function

TTE may be used to assess global left ventricular (LV) function with linear and volumetric measurements, though due to the complex three-dimensional nature of the heart, each of these measurements has limitations (1). Table 7.2 summarizes various techniques that may be used to assess LV function.

TABLE 7.1 Summary of the Rapid Ultrasound for Shock and Hypotension (RUSH) Protocol for Diagnosing the Type of Shock

Exam	Hypovolemic shock	Cardiogenic shock	Distributive shock	Obstructive shock
Pump (cardiac function)	Hypercontractile heart	Hypocontractile heart	Hypercontractile heart (early sepsis)	Pericardial effusion
	Small heart size	Dilated heart size	Hypocontractile heart (late sepsis)	RV strain
Tank (intravascular volume)	Flat IVC	Distended VC	Normal or small IVC	Distended IVC
	Flat IJV	Distended IJV	Normal or small IJV	Distended IJV
	Peritoneal fluid	B-lines (lung)	Pleural fluid	Absent lung sliding
	Pleural fluid	Pleural effusions	Peritoneal fluid	
Pipes (vascular assessment)	Aortic dissection	Normal	Normal	Deep vein thrombosis
	Aortic aneurysm			

IVC = inferior vena cava; IJV = internal jugular vein; RV = right ventricle.

Adapted from Perera P, Mailhot T, Riley D, Mandavia D. The RUSH exam: rapid ultrasound in shock in the evaluation of the critically ill. Emerg Med Clin North Am 2010;28(1):29-56.

TABLE 7.2 Quantitative Left Ventricular Assessment Methods

Technique	Fractional Shortening (FS)	Teichholz (Ejection Fraction)	Fractional Area of Change (FAC)	E-Point Septal Separation (EPSS)
Formula	FS (%) = $\frac{LVIDd - LVIDs}{LVIDd} \times 100$	EF (%) = $\frac{LVEDV - LVESV}{LVEDV} \times 100$	FAC (%) = $\frac{LVEDA - LVESA}{LVEDA} \times 100$	None
Measurement	Parasternal long-axis view M-mode, 2D echo with linear calipers LV diameter measured at mitral leaflet tips	Parasternal long-axis view LV diameter measured at mitral leaflet tips	Parasternal short-axis view at level of papillary muscles Tracing of endocardial borders (including papillary muscles)	Parasternal long-axis view M-mode, distance from anterior mitral leaflet tip in early diastole and the interventricular septum
Normal value	21–43% for men 27–45% for women	52–72% for men 54–74% for women	35–65%	>7 mm abnormal >18 mm severely abnormal
Limitations	Errors common with regional wall abnormalities (i.e., myocardial infarction) Chamber enlargement may overestimate or underestimate values	Errors common with regional wall abnormalities (i.e., myocardial infarction) Chamber enlargement may overestimate or underestimate values	Errors common with regional wall abnormalities (i.e., myocardial infarction) Chamber enlargement may overestimate or underestimate values Does not account for basal or apical abnormalities	Limited applicability in patients with valvular disease Does not fully account for heterogeneity associated with three-dimensional nature of the heart

LVIDd = left ventricle end-diastolic internal diameter; LVIDs = left ventricle end-systolic internal diameter; LVEDV = left ventricle end-diastolic volume; LVESV = left ventricle end-systolic volume; LVEDA = left ventricle end-diastolic area; LVSA = left ventricle end-systolic area.

MAPSE

The mitral annular plane systolic excursion (MAPSE) measurement is a validated technique that can be assessed to estimate global longitudinal LV function (9-11). To measure the MAPSE, the apical four-chamber view is obtained and displacement of the lateral or septal wall of the mitral annulus is measured in relation to the ventricular apex in M-mode. MAPSE >10 mm suggests a preserved ejection fraction (i.e., >50%), whereas values <7 mm indicate severely impaired function (i.e., <30%) (9-11). Another method for estimating LV function is e-point septal separation (EPSS) (Figure 7.1). Using M-mode and a parasternal long-axis view, EPSS >18 mm has been correlated with a low (<30%) ejection fraction (12-13).

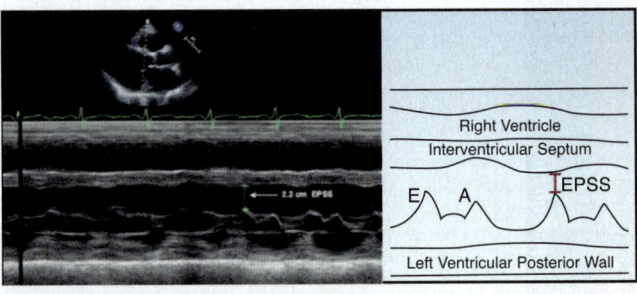

FIGURE 7.1. E-point septal separation (EPSS). This long-axis view of the heart demonstrates EPSS of 2.3 cm, consistent with severe left ventricular dysfunction. (Adapted from McKaigney CJ, Krantz MJ, La Rocque CL, et al. E-point septal separation: a bedside tool for emergency physician assessment of left ventricular ejection fraction. Am J Emerg Med 2014;32[6]: 493-7.)

Simpson's Method

The modified Simpson's method (biplane method of disks) is recommended for the most accurate estimations of LV ejection fraction because this method better measures the longitudinal contraction of the LV. Either apical four-chamber or two-chamber views can be utilized to trace the endocardial border of the left ventricle in both systole and diastole. Each tracing is divided into a predetermined number of disks (i.e., typically 20) and the volume of each disk is calculated to estimate the LV cavity volume. Modern ultrasound machines with the appropriate echocardiographic software can use the calculated volumetric data to estimate the ejection fraction.

Right Ventricular Function

The crescent-shaped right ventricle (RV) has far less mass compared to the left ventricle and functions to propel blood from the heart to the low-impedance pulmonary vasculature (1,14). The RV receives blood flow throughout the entire cardiac cycle and has lower oxygen consumption, thus making the RV less vulnerable to myocardial ischemia; however, acute increases in afterload or pulmonary arterial pressure can result in RV ischemia and failure (14). RV failure may be difficult to diagnose in the ICU, and TTE is the quickest, most non-invasive modality to rapidly assess RV function.

RV Views

Both qualitative and quantitative assessments of the RV are possible with TTE. Using a four-chamber view at the end of diastole, the RV can be qualitatively compared to the LV. The end-diastolic area of the RV should be two-thirds the volume of the LV with an RV/LV ratio >1 indicating RV enlargement. The RV should not "own" the apex of the heart; the apex should be comprised predominantly by the LV. When the RV is enlarged, the RV may encroach upon the apex, indicating susceptibility to RV dysfunction. Flattening of the interventricular septum towards the LV is another indication of RV enlargement (1). While an in-depth review of quantitative measurements is beyond the scope of this text, several useful reference values are listed in Table 7.3.

TAPSE

Among the quantitative TTE assessments for RV function, the tricuspid annular plane systolic excursion (TAPSE) is

TABLE 7.3 Quantitative Right Ventricular Transthoracic Echocardiographic Measurements for Assessing Dysfunction

Measurement	Best Echocardiographic View	Abnormal Value Threshold
Tricuspid annular plane systolic excursion (TAPSE)	Apical four chamber	<1.7 cm (17 mm)
Right ventricular wall thickness	Subcostal view Parasternal long axis	>5 mm
RV to LV end-diastolic areas	Apical four chamber Subcostal	>0.6
Peak tissue Doppler velocity (at tricuspid valve annulus)	Apical four chamber	<10 cm/s
Right atrial area	Apical four chamber	>18 cm^2
RV fractional areas of change (FAC)	Apical four chamber	<17 %

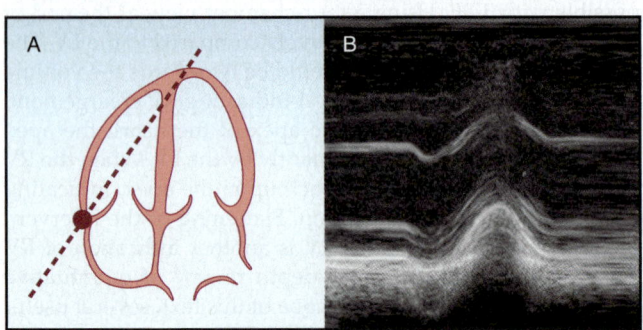

FIGURE 7.2. Tricuspid annular plane systolic excursion (TAPSE). (A) An apical four chamber view is obtained. A tracing is made from the lateral tricuspid annulus along the right ventricular free wall extending to the apex of the heart. (B) M-mode is used to measure the displacement of the tricuspid annulus in relation to the right ventricular apex. A TAPSE <17 mm indicates right ventricular systolic dysfunction.

frequently used by intensivists. Using M-mode, the systolic excursion of the tricuspid annulus can be measured (see Figure 7.2). A value <17 mm is specific for depressed RV function although this technique may not account for regional wall abnormalities in cases of isolated RV myocardial infarction (15).

Pericardium

Pericardial effusion

The pericardium normally contains <50 mL of fluid (16). TTE can be used to assess fluid in the pericardial space. The greatest amount of fluid usually accumulates posterior to the LV in a supine patient. Table 7.4 lists the criteria for quantifying pericardial effusions (16).

TABLE 7.4	Semiquantitative Thresholds for Classifying the Size of Pericardial Effusions Using Transthoracic Echocardiography	
Size	Pericardial Layer Separation (cm)*	Approximate Volume (mL)
Small	<0.5	100-200
Moderate	0.5-2.0	>5 mm
Large**	>2	>0.6

*The pericardial layer separation is defined as the distance between pericardial layers caused by the presence of fluid.

**Large effusions are usually circumferential.

Multiple TTE views are required to assess the size of pericardial effusions because single views are often imprecise (16-17). Measurements should be obtained during diastole, and using the view where the pericardial effusion is most pronounced.

Pericardial Tamponade

Pericardial tamponade is defined as a life-threatening condition caused by accumulation of fluid in the pericardial space

(1). Echocardiographic findings that can be used to confirm the diagnosis are listed in Table 7.5.

TABLE 7.5	Echocardiographic Findings Associated with Pericardial Tamponade
Echocardiographic Finding	**Comment**

Size of effusion	• Linear measurement at end diastole
	• Classification:
	    10 mm - small
	    10-20 mm - medium
	    >20 mm - large
	• Note: sizing is subject to errors due to variations in heart size, shifts of fluid during the cardiac cycle, and asymmetrical distributions of fluid

Increased right ventricular diameter with inspiration	Can be measured in M-mode
Plethoric inferior vena cava	>2 cm diameter in long axis view
25% inspiratory decrease in mitral E wave velocity	Doppler used to compare mitral E wave velocity between expiration and inspiration
Peak tricuspid E wave larger during expiration	A threshold of >40% is typically used
End-diastolic collapse	The absence of collapse of any cardiac chamber at the end of diastole (i.e., end of T wave on ECG) is associated with a very high negative predictive value for tamponade

PHYSIOLOGICAL ASSESSMENTS

Hypovolemia and Hypervolemia

TTE can be used to assess for hypovolemia and the expected response (i.e., increased stroke volume) to a fluid challenge.

Multiple parameters should be assessed, as none are sufficiently sensitive and specific. Echocardiographic parameters associated with increased stroke volume following administration of fluid are listed in Table 7.6 (18-20).

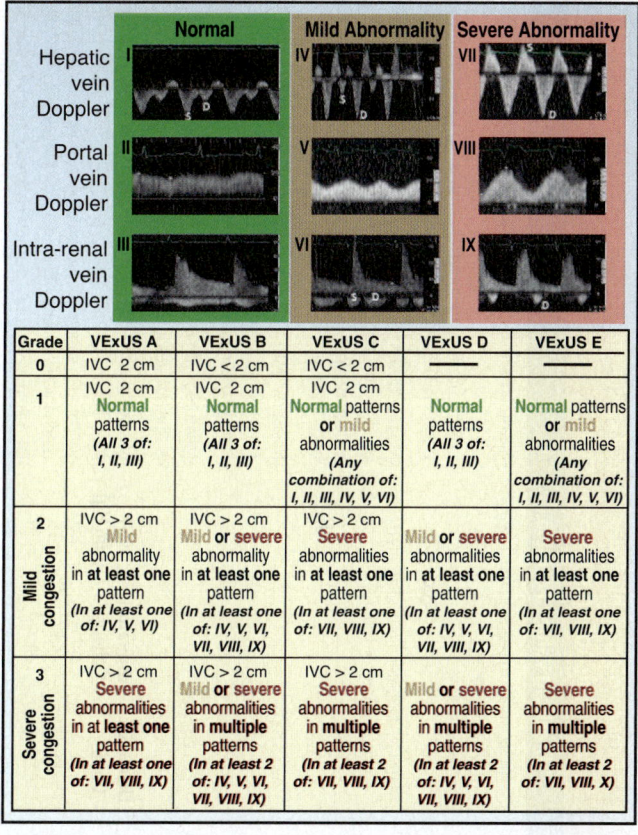

FIGURE 7.3. The VExUS score. Different profiles (i.e., A, B, C…) represent different degrees of venous congestion. (From Beaubien-Souligny W, Rola P, Haycock K, et al. Quantifying systemic congestion with Point-Of-Care ultrasound: development of the venous excess ultrasound grading system. Ultrasound J 2020;12[1]:16.)

TABLE 7.6 Echocardiographic Parameters Associated with an Increase in Stroke Volume Following Administration of Fluid

Parameter	Threshold Value / Formula	Comment
Superior vena cava collapsibility index (SVC–CI)	• [max. area − min. area] / max. area during 6-s cycle • SVC-CI >30 %	• Measured with a longitudinal axis via an upper esophageal TEE view • SVC-CI cut-offs for volume responsiveness vary in the literature; values between 31-36% have been associated with an increase in stroke volume
Inferior vena cava (IVC) distensibility index	• [max. diameter − min. diameter] / min. diameter × 100 • >18%	• Measured with a TTE subcostal longitudinal view, 1-2 cm within the right atrial-IVC junction • Validated in patients on controlled mechanical ventilation (>8 mL/kg ideal body weight)
IVC end-expiratory diameter	• <13 mm	• Measured with a TTE subcostal longitudinal view, 1-2 cm within the right atrial-IVC junction • Limited use in patients with elevated intra-abdominal pressure
LV end-diastolic area	• <5 cm²/m²	• Measured with a short axis TTE view at the end of diastole • A small LV area is highly associated with hypovolemia
IVC diameter and collapsibility	**Diameter (mm)** / **Inspiratory Collapse** / **CVP (mm Hg)** >20 / none / ≥20 >20 / <50% / 15 <20 / <50% / 10 <20 / >50% / ≤5 >20 / >50% / >15	• Measured with a TTE subcostal longitudinal view, 1-2 cm within the right atrial-IVC junction • Validated in spontaneously breathing patients; limited utility for patients on mechanical ventilation due to a high prevalence of IVC dilation • IVC >20 mm without a diameter decrease by more than 50% with inspiration (i.e., "sniffing") may indicate elevated right atrial pressure

Ultrasonography may be used to assess for signs of hypovolemia by using the the VExUS score (Figure 7.3). The VExUS score uses Doppler ultrasound to interrogate the IVC, the hepatic, portal, and renal veins to make an assessment regarding venous congestion (18,21).

Hemodynamics

TTE can be used to estimate the cardiac output and cardiac index. TTE measurements of the left ventricular outflow tract (LVOT) diameter and pulsed wave Doppler LVOT velocity-time integral (VTI) can be used to calculate stroke volume (1). Stroke volume can be calculated using the following equation:

$$\text{Stroke volume (mL)} = \text{VTI}_{LVOT} \text{ (cm)} \times \pi (d^2/2) \text{ (cm}^2)$$

Figure 7.4 depicts techniques for correctly measuring the LVOT and LVOT VTI.

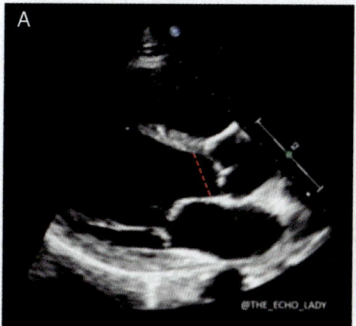
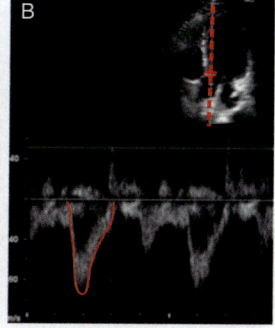

FIGURE 7.4. LVOT and LVOT VTI measurements. A. Parasternal long axis TTE view, demonstrating the LVOT diameter measurement. The LVOT should be measured in mid-systole, from the endothelial border to within 1 cm from the insertion of the aortic leaflets. B. LVOT VTI measurement. An apical 5-chamber view is obtained. Apical pulse wave Doppler is activated and positioned just proximal to the aortic annulus. The Doppler envelope is observed on M-mode and the white envelope is traced beginning at systole and ending at the closure of the aortic valve. Ultrasound enables the use of this measurement to calculate the VTI.

Once the stroke volume (mL) is determined, this value is multiplied by the heart rate to determine cardiac output (mL/min). It is important to obtain accurate measurements when using this technique because errors in measuring the LVOT will result in radius errors magnified by the square (see the equation referenced above). Off-axis measurement for either the LVOT or VTI may underestimate or overestimate stroke volume. Nevertheless, use of echocardiography has been shown to correlate well with more invasive techniques, such as pulmonary artery thermodilution (22). Once stroke volume is obtained, a series of additional physiological calculations may be made (Table 7.7).

TABLE 7.7 Stroke Volume, Cardiac Output, and Other Echocardiographic Physiological Measurements

Parameter	Formula	Normal Value
Stroke Volume (SV)	VTI_{LVOT} (cm) × $\pi(d^2/2)$ (cm^2)	60-100 mL
Cardiac Output (CO)	Stroke volume (mL) × heart rate (bpm)	4.0-8.0 mL/min
Cardiac Index (CI)	CO / BSA (m^2)	2.5-4.0 L/min/m^2
Systemic Vascular Resistance (SVR)	80 × MAP (mm Hg) − RAP (mm Hg) / CO (mL/min)	800-1,200 dynes·sec·cm^{-5}
Stroke Volume Indexed (SVI)	Stroke volume (mL) / BSA (m^2)	34-47 ml/m^2/beat
Systemic Vascular Resistance index (SVRI)	[MAP (mm Hg) − CVP (mm Hg) × 80] / CI (L/min/m^2)	1,970-2,390 dynes·sec / cm^{-5}·m^2

CO = Cardiac output; BSA = body surface area; MAP = Mean arterial pressure; RAP = Right atrial pressure; CVP = Central venous pressure; CI = Cardiac index.

TRANSESOPHAGEAL ECHOCARDIOGRAPHY

Transesophageal echocardiography (TEE) may be useful when TTE views are unobtainable (i.e., large chest wounds, obesity) or poor sonographic windows. TEE has been shown to be safe, feasible, and easy for intensivists to learn (23). Not all TEE views need to be obtained, and compared to cardiology-conducted exams, critical care echocardiography has been shown to have high specificity, sensitivity, and accuracy for ascertaining a primary diagnosis in the ICU (24). Figure 7.5 compares TTE and TEE short axis LV views with corresponding anatomical blood supply distributions.

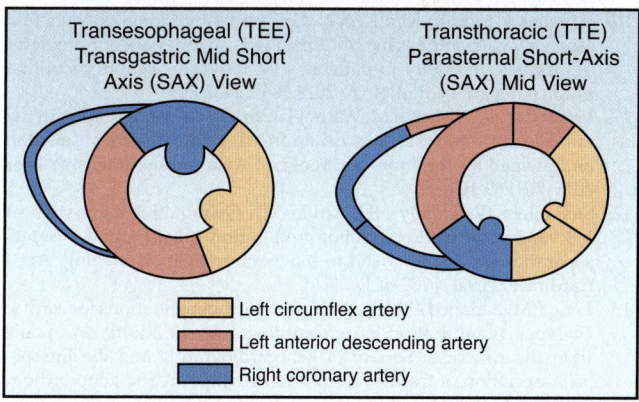

FIGURE 7.5. Coronary artery territories on middle parasternal short-axis (TTE) and transgastric short axis views (TEE).

References

1. Diaz-Gomez JL, Nikravan S, Conlon T, eds. *Comprehensive Critical Care Ultrasound*. Society of Critical Care Medicine; 2020.
2. Denault AY, Vegas A, Lamarche Y, et al, eds. *Basic Transesophageal and Critical Care Ultrasound*. Taylor & Francis Group; 2018.
3. Levitov A, Mayo P, Slonim A, eds. *Critical Care Ultrasonography*. 2nd ed. McGraw Hill; 2014:1-368.

4. Walden A, Campbell A, Miller A, Wise M, eds. *Ultrasound in the Critically Ill: A Practical Guide.* Springer Nature; 2022.
5. Seif D, Perera P, Mailhot T, et al. Bedside ultrasound in resuscitation and the rapid ultrasound in shock protocol. Crit Care Res Pract 2012;2012:503254.
6. Jensen MB, Sloth KM, Larsen M, Schmidt MB. Transthoracic echocardiography for cardiopulmonary monitoring in intensive care. Eur J Anaesthesiol 2004;21(9):700-7.
7. Ferrada P, Murthi S, Anand J, et al. Transthoracic focused rapid echocardiographic examination: real-time evaluation of fluid status in critically ill trauma patients. J Trauma 2011;70(1):56-64.
8. Perera P, Mailhot T, Riley D, Mandavia D. The RUSH exam: rapid ultrasound in shock in the evaluation of the critically ill. Emerg Med Clin N Am 2010;28(1):29-56.
9. Hu K, Liu D, Herrmann S, et al. Clinical Implication of Mitral Annular Plane Systolic Excursion for Patients with Cardiovascular Disease. Eur Heart J Cardiovasc Imaging 2012;14(3):205-12.
10. Romano S, Judd R, Kim R, et al. Left ventricular long-axis function assessed with cardiac cine MR imaging is an independent predictor of all-cause mortality in patients with reduced ejection fraction: a multicenter study. Radiology 2018;286(2):452-60.
11. Vermeiren G, Malbrain M, Walpot J. Cardiac ultrasonography in the critical care setting: a practical approach to asses cardiac function and preload for the "non-cardiologist." Anaesthesiol Intensive Ther 2015;47(J):89-104.
12. Silverstein JR, Laffely NH, Rifkin RD. Quantitative estimation of left ventricular ejection fraction from mitral valve E-point to septal separation and comparison to magnetic resonance imaging. Am J Cardiol 2006;97(1):137-40.
13. Lang RM, Badano LP, Mor-Avi V, et al. Recommendations for cardiac chamber quantification by echocardiography in adults: an update from the American Society of Echocardiography and the European Association of Cardiovascular Imaging. J Am Soc Echocardiogr 2015;28(1):1-39.e14.
14. Bernal-Ramirez J, Díaz-Vesga MC, Talamilla M, et al. Exploring functional differences between the right and left ventricles to better understand right ventricular dysfunction. Oxid Med Cell Longev 2021;2021:9993060.
15. Genovese D, Mor-Avi V, Palermo C, et al. Comparison between four-chamber and right ventricular-focused views for the quantitative evaluation of right ventricular size and function. J Am Soc Echocardiogr 2019;32(4):484-94.
16. Klein AL, Abbara S, Agler DA, et al. American Society of Echocardiography clinical recommendations for multimodality cardiovascular imaging of patients with pericardial disease: endorsed by

the Society for Cardiovascular Magnetic Resonance and Society of Cardiovascular Computed Tomography. J Am Soc Echocardiogr 2013;26(9):965-1012.e15.
17. DeMaria DM, Waring AA, Gregg DE, Litwin SE. Echocardiographic assessment of pericardial effusion size: time for a quantitative approach. J Am Soc Echocardiogr 2019;32(12):1615-1617.e1.
18. Longino AA, Martin KC, Douglas IS. Monitoring the venous circulation: novel techniques and applications. Curr Opin Crit Care 2024;30(3):260-7.
19. Barbier C, Loubières Y, Schmit C, et al. Respiratory changes in inferior vena cava diameter are helpful in predicting fluid responsiveness in ventilated septic patients. Intensive Care Med 2004;30(9):1740-6.
20. Furtado S, Reis L. Inferior vena cava evaluation in fluid therapy decision making in intensive care: practical implications. Rev Bras Ter Intensiva 2019;31(2):240-7.
21. Beaubien-Souligny W, Rola P, Haycock K, et al. Quantifying systemic congestion with Point-Of-Care ultrasound: development of the venous excess ultrasound grading system. Ultrasound J 2020;12(1):16.
22. Olivieri PP, Patel R, Kolb S, et al. Echo is a good, not perfect, measure of cardiac output in critically ill surgical patients. J Trauma Acute Care Surg 2019;87(2):379-85.
23. Mayo PH, Narasimhan M, Koenig S. Critical care transesophageal echocardiography. Chest 2015;148(5):1323-32.
24. Lau V, Priestap F, Landry Y, et al. Diagnostic accuracy of critical care transesophageal echocardiography vs cardiology-led echocardiography in ICU patients. Chest 2019;155(3):491-501.

Oximetry and Capnography — Chapter 8

Oximetry is the application of spectrophotometry to measure oxygen saturation in the blood. Known absorption patterns of light waves can be used to measure oxygenated and deoxygenated hemoglobin.

PULSE OXIMETRY

The oxygen saturation of blood can be measured by shining specific light waves through capillary and arteriolar tissue beds. Oxygenated and deoxygenated hemoglobin absorb different wavelengths of light, specifically 940 nanometers (nm) for oxygenated blood and 660 nm for deoxygenated blood (1). Light-emitting diodes emit monochromic light waves (940 nm and 660 nm) through tissue and are sensed by a photodetector, resulting in a photoplethysmography tracing. The intensity of light transmission during the systolic portion of the photoplethysmography tracing is used as a reflection of the deoxygenated hemoglobin (Hb at 660 nm) and oxygenated hemoglobin (HbO_2 at 940 nm) in arterial blood (Figure 8.1). The ratio of HbO_2 to total hemoglobin (HbO_2 + Hb) is then used to define the fraction of hemoglobin that is saturated with oxygen.

The resulting "pulse oximeter saturation" (SpO_2) is expressed as a percentage:

$$SpO_2 = (HbO_2 / Hb + HbO_2) \times 100 \qquad (8.1)$$

Figure 8.2 demonstrates pulse oximetry using a fingertip probe. The pulsatile photoplethysmography tracing is shown in the bottom panel.

Where to place the probe?

Multiple sites can be used for pulse oximetry including the nasal alar, lips, forehead, toenail beds, earlobes, and

CHAPTER 8 ■ Oximetry and Capnography

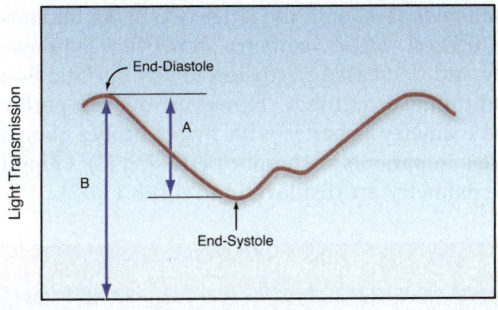

FIGURE 8.1. Photoplethysmography tracing showing the changes in light transmission resulting from the pulsatile change in arterial blood volume. A = systolic amplitude, B = baseline transmission. See text for further explanation. (From Oximetry and Capnography. In: Marino PL. *Marino's The ICU Book*. 5th ed. Wolters Kluwer; 2025:107-18. Figure 7.2)

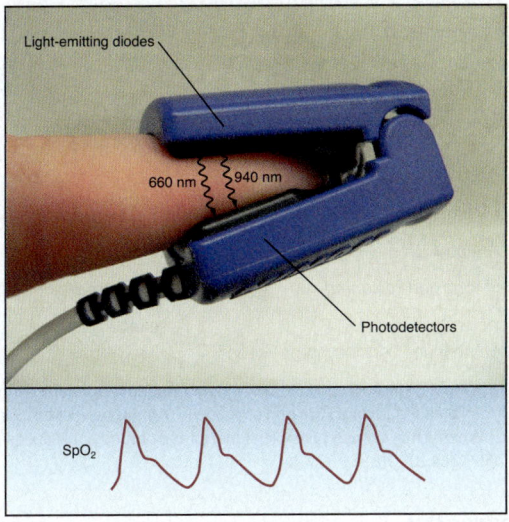

FIGURE 8.2. Pulse oximetry using a fingertip probe. The bottom panel shows the pulsatile photoplethysmography tracing. See text for explanation. (From Oximetry and Capnography. In: Marino PL. *Marino's The ICU Book*. 5th ed. Wolters Kluwer; 2025:107-18. Figure 7.3.)

fingernail beds (1-2) with the latter two being the most commonly utilized. Pulse oximetry, however, requires pulsatile flow and decreased perfusion to any specific tissue bed will compromise accuracy. However, overall performance of pulse oximetry is better with finger probes compared to other sites in patients with poor perfusion (3). Other pitfalls of pulse oximetry are displayed in Table 8.1 (1-2).

TABLE 8.1 Pitfalls of Pulse Oximetry

Error Source	Error Type
Poor Peripheral Circulation • Hypotension • Hypothermia • Vasoconstriction • Raynaud's Disease	Inability to read or false reading
Venous Pulsation • Probe too tight • Heart Failure • Severe Tricuspid Regurgitation	Falsely low reading
Dyshemoglobinemia • Carboxyhemoglobinemia • Methemoglobinemia	False readings
Light Barriers • Dark Skin • Tattoos • Nail Polish/Artificial Nails	False readings
Motion Artifacts	Falsely low reading
Severe Anemia	Falsely low reading
Carbon Monoxide Poisoning	Falsely normal or elevated
Intravenous Dyes • Methylene Blue • Indocyanine Green	False readings

From Torp KD, Modi P, Pollard EJ, and Simon LV. Pulse Oximetry. In: StatPearls. Treasure Island (FL): StatPearls Publishing; 2024 and Leppänen T, Kainulainen S, Korkalainen H, et al. Pulse oximetry: the working principle, signal formation, and applications. Adv Exp Med Biol 2022:1384:205-18.

CO-Oximetry

Standard pulse oximeters do not detect carboxyhemoglobin (COHb) or methemoglobin (metHb) in blood. This requires additional wavelengths of light, and these are available in devices called "CO-oximeters" that generate up to 8 wavelengths of light to measure all forms of hemoglobin. These devices are located in clinical laboratories and require an arterial blood sample. There is also a portable pulse CO-oximeter (Rainbow Pulse CO-oximeter, Masimo Corp) that has been used by firefighters and emergency personnel to detect carbon monoxide intoxication, but the accuracy of this device has been inconsistent (4).

Applications

Arterial Oxygenation

As a real-time, noninvasive, and constantly monitorable direct surrogate for SaO_2, SpO_2 is very useful for monitoring arterial oxygenation in the ICU patient. The most recent clinical practice guideline for oxygen therapy recommends a target SpO_2 of 90-94% for most patients, and a slightly lower target (88-92%) for patients with hypercapnic respiratory failure (5).

Venous Oxygenation

Venous oxygen saturation can be measured within the central venous circulation (superior vena cava, inferior vena cava, or the pulmonary artery) utilizing a central venous catheter for the central venous oxygen saturation ($ScvO_2$) or the mixed venous oxygen saturation (SvO_2) using a pulmonary artery catheter. The SvO_2 is the blended saturations of all venous blood returning to the heart (except for bronchial veins that drain into the azygos vein on the right side and the hemiazygos vein on the left side). This includes the venous return from the superior vena cava (SVC), the inferior vena cava (IVC), and the coronary sinus. The $ScvO_2$ is measured from either the SVC or IVC. Although not the same, they follow similar trends except in instances of ventricular and/or atrial septal defects.

The clinical importance of venous saturation is its reflection of the balance between oxygen delivery (DO_2) and oxygen consumption (VO_2) as described in the following equation:

$$SvO_2 = 1 - VO_2/DO_2 \quad (8.2)$$

Thus, a decrease in SvO_2 from its normal value of 70-75% indicates a decrease in O_2 delivery relative to O_2 consumption.

Dual Oximetry

The interpretive value of SvO_2 (or $ScvO_2$) can be enhanced by adding the SpO_2 from pulse oximetry. The difference $(SpO_2 - SvO_2)$ is roughly equivalent to the O_2 extraction from capillary blood (18), so the following relationships should hold:

$$VO_2 = DO_2 \times (SpO_2 - SvO_2) \quad (8.3)$$

When O_2 delivery (DO_2) begins to decline (from a decrease in cardiac output, anemia, or hypoxemia), there is an increase in O_2 extraction from capillary blood $(SpO_2 - SvO_2)$, and this helps to maintain a constant O_2 consumption (VO_2). The $(SpO_2 - SvO_2)$ increases in a linear fashion from a normal value of about 0.25 (25%) up to a value of about 0.50 (50%). Beyond this, any further decrease in DO_2 elicits less of an increase in $(SpO_2 - SvO_2)$, and this marks the onset of oxygen-limited metabolism. Therefore, the following interpretations of the $(SpO_2 - SvO_2)$ are possible:

1. An $(SpO_2 - SvO_2)$ >25% indicates that O_2 delivery is reduced (from low cardiac output, anemia, or hypoxemia) relative to O_2 consumption.
2. An $(SpO_2 - SvO_2)$ >25% but <50% indicates that O_2 delivery is reduced, but not enough to compromise aerobic metabolism.
3. An $(SpO_2 - SvO_2)$ ≥50% indicates a threat to aerobic metabolism.
4. The utility of $(SpO_2 - SvO_2)$ monitoring is demonstrated by a study showing that an $(SpO_2 - SvO_2)$ ≥50% is a valid indicator for the transfusion of packed red blood cells to correct anemia (6).

CAPNOGRAPHY AND CARBON DIOXIDE (CO_2) COLORIMETRY

Capnography is the graphic display of expired carbon dioxide concentration or "end-tidal" CO_2 ($ETCO_2$) which is quantitative, whereas CO_2 colorimetry is a chemical color change in the presence of exhaled CO_2 (qualitative) (7). Exhaled carbon dioxide can be detected qualitatively or quantitatively with multiple clinical uses.

CO_2 Colorimetric Applications

Endotracheal Intubation

Confirmation of endotracheal intubation by CO_2 detection (by capnography or colorimetry) is the "standard of care" (8) for the following reasons:

1. Unrecognized esophageal intubation (which can be fatal) is reported in one of every 18 emergency intubations in critically ill patients (9).
2. Clinical assessment, such as auscultation for breath sounds, does not always differentiate between tracheal and esophageal intubation (10).

The application of CO_2 colorimetric detection is shown in Figure 8.3.

Nasogastric Tube (NGT) Placement

CO_2 colorimetry can also be used to assist with nasogastric tube insertion to confirm that its placement is not within the trachea. After the tube is inserted, the detector is attached, and a bellows is used to apply negative pressure (aspirates the tube) assessing the presence or absence of CO_2. Color change to yellow indicates CO_2 and the incorrect location of the tube in the trachea/airways, and the tube should be

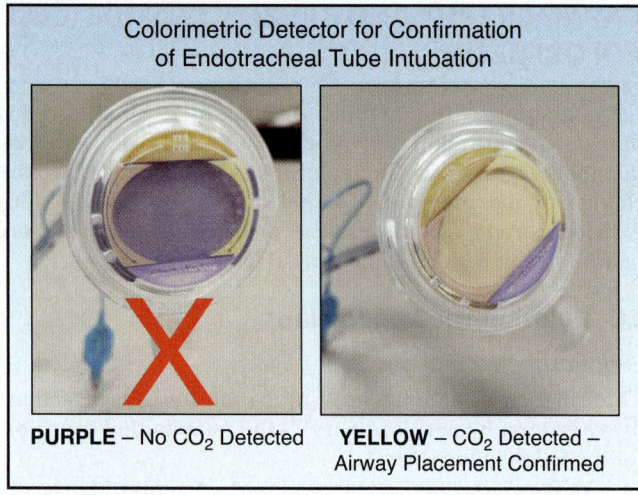

FIGURE 8.3. Colorimetric detector for confirmation of endotracheal intubation. See text for description.

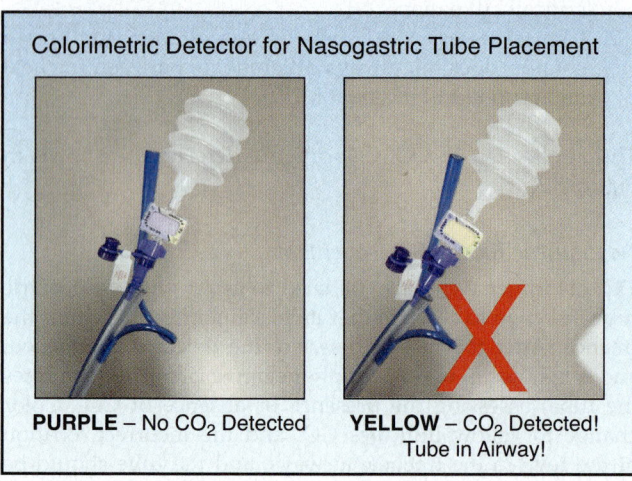

FIGURE 8.4. Colorimetric detector for nasogastric tube placement. See text for description.

immediately removed. No change from the original purple denotes positioning in the digestive tract. This may be useful in unconscious patients by avoiding accidental airway insertion and the delay of the confirmation x-ray (11). However, x-ray confirmation is still required prior to infusing through the NGT. Colorimetric CO_2 detection for NGT placement is demonstrated in Figure 8.4.

Capnography

Monitoring Ventilation

Capnography (the continuous, quantitative monitoring of $ETCO_2$) is the standard of care for patients receiving general anesthesia (12). Along with concomitant pulse oximetry, capnography gives information about both the respiratory and metabolic condition of the patient. Such continuous monitoring is decreasing blood use in mechanically ventilated patients.

Procedural Sedation

The sedation and analgesia used for a variety of procedures creates a risk of hypoventilation. Hypoventilation causes an increase in $ETCO_2$, and this change occurs before the decrease in SpO_2. Capnography has proven superior to oximetry for detecting hypoventilation during procedural sedation (13-14); as a result, monitoring $ETCO_2$ is recommended in all instances where procedural sedation is used (15).

Changes in Cardiac Output

One of the most promising applications of $ETCO_2$ monitoring is the detection of acute changes in cardiac output. The correlation between changes in $ETCO_2$ and changes in cardiac output are demonstrated in Figure 8.5 (16). This relationship suggests that $ETCO_2$ monitoring might be valuable for detecting cardiac output responses to interventions such as volume loading. In this context, the available studies have shown that changes in $ETCO_2$ are predictive of fluid responsiveness in mechanically ventilated patients (17), but not in spontaneously breathing healthy patients (18). $ETCO_2$ has also been found to be closely associated with $ScvO_2$ in hemorrhagic shock (19). The relationship of $ETCO_2$ and cardiac output is shown in Figure 8.5.

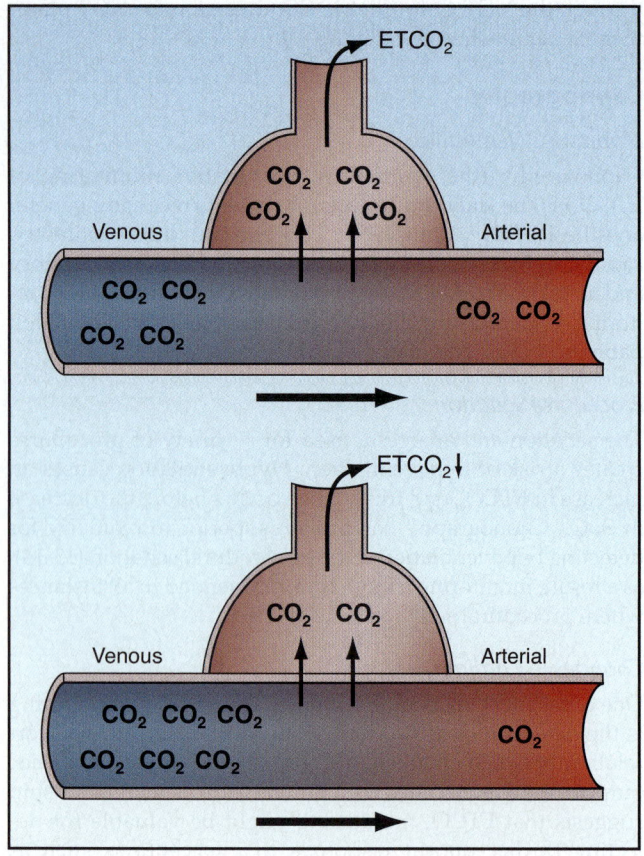

FIGURE 8.5. The association of $ETCO_2$ and cardiac output. See text for description.

Venous return to the heart delivers CO_2 to the lungs and is exhaled ($ETCO_2$). As cardiac output decreases so does the delivery of CO_2 resulting in a decrease in $ETCO_2$ as CO_2 accumulates in the venous blood (20-21).

Cardiopulmonary Resuscitation (CPR)

The relationship of $ETCO_2$ and cardiac output are also valid during CPR (22-23):

1. The efficiency of chest compressions is poor if the $ETCO_2$ is <10 mm Hg and is preferable >20 mm Hg (24).
2. A dramatic increase in $ETCO_2$ during CPR denotes a return of spontaneous circulation (23-24).

TABLE 8.2	Conditions that Alter the Relationship Between Arterial and End-Tidal PCO_2
$ETCO_2 < PaCO_2$	$ETCO_2 > PaCO_2$
• Leaky Ventilator Circuit	• Hypermetabolism
• Excessive Lung Inflation	• Metabolic Acidosis
• Pneumonia	• Hyperoxia
• Obstructive Lung Disease	
• Pulmonary Edema	
• Pulmonary Embolism	
• Acute Decrease in Cardiac Output	

From Oximetry and Capnography. In: Marino PL. *Marino's The ICU Book*. 5th ed. Wolters Kluwer; 2025:107-18. Table 7.1.

$ETCO_2$ – $PaCO_2$ Difference

In healthy subjects, the $ETCO_2$ is essentially equivalent to the arterial PCO_2 ($PaCO_2$). Conditions that alter the $ETCO_2$ – $PaCO_2$ difference is shown in Table 8.2.

References

1. Torp KD, Modi P, Pollard EJ, and Simon LV. Pulse Oximetry. In: StatPearls. Treasure Island (FL): StatPearls Publishing; 2024.
2. Leppänen T, Kainulainen S, Korkalainen H, et al. Pulse oximetry: the working principle, signal formation, and applications. Adv Exp Med Biol 2022;1384:205-18.
3. Clayton DG, Webb RK, Ralston AC, et al. Pulse oximeter probes. A comparison between finger, nose, ear and forehead probes under conditions of poor perfusion. Anaesthesia 1991;46:260-5.
4. Nitzan M, Romem A, Koppel R. Pulse oximetry: fundamentals and technology update. Med Devices (Auckl) 2014;7:231-9.
5. Siemieniuk RAC, Chu DK, Kim LH, et al. Oxygen therapy for acutely ill medical patients: a clinical practice guideline. BMJ 2018;363:k4169.
6. Levy PS, Chavez RP, Crystal GJ, et al. Oxygen extraction ratio: a valid indicator of transfusion need in limited coronary vascular reserve? J Trauma 1992;32:769-73; discussion 73-4.
7. Canelli R, Ortega R. Colorimetric capnography: a misnomer worth correcting. J Clin Monit Comput 2021;35:951.
8. Chrimes N, Higgs A, Hagberg CA, et al. Preventing unrecognised oesophageal intubation: a consensus guideline from the Project for Universal Management of Airways and international airway societies. Anaesthesia 2022;77:1395-415.
9. Russotto V, Myatra SN, Laffey JG, et al. Intubation practices and adverse peri-intubation events in critically ill patients from 29 countries. JAMA 2021;325:1164-72.
10. Mizutani AR, Ozaki G, Benumof JL, Scheller MS. Auscultation cannot distinguish esophageal from tracheal passage of tube. J Clin Monit 1991;7:232-6.
11. Meyer P, Henry M, Maury E, et al. Colorimetric capnography to ensure correct nasogastric tube position. J Crit Care 2009;24:231-5.
12. Ortega R, Connor C, Kim S, et al. Monitoring ventilation with capnography. N Engl J Med 2012;367:e27.
13. Nassar BS, Schmidt GA. Capnography during critical illness. Chest 2016;149:576-85.
14. Waugh JB, Epps CA, Khodneva YA. Capnography enhances surveillance of respiratory events during procedural sedation: a meta-analysis. J Clin Anesth 2011;23:189-96.
15. Godwin SA, Burton JH, Gerardo CJ, et al. Clinical policy: procedural sedation and analgesia in the emergency department. Ann Emerg Med 2014;63:247-58 e18.
16. Shibutani K, Shirasaki S, Braatz T. Changes in cardiac output affect $PETCO_2$, CO_2 transport, and O_2 uptake during unsteady state in humans. J Clin Monit 1992;8:175-6.

17. Monge García MI, Gil Cano A, Gracia Romero M, et al. Non-invasive assessment of fluid responsiveness by changes in partial end-tidal CO_2 pressure during a passive leg-raising maneuver. Ann Intensive Care 2012;2:9.
18. Arango-Granados MC, Zarama Córdoba V, Castro Llanos AM, Bustamante Cristancho LA. Evaluation of end-tidal carbon dioxide gradient as a predictor of volume responsiveness in spontaneously breathing healthy adults. Intensive Care Med Exp 2018;6:21.
19. Wilson HH, Cunningham KW, Katzen MM, et al. Early warning: End-tidal carbon dioxide is associated with central venous oxygenation under continuous cardio-respiratory monitoring in a porcine model of hemorrhagic shock and resuscitation. Am J Surg 2023;226:912-6.
20. Karlsson J, Lönnqvist PA. Capnodynamics-measuring cardiac output via ventilation. Paediatr Anaesth 2022;32:255-61.
21. Williams KB, Christmas AB, Heniford BT, et al. Arterial vs venous blood gas differences during hemorrhagic shock. World J Crit Care Med 2014;3:55-60.
22. American Heart Association. *Advanced Cardiovascular Life Support: Provider Manual.* American Heart Association; 2020.
23. Kodali BS, Urman RD. Capnography during cardiopulmonary resuscitation: current evidence and future directions. J Emerg Trauma Shock 2014;7:332-40.
24. Sandroni C, De Santis P, D'Arrigo S. Capnography during cardiac arrest. Resuscitation 2018;132:73-7.

The Pulmonary Artery Catheter

Chapter 9

Over 50 years ago, the pulmonary artery (PA) catheter was introduced, revolutionizing bedside hemodynamic monitoring (1). The PA catheter allows for direct and indirect (calculated) measurements of hemodynamic parameters and oxygen transport which can be helpful diagnostically as well as guiding therapies. The most frequent indications for placement of a PA catheter are shown in Table 9.1 (2-3).

TABLE 9.1 Indications for PA Catheter Placement

- Management or diagnosis of pulmonary hypertension
- Severe cardiogenic shock
- Unexplained shock
- Severe underlying cardiopulmonary disease (e.g., intracardiac shunts, severe valvular disease)
- Assessment of volume status in shock

PA = pulmonary artery.

Adapted from Rodriguez-Ziccardi M, Khalid N. Pulmonary Artery Catheterization. In: StatPearls. Treasure Island (FL): StatPearls Publishing; 2025 and Weinhouse GL. Pulmonary artery catheterization: Indications, contraindications, and complications in adults. In: Connor RF, ed. UpToDate: Wolters Kluwer; 2017.

CATHETER BASICS

The PA catheter (Figure 9.1) is 110 cm in length (about 5-6 times longer than a central venous catheter) and has an outside diameter of 8 French.

There are three internal channels:

1. A distal channel at the end of the catheter allows for PA pressure monitoring and acquisition of PA blood for SVO_2 measurement.

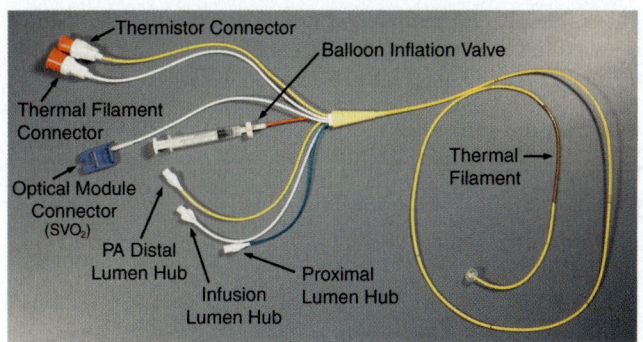

FIGURE 9.1. Pulmonary artery catheter. See text for further explanation.

2. The second channel emerges 30 cm proximal to the catheter tip (and should be situated in the right atrium when the catheter is properly positioned). The right atrial pressures can be continuously measured and are essentially equal to the CVP in most circumstances.
3. A third channel is positioned in the superior vena cava for infusion.

For insertion, the distal end of the catheter has an inflatable balloon (1.5 mL capacity) that allows venous flow to carry the catheter through the right heart into a pulmonary artery.

A small thermistor (a temperature-sensing transducer) is located near the tip of the catheter, and this allows measurement of the cardiac output by the thermodilution method. The catheter shown (Figure 9.1) has a thermal filament that allows for continuous cardiac output monitoring.

There is an optical module connector at the proximal end of the PA catheter that sends and receives fiberoptic signals from a LED photodetector at the distal end of the catheter to measure continuous SVO_2 (4).

Insertion and Placement

The *balloon flotation* principle allows catheterization of the right heart and pulmonary arteries without fluoroscopic guidance. The PA catheter is inserted through a protective sleeve, then through an introducer sheath that can accept the 8 French PA catheter (Figure 9.2).

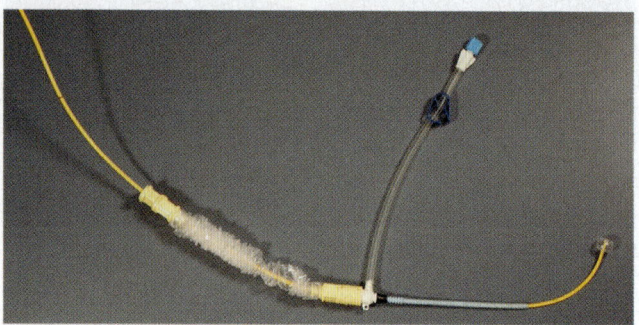

FIGURE 9.2. Pulmonary artery catheter. See text for further explanation.

The introducer sheath is first inserted into the subclavian vein or internal jugular vein. The sleeve can expand and is designed to keep the catheter "sterile' allowing for later manipulations after its initial placement. However, it does not *remain* sterile, and the PA catheter may be withdrawn a distance but never re-advanced into the sheath (5). The distal lumen of the catheter is attached to a pressure transducer to guide catheter placement. When the catheter emerges from the introducer sheath and enters the superior vena cava, a venous pressure waveform appears. The balloon is then inflated, and the catheter is advanced, using pressure tracings to determine the location of the catheter tip, as shown in Figure 9.3.

When the catheter moves across the pulmonic valve and enters a main pulmonary artery, the pressure waveform shows a sudden rise in diastolic pressure with no change in the systolic pressure. The rise in diastolic pressure is caused by resistance to flow in the pulmonary circulation. As the catheter is advanced along the pulmonary artery, the pulsatile waveform eventually disappears, leaving a non-pulsatile pressure (which is typically at the same level as the diastolic

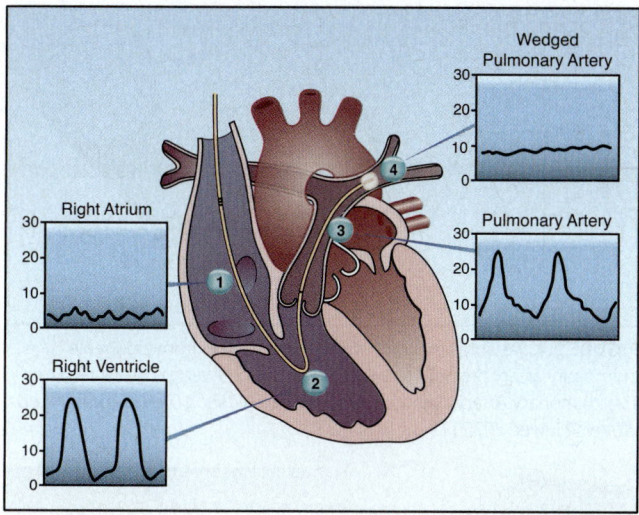

FIGURE 9.3. Pressure waveforms along the normal course of a pulmonary artery catheter. (From The Pulmonary Artery Catheter. In: Marino PL. *Marino's The ICU Book*. 5th ed. Wolters Kluwer; 2025:119-33. Figure 8.2.)

pressure of the pulsatile waveform). This is the *pulmonary artery occlusion pressure*, also called the *wedge pressure*, and it reflects the filling pressure of the left side of the heart. The balloon is then deflated, and the pulsatile pressure waveform should reappear. The catheter is then secured in place. The wedge pressure represents the venous pressure on the left side of the heart, and the magnified section of the wedge pressure in Figure 9.4 shows a contour that is similar to the venous pressure on the right side of the heart.

In about 25% of cases, the pulsatile PA pressure never disappears despite advancing the PA catheter maximally (6). When this occurs, the PA diastolic pressure can be used as a surrogate measure of the wedge pressure, except in the presence of pulmonary hypertension (when the wedge pressure is lower than the PA diastolic pressure). Once secured, a chest x-ray should be performed to confirm proper position in the pulmonary artery (Figure 9.5).

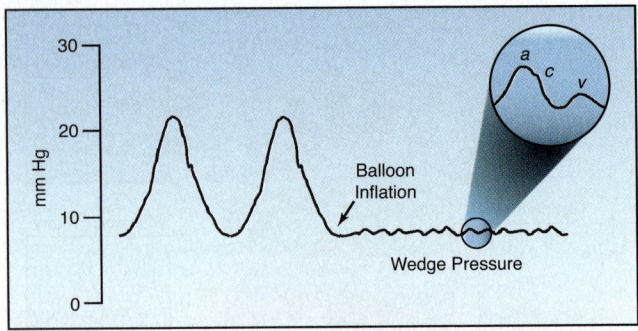

FIGURE 9.4. Pressure tracing showing the transition from a pulsatile pulmonary artery pressure to a balloon occlusion (wedge) pressure. (From The Pulmonary Artery Catheter. In: Marino PL. *Marino's The ICU Book*. 5th ed. Wolters Kluwer; 2025:119-33. Figure 8.3.)

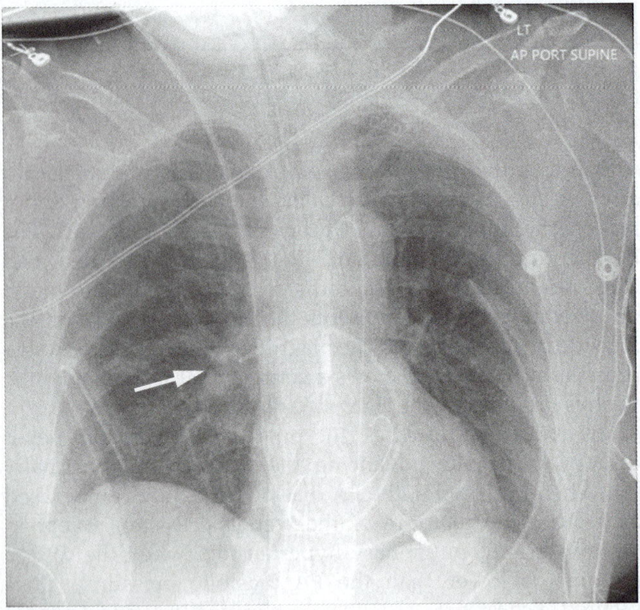

FIGURE 9.5. Post placement chest x-ray showing tip of PA catheter positioned in the right pulmonary artery (*arrow*).

THE WEDGE PRESSURE

The Principle

The principle of the wedge pressure measurement is illustrated in Figure 9.6.

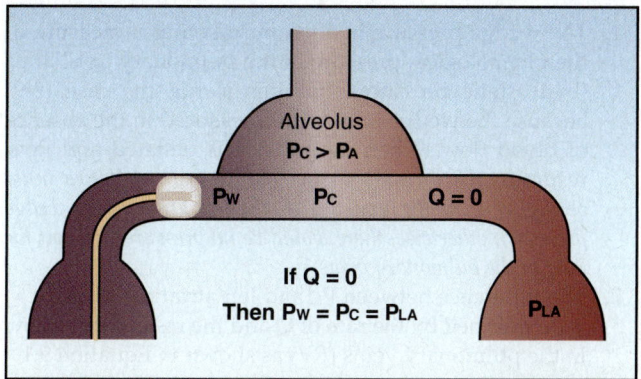

FIGURE 9.6. The basis of the wedge pressure measurement. When flow ceases because of balloon inflation (Q = 0), the wedge pressure (Pw) is equivalent to the pulmonary capillary pressure (Pc) and the pressure in the left atrium (PLA). This occurs only when the pulmonary capillary pressure is greater than the alveolar pressure (Pc > PA). (From The Pulmonary Artery Catheter. In: Marino PL. *Marino's The ICU Book*. 5th ed. Wolters Kluwer; 2025:119-33. Figure 8.4.)

Inflation of the balloon on the PA catheter obstructs blood flow (Q) in the pulmonary artery, and this creates a static column of blood between the tip of the catheter and the left atrium. In this situation, the "wedged" pressure at the tip of the catheter (Pw) is the same as the pulmonary capillary pressure (Pc) and the pressure in the left atrium (PLA); that is, if Q = 0, then Pw = Pc = PLA.

The wedge pressure will reflect left atrial pressure only if the pulmonary capillary pressure is greater than the alveolar pressure (Pc > PA). This condition is not satisfied when the wedge pressure varies with the respiratory cycle (7).

If the mitral valve is behaving normally, the left atrial pressure (Pw) is equivalent to the end-diastolic pressure (the filling pressure) of the left ventricle. Therefore, in the absence of mitral valve disease, the wedge pressure is a measure of left ventricular filling pressure.

Wedge vs. Pulmonary Capillary Pressure

1. The wedge pressure is often mistaken as a measure of the physiological pressure in the pulmonary capillaries (hydrostatic pressure), but this is not the case (8-9) because the wedge pressure is measured in the absence of blood flow. When the balloon is deflated and flow resumes, *the pressure in the pulmonary capillaries must be higher than the pressure in the left atrium (the wedge pressure); otherwise, there would be no pressure gradient for flow in the pulmonary veins.*

2. The difference between Pc and left atrial pressure (P_{LA}) is determined by the rate of Q and the resistance to flow in the pulmonary veins (RV) as shown in Equation 9.1.

$$P_C - P_{LA} = Q \times RV \tag{9.1}$$

Since the wedge pressure (Pw) is equivalent to the left atrial pressure, Equation 9.1 can be restated as follows:

$$P_C - P_W = Q \times RV \tag{9.2}$$

3. Therefore, *in the presence of blood flow, the wedge pressure will always underestimate the pulmonary capillary pressure*. The magnitude of the ($P_C - P_W$) difference is not possible to determine in individual patients because it is not possible to measure RV. However, this difference will be magnified by conditions that promote pulmonary venoconstriction, such as hypoxemia, endotoxemia, and the acute respiratory distress syndrome (ARDS) (10-11).

THERMODILUTION CARDIAC OUTPUT

The PA catheter shown in Figure 9.1 is equipped with a thermal filament and a thermistor that allows the measurement of cardiac output by the thermodilution method. The thermal filament generates pulses of heat. The distal thermistor detects the change in blood temperature with time. The area under the temperature-time curve is inversely proportional to the flow rate in the pulmonary artery, and this flow rate is equivalent to the cardiac output. This method is comparable with the gold standard of the intermittent bolus technique (12).

Sources of Error

Tricuspid Regurgitation

Regurgitant flow across the tricuspid valve (which can be common during positive-pressure mechanical ventilation) causes the indicator fluid to be recycled, producing a prolonged, low-amplitude thermodilution curve similar to the one produced by a low cardiac output. Therefore, tricuspid regurgitation produces a spuriously low cardiac output measurement (13).

Intracardiac Shunts

In right-to-left shunts, a portion of the warmed blood passes the thermistor, creating an abbreviated thermodilution curve similar to the one produced by a high-cardiac output.

In left-to-right shunts, the thermodilution curve is also abbreviated, because the shunted blood mixes with the normal flow through the right heart, reducing the change in blood temperature measured at the distal thermistor.

CARDIOVASCULAR AND OXYGEN TRANSPORT PARAMETERS

The PA catheter provides a wealth of information about cardiovascular function and systemic oxygen transport.

The measurements available with PA catheters are shown in Table 9.2.

TABLE 9.2 Cardiovascular and Oxygen Transport Variables Measurements Available with PA Catheters

Parameter	Abbreviation	Normal Range
Central Venous Pressure	CVP	0-5 mm Hg
Pulmonary Artery Wedge Pressure	PAWP	6-12 mm Hg
Cardiac Index	CI	2.4-4.0 L/min/m^2
Stroke Index	SI	20-40 mL/m^2
Systemic Vascular Resistance Index	SVRI	25-30 Wood Units†
Pulmonary Vascular Resistance Index	PVRI	1-2 Wood Units†
Mixed Venous O$_2$	SvO$_2$	70-75%
Oxygen Delivery (Index)	DO$_2$	520-570 mL/min/m^2
Oxygen Uptake (Index)	VO$_2$	110-160 mL/min/m^2
Oxygen Extraction Ratio	O$_2$ER	0.2-0.3

†mm Hg /L/min/m^2

PA = pulmonary artery.

From The Pulmonary Artery Catheter. In: Marino PL. *Marino's The ICU Book*. 5th ed. Wolters Kluwer; 2025:119-33. Table 8.1.

Cardiac Filling Pressures

Central Venous Pressure

When the PA catheter is properly placed, the proximal port of the catheter should be situated in the right atrium, and the pressure recorded from this port should be the mean right atrial pressure, also known as the *central venous pressure* (CVP). This pressure is equivalent to the right ventricular end-diastolic pressure (RVEDP) when tricuspid valve function is normal.

$$CVP = RVEDP \tag{9.3}$$

The CVP is normally a low pressure (0-5 mm Hg), which helps to promote venous return to the right side of the heart.

Pulmonary Artery Wedge Pressure

The pulmonary artery wedge pressure (PAWP), described earlier in the chapter, is equivalent to the left ventricular end-diastolic pressure (LVEDP) when mitral valve function is normal.

$$PAWP = LVEDP \tag{9.4}$$

The normal PAWP (6-12 mm Hg) is slightly higher than the CVP, and this pressure difference keeps the foramen ovale closed (which prevents intracardiac right-to-left shunts).

Variability. There is an inherent variability in the wedge pressure, which does not exceed 4 mm Hg in most patients (14). Therefore, *a recorded change in the wedge pressure should exceed 4 mm Hg to be considered a clinically significant change.*

Respiratory Fluctuations

Changes in intrathoracic pressure can be transmitted into blood vessels in the thorax producing respiratory fluctuations in the CVP or wedge pressure, as shown in Figure 9.7. These changes in intrathoracic pressure are misleading because the *transmural pressure* (i.e., the physiologically important pressure) is not changing.

Therefore, *when respiratory variations are evident in the CVP or wedge pressure, the pressure should be measured at the end of expiration*, when intrathoracic pressure is closest to atmospheric (zero reference) pressure. This is at the bottom of the wave during positive pressure ventilation, and the top of the wave during spontaneous, unassisted ventilation (15).

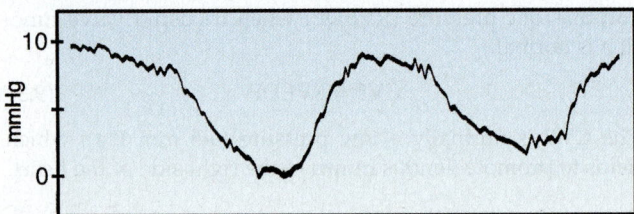

FIGURE 9.7. Respiratory variation in the central venous pressure (CVP) during mechanical ventilation. The CVP should be measured at the end of expiration, which corresponds to the lowest points in the pressure undulations. See text for further explanation. (From The Pulmonary Artery Catheter. In: Marino PL. *Marino's The ICU Book.* 5th ed. Wolters Kluwer; 2025:119-33. Figure 8.5.)

Cardiac Index

The thermodilution cardiac output (CO) is expressed in relation to body size using the body surface area (BSA). The size-adjusted cardiac output is called the *cardiac index* (CI). Normal CI is 2.4-4 L/min/m^2.

$$CI = CO/BSA \quad (9.5)$$

Stroke Index

The stroke volume (the volume of blood ejected by the ventricle during systole) is a more direct measure of intrinsic cardiac performance than the cardiac output. The *stroke index* (SI) is an expression of the stroke volume when CI is used instead of cardiac output (and where HR is the heart rate):

$$SI = CI/HR \quad (9.6)$$

Vascular Resistance

The resistance to flow in the systemic and pulmonary circulations is not a clinically measurable quantity because resistance is flow dependent, and blood vessels are compressible and not rigid. The following measures of vascular resistance are simply expressions of the relationship between averaged flow rates (cardiac output) and intravascular pressure gradients.

Systemic Vascular Resistance Index

The *systemic vascular resistance index* (SVRI) is calculated as the difference between mean arterial pressure (MAP) and CVP, divided by the CI.

$$\text{SVRI} = (\text{MAP} - \text{CVP})/\text{CI} \tag{9.7}$$

The SVRI is expressed in Wood units (mm Hg/L/min/m^2), which can be multiplied by 80 to convert to conventional units of resistance (dynes•sec^{-1}•cm^{-5}/m^2) (16). SVRI plays a vital role regarding cardiac output (as afterload) and blood pressure (17), mathematically expressed as:

$$\text{MAP} = \text{CI} \times \text{SVRI} \tag{9.8}$$

Pulmonary Vascular Resistance Index

The *pulmonary vascular resistance index* (PVRI) is calculated as the difference between the mean pulmonary artery pressure (MPAP) and the mean left atrial pressure, or PAWP, divided by the CI.

$$\text{PVRI} = (\text{MPAP} - \text{PAWP})/\text{CI} \tag{9.9}$$

The PVRI has the same units (mm Hg/L/min/m^2) as the SVRI and has the same limitations as described for the SVRI.

OXYGEN TRANSPORT PARAMETERS

Oxygen transport parameters are global measures of systemic oxygen supply and oxygen consumption, and they provide an indirect assessment of tissue oxygenation. These parameters are expressed in relation to body size, and the normal range for each parameter is shown in Table 9.2.

Oxygen Delivery

The rate of oxygen transport in arterial blood is known as *oxygen delivery* (DO_2) and is equivalent to the product of the CI and the O_2 content in arterial blood (CaO_2) as shown as Equation 9.10.

$$DO_2 = CI \times CaO_2 \times 10 \qquad (9.10)$$

1. The CaO_2 is expressed as mL O_2 per 100 mL blood (mL/100 mL), and the multiplier of 10 is used to convert the units to mL/L.
2. CaO_2 is equivalent to the product of the hemoglobin concentration [Hb] (g/100 mL), the O_2 binding capacity of Hb (1.34 mL/g/100 mL), and the saturation of Hb with O_2 in arterial blood (SaO_2). Therefore, Equation 9.10 can be restated as follows:

$$DO_2 = CI \times (1.34 \times [Hb] \times SaO_2) \times 10 \qquad (9.11)$$

3. DO_2 is expressed as mL/min/m², and the normal range is 520-600 mL/min/m².

Oxygen Uptake

Oxygen uptake (VO_2) is the rate at which O_2 is taken up from the systemic capillaries into the tissues. Since O_2 is not stored in tissues, VO_2 *is equivalent to O_2 consumption*. The VO_2 is calculated as the product of the CI and the difference in O_2 content between arterial and venous blood ($CaO_2 - CvO_2$).

$$VO_2 = CI \times (CaO_2 - CvO_2) \times 10 \qquad (9.12)$$

(The multiplier of 10 is included for the same reason as explained for the DO_2.) Equation 9.12 is a modified version of the Fick equation for cardiac output ($CO = VO_2 / [CaO_2 - CvO_2]$).

1. If the CaO_2 and CvO_2 are each broken down into their component parts, Equation 9.12 can be rewritten as:

$$VO_2 = CI \times 1.34 \times [Hb] \times (SaO_2 - SvO_2) \times 10 \quad (9.13)$$

where SaO_2 and SvO_2 are the oxyhemoglobin saturations in arterial and venous blood, respectively. (Venous blood in this instance is "mixed" venous blood in the pulmonary arteries.)

2. VO_2 is expressed as mL/min/m², and the normal range is 110-160 mL/min/m². A subnormal VO_2 in critically ill patients (who rarely have a low metabolic rate) is reasonable evidence of impaired tissue oxygenation.

3. The inherent variability of the calculated VO_2 is high (±18%) because it represents the summed variability of the 4 component measurements (14,18-19).

4. The calculated VO_2 from the modified Fick equation is not the whole body VO_2 because it does not include the O_2 consumption of the lungs. The VO_2 of the lungs normally accounts for less than 5% of the whole body VO_2 (1), but it can make up 20% of the whole body VO_2 when there is inflammation in the lungs (which is common in ICU patients) (20).

Oxygen Extraction Ratio

The balance between DO_2 and VO_2 is expressed by the oxygen extraction ratio (O_2ER), which is equivalent to the VO_2/DO_2 ratio and is often multiplied by 100 to express it as a percent (21).

$$O_2ER = VO_2/DO_2 \quad (9.14)$$

The normal O_2ER is 0.2-0.3, which means that only 20-30% of the O_2 delivered to the systemic capillaries is taken up into the tissues. The O_2ER can increase up to 0.5-0.6 when O_2 delivery is reduced, and this helps to maintain tissue oxygenation despite a declining O_2 supply.

References

1. Swan HJ, Ganz W, Forrester J, et al. Catheterization of the heart in man with use of a flow-directed balloon-tipped catheter. N Engl J Med 1970;283:447-51.
2. Rodriguez Ziccardi M, Khalid N. Pulmonary Artery Catheterization. In: StatPearls. Treasure Island (FL): StatPearls Publishing; 2025.
3. Weinhouse GL. Pulmonary artery catheterization: Indications, contraindications, and complications in adults. In: Connor RF, ed. UpToDate: Wolters Kluwer; 2017.
4. Lee CP, Bora V. Anesthesia Monitoring of Mixed Venous Strain. In: StatPearls. Treasure Island (FL): StatPearls Publishing; 2025.
5. Corcoran TB, Grape S, Duff O, et al. The pulmonary artery catheter sleeve—protective or infective? Anaesth Intensive Care 2009;37:290-5.
6. Swan HJ. The pulmonary artery catheter. Dis Mon 1991;37:473-543.
7. O'Quin R, Marini JJ. Pulmonary artery occlusion pressure: clinical physiology, measurement, and interpretation. Am Rev Respir Dis 1983;128:319-26.
8. Cope DK, Grimbert F, Downey JM, Taylor AE. Pulmonary capillary pressure: a review. Crit Care Med 1992;20:1043-56.
9. Pinsky MR. Hemodynamic monitoring in the intensive care unit. Clin Chest Med 2003;24:549-60.
10. Kloess T, Birkenhauer U, Kottler B. Pulmonary pressure-flow relationship and peripheral oxygen supply in ARDS due to bacterial sepsis. Prog Clin Biol Res 1989;308:175-80.
11. Tracey WR, Hamilton JT, Craig ID, Paterson NA. Effect of endothelial injury on the responses of isolated guinea pig pulmonary venules to reduced oxygen tension. Am Rev Respir Dis 1989;140:68-74.
12. Lorsomradee S, Lorsomradee SR, Cromheecke S, De Hert SG. Continuous cardiac output measurement: arterial pressure analysis versus thermodilution technique during cardiac surgery with cardiopulmonary bypass. Anaesthesia 2007;62:979-83.
13. Balik M, Pachl J, Hendl J. Effect of the degree of tricuspid regurgitation on cardiac output measurements by thermodilution. Intensive Care Med 2002;28:1117-21.
14. Sasse SA, Chen PA, Berry RB, et al. Variability of cardiac output over time in medical intensive care unit patients. Crit Care Med 1994;22:225-32.
15. Nair R, Lamaa N. Pulmonary Capillary Wedge Pressure. In: StatPearls. Treasure Island (FL): StatPearls Publishing; 2025.
16. Bartlett RH. Critical Care Physiology. New York: Little, Brown & Co.; 1996.
17. Trammel JE, Sapra A. Physiology, Systemic Vascular Resistance. In: StatPearls. Treasure Island (FL): StatPearls Publishing; 2025.

18. Bartlett RH, Dechert RE. Oxygen kinetics: pitfalls in clinical research. J Crit Care 1990;5:77-80.
19. Schneeweiss B, Druml W, Graninger W, et al. Assessment of oxygen-consumption by use of reverse Fick-principle and indirect calorimetry in critically ill patients. Clin Nutr 1989;8:89-93.
20. Jolliet P, Thorens JB, Nicod L, et al. Relationship between pulmonary oxygen consumption, lung inflammation, and calculated venous admixture in patients with acute lung injury. Intensive Care Med 1996;22:277-85.
21. Hess AS. Oxygen extraction ratios to guide red blood cell transfusion. Transfus Med Rev 2024;38:150834.

SECTION III
RESUSCITATION FLUIDS

Chapter 10
Colloid and Crystalloid Fluids

First-line resuscitation fluids are crystalloid and colloid fluids. This chapter reviews common crystalloid and colloid fluids used for resuscitation and describes the salient features of each.

CRYSTALLOID FLUIDS

Crystalloid fluids are electrolyte solutions that move freely from the plasma to the interstitial space. The principal ingredient in crystalloid fluids is the inorganic salt, sodium chloride (NaCl).

Volume Distribution

Understanding body fluid compartments and the concept of "volume distribution" is critical to the understanding of the use of fluids for "maintenance" as opposed to "resuscitation" (Figure 10.1).

Crystalloid fluids distribute uniformly in extracellular fluid, i.e., plasma and interstitial fluid. Since plasma volume is 25% of the extracellular fluid volume, then 75% of an infused crystalloid fluid bolus will leave the intravascular space and equilibrate into the interstitial space expanding the interstitial fluid space (1). This effect occurs in approximately 60 minutes (2). Thus, *the principal effect of crystalloid fluids is to expand the interstitial fluid volume, not the plasma volume*. Therefore, it is critical to understand that during resuscitation, crystalloids must be rapidly infused to achieve a hemodynamic benefit (*increased preload*). This "equilibration" explains the frequent transient impact of a crystalloid bolus (Figure 10.2).

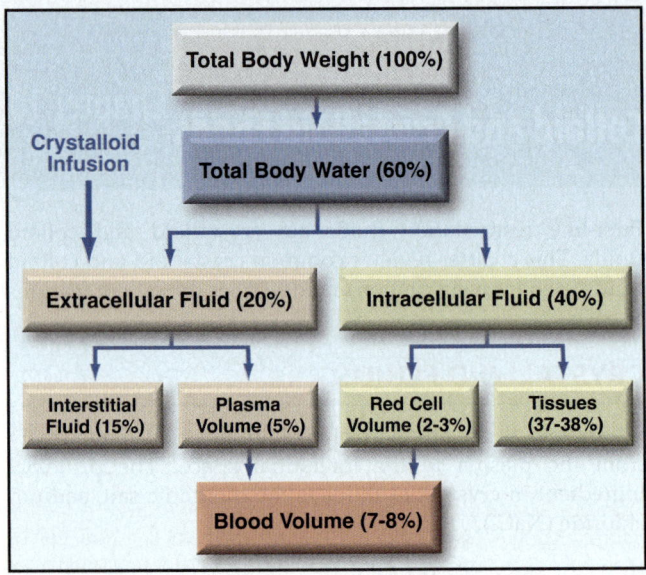

FIGURE 10.1. Body fluid compartments.

Note that measured osmolality compared to the calculated osmolality provides a more accurate reflection of *in vivo* osmotic activity, i.e., the contribution to plasma volume rather than the calculated osmolalities (which are the summed concentrations of all osmotically active species in a fluid). See Table 10.1.

The measured osmotic activities are lower than the calculated (predicted) activities. This discrepancy is caused by electrostatic interactions between ions in the fluid, which reduces the number of osmotically active particles. This deserves mention because the manufacturers of crystalloid fluids use the calculated osmotic activity to describe the *in vivo* behavior of the fluid.

Isotonic Saline

The most widely used crystalloid fluid is 0.9% NaCl, more commonly known as *normal saline*, a misnomer, as will be explained.

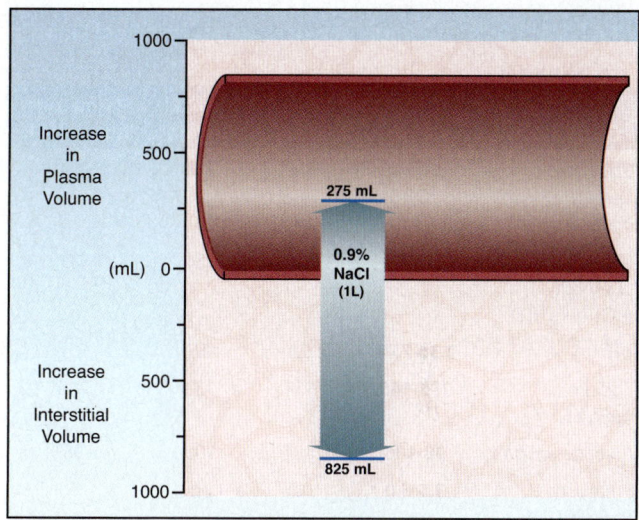

FIGURE 10.2. The effects of 0.9% NaCl on plasma and interstitial volume. Infusion volume shown in parentheses. (Modified from Intravenous Fluids. In: Marino PL. *Marino's The ICU Book*. Wolters Kluwer; 2025:153-69. Figure 10.1.)

Features

When compared to plasma (also included in Table 10.1), 0.9% NaCl has a higher sodium concentration (154 vs 140 mEq/L), a much higher chloride concentration (154 vs 103 mEq/L), and a lower pH (5.7 vs 7.4). The only feature of 0.9% NaCl that matches plasma is the measured osmolality. These comparisons show that *normal saline is not normal* chemically, *but it is relatively isotonic with plasma*. Therefore, *the appropriate name for this fluid is isotonic saline*, not normal saline.

Volume Effects

The volume effects of 0.9% NaCl in plasma and interstitial fluid are illustrated in Figure 10.2. Approximately 825 mL of a one-liter intravenous infusion of 0.9% NaCl will distribute into the interstitial space, and 275 mL will remain in the plasma volume (1-2). This is the volume distribution expected

TABLE 10.1 Comparison of Isotonic Crystalloid Fluids with Human Plasma

Components	Plasma	0.9% Saline	Lactated Ringer's	Plasma-Lyte/ Normosol-R
Calculated Osmolarity (mOsm/L)	**280-300**	308	273	294
Measured Osmolality mOsm/kg H₂O	**287**	286	256	271
pH	**7.36-7.44**	5.0	6.5	7.4
Sodium (mEq/L)	**135-145**	154	130	140
Chloride (mEq/L)	**98-106**	154	109	98
Potassium (mEq/L)	**3.5-5.0**	0	4	5
Buffer (mmol/L)	**23-28 (bicarbonate)**	0	28 (lactate)	27 (acetate) 23 (gluconate)
Ionized Calcium (mg/dL)	**3.0-4.5**	0	2.7	0
Magnesium (mg/dL)	**1.8-3.0**	0	0	3
Glucose (mg/dL)	**77-99**	0	0	0

Crystalloid data from Baxter Healthcare Corporation, Deerfield, IL.

from a crystalloid fluid based on its osmotic characteristics. Note that the total increase in extracellular volume in Figure 10.2 (1,100 mL) is slightly greater than the infused volume. The additional 100 mL of extracellular fluid is the result of a fluid shift from intracellular to extracellular fluid compartments, prompted by the excess sodium in 0.9% NaCl.

Adverse Effects

Interstitial edema is a risk with all crystalloid fluids, but the risk is greatest with isotonic saline (3) because the sodium load exceeds that in other crystalloid fluids (and sodium is the principal determinant of extracellular volume) (4). Infusions of isotonic saline are accompanied by a decrease in renal perfusion, presumably as a result of chloride-mediated renal vasoconstriction (5). Rapid or large-volume infusions of isotonic saline are often accompanied by a *hyperchloremic metabolic acidosis* (6-7), which is attributed to the excess chloride in isotonic saline. Whereas some trials have shown no evidence of a causal link between isotonic saline and acute kidney injury (AKI) (5-6,8), more compelling evidence demonstrates an increased AKI requiring renal replacement therapy (RRT) and mortality in critically ill patients (9-11).

Balanced Crystalloid Solutions

Crystalloid solutions with compositions closer to human plasma, termed "balanced crystalloids" such as Lactated Ringer's (LR) and Plasma-Lyte/Normosol-R, are isotonic alternatives to 0.9% NaCl. The use of balanced crystalloids has demonstrated improved mortality rates, lower AKI requiring RRT, and less persistent renal dysfunction compared with 0.9% NaCl (10,12-13).

Lactated Ringer's

LR solution (introduced in 1880 by Sydney Ringer, a British physician) is an isotonic solution that contains potassium and calcium (which were added to promote the viability of frog heart preparations, a research interest of Dr. Ringer). Lactate was later added as a buffer (by Alexis Hartmann, an American pediatrician) to create *LR solution* (also known as *Hartmann's solution*).

Features

The chemical features of LR are included in Table 10.1. The following comparisons with 0.9% NaCl are significant:

- The addition of potassium and calcium (in concentrations that approximate the free or ionized levels in plasma) is

balanced by a reduction in the sodium concentration (to 130 mEq/L) to maintain electrical neutrality.
- Lactate is added (as sodium lactate) as a buffer and is metabolized to bicarbonate in the liver. The chemical reaction is as follows:

$$CH_2 - CHOH - COO^- = 2CO_2 + 2H_2O + HCO_3^- \quad (10.1)$$

- Note that oxygen is required for this reaction, which means that *lactate will not act as a buffer source when tissue hypoxia is present* (i.e., in circulatory shock) (14).
- The addition of lactate requires a reduction in chloride concentration for electrical neutrality. *The chloride concentration in LR is close to that in plasma*, which *decreases the risk of hyperchloremic metabolic acidosis*.
- The osmolality of LR is significantly lower than plasma and is the lowest of the "isotonic" crystalloid fluids. This hypotonicity makes LR the least desirable crystalloid fluid for patients with cerebral edema, or those at risk for cerebral edema (e.g., traumatic head injuries).

Adverse Effects

- The calcium in LR can bind to the citrated anticoagulant in blood products. For this reason, *LR are contraindicated as diluent fluids for the transfusion of packed red blood cells (RBCs)* (14). However, clot formation does not occur if the volume of LR does not exceed 50% of the volume of packed RBCs, or if the fluid is infused rapidly (15-16).
- The lactate content in LR (28 mmol/L) is sodium lactate and not lactic acid. It can however increase serum lactate levels, (7,17) especially when lactate metabolism is impeded (i.e., in liver failure or circulatory shock). This risk was evident in a study of burn patients, where hyperlactatemia was common when LR was used for fluid management, but not when a lactate-free Ringer's solution was used (18).
- When considering this risk of hyperlactatemia, the diagnostic and prognostic value of serum lactate levels

in critically ill patients may be impacted; e.g., blood samples withdrawn through catheters being used for LR infusions can yield spuriously high lactate levels (19).

Normal pH Fluids

There are two crystalloid fluids with a pH in the normal, physiological range: *Normosol-R* and *Plasma-Lyte*. The composition of these fluids is identical.

Features

The chloride concentration in these fluids (98 mEq/L) is within the normal physiological range, and they contain magnesium (3 mg/dL) instead of calcium. These fluids contain both acetate (27 mmol/L), and gluconate (23 mmol/L) as buffers. Gluconate is a weak alkalinizing agent that adds little to the buffer capacity (2), but acetate is rapidly metabolized to bicarbonate in skeletal muscle via the following oxidation reaction:

$$CH_3 - COO^- + 2O_2 = CO_2 + H_2O + HCO_3^- \quad (10.2)$$

Note that O_2 is required for this reaction, which means that acetate may not serve as a buffer source when tissues are hypoxic (e.g., in circulatory shock), similar to lactate (see Equation 10.1).

Advantages

These fluids offer the following advantages over other crystalloid fluids:

- The physiological chloride concentration decreases the risk of hyperchloremia (hyperchloremic metabolic acidosis), even compared with other balanced crystalloid solutions (20).
- The absence of lactate eliminates the risk of spurious elevated lactate levels in patients with liver failure or circulatory shock. In addition, acetate is considered

superior to lactate as a buffer source because it is more rapidly converted to bicarbonate (2). Plasma-Lyte/Normosol-R results in an elevated base excess compared with LR (20).
- The absence of calcium makes these fluids suitable for use with blood transfusions.
- In studies comparing isotonic saline and Plasma-Lyte, the latter showed less tendency for interstitial edema, and was associated with improved outcomes (3,21).

Hypertonic Saline

Concentrated NaCl (hypertonic saline) solutions have been used in the management of traumatic shock, traumatic brain injury, and symptomatic hyponatremia. The most commonly used hypertonic saline solutions are shown in Table 10.2.

TABLE 10.2 Hypertonic Saline

Solution	Sodium (mEq/L)	Chloride (mEq/L)	Osmolarity[†] (mOsm/L)	pH
3% NaCl	513	513	1,026	5.0
5% NaCl	856	856	1,712	5.0
7.5% NaCl	1,283	1,283	2,566	5.7
23.4% NaCl	4,004	4,004	8,008	5.0

Baxter International offers 3% and 5% NaCl in 500 mL unit sizes. Hospital pharmacists make 7.5% NaCl upon request, however it is not commercially available.

[†]Calculated as the sum of the Na and Cl concentrations.

Volume Effects

- Small volumes of hypertonic saline are more effective for *expanding* the plasma volume than larger volumes of isotonic saline. This is demonstrated in Figure 10.3.
- Note that 250 mL of 7.5% NaCl produces a 535 mL increment in plasma volume and a 700 mL increase in interstitial fluid (total volume increment = 1,235 mL),

whereas 1 L of 0.9% NaCl produces only a 275 mL increase in plasma volume.
- Intracellular fluid shifts are responsible for the extracellular volume expansion, with RBCs and endothelial cells contributing to the increment in plasma volume.
- The colloid oncotic pressure from the tonicity increase in the blood causes a swift fluid shift across the blood–brain barrier (cerebrospinal fluid to blood), resulting in rapid decrease in intracranial pressure.

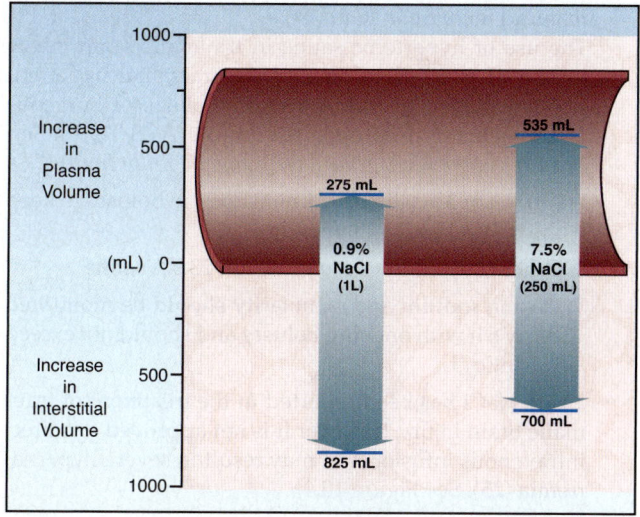

FIGURE 10.3. The effects of 0.9% NaCl and 7.5% NaCl on plasma and interstitial volume. Infusion volume shown in parentheses. (Modified from Intravenous Fluids. In: Marino PL. *Marino's The ICU Book*. Wolters Kluwer; 2025:153-69. Figure 10.1.)

Traumatic Shock

Despite numerous physiological benefits (22), resuscitation of trauma-related hemorrhagic shock with hypertonic saline (500 mL of 5% saline or 250 mL of 7.5% saline) has demonstrated no consistent survival benefit over resuscitation with isotonic fluids (23). Nevertheless, small-volume resuscitation with hypertonic saline has a continuing appeal for early resuscitation of combat injuries in the field (where large volumes of resuscitation fluids are not immediately available).

Traumatic Brain Injury

- In cases of post-traumatic intracranial hypertension, hypertonic saline has proven effective in reducing intracranial pressure (ICP) and offers some advantages over conventional therapy with mannitol (i.e., greater magnitude of ICP reduction, longer duration of action, and no rebound increase in ICP) (24).
- The use of hypertonic saline in traumatic brain injury is part of a tiered response for intracranial hypertension developed by the American College of Surgeons Trauma Quality Improvement Project (ACS-TQIP): *Best Practices in the Management of Traumatic Brain Injury*:
    1. 250 mL of 3% saline is administered in boluses to keep the ICP below 20-25 mm Hg
    2. Other concentrations, e.g., 30 mL 23.5% saline
    3. Plasma sodium and osmolarity should be monitored every 6 h with ongoing boluses and should not exceed 160 mEq/L
- 23.4% NaCl has been reported in the treatment of traumatic brain injury, however it is not approved for direct intravenous infusion and may result in severe hypernatremia (25). See Figure 10.4.

5% DEXTROSE SOLUTIONS

Protein-Sparing Effect

- Prior to the standard use of enteral tube feedings and total parenteral nutrition (TPN), 5% dextrose solutions were used to provide calories in patients who were unable to eat.
- One gram of dextrose provides 3.4 kilocalories (kcal) when fully metabolized, so a 5% dextrose solution (50 g/L) provides 170 kcal/L.

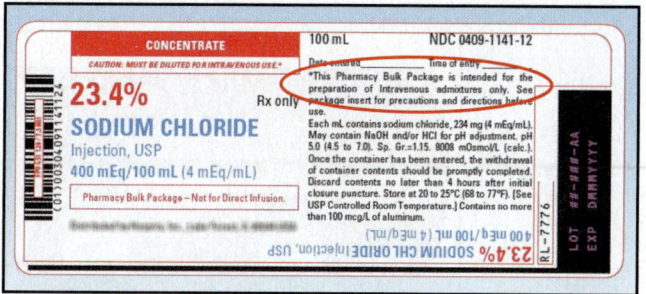

FIGURE 10.4. Label showing 23.4% NaCl is not approved for direct intravenous infusion.

- Daily infusion of 3 L of a 5% dextrose (D_5) solution provides about 500 kcal per day, which is enough nonprotein calories to limit the breakdown of endogenous proteins to meet daily caloric requirements. This protein-sparing effect is responsible for the early popularity of dextrose-containing fluids.
- The current availability of enteral and parenteral nutrition regimens obviates the need for dextrose-containing fluids.

Volume Effects

The addition of dextrose to intravenous fluids increases osmolality, i.e., 50 g of dextrose adds 278 mOsm/L to an intravenous fluid. For a 5% dextrose-in-water solution (D_5W), the added dextrose brings the osmolality close to that of plasma. However, since the dextrose is taken up by cells and metabolized, this osmolality effect rapidly declines, and the added water then moves into the intracellular compartment. This is shown in Figure 10.5, in the arrow marked D_5W, where the combined increments in plasma volume (100 mL) and interstitial fluid volume (250 mL) are far less than the volume infused (1,000 mL). This difference (650 mL) is the result of fluid movement into cells, which means that *D_5W primarily expands the intracellular volume, and despite being relatively isotonic it should never be used for plasma volume resuscitation.*

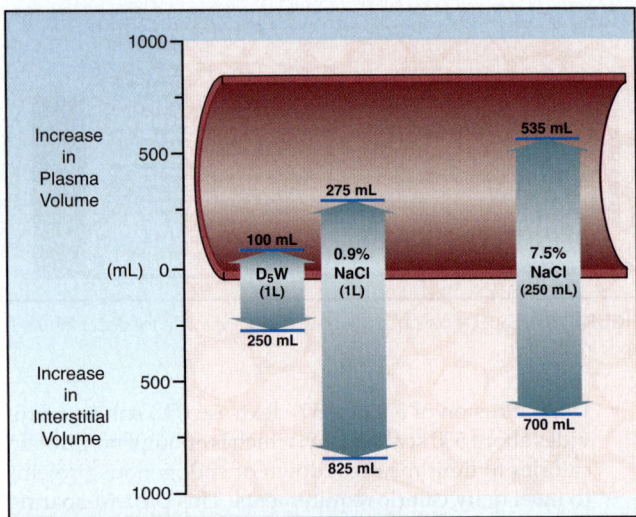

FIGURE 10.5. The effects of D_5W on plasma and interstitial volume compared with 0.9% and 7.5% NaCl. Infusion volume shown in parentheses. (Modified from Intravenous Fluids. In: Marino PL. *Marino's The ICU Book*. Wolters Kluwer; 2025:153-69. Figure 10.1.)

Adverse Effects

Enhanced Lactate Production

In healthy subjects, only 5% of an infused glucose load will be metabolized to lactate, but in critically ill patients with tissue hypoperfusion, as much as 85% of glucose metabolism is diverted to lactate production (26). Studies in patients with compromised circulatory flow have shown that infusion of 5% dextrose solutions produces significant increases in serum lactate levels (27).

Hyperglycemia

Infusion of D_5W increases the risk of hyperglycemia, which has several undesirable effects in critically ill patients, including immune suppression (28), aggravation of ischemic brain injury (see Chapter 42: Disorders of Consciousness), and an association with increased mortality (29).

COLLOID FLUIDS

Colloid solutions contain large molecules that increase the colloid osmotic pressure (or oncotic pressure) and remain within the intravascular compartment longer than crystalloid solutions.

Colloid Osmotic Pressure

- This promotes the retention of water within the vascular compartment.
- The following relationship identifies the role of the colloid osmotic pressure in capillary fluid exchange.

$$Q \sim (P_c - COP) \tag{10.3}$$

Q is the flow rate across the capillaries. P_c is the hydrostatic pressure in the capillaries. COP is the colloid osmotic pressure of plasma. About 80% of the COP is attributed to the albumin concentration in plasma.

- The two pressures (P_c and COP) act in opposition: P_c favors the movement of fluid out of the capillaries, and COP favors movement into the capillaries.
- In the supine position, the normal P_c averages 25 mm Hg, and the normal COP is about 28 mm Hg (30), so the two forces are roughly matched.
- The volume distribution of both crystalloid and colloid fluids can be explained by their effect on the COP of plasma.
  - Crystalloid fluids reduce the plasma COP (dilutional effect), which favors the movement of these fluids out of the bloodstream.
  - Colloid fluids tend to preserve the plasma COP, which favors the retention of these fluids in the bloodstream.

Volume Effects

- The effect of colloid fluid resuscitation on plasma and interstitial fluid volumes is shown in Figure 10.6. The colloid fluid in this case is a 5% albumin solution; infusion of 1 L adds 700 mL to the plasma and 300 mL to the interstitial fluid. Thus, 70% of the infused colloid fluid is retained in the vascular compartment compared with 25% with 0.9% NaCl. Comparing the effects of the colloid and crystalloid fluids on plasma volume in Figure 10.6 reveals that *colloid fluids are about three times more effective than crystalloid fluids for increasing the plasma volume* (1,31-32).

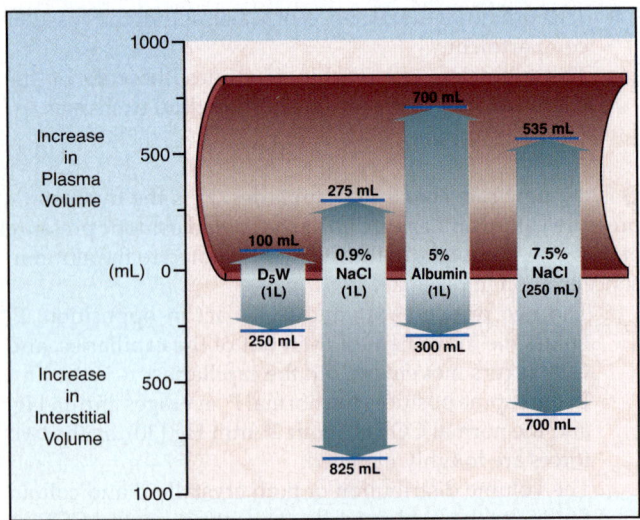

FIGURE 10.6. The effects of selected intravenous fluids on plasma volume and interstitial volume. Infusion volume shown in parentheses. (From Intravenous Fluids. In: Marino PL. *Marino's The ICU Book*. Wolters Kluwer; 2025:153-69. Figure 10.1.)

Albumin Solutions

Albumin solutions are heat-treated preparations of human serum albumin that are available as a 5% solution

(50 g/L) and a 25% solution (250 g/L) in 0.9% NaCl (Figure 10.7).

The salient features of these fluids are shown in Table 10.3.

Volume Effects

- The 5% albumin solution is a *hypo-oncotic* fluid (i.e., the COP is 20 mm Hg, which is less than the COP of plasma). It is given in aliquots of 250 mL, and the volume effect (at least 70% retention in plasma, as indicated in Table 10.3) begins to dissipate at 6 h and is lost after 12 h (1,31).
- The 25% albumin solution is a *hyperoncotic* fluid (i.e., the COP is 70 mm Hg, about 2.5 times that of plasma). It is given in aliquots of 50 or 100 mL, and the increment in plasma volume is about 3-4 times the infused volume, as shown in Table 10.3. (This volume is drawn from interstitial fluid.) The duration of effect is similar to 5% albumin.
- Because 25% albumin does not replace lost volume, but instead shifts fluid from one compartment to another, it *should not be used for volume resuscitation in cases of acute blood loss*. The principal role for 25% albumin is in patients with hypoalbuminemia and edema who are either hypotensive or resistant to diuretic therapy. (In both instances, 25% albumin can increase plasma volume in an attempt to correct the problem without infusing relatively large volumes of isotonic crystalloid fluids.)
- Following paracentesis, hypoalbuminemia is associated with increased morbidity and mortality across multiple patient populations, e.g., medical and surgical, however, replacement therapy does not improve outcomes (33).

Safety

- Multiple clinical studies, including randomized controlled trials demonstrated a better hemodynamic response with albumin over crystalloids regarding mean arterial blood pressure and cardiac output (34). Although the Saline versus Albumin Fluid Evaluation

(SAFE) Study (35-36) was associated with an improvement in mortality in sepsis, a more recent meta-analysis of over 50 randomized controlled trials (RCTs) did not show a mortality benefit (34).
- Early claims of increased mortality attributed to albumin solutions have not been corroborated in more recent studies (35,37). In fact, the use of albumin in sepsis is supported by the "Surviving Sepsis Campaign"(38).
  - 5% albumin is safe to use as a resuscitation fluid, with the exception of patients with traumatic head injury, i.e., the SAFE trial demonstrated "less favorable" neurologic outcomes and a trend towards a higher mortality in patients with traumatic brain injury who were resuscitated with albumin instead of isotonic saline) (36,39).

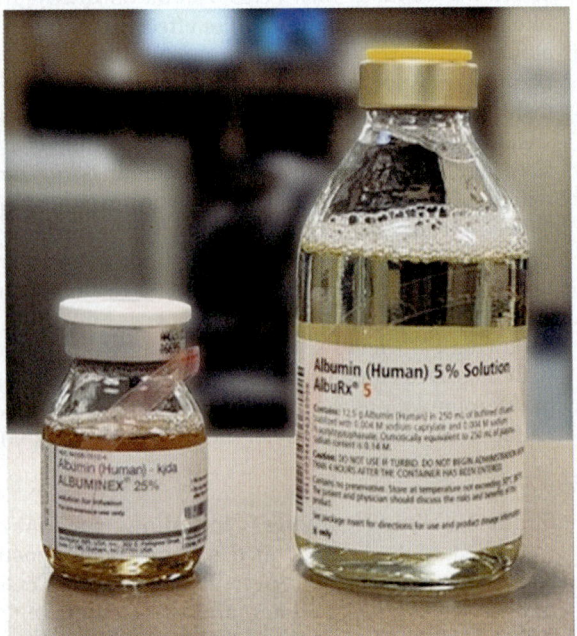

FIGURE 10.7. 25% and 5% albumin.

TABLE 10.3 Colloid Fluid Comparisons

Fluid	COP (mm Hg)	Δ Plasma to Infusate Volume	Duration of Effect
5% Albumin	20	0.7-1.3	12 h
6% Hetastarch	30	1.0-1.3	24 h
10% Dextran-40	40	1.0-1.5	6 h
25% Albumin	70	3.0-4.0	12 h

Data from References 1, 31-32, 40.

Hydroxyethyl Starch (HES) aka "Hetastarch"

HES is a chemically modified starch polymer that is available as a 6% solution in isotonic saline. There are three FDA-approved HES products available: 1. Hextend (6% HES in lactated electrolyte solution; BioTime, Inc.); 2. Voluven (6% HES in 0.9% NaCl; Fresenius Kabi); and 3. Hespan (6% HES in 0.9% NaCl; B. Braun Medica, Inc.).

Features

HES has a higher COP than 5% albumin and is slightly more effective as a plasma volume expander (see Table 10.3) (31,40). The volume effects of hetastarch also last longer (up to 24 h) than those of 5% albumin (40).

Safety

- There is increasing evidence that critically ill and surgical patients who receive hetastarch have an increased risk of renal failure requiring hemodialysis, an increased mortality rate and excess bleeding risk (FDA.gov vaccines-blood-biologics July 7, 2021).
- Because of these findings, *the FDA issued a statement in July 2021 against the use of hetastarch unless adequate alternative treatment is not available.*

Dextrans

The dextrans are glucose polymers that were first introduced as plasma volume expanders in the 1940s. The two most common dextran preparations are 10% dextran-40 and 6% dextran-70.

Features

- Both dextran preparations have a COP of 40 mm Hg (i.e., hyperoncotic fluids), and produce a greater increase in plasma volume than either 5% albumin or 6% hetastarch (see Table 10.3). Dextran-70 may be preferred because the duration of action (12 h) is longer than that of dextran-40 (6 h) (31).
- Dextrans purportedly improve microcirculatory flow by decreasing blood viscosity and inhibiting platelet aggregation (see *Disadvantages* in the section that follows). Outcomes in reimplantations have not demonstrated benefits (41).

Disadvantages

- Dextrans produce a dose-related bleeding tendency that involves impaired platelet aggregation, decreased levels of Factor VIII and von Willebrand factor, and enhanced fibrinolysis (42-43).
- Dextrans coat the surface of red blood cells and can interfere with the ability to crossmatch blood. Red cell preparations must be washed to eliminate this problem. Another consequence of this interaction with red blood cells is an increase in the erythrocyte sedimentation rate (43).
- Dextrans have been associated with a hyperoncotic renal injury similar to that reported with hetastarch (44). However, this is a rare occurrence.
- Anaphylactic reactions were once common with dextrans but are now reported in only 0.03% of infusions (43).

THE COLLOID-CRYSTALLOID DEBATE

The Debate

There is a longstanding debate concerning which type of fluid (colloid or crystalloid) is most appropriate for correcting hypovolemia. The essential arguments are as follows:

1. Proponents of crystalloid resuscitation cite the lack of a proven survival benefit with colloid resuscitation (45) and the lower cost of crystalloid fluids.
2. Proponents of colloid resuscitation cite the relatively large volume of crystalloid fluids needed to expand the plasma volume (at least 3 times the volume of colloid fluids), thereby promoting edema formation and a positive fluid balance, both of which are associated with increased morbidity and mortality in critically ill patients (21,46).

As in all longstanding debates, the truth is somewhere in the middle.

Resolution

The fallacy in the colloid-crystalloid debate is the assumption that one type of fluid is best for all the conditions associated with hypovolemia. The following examples demonstrate that *tailoring the type of resuscitation fluid to the specific cause of hypovolemia is a more logical approach than using the same type of fluid for all cases of hypovolemia.*

1. In cases of hypovolemic shock (where prompt restoration of intravascular volume is a priority), a colloid fluid like 5% albumin (which is much more effective for increasing plasma volume than crystalloid fluids) is physiologically the best choice with the exception of traumatic brain injury (36,39).
2. In cases of hypovolemia due to dehydration (where there is uniform loss of interstitial fluid and plasma), a balanced crystalloid solution (which is distributed uniformly throughout the extracellular fluid) is most appropriate.
3. In cases of hypovolemia where hypoalbuminemia is implicated (causing fluid shifts from plasma to interstitial fluid) small volumes of a hyperoncotic colloid fluid like 25% albumin (which will shift fluid back from interstitium to plasma) is an appropriate choice.

De-resuscitation

As fluid resuscitation is typically aggressive in unstable patients, along with the limited time of intravascular volume expansion of all fluids, excess resuscitation can lead to interstitial edema with resultant adverse events in multiple organ systems. Thus, the concept of "de-resuscitation" should begin as soon as the resuscitation phase is completed (47).

References

1. Imm A, Carlson RW. Fluid resuscitation in circulatory shock. Crit Care Clin 1993;9:313-33.
2. Hahn RG, Lyons G. The half-life of infusion fluids: an educational review. Eur J Anaesthesiol 2016;33:475-82.
3. Chowdhury AH, Cox EF, Francis ST, Lobo DN. A randomized, controlled, double-blind crossover study on the effects of 2-L infusions of 0.9% saline and plasma-lyte 148 on renal blood flow velocity and renal cortical tissue perfusion in healthy volunteers. Ann Surg 2012;256:18-24.
4. Hoenig MP, Zeidel ML. Homeostasis, the milieu interieur, and the wisdom of the nephron. Clin J Am Soc Nephrol 2014;9:1272-81.
5. Young P, Bailey M, Beasley R, et al. Effect of a buffered crystalloid solution vs saline on acute kidney injury among patients in the intensive care unit: the SPLIT randomized clinical trial. JAMA 2015;314:1701-10.
6. Orbegozo Cortes D, Rayo Bonor A, Vincent JL. Isotonic crystalloid solutions: a structured review of the literature. Br J Anaesth 2014;112:968-81.
7. Ross SW, Christmas AB, Fischer PE, et al. Impact of common crystalloid solutions on resuscitation markers following class I hemorrhage: a randomized control trial. J Trauma Acute Care Surg 2015;79:732-40.
8. Self WH, Semler MW, Wanderer JP, et al. Balanced crystalloids versus saline in noncritically ill adults. N Engl J Med 2018;378:819-28.
9. Neyra JA, Canepa-Escaro F, Li X, et al. Association of hyperchloremia with hospital mortality in critically ill septic patients. Crit Care Med 2015;43:1938-44.
10. Semler MW, Self WH, Wanderer JP, et al. Balanced crystalloids versus saline in critically ill adults. N Engl J Med 2018;378:829-39.
11. Yunos NM, Bellomo R, Hegarty C, et al. Association between a chloride-liberal vs chloride-restrictive intravenous fluid admin-

istration strategy and kidney injury in critically ill adults. JAMA 2012;308:1566-72.
12. Beran A, Altorok N, Srour O, et al. Balanced crystalloids versus normal saline in adults with sepsis: a comprehensive systematic review and meta-analysis. J Clin Med 2022;11.
13. Brown RM, Wang L, Coston TD, et al. Balanced crystalloids versus saline in sepsis. A secondary analysis of the SMART clinical trial. Am J Respir Crit Care Med 2019;200:1487-95.
14. Reddy S, Weinberg L, Young P. Crystalloid fluid therapy. Crit Care 2016;20:59.
15. Albert K, van Vlymen J, James P, Parlow J. Ringer's lactate is compatible with the rapid infusion of AS-3 preserved packed red blood cells. Can J Anaesth 2009;56:352-6.
16. Lorenzo M, Davis JW, Negin S, et al. Can Ringer's lactate be used safely with blood transfusions? Am J Surg 1998;175:308-10.
17. Zitek T, Skaggs ZD, Rahbar A, et al. Does intravenous Lactated Ringer's solution raise serum lactate? J Emerg Med 2018;55:313-8.
18. Gille J, Klezcewski B, Malcharek M, et al. Safety of resuscitation with Ringer's acetate solution in severe burn (VolTRAB)—an observational trial. Burns 2014;40:871-80.
19. Jackson EV Jr, Wiese J, Sigal B, et al. Effects of crystalloid solutions on circulating lactate concentrations: part 1. Implications for the proper handling of blood specimens obtained from critically ill patients. Crit Care Med 1997;25:1840-6.
20. Curran JD, Major P, Tang K, et al. Comparison of balanced crystalloid solutions: a systematic review and meta-analysis of randomized controlled trials. Crit Care Explor 2021;3:e0398.
21. Shaw AD, Bagshaw SM, Goldstein SL, et al. Major complications, mortality, and resource utilization after open abdominal surgery: 0.9% saline compared to Plasma-Lyte. Ann Surg 2012;255:821-9.
22. Galvagno SM Jr, Mackenzie CF. New and future resuscitation fluids for trauma patients using hemoglobin and hypertonic saline. Anesthesiol Clin 2013;31:1-19.
23. Bunn F, Roberts I, Tasker R, Akpa E. Hypertonic versus near isotonic crystalloid for fluid resuscitation in critically ill patients. Cochrane Database Syst Rev 2004;2004:CD002045.
24. Mangat HS, Hartl R. Hypertonic saline for the management of raised intracranial pressure after severe traumatic brain injury. Ann N Y Acad Sci 2015;1345:83-8.
25. Traficante D, Galaktionova D, Marseille U, et al. Comparison of 3% vs. 23.4% hypertonic saline in traumatic brain injury. J Curr Surg 2019;9:39-44.
26. Gunther B, Jauch KW, Hartl W, et al. Low-dose glucose infusion in patients who have undergone surgery. Possible cause of a muscular energy deficit. Arch Surg 1987;122:765-71.

27. Degoute CS, Ray MJ, Manchon M, et al. Intraoperative glucose infusion and blood lactate: endocrine and metabolic relationships during abdominal aortic surgery. Anesthesiology 1989;71:355-61.
28. Turina M, Fry DE, Polk HC Jr. Acute hyperglycemia and the innate immune system: clinical, cellular, and molecular aspects. Crit Care Med 2005;33:1624-33.
29. van den Berghe G, Wouters P, Weekers F, et al. Intensive insulin therapy in critically ill patients. N Engl J Med 2001;345:1359-67.
30. Hall JE. *Guyton and Hall Textbook of Medical Physiology*. 13th ed. Elsevier; 2016:192-3.
31. Griffel MI, Kaufman BS. Pharmacology of colloids and crystalloids. Crit Care Clin 1992;8:235-53.
32. Kaminski MV Jr, Haase TJ. Albumin and colloid osmotic pressure implications for fluid resuscitation. Crit Care Clin 1992;8:311-21.
33. Melia D, Post B. Human albumin solutions in intensive care: a review. J Intensive Care Soc 2021;22:248-54.
34. Martin GS, Bassett P. Crystalloids vs. colloids for fluid resuscitation in the intensive care unit: a systematic review and meta-analysis. J Crit Care 2019;50:144-54.
35. Finfer S, Bellomo R, Boyce N, et al. A comparison of albumin and saline for fluid resuscitation in the intensive care unit. N Engl J Med 2004;350:2247-56.
36. The SAFE study investigators. Saline or albumin for fluid resuscitation in patients with traumatic brain injury. N Engl J Med 2007;357:874-84.
37. Wilkes MM, Navickis RJ. Patient survival after human albumin administration. A meta-analysis of randomized, controlled trials. Ann Intern Med 2001;135:149-64.
38. Evans L, Rhodes A, Alhazzani W, et al. Surviving sepsis campaign: international guidelines for management of sepsis and septic shock 2021. Crit Care Med 2021;49:e1063-e143.
39. Cooper DJ, Myburgh J, Heritier S, et al. Albumin resuscitation for traumatic brain injury: is intracranial hypertension the cause of increased mortality? J Neurotrauma 2013;30:512-8.
40. Treib J, Baron JF, Grauer MT, Strauss RG. An international view of hydroxyethyl starches. Intensive Care Med 1999;25:258-68.
41. Retrouvey H, Solaja O, Baltzer HL. Role of postoperative anticoagulation in predicting digit replantation and revascularization failure: a propensity-matched cohort study. Ann Plast Surg 2019;83:542-7.
42. de Jonge E, Levi M. Effects of different plasma substitutes on blood coagulation: a comparative review. Crit Care Med 2001;29:1261-7.
43. Nearman HS, Herman ML. Toxic effects of colloids in the intensive care unit. Crit Care Clin 1991;7:713-23.

44. Drumi W, Polzleitner D, Laggner AN, et al. Dextran-40, acute renal failure, and elevated plasma oncotic pressure. N Engl J Med 1988;318:252-4.
45. Heming N, Lamothe L, Jaber S, et al. Morbidity and mortality of crystalloids compared to colloids in critically ill surgical patients: a subgroup analysis of a randomized trial. Anesthesiology 2018;129:1149-58.
46. Boyd JH, Forbes J, Nakada TA, et al. Fluid resuscitation in septic shock: a positive fluid balance and elevated central venous pressure are associated with increased mortality. Crit Care Med 2011;39:259-65.
47. Malbrain M, Martin G, Ostermann M. Everything you need to know about deresuscitation. Intensive Care Med 2022;48:1781-6.

Fluid Management — Chapter 11

Fluids are the vehicle for the transport of the essentials of life, from the transport of water, oxygen, nutrients, electrolytes, etc., to tissues, to the delivery of metabolic wastes to the kidneys for excretion. Fluid management can be divided into two major roles: resuscitation and maintenance. This chapter will focus on resuscitation as maintenance has been described in Chapter 10: Colloid & Crystalloid Fluids.

The driving force to circulate and deliver oxygen to the tissues is the cardiac output, of which fluid resuscitation plays a critical role. However, excessive fluid resuscitation is common and can result in increased morbidity and mortality (1-2). This chapter will discuss the physiology of fluid resuscitation, the evaluation of fluid responsiveness and problems with infusion therapy.

THE PHYSIOLOGY OF FLUID RESUSCITATION

Preload

There are four determinants of cardiac output (3):

1. Preload
2. Heart rate
3. Contractility
4. Afterload

Of these, preload is the primary determinant in a normal heart. This is founded on the understanding of the Frank-Starling law, which describes stroke volume increases in response to ventricular filling (preload) (3-4). The Frank-Starling law can be illustrated as a "curve" showing the relationship of ventricular filling (preload) and stroke volume (Figure 11.1).

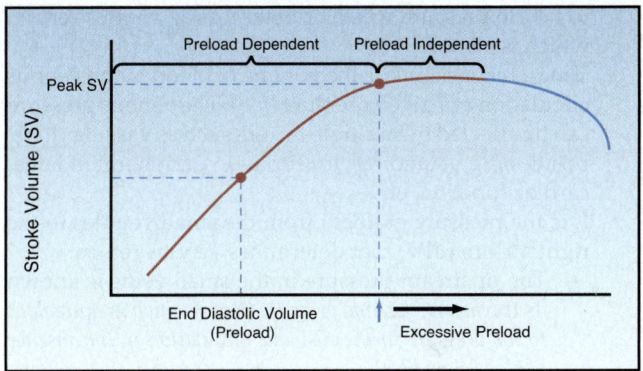

FIGURE 11.1. Frank-Starling curve.

- Stroke volume is the amount of blood ejected by the left ventricle by a single contraction.
- Stroke volume multiplied by heart rate determines the cardiac output.
- Stroke volume is preload dependent to a point, then plateaus (preload independent).
- Further preload no longer results in improved stroke volume but may result in increased hydrostatic pressure promoting interstitial edema, pulmonary edema, and eventually overstretch, leading to cardiac failure and decreased stroke volume.

Venous Return

Volume resuscitation is aimed at optimizing preload, but this fluid must get to the heart (venous return). A misunderstanding of the physiology of venous return can result in the inappropriate use of intravenous fluids.

Determinants of Venous Return
- The difference between the mean arterial pressure and the pressure in the right atrium is commonly assumed

to be the pressure gradient determining venous return, which is *incorrect!*

- Venous capacitance is the volume of blood in the venous circulation at a given pressure (5-6). The venous pressure can be affected by multiple factors such as vascular tone, positioning (standing to supine), peripheral edema, cardiac function, etc.
- It is the pressure gradient from the small venules to the right atrium (ΔPv) that determines venous return.
  - The upstream pressure in the small veins is known as the *mean systemic pressure* (Pms) *which is equivalent to the pressure in the systemic circulation in the absence of blood flow* (7-8).
  - The Pms is not easily measured.
  - Since the central venous pressure (CVP) is the clinical measure of the right atrial pressure, venous return can be described as:

  $$\text{Venous Return} = (\text{Pms} - \text{CVP})/\text{Rv} \qquad (11.1)$$

  Rv is the resistance to flow in the venous circulation.
  - Clearly, the driving pressure for venous return is distinct from the arterial pressure (9).

A Deeper Look at the Central Venous Pressure

Historically, CVP has been used as a measure of preload, however, there is no direct correlation to CVP and blood volume (or preload), and it is a poor predictor of fluid responsiveness (10). Equation 11.1 indicates that *an increase in CVP will impede venous return* (also shown in Figure 11.2).

The lines in Figure 11.2 are constructed by varying the CVP independently, i.e., without a change in blood volume, and recording the resulting changes in blood flow (venous return). Note that progressive increases in CVP above 0 are associated with a steady decline in venous return: An increase in CVP of 1 mm Hg results in an average 14% decrease in venous return (8). When venous return eventually ceases, the CVP is equivalent to the Pms, and there is no pressure gradient for venous return. Clearly, a high CVP will compromise venous return and therefore compromise preload (11). Note that changes in intravascular volume (i.e., hypovolemia and hypervolemia) are associated with the same directional change in Pms, *indicating that Pms is volume dependent.*

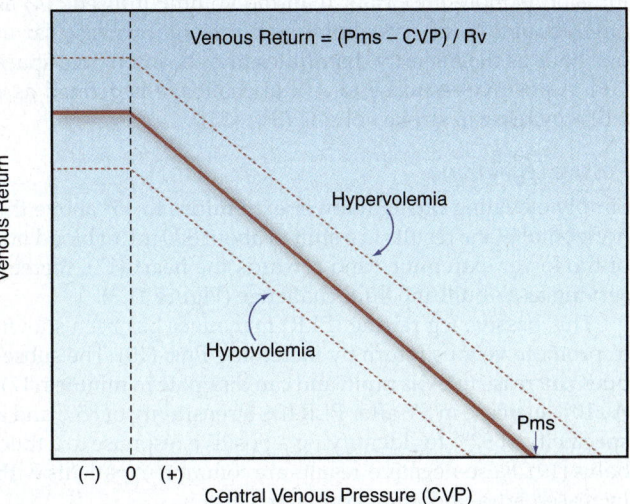

FIGURE 11.2. Graph showing the influence of central venous pressure (right atrial pressure) on venous return. The normal curve is indicated by the solid line. When venous return is zero, the central venous pressure (CVP) is equivalent to the mean systemic pressure (Pms). See text for explanation. (From Fluid Management. In: Marino PL. *Marino's The ICU Book.* 5th ed. Wolters Kluwer; 2025:170-84. Figure 11.2.)

Fluid Responsiveness

Clinical studies have consistently shown that the Pms increases in response to a fluid challenge (typically 250-500 mL) (7-8,12-13), but the increase in Pms alone does not identify a beneficial response to fluids (not if there is a similar increase in the CVP) (7). Rather, *patients who are "fluid responsive" are identified by an increase in the (Pms − CVP) gradient after a fluid challenge* (7,12), as predicted by Equation 11.1.

The Fluid Challenge

The standard method for determining fluid responsiveness is to administer a fluid bolus, which is usually *500 mL of a crystalloid fluid infused over 10-15 minutes* (14-15). The rate of infusion is more important than the volume infused (14) as only about 20% of crystalloids will remain intravascular at one hour as the majority distributes into the interstitial space (16). A positive response to a fluid challenge is defined as a >10% increase in stroke volume (SV) (15).

Passive Leg Raising

Simply elevating bilateral lower extremities to 45° above the horizontal plane results in a shift of about 300 mL of blood out of the lower extremities and towards the heart (17), thereby serving as a "built-in" fluid challenge (Figure 11.3).

This passive leg raising (PLR) maneuver has been shown to promote venous return by increasing Pms (18). The subsequent increase in SV is rapid and can dissipate in minutes (17). A ≥10% increase in SV after PLR has a sensitivity of 85% and a specificity of 92% for identifying a positive response to a fluid bolus (19). False-negative results are common in patients with increased intra-abdominal pressure (20).

Stroke Volume Variation

Stroke volume variation (SVV) is the variation (as a percentage) of SV during a mechanical ventilation cycle and assessed by the following equation:

$$SVV = (SV_{max} - SV_{min}) / SV_{mean} \quad (11.2)$$

During positive pressure mechanical ventilation, the respiratory cycle is accompanied by changes in intrathoracic pressures impacting left ventricular preload resulting in cyclic changes in the left ventricular SV. These changes are more pronounced in the presence of hypovolemia (21).

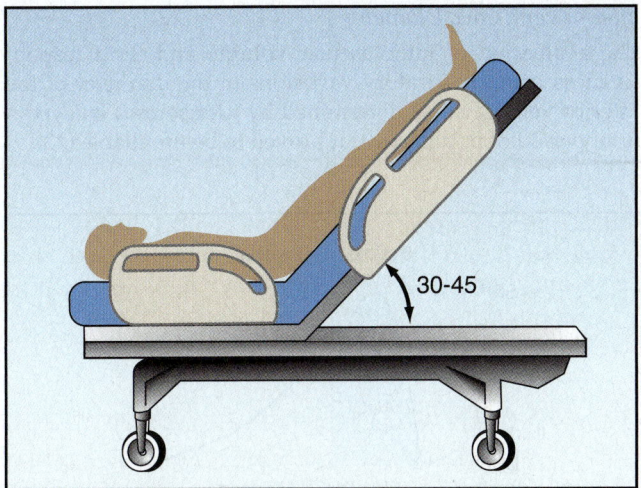

FIGURE 11.3. The passive leg raising test. (Modified from Fluid Management. In: Marino PL. *Marino's The ICU Book*. 5th ed. Wolters Kluwer; 2025:170-84. Figure 11.6.)

This SVV can be quantified as shown in Figure 11.4, and clinical studies have shown that an SVV of ≥15% can identify fluid responsiveness in 80% of cases (22).

Clinical variables impacting accurate SVV measurements are as follows:

- Must be on volume-controlled mechanical ventilation
- Cannot be spontaneously breathing
- Must have stable heart rhythm, e.g., cannot be in atrial fibrillation
- Open abdomen will reduce SVV
- Changes in lung compliance

Inferior Vena Cava Diameter

The evaluation of intravascular volume and fluid responsiveness using respiratory variations in the diameter of the inferior vena cava (as determined by ultrasound) enjoyed a brief period of popularity but proved to be unreliable (23).

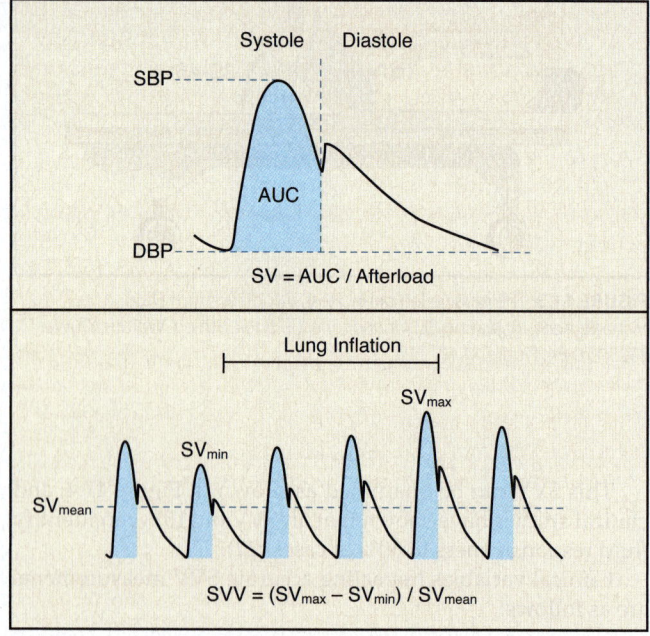

FIGURE 11.4. The upper panel shows the pulse contour method of measuring the stroke volume (SV), where the area under the curve (AUC) represents the systolic portion of the arterial pressure waveform. The lower panel demonstrates the respiratory variation in SV that occurs during mechanical ventilation and shows how this stroke volume variation (SVV) is quantified. SBP = systolic blood pressure, DBP = diastolic blood pressure. See text for further explanation. (From Fluid Management. In: Marino PL. *Marino's The ICU Book*. 5th ed. Wolters Kluwer; 2025:170-84. Figure 11.5.)

KEYS TO FLUID RESUSCITATION

- The goal is to increase preload, thereby increasing stroke volume.
- The optimal fluid may vary (Chapter 10: Colloid & Crystalloid Fluids). Clearly, with hemorrhage, blood products are required. When crystalloids are used, balanced crystalloids such as Lactated Ringer's and PlasmaLyte are preferred (24).
- Conventional clinical variables such as vital signs, CVP, pulmonary artery wedge pressure, or inferior vena cava diameter are not helpful in determining fluid responsiveness (15,17).
- Fluid responsiveness does not equate to the need for further fluid boluses (11).
- Continued boluses should balance benefit to risks of fluid overload.
- The PLR maneuver is a reliable evaluation of fluid responsiveness; however, it requires continuous cardiac output monitoring to assess (15,17).
- SVV is useful but has limitations (see previous section).

It is important to emphasize to not "over-resuscitate" with fluids beyond the preload independent point of the Frank-Starling curve as excess volume resuscitation can lead to multiple adverse effects. See Table 11.1 (1-2,15).

TABLE 11.1	Adverse Effects of Excess Fluid Resuscitation
• Increased interstitial edema • Pulmonary edema • Increased acute kidney injury • Decreased cardiac output • Increased mortality	

From References 1-2, 15.

DE-RESUSCITATION

De-resuscitation refers to the concept of actively removing excess fluid volume using diuretics or ultrafiltration (25). Once the patient is hemodynamically stabilized, no longer requiring fluid replacement for losses, and on no-to-minimal vasopressors, a "de-resuscitation" should be considered (25). This strategy should take into consideration clinical indicators of excess fluid such as pulmonary edema, pleural effusions, elevated CVP, peripheral edema, etc.

References

1. Finfer S, Myburgh J, Bellomo R. Intravenous fluid therapy in critically ill adults. Nat Rev Nephrol 2018;14:541-57.
2. Messmer AS, Zingg C, Muller M, et al. Fluid overload and mortality in adult critical care patients—a systematic review and meta-analysis of observational studies. Crit Care Med 2020;48:1862-70.
3. Vincent JL. Understanding cardiac output. Crit Care 2008;12:174.
4. O'Keefe E, Singh P. Physiology, Cardiac Preload. In: StatPearls. Treasure Island (FL): StatPearls Publishing; 2024.
5. Gelman S. Venous function and central venous pressure: a physiologic story. Anesthesiology. 2008;108:735-48.
6. Sorimachi H, Burkhoff D, Verbrugge FH, et al. Obesity, venous capacitance, and venous compliance in heart failure with preserved ejection fraction. Eur J Heart Fail 2021;23:1648-58.
7. Persichini R, Lai C, Teboul JL, et al. Venous return and mean systemic filling pressure: physiology and clinical applications. Crit Care 2022;26:150.
8. Vos JJ, Kalmar AF, Scheeren TWL. Bedside assessment and clinical utility of mean systemic filling pressure in acute care. J Emerg Crit Care Med 2020;4:25.
9. Magder S. Volume and its relationship to cardiac output and venous return. Crit Care 2016;20:271.
10. Shah P, Louis MA. Physiology, Central Venous Pressure. In: StatPearls. Treasure Island (FL): StatPearls Publishing; 2024.
11. Marik PE. Fluid responsiveness and the six guiding principles of fluid resuscitation. Crit Care Med 2016;44:1920-2.
12. Cecconi M, Aya HD, Geisen M, et al. Changes in the mean systemic filling pressure during a fluid challenge in postsurgical intensive care patients. Intensive Care Med 2013;39:1299-305.

13. Maas JJ, Pinsky MR, Geerts BF, et al. Estimation of mean systemic filling pressure in postoperative cardiac surgery patients with three methods. Intensive Care Med 2012;38:1452-60.
14. Cecconi M, Parsons AK, Rhodes A. What is a fluid challenge? Curr Opin Crit Care 2011;17:290-5.
15. Marik PE, Weinmann M. Optimizing fluid therapy in shock. Curr Opin Crit Care 2019;25:246-51.
16. Hahn RG, Lyons G. The half-life of infusion fluids: an educational review. Eur J Anaesthesiol 2016;33:475-82.
17. Monnet X, Teboul JL. Passive leg raising: five rules, not a drop of fluid! Crit Care 2015;19:18.
18. Guerin L, Teboul JL, Persichini R, et al. Effects of passive leg raising and volume expansion on mean systemic pressure and venous return in shock in humans. Crit Care 2015;19:411.
19. Cherpanath TG, Hirsch A, Geerts BF, et al. Predicting fluid responsiveness by passive leg raising: systematic review and meta-analysis of 23 clinical trials. Crit Care Med 2016;44:981-91.
20. Beurton A, Teboul JL, Girotto V, et al. Intra-abdominal hypertension is responsible for false negatives to the passive leg raising test. Crit Care Med 2019;47:e639-e47.
21. Li C, Lin FQ, Fu SK, et al. Stroke volume variation for prediction of fluid responsiveness in patients undergoing gastrointestinal surgery. Int J Med Sci 2013;10:148-55.
22. Marik PE, Cavallazzi R, Vasu T, Hirani A. Dynamic changes in arterial waveform derived variables and fluid responsiveness in mechanically ventilated patients: a systematic review of the literature. Crit Care Med 2009;37:2642-7.
23. Orso D, Paoli I, Piani T, et al. Accuracy of ultrasonographic measurements of inferior vena cava to determine fluid responsiveness: a systematic review and meta-analysis. J Intensive Care Med 2020;35:354-63.
24. Semler MW, Self WH, Wanderer JP, et al. Balanced crystalloids versus saline in critically ill adults. N Engl J Med 2018;378:829-39.
25. Malbrain M, Martin G, Ostermann M. Everything you need to know about deresuscitation. Intensive Care Med 2022;48:1781-6.

Anemia and Erythrocyte Transfusions

Chapter 12

Anemia is nearly universal in the ICU reaching as high as 66% (1) of ICU patients and over 90% in surgical intensive care units (2). Thirty to 50% of ICU patients receive red blood cells (RBC) during their hospitalization (3).

ANEMIA IN THE ICU

Definitions

Anemia is defined as a *decrease in the oxygen carrying capacity of blood*. The most accurate measure of this is the red cell mass, which is not easily obtained. As a result, the hemoglobin (Hb) and hematocrit (Hct) are used as surrogate measures of the O_2 carrying capacity of blood. (The reference ranges for red blood cell parameters are shown in Table 12.1).

TABLE 12.1 Reference Ranges for Red Cell Parameters in Adults

Hemoglobin (Hb) Males: 13.5-18 g/dL Females: 12-16 g/dL*	*Mean Cell Volume* Males: 80-100 × 10^{-15}/L Females: same
Hematocrit (Hct) Males: 40-54% Females: 38-47%	*Red Blood Cell Count* Males: 4.6-6.2 × 10^{12}/L Females: 4.2-5.4 × 10^{12}/L
Red Cell Mass Males: 26 mL/kg Females: 24 mL/kg	*Reticulocyte Count* Males: 25-75 × 10^9/L Females: same

*Normal range is 1 g/dL lower after the first trimester of pregnancy.

From Walker RH (ed.). *Technical Manual of the American Association of Blood Banks*. 10th ed. American Association of Blood Banks; 1990:649-50; Hillman RS, Finch CA. *Red Cell Manual*. 6th ed. FA Davis; 1994:46.

Hemoglobin is the protein molecule in the red blood cells, or "erythrocytes" responsible for majority of oxygen transport by blood. Its contribution to the quantitative amount of oxygen in blood is termed *oxygen content*, which is described as:

$$CaO_2 = (1.34 \times Hb \times O_2 \text{ saturation}) + (pO_2 \times 0.0031) \quad (12.1)$$

CaO_2 – the concentration of oxygen in arterial blood; CvO_2 would describe the concentration of oxygen in venous blood.

1.34 – refers to the binding of 1.34 mL O_2 to each gram of hemoglobin

pO_2 – the partial pressure of oxygen dissolved in the blood (not bound to hemoglobin)

0.0031 – refers to the constant representing the amount of oxygen dissolved in plasma per mm Hg of the pO_2; Equation 12.1 demonstrates pO_2 is a small proportion of the total amount of oxygen in blood (approximately 3%).

Hematocrit is the volume of red blood cells compared to the total blood volume (plasma, white blood cells, and platelets).

Blood Volume is the total amount of blood circulating within the entire cardiovascular system, which includes plasma volume, erythrocytes, leukocytes, and platelets.

Plasma Volume is the fluid component of blood typically accounting for approximately 55-60% of total blood volume (4) (see Figure 12.1).

The confounding factor concerning Hb and Hct as measures of O_2 carrying capacity is that they are influenced by the plasma volume. For example, an increase in plasma volume will decrease the Hb and Hct (dilution effect), thereby creating the false impression of a drop in the O_2 carrying capacity of blood (pseudoanemia). Clinical studies have shown that the *Hb and Hct, in isolation, are unreliable as markers of anemia in critically ill patients* (4-6), i.e., not a reliable surrogate for red cell mass. For example, if a subject has rapidly hemorrhaged half their blood volume and their Hb and Hct were immediately checked, they would be unchanged; however, the blood volume (red cell mass and plasma volume) would be markedly decreased.

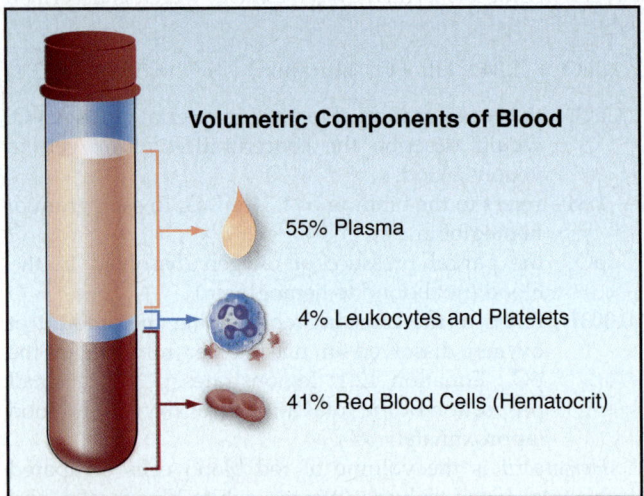

FIGURE 12.1. Volumetric components of blood.

Contributing Factors

ICU-associated anemia is attributed to two conditions: systemic inflammation and repeated phlebotomy for laboratory studies.

Inflammation

- Inflammation is responsible for the *anemia of chronic disease*, which is now called the *anemia of inflammation* (7).
- The hematologic effects of inflammation include inhibition of erythropoietin release from the kidneys, reduced marrow responsiveness to erythropoietin, iron sequestration in macrophages, and increased destruction of RBCs (8-10).
- The resulting anemia is hypochromic and microcytic, with a low plasma iron level. Inflammatory anemia

can be confused with iron-deficiency anemia but can be differentiated by measuring plasma ferritin levels (a marker of tissue iron stores) which is increased in inflammatory anemia and decreased in iron-deficiency anemia.

Phlebotomy

- The volume of blood withdrawn for laboratory tests averages 40-70 mL daily in ICU patients (9), and the cumulative loss of blood in one week can reach 500 mL (>1 unit of whole blood).
- A significant percentage of blood loss for laboratory testing is related to technique, i.e., when a blood sample is obtained from a vascular catheter, an initial aliquot of blood is withdrawn first and discarded, to eliminate interference from intravenous fluids in the catheter. The discarded volume is about 5 mL per blood draw, and returning this blood to the patient can reduce daily phlebotomy loss by 50% (8).

Physiological Effects of Anemia

Anemia elicits two responses that help to preserve tissue oxygenation: (1) an increase in cardiac output and (2) an increase in O_2 extraction from capillary blood.

Cardiac Output

Anemia affects viscosity, which can have direct impact on cardiac output as explained by the Hagen-Poiseuille equation (Figure 12.2), which shows that the flow rate of a fluid is inversely related to the viscosity of the fluid.

This equation states that steady flow (Q) through a rigid tube is directly related to the driving pressure (ΔP) for flow and the fourth power of the inner radius (r) of the tube and is inversely related to the length (L) of the tube and the viscosity (μ) of the infusate. These relationships also describe the infusion of resuscitation fluids through vascular catheters.

$$Q = \Delta P \left(\pi r^4 / 8\mu L \right)$$

FIGURE 12.2. Hagen-Poiseuille equation. See text for explanation.

Since Hct is the principal determinant of blood viscosity, a decrease in Hct will decrease blood viscosity, which will result in an increase in blood flow (cardiac output).

O_2 Extraction

O_2 extraction is the ratio of O_2 consumption (VO_2) to O_2 delivery (DO_2); i.e.,

$$O_2 \text{ Extraction} = VO_2 / DO_2 \qquad (12.2)$$

Rearranging terms in this relationship yields the following:

$$VO_2 = DO_2 \times O_2 \text{ Extraction} \qquad (12.3)$$

This relationship predicts that a decrease in DO_2 (e.g., from anemia), will not impair aerobic metabolism (VO_2) if there is a proportional increase in O_2 extraction. This type of response is demonstrated in Figure 12.3 (10).

- A progressive decrease in Hct is accompanied by a similar decrease in DO_2. However, the decrease in DO_2 is initially accompanied by an increase in O_2 extraction, and this keeps the VO_2 constant.
- When the Hct falls below 10%, the increase in O_2 extraction is no longer able to match the decrease in DO_2, and the VO_2 begins to fall. This is the *anaerobic threshold*.

- Thus, aerobic metabolism is maintained during progressive anemia because of an increase in O_2 extraction, and the Hct and Hb must fall to extremely low levels before aerobic metabolism is affected. Figure 12.3 demonstrates the influence of progressive anemia on oxygen delivery and extraction.

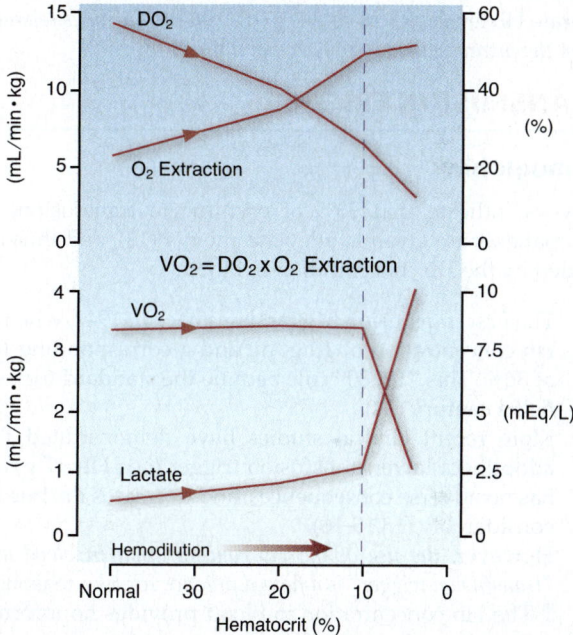

FIGURE 12.3. The influence of progressive isovolemic anemia on measures of systemic oxygenation in nonhuman primates. $DO_2 = O_2$ delivery, $VO_2 = O_2$ uptake. See text for explanation. (From Anemia and Red Blood Cell Transfusions. In: Marino PL. *Marino's The ICU Book*. 5th ed. Wolters Kluwer; 2025:187-203. Figure 12.3. Data from Wilkerson DK, Rosen AL, Gould SA, et al. Oxygen extraction ratio: a valid indicator of myocardial metabolism in anemia. J Surg Res 1987;42:629-34.)

Tolerance to Anemia

In a large study that included 300 postoperative patients, 50% of the patients survived with an Hb level of 2-3 g/dL, and 75% of the patients survived with an Hb level of 3-4 g/dL (11). Another study of progressive hemodilution in healthy adults showed that Hb levels of 5 g/dL produced no apparent harm (12). Thus, the available studies suggest that Hb levels down to 5.0 can be safe, and individual patients can tolerate Hb levels as low as 2-3 g/dL! *Severe anemia is tolerated when the intravascular volume is maintained*.

TRANSFUSION TRIGGERS

Hemoglobin

Surveys indicate that 90% of erythrocyte transfusions in ICU patients are given to alleviate anemia (13), and thus are guided by the Hb concentration in blood.

- The first transfusion trigger dates back to 1942, when an Hb concentration of 10 g/dL and a corresponding Hct of 30%. This "10/30" rule became the standard for over half a century (14).
- More recent clinical studies have demonstrated that adopting a lower transfusion trigger (i.e., Hb <7 g/dL) has no adverse consequences, and decreases the burden considerably (13,15-16).
- However, *the use of the Hb concentration in blood as a "transfusion trigger" is a flawed practice* for two reasons:
  1. The Hb concentration in blood provides no information about the state of tissue oxygenation.
  2. The Hb concentration in blood is influenced by changes in plasma volume, which means that changes in the Hb concentration in blood do not always reflect changes in the O_2 carrying capacity of blood (red cell mass of blood volume).
- The most recent guidelines on erythrocyte transfusions in critically ill patients state that the use of the Hb concentration as a "trigger" for transfusions *should be avoided*

(4). Despite this statement, the guidelines recommend that transfusion *should be considered* when the Hb is <7 g/dL in critically ill patients and <8 g/dL in acute coronary syndromes (4,16).
- A patient's ability to compensate for acute anemia, even when maintaining stable blood volume, is also influenced by the baseline hemoglobin and age (14,17).

Oxygen Extraction

As described earlier and shown in Figure 12.3, anemia elicits a compensatory increase in O_2 extraction from capillary blood, which serves to maintain a constant rate of aerobic metabolism. However, the increase in O_2 extraction reaches a maximum at about 50%, whereupon further decreases in Hb are accompanied by proportional decreases in VO_2.

Central Venous O_2 Saturation

When the arterial O_2 saturation is close to 100%, the O_2 extraction is roughly equivalent to the difference between the arterial and central venous O_2 saturations ($SaO_2 - ScvO_2$):

$$O_2 \text{ Extraction} = SaO_2 - ScvO_2 \qquad (12.4)$$

Or to simplify further:

$$O_2 \text{ Extraction} = 1 - ScvO_2 \qquad (12.5)$$

An $ScvO_2$ <70% has been proposed as a transfusion trigger and may demonstrate increasing compensatory mechanisms for inadequate oxygen delivery (18). An $ScvO_2$ of <70% in the first hours of ICU admission and 6 hours later was associated with an increased mortality (19).

ERYTHROCYTE PRODUCTS

The red blood cell (RBC) preparations available for transfusion are listed in Table 12.2 (18,20). Except for whole blood the other erythrocyte preparations lack any significant coagulation factors or platelets.

TABLE 12.2	Red Blood Cell Preparations
Preparation	Features
Packed RBCs	1. Each unit has a volume of 350 mL and hematocrit of about 60%. 2. Contains leukocytes and residual plasma (15-30 mL per unit) 3. Can be stored for 42 days with appropriate additives
Leukocyte-Reduced RBCs	1. Donor RBCs are passed through specialized filters to remove most of the leukocytes. This reduces the risk of nonhemolytic febrile reactions. 2. Indicated for patients with a history of (nonhemolytic) febrile transfusion reactions
Washed RBCs	1. Packed RBCs are saline washed to remove residual plasma, which reduces the risk of hypersensitivity reactions. 2. Indicated for patients with a history of transfusion-related allergic reactions and in patients with IgA deficiency, who are at risk for transfusion-related anaphylaxis
Whole Blood	1. Typical unit has volume of 500 mL 2. Contains plasma and coagulation factors 3. Can be stored up to 42 days refrigerated 4. Labile clotting factors V and VIII degrade rapidly during storage. 5. Platelet function declines 1-2% per day in cold storage.

From King KE, ed. *Blood Transfusion Therapy: A Physician's Handbook.* 9th ed. American Association of Blood Banks; 2008:1-18,91-5.

Whole Blood

- Whole blood is indicated for life-threatening hemorrhage (20-21). It provides red cells (oxygen carrying capacity), plasma for volume expansion and coagulation factors.

- The labile coagulation factors (V and VIII) degrade rapidly even in cold storage therefore may be inadequate for hemostasis unless used fresh (20,22).
- Platelet function degrades about 1-2% per day. Recovery of platelets from stored whole blood is acceptable up to 15 days (from donation) (23).

Packed RBCs

- Called "packed" RBCs (pRBCs) because the plasma has been removed, therefore contains less volume for the same oxygen carry capacity than a unit of whole blood A unit of packed red blood cell volume of 200 mL would be equivalent to a 450 mL unit of whole blood (20).
- The RBC fraction of donated blood is placed in a preservative fluid and stored at 1-6°C. Newer preservative solutions contain adenine, which helps to maintain ATP levels in stored RBCs, and allows storage of donor RBCs for up to 42 days (18).
- Each unit of donor RBCs, known as pRBCs, has Hct of about 60% and a volume of about 300 mL.
- pRBCs also contain 30-50 mL of residual plasma and a considerable number of leukocytes (1-3 billion leukocytes per unit of pRBCs) (24).

Leukocyte-Reduced RBCs

- The leukocytes in pRBCs can trigger an antibody response in the recipient after repeated transfusions, and this is responsible for *febrile nonhemolytic transfusion reactions* (see section that follows).
- To reduce the risk of this reaction, donor RBCs are passed through specialized filters to remove most of the leukocytes. This is performed routinely in many blood banks, but universal leukocyte reduction has yet to be adopted in the United States.
- Leukocyte-reduced RBCs are recommended for patients with prior febrile nonhemolytic transfusion reactions (25).

Washed RBCs

- Donor RBCs can be washed with isotonic saline to remove residual plasma. This reduces the risk of hypersensitivity reactions by removing 98-99% of the plasma constituents that can lead to anaphylaxis caused by prior sensitization to plasma proteins in donor blood.
- Washed RBCs are recommended for patients with a history of hypersensitivity reactions to blood transfusions, and for patients with immunoglobulin A deficiency, who have an increased risk of transfusion-related anaphylaxis (24).
- Washed pRBC units contain 105-20% less RBCs than original units and are depleted of 99% of plasma proteins and 85% of white blood cells (26).
- Stored pRBC accumulated biochemical and structural changes known as *red blood cell storage lesions*. These "lesions" are thought to contribute to inflammatory events associated with older pRBCs. Washing decreases these lesions and may lessen the sequelae (27).

UNDERSTANDING THE BLOOD BANK

Ordering

- *Type and Hold* – the patient's blood type (ABO and Rh factor) is determined but no further testing. The blood specimen is "held" in the blood bank and can be cross matched if a transfusion becomes necessary.
- *Type and Screen* – performed when transfusion not emergent, determines ABO and Rh factor and screens for atypical antibodies. Allows for more rapid cross matching if transfusion becomes necessary.
- *Type and Cross* – directly tests patient blood with specific donor units reserving these units for the specific patient. A complete crossmatch takes 45 minutes.

RBC Compatibility

Blood Groups

There are four major blood groups, based on the presence or absence of two antigens (A and B) on the surface of red blood cells (A, B, AB, and no antigens, designated O). Each blood group is classified further by the presence or absence of another surface antigen, the Rh factor.

Plasma contains antibodies to antigens that are absent on the RBCs. For example, type O blood has no A or B antigens on the RBCs, and the plasma contains anti-A and anti-B antibodies.

Universal Donor RBCs

Life-threatening hemolytic transfusion reactions are the result of anti-A, anti-B, or anti-Rh antibodies in the recipient that react with their corresponding antigens on donor RBCs. Transfusing antigen-free PRBCs (i.e., type-O, Rh-negative) eliminates the risk of hemolytic transfusion reactions. Therefore, type-O, Rh-negative blood is called the *universal red cell donor*.

Uncrossmatched type-O Rh-positive RBCs are often used in cases of acute hemorrhage. In a study of over 500 transfusions of type-O Rh-positive RBCs, only one Rh-negative patient developed anti-Rh antibodies after transfusion (24).

Rh Immunoglobulin

If an Rh-negative woman receives Rh-positive RBCs, anti-Rh antibodies may be formed, and these antibodies can cross the placenta during pregnancy and cause hemolysis in an Rh-positive fetus. Rh immunoglobulin (RhoGAM, Kedrion Biopharma) can prevent the formation of anti-Rh antibodies in response to an Rh-positive transfusion.

In women of childbearing age who are Rh-negative, an injection of Rh immunoglobulin should be given within 72 hours of a transfusion with Rh-positive pRBCs (28).

Blood Filters

Standard blood filters (pore size 170-260 microns) are required for the transfusion of all blood products. These filters trap blood clots and other debris, but they do not trap leukocytes and are not effective for leukocyte reduction (18). These filters can become an impediment to flow as they collect trapped debris, and sluggish infusion rates should prompt replacement of the filter.

Physiologic Effects

- In an average sized adult, one unit of pRBCs is expected to raise the Hb concentration and Hct by 1 g/dL and 3%, respectively (18).
- Prolonged storage of RBCs can actually impair tissue oxygenation after transfusion (29). These studies have prompted the following statement in the guidelines for RBC transfusions (4):

    RBC transfusion should not be considered an absolute method to improve tissue oxygenation in critically ill patients.

TRANSFUSION RISKS

The spectrum of adverse events associated with blood transfusions are shown in Table 12.3, along with the incidence of each event expressed in relation to the number of units transfused (18,30-36). Note that human errors with transfusions are much more frequent than the feared transmission of HIV or the hepatitis B virus. The following is a brief description of the principal transfusion reactions.

Acute Hemolytic Reactions

Acute hemolytic reactions are prompted by the transfusion of RBCs that are ABO-incompatible with the recipient. When this occurs, antibodies in recipient blood bind to ABO antigens on the donor RBCs, and the ensuing RBC lysis triggers a systemic inflammatory response that can lead to hypotension

TABLE 12.3 Adverse Events Associated with RBC Transfusions*

Immune-Related	Others
Nonhemolytic fever (1:60)	Circulatory Overload (1:100)†
Hypersensitivity Reactions:	Transmitted Infections:
Urticaria (1:100)	Bacterial (1:500,000)
Anaphylaxis (1:1,000)	Hepatitis B virus (1:1.2 million)
Anaphylactic shock (1:50,000)	Hepatitis C virus (1:1.5 million)
Acute lung injury (1:12,000)	HIV (1:1.5 million)
Nosocomial Infections (?)	Transfusion Errors:
Acute hemolysis (1:35,000)	Wrong person transfused (1:15,000)
Fatal hemolysis (1:1.9 million)	Incompatible transfusion (1:33,000)

*Per units transfused.
†Estimated risk per recipients rather than units.
From References 18, 31, 33-36.

and multiorgan failure. These reactions are usually the result of human error.

Clinical Features

The hallmark of acute hemolytic reactions is the abrupt onset of fever, dyspnea, chest pain, low back pain, and hypotension, within minutes after starting the transfusion. Severe reactions are accompanied by a consumptive coagulopathy and progressive multiorgan dysfunction.

Management

- If a hemolytic reaction is suspected, STOP the transfusion immediately and verify that the correct blood was given to the correct patient. It is imperative to stop the transfusion as soon as possible because the severity of hemolytic reactions is a function of the volume of blood transfused (31).
- If the donor blood is correctly matched to the patient, an acute hemolytic reaction is unlikely. However, the blood bank must be notified, and they will ask for blood

samples to perform a plasma free hemoglobin determination (for evidence of intravascular hemolysis) and a direct Coombs' test (for evidence of the anti-ABO antibodies).
- If an acute hemolytic reaction is confirmed, support blood pressure and ventilation as needed. The management of severe hemolytic reactions is similar to septic shock (i.e., volume resuscitation and a vasopressor, if necessary). Most patients should survive the illness.

Febrile Nonhemolytic Reactions

Clinical Features
- A febrile, nonhemolytic transfusion reaction is defined as a temperature elevation >1°C (1.8°F) that occurs during transfusion or up to 6 hours after transfusion and is not attributed to another cause (18).
- The fever typically does not appear in the first hour after the start of transfusion (unlike the fever associated with acute hemolytic reactions), but it can be accompanied by rigors.
- The culprit is the presence of anti-leukocyte antibodies in recipient blood that react with antigens on donor leukocytes. This triggers the release of endogenous pyrogens from phagocytes, which is the source of the fever.
- This reaction is reported in 0.5% of RBC transfusions and occurs in patients who have received prior transfusions and in multiparous women.
- Transfusion of leukocyte-reduced RBCs reduces, but does not eliminate, the risk of this reaction (18).

Management
The initial approach to transfusion-related fever is the same as described for hemolytic transfusion reactions. The diagnosis is confirmed by excluding the presence of hemolysis with the tests described previously. The blood bank will perform a gram stain on the donor blood and may request blood

cultures on the recipient. This is usually unrewarding because microbial contamination in stored blood is rare (1 per 5,000,000 units).

Future Transfusions
- More than 75% of patients with a nonhemolytic fever will not experience a similar reaction to subsequent transfusions (32). Therefore, no special precautions are needed for future transfusions.
- If a second febrile reaction occurs, leukocyte-reduced RBCs are advised for all subsequent transfusions.

Hypersensitivity Reactions

Hypersensitivity reactions are the result of sensitization to plasma proteins in donor blood from prior transfusions. Patients with IgA deficiency are prone to hypersensitivity transfusion reactions, and prior exposure to plasma products is not required.

Clinical Features
- The most common hypersensitivity reaction is urticaria, which is reported in one of every 100 units transfused (32), and appears during the transfusion.
- The abrupt onset of dyspnea during a transfusion could represent laryngeal edema or bronchospasm from anaphylaxis, and hypotension from anaphylactic shock can be mistaken for an acute hemolytic reaction.

Management
- Mild urticaria without fever does not require interruption of the transfusion. However, the popular practice is to stop the transfusion temporarily and administer an antihistamine for symptom relief (e.g., *diphenhydramine*, 25-50 mg PO, IM, or IV).
- The transfusion should be stopped immediately if anaphylaxis is suspected.

- Washed RBCs should be used for all future transfusions in patients with hypersensitivity reactions. However, in patients with anaphylactic reactions, future transfusions are risky, even with washed RBCs, and should be avoided unless absolutely necessary.
- Patients who develop hypersensitivity reactions should be tested for an underlying IgA deficiency.

Transfusion-Associated Circulatory Overload (TACO)

Etiology

Similar to transfusion related acute lung injury (discussed below) there is a hypothesis that TACO may also have a "two hit" etiology rather than just volume overload with however the presentation is typically combined with underlying cardiovascular or renal disease (37-38).

TACO has been reported after single blood component transfusion associated with acute hypertension, the acutely elevated systemic vascular resistance can lead to increased cardiac filling pressures and pulmonary pressures leading to hydrostatic pulmonary edema in absence of significant volume expansion (37).

Clinical Features

Acute onset of respiratory distress within 6 hours of blood transfusion. Physical exam and radiologic findings are consistent with circulatory overload. B-type natriuretic protein is elevated.

Management

Immediate discontinuation of transfusion if applicable. Supportive care and treatment of circulatory overload, i.e., upright positioning, supplemental oxygen, consideration of diuresis with cardiac evaluation of function. Laboratory analysis to include B-type natriuretic peptide.

Future Transfusions

There are no recommendations regarding future transfusions.

Transfusion-Related Acute Lung Injury

Transfusion-related acute lung injury (TRALI) is an inflammatory lung injury associated with blood produce transfusions including RBCs, plasma, cryoprecipitate, platelets, and even immune globulins (39-40). TRALI resembles the acute respiratory distress syndrome (ARDS), a non-cardiogenic cause of pulmonary edema. *TRALI is the leading cause of transfusion-related deaths* (16,38-39).

Pathophysiology

TRALI is believed to be the result of a "two-hit" phenomenon, the first hit being shock. Shock leads to activation of the pulmonary endothelium along with primed neutrophils (39-40). The second "hit" is anti-leukocyte antibodies in donor blood that bind to antigens on circulating neutrophils in the recipient. This triggers neutrophil activation, and the activated neutrophils become sequestered in pulmonary capillaries and migrate into the lungs to produce the inflammatory injury (40).

Clinical Features

- Signs of respiratory compromise (dyspnea, tachypnea, hypoxemia, etc.) typically appear within 6 hours after the start of a transfusion, but they usually appear within the first hour after the transfusion begins (38,40). Unlike TACO, TRALI is not associated with volume overload.
- Radiologic features are similar to ARDS exhibiting alveolar and interstitial infiltrates (Figure 12.4).
- Fever is common, and the chest x-ray typically shows diffuse infiltrates in both lungs.
- TRALI can be severe at the outset, and often requires mechanical ventilation, but the condition typically resolves within 96 hours (40).

Management

- If the transfusion is not completed, it should be stopped at the first signs of respiratory difficulty. The blood bank should be notified for all cases of TRALI. (Assays for anti-leukocyte antibodies are available but are not currently used in the diagnostic evaluation of TRALI.)
- The management of TRALI is supportive and is very similar to the management of ARDS.

Future Transfusions

There are no firm recommendations regarding future transfusions in patients who develop TRALI. Some recommend

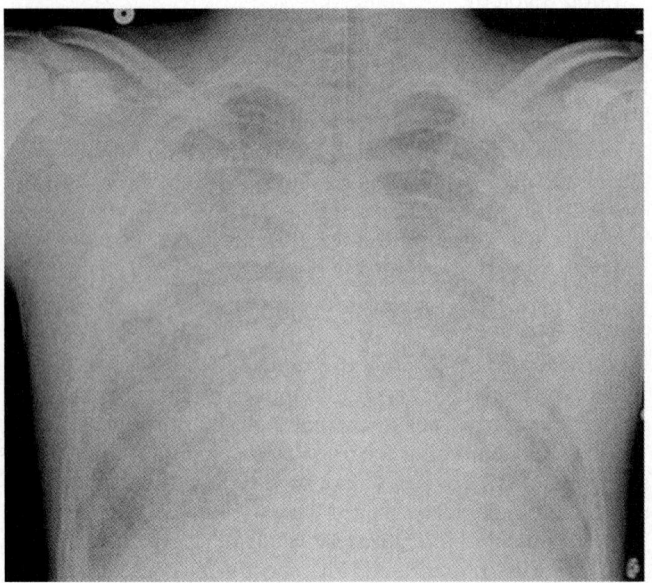

FIGURE 12.4. Portable chest film from a patient with transfusion-related acute lung injury. Note the homogeneous pattern of infiltration in the lungs, which is a characteristics of inflammatory lung injury. (From Anemia and Red Blood Cell Transfusions. In: Marino PL. *Marino's The ICU Book*. 5th ed. Wolters Kluwer; 2025:187-203. Figure 12.5.)

using washed RBCs to remove antibodies from donor blood, but the effectiveness of this measure is not known (41). A side-to-side comparison of TRALI with TACO is shown in Table 12.4 (42).

Nosocomial Infections

RBC transfusions have an immunosuppressant effect (43), and several clinical studies have shown that patients who receive blood transfusions have a higher incidence of nosocomial infections (44-45). Furthermore, at least 22 studies have shown that blood transfusion is an independent risk factor for nosocomial infections (46).

TABLE 12.4 Comparison of TRALI and TACO

TRALI	TACO*
• Acute respiratory distress within 6 hours of blood transfusion	• Acute respiratory distress within 6 hours of blood transfusion

• Hypoxemia:
  - PaO_2 / FiO_2 <300, or
  - SpO_2 <90% on room air
	• Radiographic evidence of pulmonary edema

• Bilateral infiltrates on chest radiography	• Elevated CVP
• No evidence of circulatory overload	• Evidence of left heart failure
• No pre-existing ALI prior to blood transfusion	• Elevated B-type natriuretic peptide (BNP)
• Absence of alternate ARDS risk factors	• Positive fluid balance
• No temporal relationship to alternative risk if ALI	

T.R.A.L.I. = transfusion-related acute lung injury; T.A.C.O. = transfusion-associated cardiac overload; ALI = acute lung injury.

*3 or more criteria.

From Roubinian N. TACO and TRALI: biology, risk factors, and prevention strategies. Hematology Am Soc Hematol Educ Program 2018;2018:585-94.

More Risk than Benefit

A review of 45 clinical studies evaluating RBC transfusions in critically ill patients, which included 272,596 patients, revealed the following findings (46):

- In 42 of the 45 studies, the adverse effects of RBC transfusions outweighed any benefits.
- Only 1 of 45 studies showed that the benefits of RBC transfusions outweighed the adverse effects.
- Eighteen studies evaluated the relationship between RBC transfusions and survival, and 17 of the 18 studies showed that RBC transfusions were an independent risk factor for death. The likelihood of a fatal outcome was, on average, 70% higher in patients who received an RBC transfusion.

References

1. Czempik PF, Krzych LJ. Anemia of critical illness: a narrative review. Acta Haematol Pol 2022;53:249-57.
2. Wubet HB, Mengistu LH, Gobezie NZ, et al. The incidence and factors associated with anemia in elective surgical patients admitted to a surgical intensive care unit: a retrospective cohort study. Eur J Med Res 2024;29:290.
3. Cable CA, Razavi SA, Roback JD, Murphy DJ. RBC transfusion strategies in the ICU: a concise review. Crit Care Med 2019;47:1637-44.
4. Napolitano LM, Kurek S, Luchette FA, et al. Clinical practice guideline: red blood cell transfusion in adult trauma and critical care. Crit Care Med 2009;37:3124-57.
5. Jones JG, Holland BM, Hudson IR, Wardrop CA. Total circulating red cells versus haematocrit as the primary descriptor of oxygen transport by the blood. Br J Haematol 1990;76:288-94.
6. Society of Thoracic Surgeons Blood Conservation Guideline Task F, Ferraris VA, Ferraris SP, et al. Perioperative blood transfusion and blood conservation in cardiac surgery: the Society of Thoracic Surgeons and The Society of Cardiovascular Anesthesiologists clinical practice guideline. Ann Thorac Surg 2007;83:S27-86.
7. Weiss G, Ganz T, Goodnough LT. Anemia of inflammation. Blood 2019;133:40-50.
8. Silver MJ, Li YH, Gragg LA, et al. Reduction of blood loss from diagnostic sampling in critically ill patients using a blood-conserving arterial line system. Chest 1993;104:1711-5.

9. Smoller BR, Kruskall MS. Phlebotomy for diagnostic laboratory tests in adults. Pattern of use and effect on transfusion requirements. N Engl J Med 1986;314:1233-5.
10. Wilkerson DK, Rosen AL, Gould SA, et al. Oxygen extraction ratio: a valid indicator of myocardial metabolism in anemia. J Surg Res 1987;42:629-34.
11. Carson JL, Noveck H, Berlin JA, Gould SA. Mortality and morbidity in patients with very low postoperative Hb levels who decline blood transfusion. Transfusion 2002;42:812-8.
12. Weiskopf RB, Viele MK, Feiner J, et al. Human cardiovascular and metabolic response to acute, severe isovolemic anemia. JAMA 1998;279:217-21.
13. Hebert PC, Yetisir E, Martin C, et al. Is a low transfusion threshold safe in critically ill patients with cardiovascular diseases? Crit Care Med 2001;29:227-34.
14. Mahecic TT, Dunser M, Meier J. RBC transfusion triggers: is there anything new? Transfus Med Hemother 2020;47:361-8.
15. Hebert PC, Wells G, Blajchman MA, et al. A multicenter, randomized, controlled clinical trial of transfusion requirements in critical care. Transfusion Requirements in Critical Care Investigators, Canadian Critical Care Trials Group. N Engl J Med 1999;340:409-17.
16. Rawal G, Kumar R, Yadav S, Singh A. Anemia in intensive care: a review of current concepts. J Crit Care Med (Targu Mures) 2016;2:109-14.
17. Karkouti K, Wijeysundera DN, Yau TM, et al. The influence of baseline hemoglobin concentration on tolerance of anemia in cardiac surgery. Transfusion 2008;48:666-72.
18. King KE, Bandarenko N, Campbell-Lee SA, et al. *Blood Transfusion Therapy: A Physician's Handbook.* 9th ed: American Association of Blood Banks; 2008.
19. Boulain T, Garot D, Vignon P, et al. Prevalence of low central venous oxygen saturation in the first hours of intensive care unit admission and associated mortality in septic shock patients: a prospective multicentre study. Crit Care 2014;18:609.
20. Association for the Advancement of Blood & Biotherapies. Whole Blood and Red Blood Cell Components. Accessed March 14, 2025. https://www.aabb.org/regulatory-and-advocacy/regulatory-affairs/regulatory-for-blood/whole-blood-and-red-blood-cell-components#:~:text=Whole%20blood%20transfusion%20may%20be,and%20non%2Dlabile%20clotting%20factors
21. Cap AP, Beckett A, Benov A, et al. Whole blood transfusion. Mil Med 2018;183:44-51.
22. Simon TL. Changes in plasma coagulation factors during blood storage. Plasma Ther Transfus Technol 1988;9:309-15.
23. van der Meer PF, Klei TR, de Korte D. Quality of platelets in stored whole blood. Transfus Med Rev 2020;34:234-41.

24. Dutton RP, Shih D, Edelman BB, et al. Safety of uncrossmatched type-O red cells for resuscitation from hemorrhagic shock. J Trauma 2005;59:1445-9.
25. Kim Y, Xia BT, Chang AL, Pritts TA. Role of leukoreduction of packed red blood cell units in trauma patients: a review. Int J Hematol Res 2016;2:124-9.
26. Keir AK, Wilkinson D, Andersen C, Stark MJ. Washed versus unwashed red blood cells for transfusion for the prevention of morbidity and mortality in preterm infants. Cochrane Database Syst Rev 2016;2016:CD011484.
27. Pulliam KE, Joseph B, Makley AT, et al. Washing packed red blood cells decreases red blood cell storage lesion formation. Surgery 2021;169:666-70.
28. Qureshi H, Massey E, Kirwan D, et al. BCSH guideline for the use of anti-D immunoglobulin for the prevention of haemolytic disease of the fetus and newborn. Transfus Med 2014;24:8-20.
29. Kiraly LN, Underwood S, Differding JA, Schreiber MA. Transfusion of aged packed red blood cells results in decreased tissue oxygenation in critically injured trauma patients. J Trauma 2009;67:29-32.
30. Goodnough LT. Risks of blood transfusion. Crit Care Med 2003;31:S678-86.
31. Kuriyan M, Carson JL. Blood transfusion risks in the intensive care unit. Crit Care Clin 2004;20:237-53, ix.
32. Sayah DM, Looney MR, Toy P. Transfusion reactions: newer concepts on the pathophysiology, incidence, treatment, and prevention of transfusion-related acute lung injury. Crit Care Clin 2012;28:363-72, v.
33. Carson JL, Guyatt G, Heddle NM, et al. Clinical practice guidelines from the AABB: red blood cell transfusion thresholds and storage. JAMA 2016;316:2025-35.
34. Carson JL, Triulzi DJ, Ness PM. Indications for and adverse effects of red-cell transfusion. N Engl J Med 2017;377:1261-72.
35. Greenberger PA. Plasma anaphylaxis and immediate-type reactions. In: Rossi EC, Simon TL, Moss GS, editors. *Principles of Transfusion Medicine*. Philadelphia: Williams & Wilkins; 1991:635-9.
36. Rohde JM, Dimcheff DE, Blumberg N, et al. Health care-associated infection after red blood cell transfusion: a systematic review and meta-analysis. JAMA 2014;311:1317-26.
37. Roubinian NH, Hendrickson JE, Triulzi DJ, et al. Contemporary risk factors and outcomes of transfusion-associated circulatory overload. Crit Care Med 2018;46:577-85.
38. Semple JW, Rebetz J, Kapur R. Transfusion-associated circulatory overload and transfusion-related acute lung injury. Blood 2019;133:1840-53.
39. Cho MS, Modi P, Sharma S. Transfusion-Related Acute Lung Injury. In: StatPearls. Treasure Island (FL): StatPearls Publishing; 2024.

40. Gupta A, Yan M. Transfusion-related acute lung injury (TRALI). Ottawa: Canadian Blood Services; 2021. Accessed March 14, 2025. https://professionaleducation.blood.ca/en/transfusion/publications/transfusion-related-acute-lung-injury-trali
41. Benson AB, Moss M, Silliman CC. Transfusion-related acute lung injury (TRALI): a clinical review with emphasis on the critically ill. Br J Haematol 2009;147:431-43.
42. Roubinian N. TACO and TRALI: biology, risk factors, and prevention strategies. Hematology Am Soc Hematol Educ Program 2018;2018:585-94.
43. Vamvakas EC, Blajchman MA. Transfusion-related immunomodulation (TRIM): an update. Blood Rev 2007;21:327-48.
44. Agarwal N, Murphy JG, Cayten CG, Stahl WM. Blood transfusion increases the risk of infection after trauma. Arch Surg 1993;128:171-6; discussion 6-7.
45. Taylor RW, O'Brien J, Trottier SJ, et al. Red blood cell transfusions and nosocomial infections in critically ill patients. Crit Care Med 2006;34:2302-8; quiz 9.
46. Marik PE, Corwin HL. Efficacy of red blood cell transfusion in the critically ill: a systematic review of the literature. Crit Care Med 2008;36:2667-74.

Platelets and Plasma

Chapter 13

This chapter presents the usual causes of significant thrombocytopenia in the ICU setting, and then describes the indications, methods, and complications of platelet therapy. Plasma components of blood are also discussed.

THROMBOCYTOPENIA

Overview

Thrombocytopenia is the most common hemostatic disorder in critically ill patients, with a reported incidence as high as 60% (1-3). The traditional definition of thrombocytopenia is a platelet count below 150,000/µL, but the risk for coagulation-related complications increases at counts <100,000/µL; so a platelet count <100,000/µL is more appropriate for identifying clinically significant thrombocytopenia (1-2,4). *The platelet count is an imprecise predictor of bleeding*; platelet *function*, vascular integrity, and many other factors contribute to bleeding risk (see Chapter 14: Coagulopathy Management) (5). At platelet counts <20,000/µL, the risk for cerebral microbleeds increases and at counts <10,000/µL, spontaneous intracerebral hemorrhage is possible, though uncommon (5-6).

Pseudothrombocytopenia

In approximately 2% of hospitalized patients with thrombocytopenia, lower than expected platelet counts are found due to clumping of platelets from the anticoagulant (EDTA) in blood collection tubes (8). Clumped platelets are misread as leukocytes, thus resulting in a spuriously low platelet count. If suspected, a peripheral smear can discern this cause by detecting the presence of clumped platelets.

Critically Ill Patients

Systemic sepsis is the most common cause of thrombocytopenia in ICU patients (3-4) and is thought to be caused by dysregulated host immunity, increased complement signaling, and other mechanisms (4). Other less common but more life-threatening causes of thrombocytopenia are listed in Table 13.1.

TABLE 13.1 Causes of Thrombocytopenia in the Critically Ill

Nonpharmacological	Pharmacological
Cardiopulmonary Bypass	Anticonvulsants: • Phenytoin • Valproic Acid
Disseminated Intravascular Coagulation (DIC)	Antimicrobial Agents: • β-Lactams • Linezolid • Trimethoprim/sulfamethoxazole (TMP/SMX) • Vancomycin
Hemolytic Uremic Syndrome	Antineoplastic Agents
Intra-Aortic Balloon Pump (IABP)	Antithrombotic Agents: • Heparin • Enoxaparin • Glycoprotein IIb/IIIa Inhibitors
Liver Disease	Histamine H_2 Receptor Antagonists (famotidine)
Hypersplenism	Miscellaneous Drugs: • Amiodarone • Furosemide • Thiazides • Morphine
Malignancy	
Renal Replacement Therapy	
Sepsis*	
Thrombotic Thrombocytopenic Purpura (TTP)	

*Sepsis is the most common cause of thrombocytopenia in the ICU setting.

From References 2-4, 7-8.

Heparin-Induced Thrombocytopenia (HIT)

Heparin-induced thrombocytopenia (HIT) is an immune-mediated condition that is associated with life-threatening thromboses (both venous and arterial) and has a mortality rate as high as 20% if left undiagnosed (7-8). The incidence of HIT with heparin is highly variable, ranging from 0.7% to 5%, with a lower incidence (0.2%) when low-molecular-weight heparin (e.g., enoxaparin) is used (7,9).

Pathogenesis

When heparin binds to platelet factor 4 (PF4) on platelets, an antigenic complex can form, triggering the formation of IgG antibodies (7). Platelets are then activated, and thrombin is generated, leading to thrombosis.

Risk Factors

The immune response that triggers HIT is not a dose-dependent reaction and can occur with low-dose exposures to heparin (i.e., heparin flushes or heparin-coated catheters) (7,9). The risk for HIT is increased in obese patients, women, and surgical patients, especially patients who undergo orthopedic or cardiac surgery (7,9-10).

Clinical Features

HIT most often occurs between 5 and 10 days following heparin exposure (7,9-10). Severe thrombocytopenia (<20,000/µL) is uncommon in HIT; platelet counts are usually between 50,000/µL and 150,000/µL and do not typically fall by more than 50% after the first exposure to heparin. The major complication of HIT is thrombosis, not bleeding; *in up to 25% of cases, the thrombosis precedes the thrombocytopenia* (11). Venous thrombosis is more common than arterial thrombosis. Reports indicate that 17% to 55% of patients with untreated HIT develop deep vein thrombosis in the legs and/or pulmonary embolism, whereas only 1% to 3% of patients develop arterial thromboses resulting in limb ischemia, thrombotic stroke, or acute myocardial infarction (11).

Diagnosis

Risk Assessment. The 4Ts score is a risk assessment tool that can be used to assess the probability of HIT (Table 13.2) (12).

TABLE 13.2 The 4Ts Score for Estimating the Risk of HIT

Conditions	Points
Thrombocytopenia:	
• PLT fall >50% AND nadir ≥20k/μL AND no surgery past 3 days	2
• PLT fall 30-50% OR nadir = 10-19k/μL	1
• PLT fall <30% OR nadir <0k/μL	0
Timing of onset after heparin exposure:	
• Onset at 5-10 days OR ≤1 day if exposure in past 5-30 days	2
• Possible onset at 5-10 days OR >10 days OR, ≤1 day if exposure 31-100 days ago	1
• Onset <4 days without exposure in past 100 days	0
Thrombosis or other adverse reactions:	
• New thrombosis OR skin necrosis OR anaphylactoid reaction	2
• Suspected, progressive, or recurrent thrombosis	1
• None of the above	0
Other causes for thrombocytopenia:	
• None apparent	2
• Possible	1
• Definite	0

Scoring: ≤3 points = Low risk of HIT (<1%)
4-5 points = Intermediate risk (≈10%)
6-8 points = High risk (≈50%)

From Platelets and Plasma. In: Marino PL. *Marino's The ICU Book.* 5th ed. Wolters Kluwer; 2025:204-20. Table 13.2.

Laboratory Testing

Two assays are used to diagnose HIT. The most popular of these is an enzyme-linked immunosorbent assay (ELISA) for antibodies to the platelet PF4 heparin complex. This assay has a high sensitivity, but a limited specificity. A negative assay helps to exclude the diagnosis of HIT, but a positive assay does not confirm the diagnosis because HIT antibodies do not always promote thrombocytopenia or thrombosis (7,11). The serotonin release assay (SRA) is considered the "gold standard" for the diagnosis of HIT (sensitivity and specificity >95%); however, this assay is more costly, not available in many hospitals, and needs to performed by experienced laboratories (7,11,13).

Management

Heparin must be discontinued immediately in suspected cases of HIT, which includes heparin flushes and heparin-coated catheters (11). Therapeutic anticoagulation with an alternative anticoagulant listed in Table 13.3 should be started immediately, *even in cases where HIT is not accompanied by thrombosis* (7-9).

Full anticoagulation with an alternative anticoagulant is recommended until the platelet count rises above 150,000/µL (14). Thereafter, coumadin or a direct-acting oral anticoagulant (DOAC) should be started. DOACs are usually continued for 1-3 months after an episode of HIT (14). If coumadin is used, it *should not be started until the platelet count increases beyond 150,000/µL, and the initial coumadin dose should not exceed 5 mg* (14). These precautions are intended to reduce the risk of limb gangrene associated with coumadin therapy during the active phase of HIT.

Thrombotic Microangiopathies

Thrombotic microangiopathies are potentially life-threatening syndromes that are characterized by four cardinal features:

1. A consumptive thrombocytopenia
2. Microvascular thrombosis
3. Dysfunction of one or more organs
4. A nonimmunogenic microangiopathic hemolytic anemia,

TABLE 13.3 Alternative Parenteral Anticoagulants for Use in HIT

Agent	Mechanism	Dose	Comment
Argatroban	Direct thrombin inhibitor	Start infusion at 1-2 µg/kg/min and titrate dose to achieve an activated PTT of 1.5-3x normal	• For hepatic insufficiency, start at 0.5 µg/kg/min • No dose adjustment is needed for renal dysfunction • No reversal agent is available (half-life of 40-50 min)
Bivalirudin	Direct thrombin inhibitor	Start infusion at 0.15 mg/kg/h and titrate to achieve an activated PTT of 1.5-3x normal	• For patients with renal dysfunction, no dose adjustment is required when bolused, but the maintenance dose should be reduced according to creatinine clearance • An infusion of 0.25 mg/kg/h is recommended for patients undergoing dialysis • The dosage may need to be reduced in severe hepatic failure • No reversal agent is available (half-life is 25 min; prolonged in renal failure)
Fondaparinux	Antithrombin-mediated inhibition of Factor Xa	Weight-based dosing: • <50 kg: 5 mg once daily • 50-100 kg: 7.5 mg once daily • >100 kg: 10 mg once daily • (all doses are given subcutaneously)	• No routine coagulation monitoring is necessary but anti-factor Xa activity can be monitored • May possibly be reversed with Andexanet alfa • Has a longer half-life than argatroban or bivalirudin (17-21 h); the half-life is prolonged in renal failure

characterized by the presence of fragmented red blood cells (schistocytes) on a peripheral blood smear

There are four pathological entities that comprise the majority of thrombotic microangiopathies: disseminated intravascular coagulation (DIC), thrombotic thrombocytopenic purpura (TTP), the hemolytic uremic syndrome (HUS) and hemolysis, elevated liver function tests, and low platelets (HELLP). The laboratory findings found with DIC, TTP, and HUS are summarized in Table 13.4.

TABLE 13.4 Laboratory Profiles in the Thrombotic Microangiopathies

Feature	DIC	TTP	HUS
Schistocytes	Present	Present	Present
Platelets	Low	Low	Low
INR	Elevated	Normal	Normal
aPTT	Prolonged	Normal	Normal
Fibrinogen	Low	Normal	Normal
Plasma D-dimer	Elevated	Normal	Normal

DIC = disseminated intravascular coagulation; TTP = thrombotic thrombocytopenia purpura; HUS = hemolytic uremic syndrome; aPTT= activated partial thromboplastin time.

From Wheeler AP, Rice TW. Coagulopathy in critically ill patients: part 2-soluble clotting factors and hemostatic testing. Chest 2010;137:185-94.

Disseminated Intravascular Coagulation (DIC)

DIC is a secondary disorder that is triggered by conditions that produce widespread tissue injury such as multisystem trauma, severe sepsis and septic shock, and obstetric emergencies (i.e., amniotic fluid embolism, abruptio placentae, eclampsia, retained fetus syndrome).

Pathogenesis. The inciting event is release of *tissue factor* from the endothelium, which activates a series of clotting factors in the bloodstream, culminating with the formation of fibrin. This leads to widespread microvascular thrombosis and secondary depletion of platelets and clotting factors, resulting in a *consumptive coagulopathy* (15-16).

Clinical Features. Microvascular thrombosis in DIC can lead to multiorgan failure, most often involving the lungs, kidneys, and central nervous system, while depletion of platelets and coagulation factors can promote bleeding, particularly from pre-existing lesions in the GI tract such as stress ulcers. DIC can also be accompanied by symmetrical necrosis and ecchymosis involving the limbs; a condition known as *purpura fulminans* that is usually seen with overwhelming systemic sepsis, most notably with meningococcemia (17).

Diagnosis. The hematological features of DIC are summarized in Table 13.4.

What distinguishes DIC from other thrombotic microangiopathies is the depletion of clotting factors, which prolongs the INR and the aPTT. Fibrinolysis also occurs during DIC, as evidenced by the elevation of fibrin degradation products (i.e., D-dimers) in the plasma. A scoring system to diagnose overt DIC (Table 13.5) has been devised and validated by the International Society of Thrombosis and Haemostasis (18).

Management. There is no specific treatment for DIC other than treating the underlying cause (17,19). Life-threatening hemorrhage often prompts platelet and plasma transfusions, but these interventions do not stop the bleeding and may only exacerbate microvascular thrombosis. DIC is a condition with a poor prognosis. Mortality rates are 40-80%, depending on the underlying cause and degree of organ failure (20).

Thrombotic Thrombocytopenic Purpura

Thrombotic thrombocytopenic purpura (TTP) is a rare, but potentially deadly thrombotic microangiopathy.

> **TABLE 13.5** International Society of Thrombosis and Haemostasis (ISTH) Scoring Criteria for DIC
>
> 1. In a patient with an underlying disorder that may be associated with overt DIC, the following laboratory tests should be sent:
>   a. Platelet count
>   b. Prothrombin time (PT)
>   c. Fibrinogen
>   d. Fibrin-related marker (i.e., D-dimer)
> 2. Score the test results
>   a. Platelet count (>100:0, <100:1, <50:2)
>   b. Elevated levels of a fibrin-related marker (e.g., D-dimer) (no increase = 0; moderate increase = 2; strong increase = 3)
>   c. Prolonged PT (<3 s: 0, >3 but <6 s: 1, >6 s: 2)
>   d. Fibrinogen level (>1 g/L: 0, <1g/L: 1)
> 3. Calculate the score:
>   a. >5 compatible with overt DIC; repeat scoring daily

From Toh CH, Alhamdi Y, Abrams ST. Current pathological and laboratory considerations in the diagnosis of disseminated intravascular coagulation. Ann Lab Med 2016;36(6):505-12.

Pathogenesis. TTP is caused by a severe deficiency of a specific von Willebrand factor-cleaving protease (ADAMTS13) (21). TTP is most often immune-mediated in adults and may follow a nonspecific viral illness. Women are two to three times more likely to develop TTP (21).

Clinical Features. TTP was historically described by a characteristic *pentad* of clinical manifestations that included fever, altered mental status, acute renal failure, thrombocytopenia, and microangiopathic hemolytic anemia. However, all five elements are *not* necessary to prompt consideration of the diagnosis of TTP. In patients with thrombocytopenia and evidence of a microangiopathic hemolytic anemia (e.g., schistocytes in the peripheral blood smear), TTP should be considered as a priority diagnosis (21). TTP can be distinguished from DIC because clotting factors are not depleted in TTP, so *the INR, aPTT, and fibrinogen levels are normal in TTP.*

Moreover, when compared to HUS, the degree of renal insufficiency is typically mild in TTP (22).

Diagnosis and Management. TTP is definitively diagnosed by detecting ADAMTS13 activity <10%, but in any patient with suspected TTP, treatment must be commenced without delay. *The front-line therapy for TTP is plasma exchange*, where blood from the patient is diverted to a device that separates and discards the patient's plasma and reinfuses plasma from a healthy donor (21-22). Plasma exchange is continued until 1.5 times the normal plasma volume is exchanged, and this process is repeated daily for 3-7 days. There is no optimal duration of therapy, and plasma exchange is often continued until a positive clinical response is achieved (21). If plasma exchange is started early (within 48 h of symptom onset), as many as 90% of patients can survive the illness (22). Steroids and immunosuppressive agents (i.e., rituximab, caplacizumab) are also used in conjunction with plasma exchange, given the autoimmune nature of most cases of TTP (21).

Hemolytic Uremic Syndrome

HUS is defined by the simultaneous combination of a microangiopathic hemolytic anemia, thrombocytopenia, and acute kidney injury (23). HUS can be caused by a variety of disorders, but infections with Shiga toxin-producing *Escherichia coli*, *Streptococcus pneumoniae*, influenza, or the human immunodeficiency virus account for most cases (23). Patterns of disease consistent with HUS can also occur in autoimmune disorders (e.g., lupus), pregnancy, malignancy, or following exposure to drugs (i.e., chemotherapy agents, clopidogrel, antibiotics, immunosuppressives, or illicit drugs) (23).

Clinical Features. HUS is defined clinically by the triad of thrombocytopenia, microangiopathic hemolytic anemia, and acute kidney injury. Acute kidney injury may range from hematuria and proteinuria to severe failure in nearly 50% of cases. Renal failure is often more severe in HUS compared to TTP. Unlike TTP, clotting factors are not consumed, so coagulation tests are normal, and fibrinolysis is not enhanced.

Management. Management of HUS is supportive. Red blood cell transfusions are only required when hemoglobin levels drop below 7 g/dL and platelet transfusions are only indicated for severe bleeding. Dialysis may be required in severe cases. For atypical (noninfectious) causes of HUS, eculizumab, an IgG antibody, may be used to bind the C5 complement protein, thereby blocking the prothrombotic effects of complement activation (24). Plasma exchange may also be considered for atypical cases.

HELLP Syndrome

HELLP syndrome is a thrombotic microangiopathy that occurs late in pregnancy or in the early postpartum period (25). About 20% of cases are associated with severe preeclampsia, and there is also an association between HELLP and the antiphospholipid syndrome.

Pathogenesis. HELLP is part of the pathophysiological spectrum of preeclampsia (25). Abnormal placentation is thought to be the predominant pathogenic factor, followed by a hepatic inflammatory response and intense activation of clotting factors and platelets.

Clinical Features. HELLP is defined by a characteristic triad of hemolysis, thrombocytopenia, and elevated liver enzymes. The most common symptom is abdominal pain. HELLP can be confused with DIC (which can occur in similar clinical settings), but the INR and aPTT are usually normal in HELLP because there is no depletion of clotting factors, and this feature should distinguish HELLP from DIC.

Management. The HELLP syndrome is described here as an example of a thrombotic microangiopathy, but this condition is an obstetric emergency, and an informed description of the management of HELLP is beyond the scope of this text. In cases where multiorgan dysfunction is present requiring critical care support, prompt delivery of the fetus is mandatory, regardless of gestational age (25). Following delivery, treatment is supportive, and steroids or other pharmacological adjuncts are not recommended (25-30).

PLATELET TRANSFUSIONS

Indications

Recommendations for platelet transfusions are listed in Table 13.6. Platelet transfusions are not recommended in thrombotic microangiopathies because platelet transfusions can exacerbate the microvascular thrombosis. These recommendations have not been rigorously validated and most of the data is derived from retrospective studies.

Platelet Products

Pooled Platelets

Platelets are separated from fresh whole blood by differential centrifugation, and the resulting platelet concentrates from 5 or 6 individual donors are pooled together prior to storage (i.e., a "six pack" of platelets). The pooled platelet concentrate contains about 38×10^{10} platelets in 260 mL plasma, which is equivalent to a platelet count of about $130 \times 10^9/\mu L$. This is six orders of magnitude higher than the normal platelet count in blood ($150\text{-}400 \times 10^3/\mu L$).

Apheresis Platelets

Apheresis platelets are collected from a single donor and have a platelet count and volume that is equivalent to the pooled platelet concentrates from 5-6 donors. The presumed benefit of single-donor platelet transfusions is a lower risk of transmitted infections and a lower incidence of platelet *alloimmunization* (i.e., developing antibodies to donor platelets, which reduces the effect of platelet transfusions).

TABLE 13.6 Indications for Platelet Transfusions

Procedure / Indication	Platelet Count Threshold
Critically ill patients	≤10,000/ μL
Central line insertion	≤20,000/ μL
Bronchoscopy with bronchoalveolar lavage	≤20,000/ μL
Elective non-neuraxial surgery	≤50,000/ μL
Lumbar puncture	≤50,000/ μL (lower thresholds may be considered for patients with malignancy or in patients with immune thrombocytopenia)
Endoscopic procedures	≤50,000/ μL (≤20,000 μL for low-risk procedures)
Neuraxial analgesia (i.e., epidural catheter placement)	≤80,000/ μL
Neurosurgery or eye surgery	≤100,000/ μL

From References 26-30.

Nonetheless, neither of these proposed benefits has been documented in clinical trials (31-32).

Leukoreduction

Leukocytes in donor blood have been implicated in several adverse reactions to blood transfusions, and leukocyte removal using specialized filters is now a routine practice (see Chapter 9: The Pulmonary Artery Catheter). Leukocyte reduction for platelet transfusions reduces the incidence of febrile reactions, as well as cytomegalovirus (CMV) transmission and platelet alloimmunization (33).

Response to Transfused Platelets

In an average sized adult with no ongoing blood loss, *the infusion of one unit of platelets (either multiple-donor or aphseresed platelets) should incrementally increase the circulating platelet count by approximately 30,000/μL (34-35).* The increment in platelet count declines with multiple transfusions—a phenomenon known as "platelet refractoriness." Platelet refractoriness is thought to be the result of antiplatelet antibodies in the recipient directed at ABO antigens on donor platelets. This effect can be mitigated by transfusing ABO-matched platelets.

Adverse Effects

The rates of adverse reactions to platelet transfusions are listed in Table 13.7. Although overall reaction rates are low, rates are slightly higher in single-donor preparations.

TABLE 13.7 Adverse Reactions to Different Platelet Preparations (Rate per 100,000 Units Transfused)

Adverse Reaction	Multiple-Donor Preparations	Single-Donor Preparations	p value
Nonhemolytic Fever	37	136	<0.01
Allergic Reaction	27	325	<0.01
Acute Lung Injury	1	22	<0.05
Circulatory Overload	7	8	NS
Acute Hemolysis	0.2	1.8	<0.01
Bacterial Transmission	0.8	1.4	NS
Viral Transmission	0	0	NS
Total Reactions	70	478	<0.01

NS = not significant.

From Mowla SJ, Kracalik IT, Sapiano MRP, et al. A comparison of transfusion-related adverse reactions among apheresis platelets, whole blood-derived platelets, and platelets subjected to pathogen reduction technology as reported to the National Healthcare Safety Network Hemovigilance Module. Transfus Med Rev 2021;35(2):78-84.

Nonhemolytic Fever. Fevers associated with platelet transfusions are caused by a reaction between anti-leukocyte antibodies in recipient blood and antigens on leukocytes in donor blood. This reaction triggers the release of endogenous pyrogens from phagocytes. The use of leukoreduction has significantly reduced, but not eliminated this reaction.

Bacterial and Viral Transmission. Bacteria are much more likely to flourish in platelet concentrates than in RBC concentrates (packed cells) because platelets are stored at room temperature (22° C) while RBCs are refrigerated at about 4° C. However, the rate of transmission, as shown in Table 13.7, is low. The use of nucleic acid testing has virtually eliminated the risk of transmission of HIV and hepatitis viruses.

Allergic Reactions. Hypersensitivity reactions (urticaria, anaphylaxis, anaphylactic shock) are the result of sensitization to plasma proteins in donor blood. The risk is higher with single-donor platelets because these preparations have a higher plasma volume.

Acute Lung Injury. Transfusion-related acute lung injury (TRALI) is described in Chapter 25: Acute Respiratory Distress Syndrome. This condition is the result of anti-leukocyte antibodies in donor plasma that bind to antigens on circulating neutrophils in the recipient. While more common with erythrocyte transfusions, TRALI may also occur with platelet transfusions.

PLASMA PRODUCTS

Fresh Frozen Plasma

Preparation

Plasma is separated from donor blood and frozen at –18° C within 8 h of blood collection. This *fresh frozen plasma* (FFP) has a volume of about 230 mL and can be stored for one year. Once thawed, FFP can be stored at 1 to 6° C for up to 5 days. Each unit must be ABO compatible, but the Rh factor need not be considered (see Chapter 12: Anemia and Erythrocyte Transfusions).

Indications

Massive Blood Loss. For patients requiring massive transfusion, units of blood products are transfused in a 1:1:1 ratio (RBCs:FFP:platelets) (36). FFP requires time to thaw, and once thawed, FFP products have a limited shelf-life which may lead to wasting of the product. Newer preparations of FFP include liquid plasma (which can be stored at 1-6° C [34-43° F]) and stored for up to 5 days), freeze dried plasma, and lyophilized plasma. As these preparations undergo further study, they may be more readily available and may help reduce the waste associated with FFP (37-38).

Prophylactic FFP. FFP is frequently used to reduce an elevated INR in coagulopathic, *nonbleeding* ICU patients; however, there is no evidence that *prophylactic* FFP prevents bleeding or provides any other clinical benefit (39).

Reversal of Warfarin Anticoagulation. Warfarin is associated with an increased risk for bleeding in ICU patients, especially in patients with INR values >5 (40). Since warfarin acts by inhibiting vitamin K-dependent clotting factors (i.e., factors II, VII, IX, X), vitamin K must be administered concomitantly to block ongoing anticoagulant activity. Vitamin K is given as 10 mg IV over 10 mi, diluted in 50 mL of IV fluid. Clotting factors are then replenished, and this has traditionally involved the infusion of FFP at a volume of 10-15 mL/kg (41). There are two shortcomings with the use of FFP in this setting: the time to normalize the INR can be prolonged, and the volume of fluid required can aggravate the bleeding. Prothrombin concentrates are an alternative to PCCs for warfarin reversal and are discussed in the next chapter (Chapter 14: Coagulopathy Management).

Adverse Effects

The adverse effects associated with FFP are listed in Table 13.8.

TABLE 13.8	Risks Associated with Fresh Frozen Plasma
Adverse Event	Odds per Transfusion
Urticaria	1-3 in 100
Anaphylaxis	1 in 20,000
Transfusion Associated Lung Injury (TRALI)	1 in 12,000 *
Transfusion Associated Circulatory Overload (TACO)	1 in 70 **
HIV infection	1 in 1.6 million
HBV infection	1 in 280,000
HCV infection	1 in 1.2 million

*TRALI rates are highly variable; some studies have reported far lower risk (1 in 250,000) with contemporary blood bank mitigation efforts (i.e., excluding use from multiparous women donors who have more leukocyte antibodies).

**With active surveillance. Lower odds (1 in 1,500) have been observed with other surveillance methods.

From Pandey S, Vyas GN. Adverse effects of plasma transfusion. Transfusion 2012;52 Suppl 1(Suppl 1):65S-79S.

Urticaria is the most common side effect associated with FFP. The risk of infectious disease transmission has been dramatically reduced with advances in donor testing and pathogen reduction techniques (41). Leukocyte-associated complications (i.e., graft versus host disease, WBC alloimmunization, etc.) and RBC alloimmunization are not typically associated with FFP transfusions since FFP is considered non-cellular (41).

Cryoprecipitate

Preparation

When FFP is allowed to thaw at 4° C, a milky residue forms that is rich in cold-insoluble proteins (cryoglobulins) to include fibrinogen, von Willebrand factor, and factor VIII. This *cryoprecipitate* can be separated from plasma and stored at

−18° C for up to one year. One unit of cryoprecipitate per 10 kg body weight will increase the plasma fibrinogen level by about 50 mg/dL (42). The goal is a serum fibrinogen level above 100 mg/dL.

Indications

Cryoprecipitate is used frequently in massive blood loss from trauma or postpartum hemorrhage because both clinical scenarios are associated with fibrinogen depletion. The use of cryoprecipitate in the ICU may also be considered for uremic bleeding and selected cases of hypofibrinogenemia. Cryoprecipitate can also be used as a source of fibrinogen in bleeding episodes associated with fibrinogen deficiency, such as variceal bleeding from liver failure.

References

1. Jonsson AB, Rygard SL, Hildebrandt T, et al. Thrombocytopenia in intensive care unit patients: A scoping review. Acta Anaesthesiol Scand 2021;65:2-14.
2. Parker RI. Etiology and significance of thrombocytopenia in critically ill patients. Crit Care Clin 2012;28:399-411.
3. Rice TR, Wheeler RP. Coagulopathy in critically ill patients. Part 1: Platelet disorders. Chest 2009;136:1622-30.
4. Leone M, Nielsen ND, Russel L. Ten tips on sepsis-induced thrombocytopenia. Intensive Care Med 2024;50:1157-60.
5. Uhl L, Assmann SF, Hamza TH, et al. Laboratory predictors of bleeding and the effect of platelet and RBC transfusions on bleeding outcomes in the PLADO trial. Blood 2017;130(10):1247-58.
6. Malhotra P, Prasad H, Jain A, et al. Variables affecting the presence of occult cerebral microbleeds and subsequent spontaneous intracranial haemorrhage in adult patients with severe thrombocytopenia. Br J Haematol 2021;194(3):e67-e70.
7. Greinacher A. Clinical practice. Heparin-induced thrombocytopenia. N Engl J Med 2015;373(3):252-61.
8. Greinacher A, Selleng S. How I evaluate and treat thrombocytopenia in the intensive care unit patient. Blood 2016;128(26):3032-42.
9. Arepally GM, Padmanabhan A. Heparin-induced thrombocytopenia: A focus on thrombosis. Arterioscler Thromb Vasc Biol 2021; 41(1):141-52.

10. Warkentin TE, Sheppard JA, Sigouin CS, et al. Gender imbalance and risk factor interactions in heparin-induced thrombocytopenia. Blood 2006;108(9):2937-41.
11. Laster J, Silver D. Heparin-coated catheters and heparin-induced thrombocytopenia. J Vasc Surg 1988;7:667-72.
12. Lo GK, Juhl D, Warkentin TE, Sigouin CS, et al. Evaluation of pre-test clinical score (4 T's) for the diagnosis of heparin-induced thrombocytopenia in two clinical settings. J Thromb Haemost 2006;4(4): 759-65.
13. Warkentin TE. Platelet count monitoring and laboratory testing for heparin-induced thrombocytopenia. Arch Pathol Lab Med 2002; 126(11):1415-23.
14. Linkins LA, Dans AL, Moores LK, et al. Treatment and prevention of heparin-induced thrombocytopenia: antithrombotic therapy and prevention of thrombosis, 9th ed: American College of Chest Physicians evidence-based clinical practice guidelines. Chest 2012; 141(Suppl):495S-530S.
15. Senno SL, Pechet L, Bick RL. Disseminated intravascular coagulation (DIC). Pathophysiology, laboratory diagnosis, and management. J Intensive Care Med 2000;15:144-58.
16. DeLoughery TG. Critical care clotting catastrophes. Crit Care Clin 2005;21:531-62.
17. Kalpatthi R, Kiss JE. Thrombotic thrombocytopenic purpura, heparin induced thrombocytopenia, and disseminated intravascular coagulation. Crit Care Clin 2020;36(2):357-77.
18. Toh CH, Alhamdi Y, Abrams ST. Current pathological and laboratory considerations in the diagnosis of disseminated intravascular coagulation. Ann Lab Med 2016;36(6):505-12.
19. Levy M. Disseminated intravascular coagulation. Crit Care Med 2007;35:2191-5.
20. Adelborg K, Larsen JB, Hvas AM. Disseminated intravascular coagulation: epidemiology, biomarkers, and management. Br J Haematol 2021;192(5):803-18.
21. Sukumar S, Lämmle B, Cataland SR. Thrombotic thrombocytopenic purpura: pathophysiology, diagnosis, and management. J Clin Med 2021;10(3):536.
22. Rock GA, Shumack KH, Buskard NA, et al. Comparison of plasma exchange with plasma infusion in the treatment of thrombotic thrombocytopenia purpura. N Engl J Med 1991;325:393-7.
23. Sheerin NS, Glover E. Haemolytic uremic syndrome: diagnosis and management. F1000Res 2019;8:F1000 Faculty Rev-1690.
24. Legendre CM, Licht C, Muus P, et al. Terminal complement inhibitor eculizumab in atypical hemolytic-uremic syndrome. N Engl J Med 2013;368(23):2169-81.

25. Giannubilo SR, Marzioni D, Tossetta G, Ciavattini A. HELLP syndrome and differential diagnosis with other thrombotic microangiopathies in pregnancy. Diagnostics (Basel) 2024;14(4):352.
26. van Veen JJ, Nokes TJ, Makris M. The risk of spinal haematoma following neuraxial anaesthesia or lumbar puncture in thrombocytopenic individuals. Br J Haematol 2010;148(1):15-25.
27. Nandagopal L, Veeraputhiran M, Jain T, et al. Bronchoscopy can be done safely in patients with thrombocytopenia. Transfusion 2016; 56(2):344-8.
28. Zeidler K, Arn K, Senn O, et al. Optimal preprocedural platelet transfusion threshold for central venous catheter insertions in patients with thrombocytopenia. Transfusion 2011;51(11):2269-76.
29. Vavricka SR, Walter RB, Irani S, et al. Safety of lumbar puncture for adults with acute leukemia and restrictive prophylactic platelet transfusion. Ann Hematol 2003;82(9):570-3.
30. Soff G, Leader A, Al-Samkari H, et al. Management of chemotherapy-induced thrombocytopenia: guidance from the ISTH Subcommittee on Hemostasis and Malignancy. J Thromb Haemost 2024;22(1):53-60.
31. Slichter SJ. Platelet transfusion therapy. Hematol Oncol Clin N Am 2007;21:697-729.
32. Mowla SJ, Kracalik IT, Sapiano MRP, et al. A comparison of transfusion-related adverse reactions among apheresis platelets, whole blood-derived platelets, and platelets subjected to pathogen reduction technology as reported to the National Healthcare Safety Network Hemovigilance Module. Transfus Med Rev 2021;35(2): 78-84.
33. Slichter SJ. Evidence-based platelet transfusion guidelines. Hematol 2007;2007:172-8.
34. Simon TL, McCullough J, Snyder EL, et al. *Rossi's Principles of Transfusion Medicine*, 5th ed., Wiley-Blackwell: United States; 2016.
35. Lieberman L, Bercovitz RS, Sholapur NS, et al. Platelet transfusions for critically ill patients with thrombocytopenia. Blood 2014;123:1146-51.
36. Holcomb JB, Tilley BC, Baraniuk S, et al.; PROPPR Study Group. Transfusion of plasma, platelets, and red blood cells in a 1:1:1 vs a 1:1:2 ratio and mortality in patients with severe trauma: the PROPPR randomized clinical trial. JAMA 2015;313(5):471-82.
37. Sheffield WP, Singh K, Beckett A, Devine DV. Prehospital freeze-dried plasma in trauma: a critical review. Transfus Med Rev 2024;38(1):150807.
38. Mok G, Hoang R, Khan MW, et al. Freeze-dried plasma for major trauma - Systematic review and meta-analysis. J Trauma Acute Care Surg 2021;90(3):589-602.

39. Müller MC, Straat M, Meijers JC, et al. Fresh frozen plasma transfusion fails to influence the hemostatic balance in critically ill patients with a coagulopathy. J Thromb Haemost 2015;13(6):989-97.
40. European Atrial Fibrillation Trial Study Group. Optimal oral anticoagulant therapy in patients with nonrheumatic atrial fibrillation and recent cerebral ischemia. N Engl J Med 1995;333(1):5-10.
41. Pandey S, Vyas GN. Adverse effects of plasma transfusion. Transfusion 2012;52 Suppl 1(Suppl 1):65S-79S.
42. Nair PM, Rendo MJ, Reddoch-Cardenas KM, et al. Recent advances in use of fresh frozen plasma, cryoprecipitate, immunoglobulins, and clotting factors for transfusion support in patients with hematologic disease. Semin Hematol 2020;57(2):73-82.

Coagulopathy Management — Chapter 14

This chapter presents an overview of viscoelastic monitoring, which is being increasingly used to detect and treat coagulopathy in critically ill patients. Hemostatic adjuncts for reversal of anticoagulation and treatment of coagulopathy are discussed next, including prothrombin concentrates, antifibrinolytics, and other commonly used agents.

VISCOELASTIC MONITORING

Thromboelastography (TEG) and rotational thromboelastometry (ROTEM) are viscoelastic tests (VET) that provide near real-time information regarding the three stages of blood clot formation: *initiation*, *amplification*, and *propagation* (1). Figure 14.1 depicts a representative TEG or ROTEM tracing superimposed on the *modern* coagulation cascade (1).

Thromboelastography (TEG)

A TEG requires a small sample of blood which is placed in a cylindrical cup that has a central pin suspended in the sample. The cup is then rotated in an alternating clockwise and counterclockwise direction, and torque is produced as the blood coagulates. A kaolin-cephalin agent is added to the sample to initiate the coagulation cascade; in "rapid" TEG (r-TEG), kaolin is replaced by tissue factor, facilitating faster activation of the coagulation cascade, with results available within 15 min (1-3). A representative TEG is shown in Figure 14.2.

Findings are displayed both numerically and graphically as a *thromboelastograph* (1-3). Additional TEG assays, including platelet mapping, provide information about specific aspects of the coagulation cascade. Platelet mapping uses the addition of arachidonic acid and adenosine diphosphate to assess platelet aggregation (i.e., function) (4).

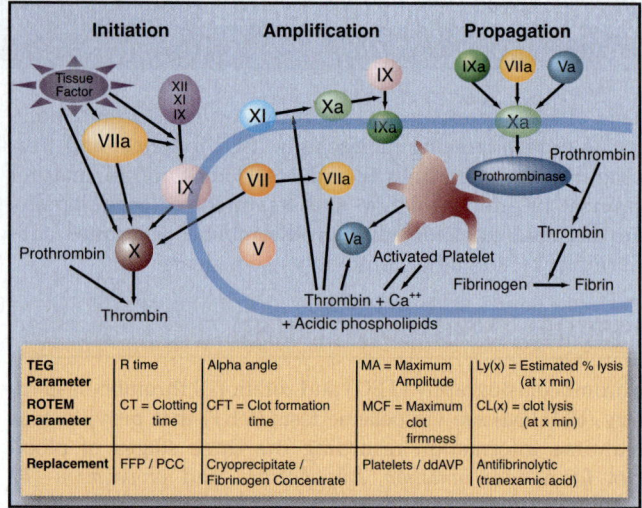

FIGURE 14.1. Correlation of thromboelastogram (TEG) and rotational thromboelastometry (ROTEM) findings with the cell-based "modern" coagulation cascade. A representative TEG or ROTEM tracing is superimposed upon the coagulation cascade. FFP = fresh frozen plasma; PCC = prothrombin concentrates; ddAVP = desmopressin.

Rotational Thromboelastometry (ROTEM)

ROTEM is a VET like TEG but uses a stationary cup and a rotating pin (4). Several independent assays can be performed to provide a comprehensive assessment of a patient's coagulation status.

INTEM Assay

The INTEM assay uses kaolin or ellagic acid to activate the intrinsic pathway, providing information similar to the activated partial thromboplastin time (aPTT) (5).

EXTEM Assay

The EXTEM assay uses tissue factor as a reagent, activating the extrinsic pathway of the coagulation cascade, providing information similar to the prothrombin time (PT) (5).

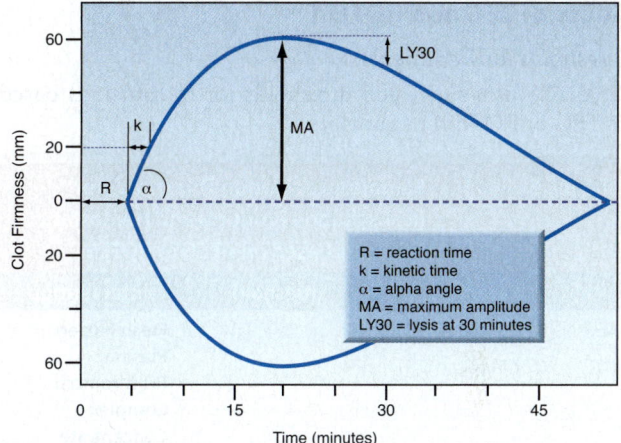

FIGURE 14.2. A thromboelastography tracing with identified components. (From Hemorrhagic Shock. In: Marino PL. *Marino's The ICU Book*. 5th ed. Wolters Kluwer; 2025:242-56. Figure 15.5.)

FIBTEM Assay

The FIBTEM assay uses cytochalasin as an additive reagent, which inhibits platelet-mediated clot retraction. This test correlates highly with fibrinogen activity and provides results more rapidly (<5 min) than the conventional Clauss fibrinogen assay (30-60 min) (4-5).

APTEM Assay

The APTEM assay uses aprotinin, a plasmin inhibitor, as a reagent to assess whether clot amplitude is affected by fibrinolysis (5).

HEPTEM Assay

The HEPTEM assay is used in heparinized patients because the INTEM assay is affected by heparin. Heparin is inhibited by heparinase with the HEPTEM assay (TEG also has a heparinase assay to neutralize the effect of heparin).

Utility of TEG and ROTEM

Thresholds for Treatments

Table 14.1 lists suggested thresholds for transfusions based on TEG or ROTEM parameters.

TABLE 14.1 Sample Intervention Thresholds for Resuscitation Products and Hemostatic Adjuncts Based on r-TEG or ROTEM

	Parameter	Threshold	Intervention
r-TEG	Reaction Time (R)	>1.1 cm	**Fresh Frozen Plasma/ Prothrombin Complex Concentrate**
ROTEM	Clotting Time (CT)	>74 s	
r-TEG	Alpha Angle (α)	<56°	**Cryoprecipitate/ Fibrinogen Concentrate**
ROTEM	Clot Formation Time (CFT)	EXTEM CT >80 s	
	FIBTEM CA10 (clot amplitude at 10 min)	FIBTEM CA10 <7 mm	
r-TEG	Maximum Amplitude (MA)	<55 mm	**Platelets/ddAVP***
ROTEM	Maximum Clot Firmness (MCF)	MCF >71 mm	
	EXTEM CA10 (clot amplitude at 10 min)	EXTEM CA10 <40 mm	
r-TEG	LY30 (% fibrinolysis at 30 min)	>3%	**Antifibrinolytics (Tranexamic Acid/ Aminocaproic Acid)**
ROTEM	EXTEM ML (% maximum lysis)	>15%	
	EXTEM/APTEM CT (clotting time)	EXTEM CT > APTEM CT	

r-TEG = rapid thromboelastography; ROTEM = rotational thromboelastometry.

*Desmopressin (ddAVP) may be considered at lower MA (48-54 mm) or MCF thresholds.

From References 6 and 8.

Figure 14.3 illustrates visual patterns associated with coagulation disorders.

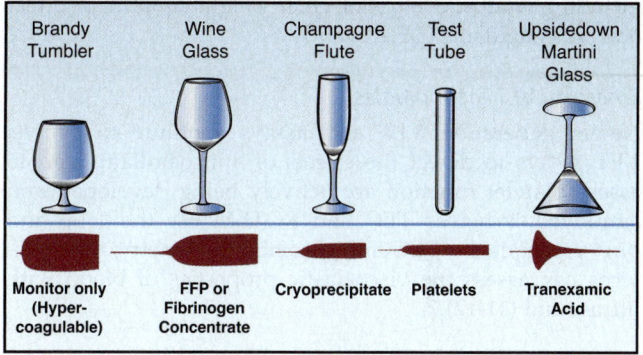

FIGURE 14.3. Visual patterns encountered in thromboelastogram (TEG) and rotational thromboelastometry (ROTEM).

Evidence Base

VET have been studied in several patient populations. In general, in surgical and orthopedic populations (including liver transplant surgery), the use of VET has been associated with reductions in red blood cell (RBC), fresh frozen plasma (FFP), and possibly platelet transfusions compared with the use of conventional coagulation tests (3). In trauma patients, results are conflicting. While one 2015 Cochrane systematic review concluded that VET should only be used for research in trauma, other reviews have demonstrated that TEG and ROTEM can predict massive transfusion better than clinical judgment, guide resuscitation for the reversal of pathophysiological coagulation derangements, and potentially replace conventional coagulation tests (6-9). In cardiac surgery, VET did not improve clinical outcomes but was associated with statistically significantly fewer RBC and platelet transfusions (10).

Limitations

Neither TEG or ROTEM is sensitive to the effect of platelet inhibitors such as aspirin or clopidogrel, unless additional platelet assays are used. TEG and ROTEM do not detect the effect of von Willebrand factor, and a normal TEG or ROTEM does not reliably exclude the presence of oral anticoagulants, including warfarin, low molecular weight heparin, or direct oral anticoagulants (DOAC).

Emerging VET Technologies

Newer generation VET and assays continue to evolve. VET assays to detect the effects of anticoagulants and to assess platelet function are actively being developed and employed. Whereas TEG and ROTEM use the "cup and pin" principle for TEG and thromboelastometry, other devices can assess the viscoelastic properties of blood with ultrasound (11-12).

HEMOSTATIC ADJUNCTS

Prothrombin Complex Concentrate (PCC)

Preparations

Prothrombin complex concentrate (PCC) contain vitamin K-dependent clotting factors; four-factor PCC contain factors II, VII, IX, and X. Three-factor PCC do not contain factor VII, so coadministration of factor VII or FFP is required. Activated prothrombin complex concentrate (aPCC) contain factors II, VII, IX, and X, but factor VII is present in an activated form, which is more prothrombotic. In the United States, Factor Eight Inhibitor Bypassing Activity (FEIBA) is the only available aPCC. FEIBA is not recommended for reversal of warfarin because of the greater thrombotic risk (13-14).

Indications and Administration

PCC are packaged as a lyophilized powder that is quickly reconstituted, thereby avoiding the time delays involved in thawing FFP, and greatly decreasing the volume of infusion. Table 14.2 lists specific antidotes and hemostatic agents that can be used for reversal of DOAC. PCC figure prominently

TABLE 14.2 Antidotes and Hemostatic Agents (PCC) for Non-Severe and Severe Bleeding Associated with DOAC

DOAC	Antidote	PCC/aPCC dosage
Apixaban	Low dose: Andexanet alfa 400 mg IV bolus over 15 min followed by 480 mg IV infusion over 2 h High dose: Andexanet alfa 800 mg IV bolus over 30 min followed by 960 mg IV infusion over 2 h	25-50 IU/kg
Dabigatran	Idarucizumab, 5 g over 5-10 min × 2 infusions, each infusion separated by 10 min	25-50 IU/kg
Edoxaban	No currently approved antidote	50 IU/kg (may only result in partial reversal)
Rivaroxaban	Low dose: Andexanet alfa 400 mg IV bolus over 15 min followed by 480 mg IV infusion over 2 h High dose: Andexanet alfa 800 mg IV bolus over 30 min followed by 960 mg IV infusion over 2 h	25-50 IU/kg

DOAC = direct oral anticoagulants; PCC = prothrombin complex concentrate; aPCC = activated prothrombin complex concentrate.

From Grottke O, Afshari A, Ahmed A, et al. Clinical guideline on reversal of direct oral anticoagulants in patients with life threatening bleeding. Eur J Anaesthesiol 2024; 41:327-50.

in the management strategy as these agents can be rapidly administered.

Warfarin reversal with FFP was discussed previously in Chapter 10: Colloid and Crystalloid Fluids, but four-factor

PCC, while significantly more expensive, are recommended as first-line reversal agents due to greater efficacy and less risk for volume overload (15). Table 14.3 lists protocols for rapid reversal of warfarin anticoagulation in cases of severe bleeding (i.e., intracerebral hemorrhage, post-surgical bleeding, severe trauma-induced coagulopathy). (See also Figure 14.4.)

TABLE 14.3 Rapid Reversal of Warfarin Anticoagulation*

Vitamin K: 10 mg over 10 min (diluted in 50 mL IV fluid)		
AND		
Four-factor prothrombin complex concentrate (PCC)	1,500-2,000 U IV over 10 min	If INR not <1.5 15 min after administration, give additional four-factor PCC.
OR		
Three-factor prothrombin complex concentrate (PCC) AND Factor VIIa	1,500-2,000 U IV over 10 min AND 20 µg/kg IV factor VIIa	If INR not <1.5 15 min after administration, give additional three-factor PCC.
OR		
FFP	2 U IV rapid infusion	If INR >1.5, administer 2 more U FFP; repeat until INR <1.5.

*For life-threatening hemorrhage.

From Alwakeal A, Maas MB, Naidech AM, et al. Fixed- versus variable-dose prothrombin complex concentrate for the emergent reversal of vitamin K antagonists: a systematic review and meta-analysis. Crit Care Med 2024;52(5):811-20.

Desmopressin (ddAVP)

Mechanism and Indications

Desmopressin (ddAVP) is a vasopressin analogue that is capable of increasing plasma concentrations of von Willebrand factor. This adjunct is used most frequently in patients with renal failure who are at risk for uremic

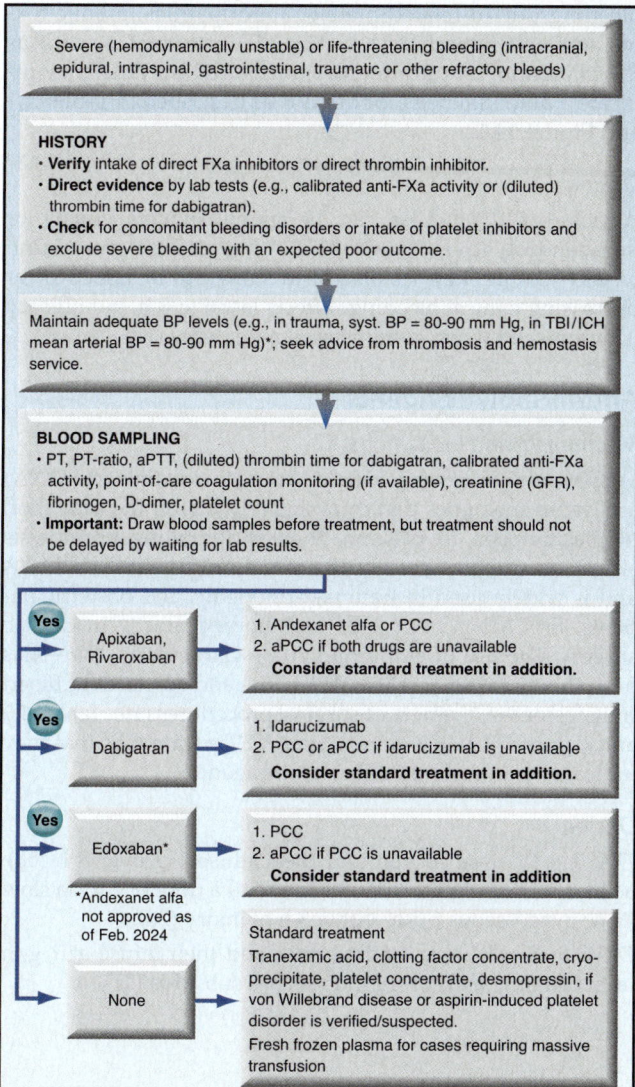

FIGURE 14.4. Treatment algorithm for the management of severe bleeding, including patients on direct oral anticoagulants (DOAC). (From Reference 13.)

bleeding due to related platelet abnormalities, uremic toxins, and other mechanisms (16). VET parameters, such as the maximum amplitude (MA) measured by TEG, may indicate a potential need for ddAVP, as described in Table 14.1 and Figure 14.1.

Dosing

A dose of 0.3 µg/kg can be given subcutaneously or intravenously (over 30 min) (17). A higher dose given intranasally (3.0 µg/kg) has also been shown to be effective for decreasing clinical bleeding. Effects last 6 to 8 h, but efficacy is diminished when administered repeatedly (17).

Antifibrinolytic Agents

Mechanism and Indications

Epsilon-aminocaproic acid (EACA) and tranexamic acid (TXA) are lysine analogues that competitively inhibit the activation of plasminogen to plasmin, thereby inhibiting fibrinolysis (18). TXA is approximately 10 times more potent than EACA and is widely used in trauma, orthopedic, and obstetric patients. EACA has been used and studied mostly in cardiac surgery. The use of antifibrinolytics—particularly TXA—has been shown to reduce clinical bleeding and the need for blood transfusions in a variety of surgical procedures (19). Table 14.1 and Figures 14.1-14.3 demonstrate VET parameters that may indicate the need for antifibrinolytic agents.

Dosing

TXA: 1 g IV over 10 min and then infuse 1 g over 8 h (18). Military trauma guidelines recommend a dose of 2 g via slow IV or intraosseous push within 3 h of injury (20).

EACA: 5-10 g IV as a loading dose and then infuse at 1 g/h until bleeding and/or fibrinolysis has subsided (21)

Adverse Effects

An increased risk for thrombosis has been suggested when antifibrinolytics are used, but in a large meta-analysis that included over 125,000 patients, a significant association with TXA and vascular occlusive events was not identified (22). Seizures are a potential risk after administration of high-dose (>4 gs) TXA though the risk is low (~1%) (23). Renal dysfunction has rarely been reported following administration of EACA during cardiac surgery (18,24).

Fibrinogen Concentrate

Fibrinogen concentrate is a product prepared using human plasma purification techniques.

Fibrinogen concentrate contains a greater amount of fibrinogen (900-1,300 mg/vial) compared to cryoprecipitate (150-250 mg/U) but is significantly more expensive (25-26). A resuscitation algorithm that emphasizes the early administration of fibrinogen concentrate or cryoprecipitate for the management of acute hemorrhage is presented in Figure 14.5.

Topical Hemostatic Agents

In the ICU, some sources of hemorrhage require local control. Examples include bleeding from tracheostomy sites (quite problematic in ECMO patients), epistaxis, and traumatic injuries. A variety of commercial topical hemostatic products are available to be applied to the sites of active bleeding for temporary or permanent hemostasis. While beyond the scope of this text, several excellent references are available to describe these agents, including two referenced here (27-28). Figure 14.6 illustrates an overview of many representative hemostatic materials and their mechanisms of action (26).

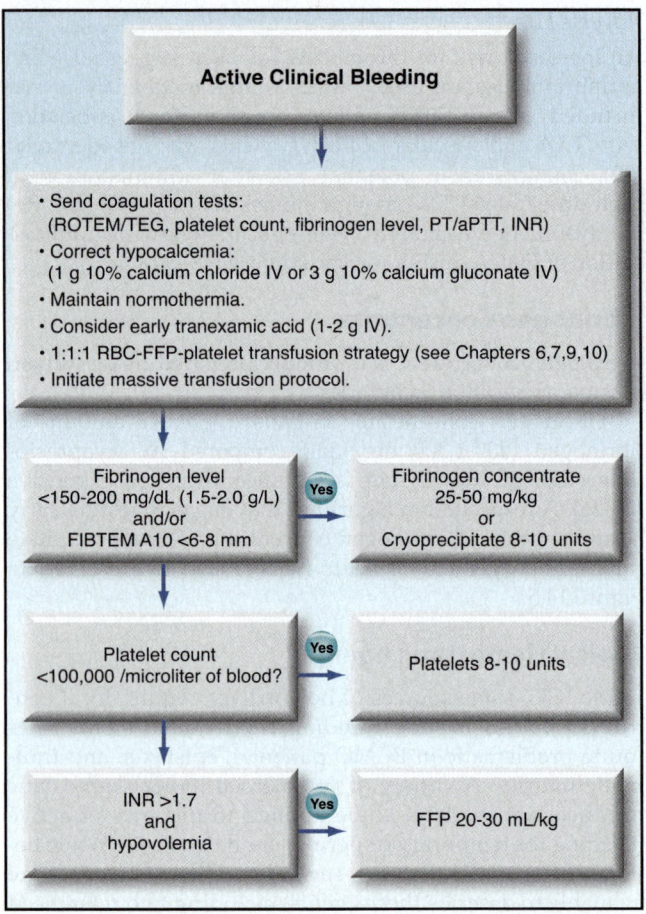

FIGURE 14.5. Management algorithm for the patient with acute hemorrhage, emphasizing the use of early fibrinogen concentrate or cryoprecipitate. FIBTEM A10 = FIBTEM amplitude at 10 min. (Adapted from Levy JH, Goodnough LT. How I use fibrinogen replacement therapy in acquired bleeding. Blood 2015;125[9]:1387-93.)

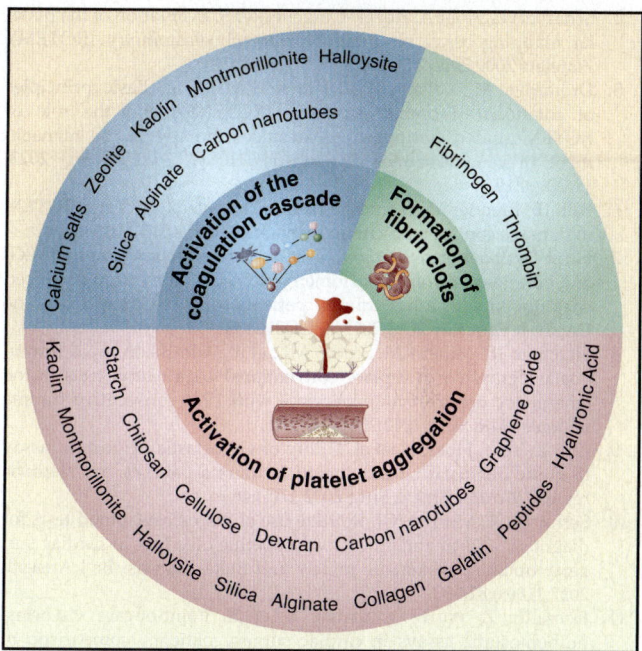

FIGURE 14.6. Hemostatic materials and their mechanisms of action. (Redrawn from Levy JH, Goodnough LT. How I use fibrinogen replacement therapy in acquired bleeding. Blood 2015;125[9]:1387-93.)

References

1. Pérez-Gómez F, Bover R. La nueva cascada de la coagulación y su posible influencia en el difícil equilibrio entre trombosis y hemorragia [The new coagulation cascade and its possible influence on the delicate balance between thrombosis and hemorrhage]. Rev Esp Cardiol 2007;60(12):1217-9.
2. Volod O, Runge A. The TEG 5000 system: system description and protocol for measurements. Methods Mol Biol 2023;2663:725-33.
3. Cotton BA, Faz G, Hatch QM, et al. Rapid thromboelastography delivers real-time results that predict transfusion within 1 hour of admission. J Trauma 2011;71(2):407-17.

4. Scharbert G, Auer A, Kozek-Langenecker S. Evaluation of the platelet mapping assay on rotational thromboelastometry (ROTEM). Platelets 2009;20(2):125-30.
5. Drotarova M, Zolkova J, Belakova KM, et al. Basic principles of rotational thromboelastometry (ROTEM®) and the role of ROTEM-guided fibrinogen replacement therapy in the management of coagulopathies. Diagnostics (Basel, Switzerland) 2023; 13(20):3219.
6. Brill JB, Brenner M, Duchesne J, et al. The role of TEG and ROTEM in damage control resuscitation. Shock 2021;56(1S):52-61.
7. Hunt H, Stanworth S, Curry N, et al. Thromboelastography (TEG) and rotational thromboelastometry (ROTEM) for trauma induced coagulopathy in adult trauma patients with bleeding. Cochrane Database Syst Rev 2015;2015(2):CD010438.
8. Holcomb JB, Minei KM, Scerbo ML, et al. Admission rapid thromboelastography can replace conventional coagulation tests in the emergency department: experience with 1974 consecutive trauma patients. Ann Surg 2012;256(3):476-86.
9. Zhu Z, Yu Y, Hong K, et al. Utility of viscoelastic hemostatic assay to guide hemostatic resuscitation in trauma patients: a systematic review. World J Emerg Surg 2022;17(1):48.
10. Serraino GF, Murphy GJ. Routine use of viscoelastic blood tests for diagnosis and treatment of coagulopathic bleeding in cardiac surgery: updated systematic review and meta-analysis. Br J Anaesth 2017;118(6):823-33.
11. Demailly Z, Wurtz V, Barbay V, et al. Point-of-care viscoelastic hemostatic assays in cardiac surgery patients: comparison of thromboelastography 6S, thromboelastometry sigma, and Quantra. J Cardiothorac Vasc Anesth 2023;37:948-55.
12. Volod O, Bunch CM, Zackariya N, et al. Viscoelastic hemostatic assays: a primer on legacy and new generation devices. J Clin Med 2022;11(3):860.
13. Grottke O, Afshari A, Ahmed A, et al. Clinical guideline on reversal of direct oral anticoagulants in patients with life threatening bleeding. Eur J Anaesthesiol 2024;41:327-50.
14. Alwakeal A, Maas MB, Naidech AM, et al. Fixed- versus variable-dose prothrombin complex concentrate for the emergent reversal of vitamin K antagonists: a systematic review and meta-analysis. Crit Care Med 2024;52(5):811-20.
15. Goldstein JN, Refaai MA, Milling TJ Jr, et al. Four-factor prothrombin complex concentrate versus plasma for rapid vitamin K antagonist reversal in patients needing urgent surgical or invasive interventions: a phase 3b, open-label, non-inferiority, randomised trial. Lancet 2015;385(9982):2077-87.
16. Kaw D, Malhotra D. Platelet dysfunction and end-stage renal disease. Semin Dial 2006 19(4):317-22.

17. Galbusera M, Remuzzi G, Boccardo P. Treatment of bleeding in dialysis patients. Semin Dial 2009;22(3):279-86.
18. Levy JH, Koster A, Quinones QJ, et al. Antifibrinolytic therapy and perioperative considerations. Anesthesiology 2018;128(3):657-70.
19. Abad-Motos A, Garcia-Erce JA, Gresele P, et al. Is tranexamic acid appropriate for all patients undergoing high risk surgery? Curr Opin Crit Care 2024;30(6):655-63.
20. Drew B, Auten JD, Cap AP, et al. The use of tranexamic acid in tactical combat casualty care: TCCC proposed change 20-02. J Spec Oper Med 2020;20(3):36-43.
21. Koster A, Faraoni D, Levy JH. Antifibrinolytic therapy for cardiac surgery: an update. Anesthesiology 2015;123(1):214-21.
22. Taeuber I, Weibel S, Herrmann E, et al. Association of intravenous tranexamic acid with thromboembolic events and mortality: a systematic review, meta-analysis, and meta-regression. JAMA Surg 2021;156(6):e210884.
23. Shi J, Zhou C, Pan W, et al. Effect of high- vs low-dose tranexamic acid infusion on need for red blood cell transfusion and adverse events in patients undergoing cardiac surgery: the OPTIMAL randomized clinical trial. JAMA 2022;328(4):336-47.
24. Manjunath G, Fozailoff A, Mitcheson D, Sarnak MJ. Epsilon-aminocaproic acid and renal complications: case report and review of the literature. Clin Nephrol 2002;58(1):63-7.
25. Stanford S, Roy A, Cecil T, et al. Differences in coagulation-relevant parameters: comparing cryoprecipitate and a human fibrinogen concentrate. PLoS One 2023;18(8):e0290571.
26. Levy JH, Goodnough LT. How I use fibrinogen replacement therapy in acquired bleeding. Blood 2015;125(9):1387-93.
27. Zhong Y, Hu H, Min N, et al. Application and outlook of topical hemostatic materials: a narrative review. Ann Transl Med 2021;9(7):577.
28. Liu Y, Zhang Y, Yao W, et al. Recent advances in topical hemostatic materials. ACS Appl Bio Mater 2024;7(3):1362-80.

SECTION IV
SHOCK SYNDROMES

Chapter 15
Approaches to Clinical Shock

Synonymous with a life-threatening and rapidly deteriorating condition, shock is best defined as inadequate cellular oxygen utilization, i.e., cellular hypoxia leading to cellular and organ dysfunction. Oxygen uptake by cells (mitochondria) is necessary to drive cellular respiration, the process by which all cells generate adenosine triphosphate (ATP) for energy. Cellular respiration consists of three stages: glycolysis, citric acid cycle, and oxidative phosphorylation. Inadequate oxygen uptake leads to the failure of cellular respiration, cellular dysfunction (i.e., shock), and death. Understanding the physiology of systemic oxygenation and uptake is critical to the understanding of shock states and their subsequent diagnoses and treatments. Often categorized into specific types such as hypovolemic shock, cardiogenic shock, obstructive shock, and distributive shock (inflammatory), all result in inadequate oxygen utilization despite different mechanisms. Not all shock fits cleanly into these categories. Furthermore, a common misconception is that all shock is a result of inadequate oxygen delivery (DO_2) while ignoring oxygen uptake/utilization. For example, DO_2 is normal to elevated in early cyanide poisoning. Cyanide inhibits the final step in oxidative phosphorylation, essentially blocking oxygen utilization.

Subsequent chapters will address specific shock states; however, it is critical to understand that shock states can frequently coincide and evolve. An extreme example would include an injured patient with spinal cord injury (neurogenic shock), tension pneumothorax (obstructive shock), and exsanguinating hemorrhage (hypovolemia/anemic shock). Prolonged and/or severe shock may then progress to vasoplegia (inflammatory/distributive shock) and even Takotsubo cardiomyopathy (cardiogenic shock).

FACTORS OF SYSTEMIC OXYGEN TRANSPORT

The normal range for measures of systemic oxygen balance is shown in Table 15.1. Note that DO_2 and oxygen consumption (VO_2) are expressed in absolute and size-adjusted terms; the body size adjustment is based on body surface area in square meters (m^2).

TABLE 15.1	Measures of Systemic Oxygen Balance	
Measure	Normal	Tissue Hypoxia
DO_2	900-1,100 mL/min or 520-600 mL/min/m^2	Variable
VO_2	200-270 mL/min or 110-160 mL/min/m^2	<200 mL/min or <110 mL/min/m^2
O_2ER	20-30%	≥50%
SvO_2	65-75%	≤50%
$ScvO_2$	70-80%	?
Lactate	1-2.2 mmol/L*	>1-2.2 mmol/L*

DO_2 = oxygen delivery; VO_2 = oxygen consumption; O_2ER = oxygen extraction ratio; SvO_2 = mixed venous oxygen saturation; $ScvO_2$ = central venous oxygen saturation.
*Normal lactate levels vary from 1.0 to 2.2 mmol/L in individual laboratories.

The amount of oxygen taken up by the body (and assumed for cellular respiration) is measured per minute as VO_2. *Note: Oxygen (O_2) is not stored in tissues.* There are two factors that determine VO_2: DO_2 and oxygen extraction (O_2EXT) (Figure 15.1).

A deficit or defect in either DO_2 or O_2EXT leading to VO_2 below an aerobic threshold (oxygenation needs) can result in anaerobic metabolism and shock.

$$VO_2 = \underbrace{CO \times \overbrace{(CaO_2 - CvO_2)}^{DO_2}}_{O_2EXT}$$

CO = cardiac output
CaO₂ = arterial oxygen content
CvO₂ = mixed venous oxygen content
DO₂ = oxygen delivery
VO₂ = oxygen consumption
O₂EXT = oxygen extraction

FIGURE 15.1. Oxygen consumption (VO_2).

Oxygen Delivery

DO_2 is the rate at which oxygen is transported through arterial blood and is a function of both arterial blood's O_2 content (CaO_2) and cardiac output (CO) (1).

$$DO_2 = CO \times CaO_2 \times 10 \text{ (mL/min)} \qquad (15.1)$$

Oxygen Content of Blood

The sum of the contributions from the O_2 bound to hemoglobin (Hb) and the O_2 dissolved in plasma determines the concentration of O_2 in blood or O_2 content.

Hemoglobin-Bound O_2. The concentration of hemoglobin-bound O_2 (HbO_2) in arterial blood is determined as (1):

$$HbO_2 = 1.34 \times Hb \times SaO_2 \text{ (mL/dL)} \qquad (15.2)$$

where Hb is the hemoglobin concentration in g/dL (grams per 100 mL), 1.34 is the O_2 binding capacity of Hb (mL/g), and SaO_2 is the O_2 saturation of Hb, expressed as a ratio (HbO_2/total Hb). When Hb is fully saturated with oxygen ($SaO_2 = 1$), each gram of Hb binds 1.34 mL of O_2 (1).

Dissolved O_2. The concentration of dissolved O_2 in plasma is determined as follows (2):

$$\text{Dissolved } O_2 = 0.003 \times PO_2 \text{ (mL/dL)} \quad (15.3)$$

PO_2 is the partial pressure of O_2 in blood (in mm Hg), and 0.003 is the solubility coefficient of O_2 in plasma (mL/dL/mm Hg) at normal body temperature (37°C). Each 1 mm Hg increment in PO_2 will increase the concentration of dissolved O_2 by 0.003 mL/dL (or 0.03 mL/L) (2). This highlights *the poor solubility of oxygen in plasma* (which is why Hb is needed as a carrier molecule) (3).

Total O_2 Content. The total O_2 content in blood (mL/dL) is determined by combining Equations 15.1 and 15.2:

$$O_2 \text{ Content} = (1.34 \times Hb \times SaO_2) + (0.03 \times PaO_2) \quad (15.4)$$

Note that the contribution of dissolved O_2 is remarkably small (3%); as a result, *the O_2 content of blood is essentially equivalent to the Hb-bound fraction.*

$$O_2 \text{ Content} = \sim 1.34 \times Hb \times SaO_2 \text{ (mL/dL)} \quad (15.5)$$

Cardiac Output

CO is the driving force delivering O_2 to the tissues.

$$DO_2 = CO \times CaO_2 \times 10 \text{ (mL/min)} \quad (15.6)$$

(The multiplier of 10 is used to convert the CaO_2 from mL/dL to mL/L.) If the CaO_2 is broken down into its components, Equation 15.7 can be rewritten as follows:

$$DO_2 = CO \times (1.34 \times Hb \times SaO_2) \times 10 \quad (15.7)$$

Note: With continuous pulse oximetry (see Chapter 8: Oximetry and Capnography) and a pulmonary artery catheter (see Chapter 9: The Pulmonary Artery Catheter), hemodynamic and oxygen transport variables (DO_2, O_2EXT, and VO_2) can be monitored continuously.

Oxygen Extraction

O_2EXT is the difference between the amount of O_2 leaving the heart to the tissues and the amount returned to the heart. The ratio of VO_2 to DO_2 is the fraction of the O_2 delivered to tissues that is used by aerobic metabolism and is expressed as the *oxygen extraction ratio* (O_2ER):

$$O_2ER = VO_2 / DO_2 \qquad (15.8)$$

(This ratio is commonly multiplied by 100 and expressed as a percentage.)

The normal range for the O_2ER is 0.2-0.3 (20-30%), which means that *in healthy adults at rest, only 20-30% of the O_2 delivered to tissues is used for aerobic metabolism.*

Mixed Venous Oxygen Saturation

Blood in the pulmonary arteries provides the global (whole-body) measurement of venous O_2 saturation (SvO_2), also known as mixed venous O_2 saturation. This measurement requires a pulmonary artery catheter (see Chapter 9: The Pulmonary Artery Catheter). The SvO_2 is an admixture of venous return from the entire body (superior vena cava [SVC], inferior vena cava [IVC], and the coronary sinus [CS]). The SVC receives venous return from the upper extremities and head; the IVC from the mesenteric circulation, kidneys, and lower extremities; and the CS from the heart.

Central Venous Oxygen Saturation

The O_2 saturation in the superior vena cava, known as the *central venous O_2 saturation* ($ScvO_2$), has become a popular surrogate for the SvO_2 because it is more readily available using a central venous catheter as opposed to a pulmonary artery catheter. $ScvO_2$ can be measured in blood samples withdrawn through a central venous catheter, or it can be monitored continuously using fiberoptic catheters (PreSep Catheters, Edwards Life Sciences, Irvine, CA). The $ScvO_2$

is higher than the SvO_2 by an average of 5% in critically ill patients (4), and this translates to a normal $ScvO_2$ of 70-80% (i.e., 5% higher than the normal range for SvO_2). However, there can be large discrepancies between the $ScvO_2$ and SvO_2, in hemodynamically unstable patients or those with left-to-right shunts (5). Changes in $ScvO_2$ correlate closely with changes in SvO_2 (4,6). The interpretation of SvO_2 and $ScvO_2$ is shown in Table 15.2

TABLE 15.2	Interpretation of SvO_2 and $ScvO_2$
Low (<65%)	Inadequate DO_2 to meet oxygen needs
Normal (65-75%)*	
High (>80%)	• Excess inotrope • Histotoxic shock (e.g., sepsis, cyanide poisoning, mitochondrial dysfunction) • Microcirculatory shunting (e.g., sepsis, hepatic failure) • Left-to-right shunts (e.g., arteriovenous (A-V) fistula, intra-cardiac shunt)

*In the setting of poor DO_2, a normal SvO_2 or $ScvO_2$ would be inappropriate, similar to a high saturation.

SYSTEMIC OXYGEN BALANCE

Control of VO_2

DO_2 and O_2ER operate to maintain a constant rate of VO_2 to maintain aerobic metabolism. The response to an increased demand will result in an increase in DO_2, primarily by increasing CO in the acute setting. Variations in O_2 supply (DO_2) are accompanied by reciprocal changes in O_2ER, i.e., decreased DO_2 will result in an increase in O_2ER. These relationships are shown by rearranging Equation 15.8:

$$VO_2 = DO_2 \times O_2ER \qquad (15.9)$$

THE INITIAL APPROACH TO SHOCK

A rapid assessment (history and physical) can frequently narrow the causation and direct initial therapies and diagnostics. For example, a recent subclavian central venous catheter insertion with acute hemodynamic deterioration is likely a tension pneumothorax (obstructive shock) which is immediately responsive to decompression. When an etiology is less clear (undifferentiated shock), further diagnostics may be required as resuscitation efforts are initiated. The fundamental objectives to approach undifferentiated shock are resuscitate, diagnose, and treat. In the rapidly deteriorating patient, these objectives are addressed concurrently. Importantly, "resuscitation" and "treatment" are not necessarily synonymous in shock (Table 15.3).

GENERAL FEATURES OF SHOCK

Signs and Symptoms

Signs and symptoms may vary depending on the mechanism and severity of shock. Terms such as *compensated shock* or *occult shock* are used to describe scenarios of hypoperfusion/hypoxia with vital signs within a normal range making early identification challenging. This is particularly problematic in young patients with strong compensatory mechanisms, or in older patients who may require higher blood pressure, or medications blocking usual responses, e.g., beta blockers (7-9).

Vital Signs
- *Heart rate* is typically elevated as a mechanism to increase CO but can be blunted by medications and heart disease. Also, paradoxical bradycardia can occur with hemorrhagic shock (10) or arterial hypoxia (11).
- *Respiratory rate*: Tachypnea is a response to acidosis and shortness of breath results from tissue hypoxia, known as "air hunger."

TABLE 15.3	Objectives for the Initial Approach to Undifferentiated Shock
Resuscitate *optimize DO$_2$*	**Hemodynamics:** blood pressure and cardiac output support (IV fluids, vasopressors, inotropes)
	Oxygenation and ventilation: supplemental oxygen and airway support (endotracheal intubation and mechanical ventilation may be required)
Diagnose *directed by history and physical (H&P) to determine the causative etiology and assess shock*	**Imaging:** chest x-ray, CT scan, ultrasonography, echocardiography, 12-lead ECG, etc.
	Laboratories: • Standard: CBC, electrolyte panel, LFTs, arterial blood gas, lactate, PT/PTT • As indicated: troponins, D-dimer, type and crossmatch, C-reactive protein, cultures (sites determined by H&P)
Treat	**Cardiogenic shock:** inotropes, diuretics (heart failure), cardioversion, anti-dysrhythmics, ECMO, etc.
	Hemorrhagic shock: stop the bleed, blood products, etc.
	Obstructive shock: thrombolysis (acute PE), needle decompression/chest tube (tension pneumothorax), etc.
	Distributive shock: source control (surgery or drainage of infection), antibiotics and corticosteroids (sepsis), antidotes for poisonings, etc.

CBC = complete blood count; CT = computed tomography; ECMO = extracorporeal membranous oxygenation; ECG = electrocardiogram; IV = intravenous; LFT = liver function testing; PE = pulmonary embolism; PT/PTT = prothrombin time/partial thromboplastin time.

- *Blood pressure* (BP) of <90 mm Hg (systolic) has been an historic threshold for diagnosing shock; however, there are numerous pitfalls to interpreting BP both diagnostically and therapeutically. The most important concept is to understand that BP is a surrogate for CO (which is the main driver for DO_2), with the other component being systemic vascular resistance (SVR) (12):

$$BP = CO \times SVR \quad (15.10)$$

- *Pitfalls of BP*
  - A compensatory increase in SVR will increase BP but not necessarily CO.
  - The elderly may require higher baseline BP, even >110 mm Hg (8,13).
  - Pharmacologic BP (vasopressors) support may not equate with increased CO (therefore, no improvement in DO_2).

- *Temperature*
  - *Fever*, commonly associated with infectious causes can occur with noninfectious etiologies. See Chapter 6: Evaluation of Fever in the ICU.
  - *Hypothermia* (<35°C), especially in hemorrhagic shock, is often the result of blood loss, poor prefusion (e.g., decrease metabolism), and environmental losses negatively impacting coagulation/hemostasis and cardiac function. CO decreases proportionally to the level of hypothermia (14-15). Core temperatures below 33°C increase cardiac irritability and the risk of ventricular fibrillation (14,16-17).

Neurological

Neurological signs include anxiety, agitation, delirium, obtundation, and coma can be nonspecific, but acute changes should prompt consideration for poor perfusion/hypoxia.

Skin

Peripheral vasoconstriction is a compensatory mechanism to maintain BP and perfusion resulting in cool extremities, delayed capillary refill (>2 s), mottled skin, and digital cyanosis.

Renal Function

A decreased urine output is indicative of decreased renal perfusion which can rapidly return with successful resuscitation. Serum creatinine is discussed in the section that follows.

Laboratory Markers of Shock

Lactate

Lactate indicates anaerobic metabolism.

Pros

1. Hyperlactatemia is universal in shock and clinically useful in assessing severity and response to therapy (18).
2. Elevated lactate levels may be seen prior to hemodynamic deterioration (occult shock) (9).
3. The clearance of lactate during resuscitation is predictive of mortality (19-20).
4. Point-of-care testing allows for rapid determination of serum levels but does require diligent quality control measures (21).

Pitfalls

1. A lactate level is a moment in time (which means it could be increasing or decreasing); therefore, serial levels should be trended to determine adequacy of resuscitation.
2. Hepatic dysfunction can delay recovery (22).
3. Lactated ringers may have a small but measurable impact on serum lactate (23).

Base Deficit

Rapidly obtained through blood gas analysis, base deficit (BD) is the amount of base (in mmol) required to titrate the blood sample to a pH of 7.40 at a PCO_2 of 40 mm Hg, essentially a quantification of acidosis.

Pros

1. Frequently used during trauma (hemorrhage) resuscitations, the BD tracks with lactic acidosis.
2. Similar to lactate, the BD can be trended to assess resuscitation response.

Pitfalls

1. Best assessed with arterial blood gas sample
2. Normal saline used for resuscitation can increase the BD (23).
3. Does not differentiate cause of acidosis

Hemoglobin

A component of the routine complete blood count, Hb is a critical component of the oxygen content of blood and therefore DO_2 (see Equations 15.2 and 15.7).

Pitfalls

1. Hb levels make take hours to equilibrate after hemorrhage or transfusion (24).
2. Hb is not equivalent to blood volume.

Serum Creatinine

Pros

1. Considered the "canary in the coal mine of shock," acute kidney injury as determined by serum creatinine has been shown to be a predictor of morbidity and mortality (25-27).
2. Changes in creatinine may occur before oliguria (28).

Pitfalls

1. Levels vary according to age and sex.
2. Elevations in serum creatinine lag behind the decrease in function.

References

1. Rhodes CE, Denault D, Varacallo MA. Physiology, Oxygen Transport. [Updated 2022 Nov 14]. In: StatPearls [Internet]. Treasure Island (FL): StatPearls Publishing; 2025 Jan-. Available from: https://www.ncbi.nlm.nih.gov/books/NBK538336/
2. Christoforides C, Hedley-Whyte J. Effect of temperature and hemoglobin concentration on solubility of o2 in blood. J Appl Physiol 1969;27:592-6.
3. Pittman RN. Oxygen transport. In: *Regulation of Tissue Oxygenation*. Morgan & Claypool Life Sciences; 2011.
4. Reinhart K, Kuhn HJ, Hartog C, Bredle DL. Continuous central venous and pulmonary artery oxygen saturation monitoring in the critically ill. Intensive Care Med 2004;30:1572-8.
5. van Beest P, Wietasch G, Scheeren T, et al. Clinical review: use of venous oxygen saturations as a goal—a yet unfinished puzzle. Crit Care 2011;15:232.
6. Dueck MH, Klimek M, Appenrodt S, Weigand C, et al. Trends but not individual values of central venous oxygen saturation agree with mixed venous oxygen saturation during varying hemodynamic conditions. Anesthesiology 2005;103:249-57.
7. Haseer Koya H, Paul M. Shock. [Updated 2023 Jul 24]. In: StatPearls [Internet]. Treasure Island (FL): StatPearls Publishing; 2025 Jan-. Available from: https://www.ncbi.nlm.nih.gov/books/NBK531492/
8. Hatton GE, McNutt MK, Cotton BA, et al. Age-dependent association of occult hypoperfusion and outcomes in trauma. J Am Coll Surg 2020;230:417-25.
9. Shehu A, Kalbas Y, Teuben MPJ, et al. Definition of occult hypoperfusion in trauma: a systematic literature review. Injury 2023;54:811-7.
10. Bell K, Elmograbi A, Smith A, Kaur J. Paradoxical bradycardia and hemorrhagic shock. Proc (Bayl Univ Med Cent) 2019;32:240-1.
11. Higgs A, Littley N, Chrimes N. Bradycardia during hypoxaemic airway crises. Does atropine treat the patient or the anaesthetist? Anaesthesia 2019;74:1482-3.
12. Trammel JE, Sapra A. Physiology, Systemic Vascular Resistance. [Updated 2023 Jul 10]. In: StatPearls [Internet]. Treasure Island (FL): StatPearls Publishing; 2025 Jan-. Available from: https://www.ncbi.nlm.nih.gov/books/NBK556075/
13. Brown JB, Gestring ML, Forsythe RM, et al. Systolic blood pressure criteria in the National Trauma Triage Protocol for geriatric trauma: 110 is the new 90. J Trauma Acute Care Surg 2015;78:352-9.
14. American College of Surgeons. *ATLS Advanced Trauma Life Support Student Course Manual*. 10th ed. American College of Surgeons; 2018.
15. Bjertnaes LJ, Naesheim TO, Reierth E, et al. Physiological changes in subjects exposed to accidental hypothermia: an update. Front Med (Lausanne) 2022;9:824395.

16. Kander T, Schott U. Effect of hypothermia on haemostasis and bleeding risk: a narrative review. J Int Med Res 2019;47:3559-68.
17. van Veelen MJ, Brodmann Maeder M. Hypothermia in trauma. Int J Environ Res Public Health 2021;18.
18. Levitt DG, Levitt JE, Levitt MD. Quantitative assessment of blood lactate in shock: measure of hypoxia or beneficial energy source. Biomed Res Int 2020;2020:2608318.
19. Marbach JA, Di Santo P, Kapur NK, et al. Lactate clearance as a surrogate for mortality in cardiogenic shock: insights from the DOREMI Trial. J Am Heart Assoc 2022;11:e023322.
20. Wang J, Ji M. The 6-hour lactate clearance rate in predicting 30-day mortality in cardiogenic shock. J Intensive Med 2024;4:393-9.
21. Larkins MC, Thombare A. Point-of-Care Testing. [Updated 2023 May 29]. In: StatPearls [Internet]. Treasure Island (FL): StatPearls Publishing; 2025 Jan-. Available from: https://www.ncbi.nlm.nih.gov/books/NBK592387/
22. Hernandez G, Bellomo R, Bakker J. The ten pitfalls of lactate clearance in sepsis. Intensive Care Med 2019;45:82-5.
23. Ross SW, Christmas AB, Fischer PE, et al. Impact of common crystalloid solutions on resuscitation markers following Class I hemorrhage: A randomized control trial. J Trauma Acute Care Surg 2015;79:732-40.
24. Elizalde JI, Clemente J, Marin JL, et al. Early changes in hemoglobin and hematocrit levels after packed red cell transfusion in patients with acute anemia. Transfusion 1997;37:573-6.
25. Griffin BR, Liu KD, Teixeira JP. Critical care nephrology: core curriculum 2020. Am J Kidney Dis 2020;75:435-52.
26. Landi A, Branca M, Leonardi S, et al. Transient vs in-hospital persistent acute kidney injury in patients with acute coronary syndrome. JACC Cardiovasc Interv 2023;16:193-205.
27. Wohlauer MV, Sauaia A, Moore EE, et al. Acute kidney injury and posttrauma multiple organ failure: the canary in the coal mine. J Trauma Acute Care Surg 2012;72:373-80.
28. Chau K, Schisler T, Er L, et al. Fluid balance, change in serum creatinine and urine output as markers of acute kidney injury post cardiac surgery: An observational study. Can J Kidney Health Dis 2014;1:19.

Hemorrhagic Shock

Chapter 16

HEMORRHAGE AND HYPOVOLEMIA

Simply stated, hemorrhagic shock is inadequate oxygen delivery (DO_2) due to blood loss. The loss of blood cells results in decreases in both components of DO_2: Cardiac output is decreased due to a reduction in blood volume (preload) and the arterial oxygen content (CaO_2) is decreased due to hemoglobin loss. Figure 16.1 illustrates the impact of blood loss on DO_2.

$$DO_2 = \text{cardiac output} \times CaO_2 \times 10 \, (\text{mL/min})$$

Arterial O_2 Content (CaO_2) ~ $1.34 \times \text{Hemoglobin} \times SaO_2$ (mL/dL)

↓ **Cardiac Output** due to decreased preload (ventricular filling)

↓ **CaO_2** due to decreased hemoglobin

FIGURE 16.1. Impact of blood loss on oxygen delivery (DO_2).

The circulatory system operates with a relatively small volume and a volume-responsive pump. This is an energy-efficient design, but it quickly falters when volume is lost. This intolerance to blood loss is the dominant concern in the bleeding patient. Although most internal organs such as the lungs, liver, and kidneys can lose as much as 75% of their functional mass without life-threatening organ failure, loss of <50% of the blood volume can be fatal. The decrease in the oxygen content of the residual blood volume contributes to the oxygen deficit.

Severity of Blood Loss

Table 16.1 outlines the classification system of The American College of Surgeons Committee on Trauma (ACS-COT) for acute blood loss based on clinical signs for estimating percentage of blood loss (1).

Class I

Loss of <15% of the blood volume (or <10 mL/kg). This degree of blood loss is usually fully compensated by interstitial fluid shifts (transcapillary refill), so that blood volume is maintained and clinical findings are minimal or absent.

Class II

Loss of 15-30% of the blood volume (or 10-20 mL/kg). This represents the compensated phase of hypovolemia, where blood pressure is maintained by systemic vasoconstriction. Postural changes in pulse rate and blood pressure may be evident, but these findings are inconsistent. The extremities become cool at this stage, and urine output falls, but does not reach oliguric levels (<0.5 mL/kg/h).

Class III

Loss of 30-40% of the blood volume (or 20-30 mL/kg). This stage marks the onset of decompensated blood loss or *hemorrhagic shock*, where the vasoconstrictor response is no longer able to sustain blood pressure and organ perfusion. Clinical findings can include supine hypotension, cold extremities, confusion, oliguria (urine output <0.5 mL/kg/h), and increased lactate levels in blood.

Class IV

Loss of >40% of blood volume (or >30 mL/kg). This degree of blood loss results in progressive hemorrhagic shock and includes *massive blood loss*, i.e., loss of >50% of the blood volume in 3 h. Clinical findings include limb cyanosis, evidence of multiorgan dysfunction (e.g., lethargy, oliguria, increased liver enzymes), and progressive lactic acidosis.

TABLE 16.1	Classification System for Acute Blood Loss			
	Class I	Class II	Class III	Class IV
Volume deficit	<15%	15-30%	31-40%	>40%
Volume loss	<10 mL/kg	10-20 mL/kg	21-30 mL/kg	>30 mL/kg
Heart rate	↔	↑	↑↑	↑↑/↓
Blood pressure	↔	↔/↓	↓	↓↓
Urine output	↔	↔/↓	↓	↓↓
Plasma lactate	↔	↔	↑	↑↑
Interpretation	Asymptomatic phase	Compensated phase	Shock phase	Advanced shock
Resuscitation	None	Crystalloid fluids	Blood	Massive transfusion

Adapted from *ATLS Advanced Trauma Life Support Student Course Manual*. 10th ed. American College of Surgeons. 2018;43-61.

CLINICAL EVALUATION

See Chapter 15: Approaches to Clinical Shock for detailed descriptions with pitfalls of clinical signs and the laboratory evaluation of shock.

RESUSCITATE, DIAGNOSE, TREAT—AT THE SAME TIME!

Acute hemorrhage involves the loss of whole blood, which is not only the oxygen carrying red blood cells but also the coagulation factors and platelets. Shock results in a systemic inflammatory response compounding the coagulopathy from the loss of coagulation factors. Prolonged shock, exposure, resuscitation with room temperature fluids, and refrigerated blood products can lead to the development of the "lethal triad" of coagulopathy, acidosis, and hypothermia (2).

The resuscitation of shock must also include the concomitant treatment of these issues to avoid the spiral to irreversible shock and death. As a priority, the source of bleeding must be controlled!

Basic Adjuncts for Resuscitation

Electrocardiographic monitoring allows real-time assessment of heart rate (response to therapy) and cardiac dysrhythmias.

Pulse oximetry allows for the continuous monitoring of arterial oxygenation, which is critical to ensure that component of DO_2 (see Chapter 8: Oximetry and Capnography).

End-tidal CO_2 monitoring not only views the adequacy of ventilation but also is an indirect assessment of cardiac output (see Chapter 8: Oximetry and Capnography).

Intravenous (IV) access. Two large-bore IVs (16 gauge or greater) are needed for rapid volume resuscitation with crystalloids and blood products. Large-bore peripheral venous access in hypovolemic patients can be challenging. Consideration to upsize to a rapid infusion catheter (can be upsized from 20 gauge) or central venous access using an introducer sheath (see Chapter 1: Central Venous Access).

Arterial line. An indwelling arterial line is critical for ongoing resuscitation of shock. Arterial lines, with real-time blood pressure data, allow for immediate assessment of the response to fluid and blood product resuscitation as well as rapid access for arterial blood gas and other laboratory analysis (3).

Nasogastric tube. Decreased mesenteric blood flow and the hyperadrenergic stress response leads to gastric dilatation, nausea, and emesis in shock (1,4). Patients in hemorrhagic shock have altered mental status due to decreased perfusion, typically require endotracheal intubation and mechanical ventilation, and are not able to protect their airway. The complication of the aspiration of gastric contents and pneumonitis in the setting of shock is frequently a lethal complication.

Urinary catheterization allows for the continuous monitoring of urine output as a measure of renal perfusion. Core temperature can also be measured in real time if a temperature probe catheter is available (Figure 16.2).

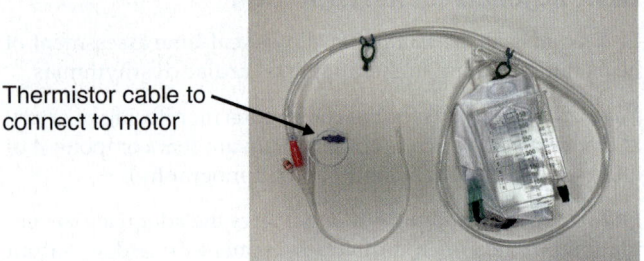

FIGURE 16.2. Urinary catheter with temperature probe and thermistor for continuous temperature monitoring.

Resuscitation

Airway and Breathing

Endotracheal intubation and mechanical ventilation are necessary as patients require adequate oxygenation and ventilation. Obtunded patients may be apneic, and agitated patients may require sedation and analgesia to allow resuscitation to proceed.

Circulation

Crystalloids (see Chapters 10: Colloid and Crystalloid Fluids and 11: Fluid Management). Isotonic crystalloids, e.g., normal saline (NS), lactated ringers (LR), and Plasma-Lyte (PL), are the preferred initial fluids for hemorrhage with balanced crystalloids (LR and PL) favored over NS (5). Crystalloids should be minimized in deference to blood products (i.e., red blood cells, fresh frozen plasma, and platelets). Large-volume crystalloid resuscitations can lead to significant adverse consequences such as dilution coagulopathy, adult respiratory distress syndrome, multi-organ dysfunction, and abdominal compartment syndrome (6). The most recent edition of the ACS-COT Advanced Trauma Life Support (ATLS) recommends blood transfusion after 1 L of crystalloid down from prior editions recommending an initial 2 L (1). Colloids offer no advantage in acute hemorrhage and are contraindicated with traumatic brain injuries (7-8).

Blood Products. Whole blood is the ideal replacement containing red blood cells, coagulation factors, and platelets but is not often available outside of major medical and trauma centers. Current resuscitation recommendations are to provide a 1:1:1 ratio of packed red blood cells, fresh frozen plasma, and platelets. See below for further discussion of the resuscitation/treatment of coagulopathy. Blood products are refrigerated and should be warmed using fluid warmer during infusion to avoid or worsen hypothermia.

Table 16.2 summarizes resuscitation fluids for blood loss.

Diagnose

Clearly, the management of hemorrhagic shock is a multidisciplinary challenge, and early surgical consultation is necessary to assist in diagnostic and treatment decisions. Other appropriate specialties should be consulted as soon as possible. For example, gastroenterology consultation for potential endoscopic intervention for gastrointestinal hemorrhage. Imaging and treatments must be triaged based on hemodynamic responses to initial fluid resuscitation.

Treat

Continuous resuscitation will fail without control of the hemorrhage. Unstable patients may require immediate surgical intervention, whereas "responders", i.e., those whose vital signs improve (even transiently) after initial fluids, may have potential nonsurgical interventions, such as endoscopic or interventional radiologic procedures. Figure 16.3 demonstrates an example of a successful angiographic embolization of a bleeding renal laceration.

TABLE 16.2 Resuscitation Fluids for Blood Loss

Type of Fluid	Products	Principal Effect	Comments
Colloid fluid	Albumin (5%, 25%) Hydroxyethyl starches, Dextrans	Expands the plasma volume	Significant cost. No mortality benefit. Contraindicated in traumatic brain injury. Dextrans and starches can contribute to coagulopathy.
Crystalloid fluid	Isotonic saline, Ringer's lactate, Normosol, Plasma-Lyte	Expands the extracellular volume	Up 75% equilibrates from intravascular space to interstitial space
RBC concentrate	Packed RBCs	Increases the O_2 content of blood	
Plasma	Fresh frozen plasma, liquid plasma	Provides procoagulant proteins	
Plasma precipitate	Cryoprecipitate, fibrinogen concentrate	Increases fibrinogen levels	
Platelet concentrate	Multiple-donor platelets, single-donor platelets	Increases circulating platelets	
Whole blood	Type-specific blood, Group O blood	All of the above	Provides: RBCs, Platelets, Coagulation factors. Not universally available

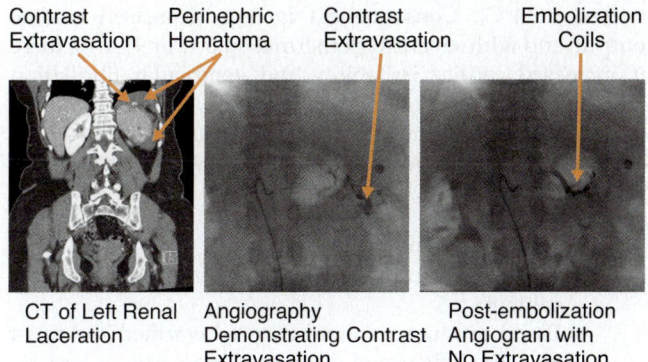

FIGURE 16.3. Computed tomography (CT) diagnosis of renal laceration with extravasation and angiographic embolization.

The Lethal Triad

Acidosis. In hemorrhagic shock, acidosis is primarily lactic acidosis due to poor tissue perfusion and oxygen uptake. Consequences of severe acidosis (pH <7.20) include hemodynamic (direct negative effects on cardiac contractility and vascular smooth muscle) (9); contribution to coagulopathy impairing activation of factors V, VIII, IX, and X (10); thrombin generation (11); and accelerating fibrinogen consumption resulting in decreased fibrinogen availability (12).

The priority of addressing acidosis is treatment of the underlying cause, i.e., blood loss and shock. There is no agreement as to which pH threshold to treat with an alkalizing agent such as sodium bicarbonate (9,13). Mortality increases as acidosis increases; however, survival is possible even with pH <7.0 with rapid resuscitation (14).

Hypothermia. Defined as a core body temperature <35°C (95°F), hypothermia is an independent predictor of mortality (11). Severe hemorrhage is accompanied by loss of thermoregulation, compounded by the infusion of blood products (stored at 4°C). Consequences include decreased cardiac output, and with severe hypothermia (<33°C or 91.4°F), there is increased cardiac irritability and ventricular fibrillation risk (1). Treatment, preferably prevention, is paramount for successful resuscitation of hemorrhagic shock.

Basic techniques for rewarming/prevention of hypothermia include the following:

- Warmed intravenous fluids
  - Crystalloids can be maintained in a fluid warmer cabinet.
  - Blood products cannot be stored warmed and must be actively warmed during infusion. This is best accomplished using a rapid infuser that can not only warm blood to 40°C but also infuse up to 1,000 mL/min via large-bore IV.
- Forced air warming air blankets. Heated air (up to 40°C) is circulated through a disposable blanket via small perforations, directly against the patient, preventing both convective and radiant heat loss. A forced air warming blanket is demonstrated in Figure 16.4.
- Ambient overhead heaters
- Simple plastic head covers

Coagulopathy. Standard laboratory testing for coagulation includes ionized calcium, prothrombin time (PT) with an

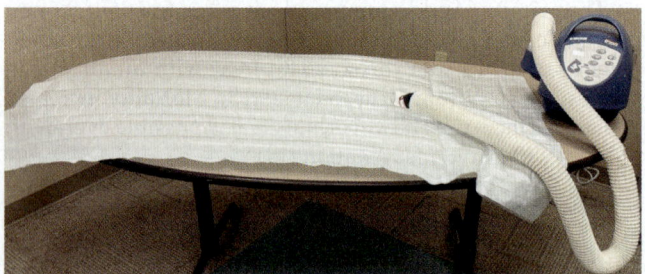

FIGURE 16.4. Forced air warming blanket.

international normalized ratio (INR), partial thromboplastin time (PTT), Clauss fibrinogen test, and a platelet count. Thromboelastography (TEG) offers a more comprehensive assessment of the entire coagulation process, including fibrinolysis, and can direct interventions (15). See Table 16.3 for interventions based on TEG. TEG is discussed in greater detail in Chapter 14: Coagulopathy Management.

TABLE 16.3 Interventions Based on Thromboelastography

Measure	Abnormal Value	Intervention
Reaction (R) time	>9 min	Transfuse plasma, or reverse anticoagulants (except warfarin)
Kinetic (k) time	>2.5 min	Transfuse plasma
Alpha (α) angle	<65°	Cryoprecipitate or fibrinogen concentrate
MA (max amplitude)	<55 mm	Transfuse platelets
LY30 (lysis at 30 min)	>3%	Tranexamic acid

From Brill JB, Brenner M, Duchesne J, et al. The role of TEG and ROTEM in damage control resuscitation. Shock 2021;56(Suppl 1):52-61.

Massive Transfusion Protocol

Massive Transfusion Protocol is a process to provide blood products to patients with active, uncontrolled hemorrhage. Transfusion of products is based on a 1:1:1 ratio of red blood cells, fresh frozen plasma, and platelet packs (16).

Calcium. Activation of multiple coagulation factors requires calcium (17). Calcium gluconate or chloride should be dosed at 1 g intravenously (gluconate or chloride) and administered every 4 U of blood to counteract the effects of the anticoagulant used for blood storage (citrate).

Cryoprecipitate or Fibrinogen Concentrate. Fibrinogen is converted to fibrin which is the main structural component of a blood clot. The target fibrinogen level should be >100 mg/dL. Hypofibrinogenemia is common in both traumatic and post-obstetrical hemorrhage and should be part of the massive transfusion protocols for these populations (15,18).

Tranexamic Acid (TXA). Shown to reduce mortality in trauma and in some localities, TXA initial dose is administered in the prehospital setting (15). Similar to trauma, TXA should be administered within 3 h of bleeding in postpartum hemorrhage (19).

TXA dosing is 1 g IV bolus (slow push) followed by 1 g IV infusion over 8 h (20).

Other bleeding scenarios have not demonstrated a benefit to empiric TXA (21). Consideration of TXA outside of trauma and postpartum hemorrhage should be based on clinical and laboratory assessment, e.g., TEG findings.

BLEEDING ON ORAL ANTICOAGULATION

Vitamin K Antagonist (VKA)-Associated Hemorrhage

Correction of VKA coagulopathy with active hemorrhage is treated with concurrent vitamin K (promoting new coagulation factor production) and four-factor prothrombin complex concentrate (4-PCC) which replaces the deficiency of factors II, VII, and X; proteins C and S; and heparin (15,22). Vitamin K is administered 10 mg intravenously. 4-PCC is weight-based and INR-based dosing (Table 16.4).

Direct Oral Anticoagulant (DOAC)-Associated Hemorrhage

DOACs are a class of anticoagulants that include direct (e.g., apixaban, rivaroxaban, and edoxaban) or the only oral direct thrombin inhibitor, dabigatran. Specific reversal agents for

TABLE 16.4	Dosage and Administration of 4-PCC (KCENTRA)		
How to calculate dosage	A single dose of 4-PCC is determined by the patient's pretreatment INR weight		
Pretreatment INR	2-<4	4-6	>6
Dose* of 4-PCC (iu+ of factor IX)/kg body weight	25	35	50
Maximum dose (unit of factor IX)	Not to exceed 2,500	Not to exceed 3,500	Not to exceed 5,000
Administer 4-PCC			

- By intravenous infusion at rate of 0.12 mL/kg/min (~3 U/kg/min) up to a maximum rate of 8.4 mL/min
- Concurrently with Vitamin K
- Through a separate infusion line
  - Repeat dosing is not supported by clinical data and is not recommended

*Dosing is based on body weight. Dose based on actual potency is stated on the vial, which will vary from 20-31 factor IX U/mL reconstitution. The actual potency for 500-U vial ranges from 400-620 U/vial. The actual potency for 1,000-U vial ranges from 800-1,240 U/vial.

4-PCC = 4-factor prothrombin complex concentrate; INR = international normalized ratio

Data from KCENTRA (Prothrombin Complex Concentrate [Human]) for Intravenous Use, Lyophilized Powder for Reconstitution Initial U.S. Approval: 2013.

DOACs are available that include andexanet alfa for direct Xa inhibitors and idarucizumab for direct thrombin inhibitor, dabigatran (15,22). However, these drugs are costly and frequently not available. 4-PCC has been shown in multiple clinical studies to be an effective alternative for the correction of coagulopathy from DOACs. Although there is no consensus on the appropriate dosing and administration, it appears that fixed dosing, e.g., 2,000 IU given via IV (as opposed to weight-based) is safe and effective (15,22-23).

GOALS OF RESUSCITATION

Many of the tissue perfusion, oxygenation, and coagulation goals have been presented elsewhere in this textbook. The overall goals of resuscitation for hemorrhagic shock are summarized in Figure 16.5.

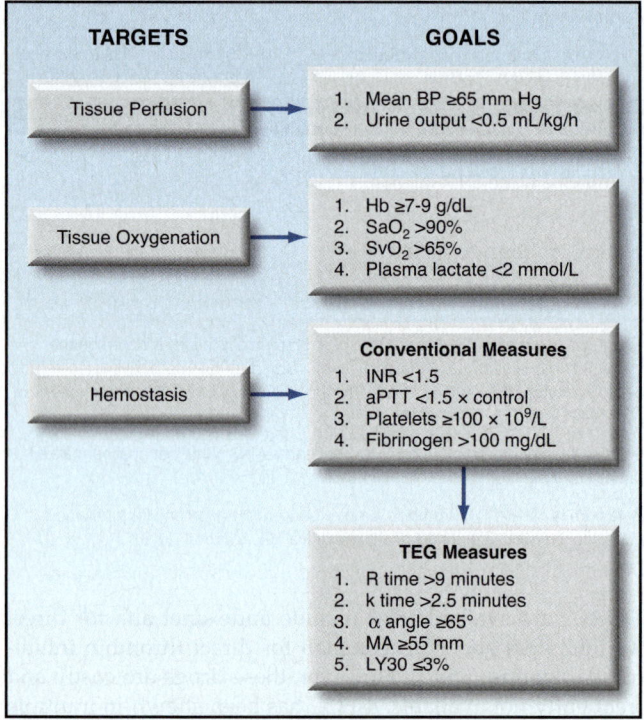

FIGURE 16.5. Summary of goals of resuscitation. aPTT = activated partial thromboplastin time; BP = blood pressure; SaO_2 = oxygen saturation in arterial blood; SvO_2 = mixed venous oxygen saturation.

References

1. Brun S. *ATLS Advanced Trauma Life Support. Student Course Manual.* 10th ed. American College of Surgeons; 2018.
2. Leibner E, Andreae M, Galvagno SM, Scalea T. Damage control resuscitation. Clin Exp Emerg Med 2020;7:5-13.
3. Williams C, Pasrija D, Pierre L, Keenaghan M. Arterial lines. [Updated 2025 Mar 23]. In: StatPearls [Internet]. Treasure Island (FL): StatPearls Publishing; 2025 Jan–.
4. Taghavi S, Nassar AK, Askari R. Hypovolemia and hypovolemic shock. [Updated 2025 Jun 1]. In: StatPearls [Internet]. Treasure Island (FL): StatPearls Publishing; 2025 Jan-.
5. Semler MW, Self WH, Wanderer JP, et al. Balanced crystalloids versus saline in critically ill adults. N Engl J Med 2018;378:829-39.
6. Chang R, Holcomb JB. Optimal fluid therapy for traumatic hemorrhagic shock. Crit Care Clin 2017;33:15-36.
7. Cooper DJ, Myburgh J, Heritier S, et al. Albumin resuscitation for traumatic brain injury: is intracranial hypertension the cause of increased mortality? J Neurotrauma 2013;30:512-8.
8. Safe Study Investigators, Australian and New Zealand Intensive Care Society Clinical Trials Group, Australian Red Cross Blood Service, et al. Saline or albumin for fluid resuscitation in patients with traumatic brain injury. N Engl J Med 2007;357:874-84.
9. Kimmoun A, Novy E, Auchet T, et al. Hemodynamic consequences of severe lactic acidosis in shock states: from bench to bedside. Crit Care 2015;19:175.
10. Martini WZ. Coagulation complications following trauma. Mil Med Res 2016;3:35.
11. van Veelen MJ, Brodmann Maeder M. Hypothermia in trauma. Int J Environ Res Public Health 2021;18.
12. Martini WZ, Holcomb JB. Acidosis & coagulopathy: the differential effects on fibrinogen synthesis and breakdown in pigs. Ann Surg 2007;246:831-5.
13. Baddam S, Tubben RE. Lactic acidosis. [Updated 2025 Apr 28]. In: StatPearls [Internet]. Treasure Island (FL): StatPearls Publishing; 2025 Jan–.
14. Ross SW, Thomas BW, Christmas AB, et al. Returning from the acidotic abyss: mortality in trauma patients with a pH < 7.0. Am J Surg 2017;214:1067-72.
15. Hofer S, Schlimp CJ, Casu S, Grouzi E. Management of coagulopathy in bleeding patients. J Clin Med 2021;11.
16. American College of Surgeons Committee on Trauma. ACS TQIP Massive Transfusion in Trauma Guidelines. Accessed June 25 2025. https://www.facs.org/media/zcjdtrd1/transfusion_guildelines.pdf

17. Potestio CP, Van Helmond N, Azzam N, et al. The incidence, degree, and timing of hypocalcemia from massive transfusion: a retrospective review. Cureus 2022;14:e22093.
18. Butwick AJ, Goodnough LT. Transfusion and coagulation management in major obstetric hemorrhage. Curr Opin Anaesthesiol 2015;28:275-84.
19. Roberts I, Brenner A, Shakur-S.till H. Tranexamic acid for bleeding: much more than a treatment for postpartum hemorrhage. Am J Obstet Gynecol MFM 2023;5:100722.
20. Chauncey JM, Patel P. Tranexamic acid. [Updated 2025 Apr 26]. In: StatPearls [Internet]. Treasure Island (FL): StatPearls Publishing; 2025 Jan–.
21. HALT-IT Trial Collaborators. Effects of a high-dose 24-h infusion of tranexamic acid on death and thromboembolic events in patients with acute gastrointestinal bleeding (HALT-IT): an international randomised, double-blind, placebo-controlled trial. Lancet 2020;395:1927-36.
22. Baugh CW, Levine M, Cornutt D, et al. Anticoagulant reversal strategies in the emergency department setting: recommendations of a multidisciplinary expert panel. Ann Emerg Med 2020;76:470-85.
23. Chiasakul T, Crowther M, Cuker A. Four-factor prothrombin complex concentrate for the treatment of oral factor Xa inhibitor-associated bleeding: a meta-analysis of fixed versus variable dosing. Res Pract Thromb Haemost 2023;7:100107.

Cardiogenic Shock

Chapter 17

Cardiogenic shock can be described as *cardiac pump failure* that results in inadequate oxygen (O_2) delivery to tissues and impaired oxidative metabolism.

ETIOLOGIES

Acute myocardial infarction (MI) has been thought to be responsible for about two-thirds of the cases of cardiogenic shock (1-3); however, in recent decades, decompensated heart failure has surpassed acute MI as the leading cause (2-3) (see Chapter 19: Acute Heart Failure[s]). The remaining cases can arise from a variety of other cardiac disorders.

Acute Myocardial Infarction

Cardiogenic shock develops in 5-10% of cases of acute MI (1), and the mechanisms involved are shown in Figure 17.1. These complications often appear within 24 h of the infarction but may also be delayed (2).

Other Causes

Causes of cardiogenic shock other than acute MI are listed in Table 17.1. Other notable conditions are summarized in the section that follows.

Dynamic Outflow Obstruction

In cases of hypertrophic cardiomyopathy, the flow of blood through the narrowed left ventricular (LV) outflow tract can create a suction effect that pulls the mitral valve leaflets anteriorly, with midsystolic contact of the mitral valve and the interventricular septum creating a "dynamic LV outflow obstruction" (4). The diagnosis of this condition is

276 SECTION IV ■ Shock Syndromes

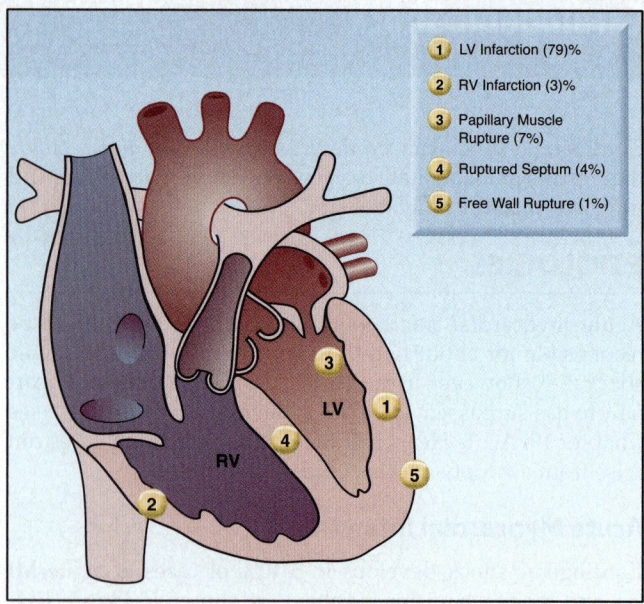

FIGURE 17.1. The mechanisms of cardiogenic shock from acute myocardial infarction. LV = left ventricle, RV = right ventricle. Percentages from Reference 1. (From Cardiogenic Shock. In: Marino PL. *Marino's The ICU Book*. 5th ed. Wolters Kluwer; 2025:257-70. Figure 16.1.)

TABLE 17.1	Causes of CS Other Than Acute MI
General	**Specific Circumstances**
Chronic heart failure with acute decompensation	Postcardiotomy shock
Acute myocarditis	Peripartum cardiomyopathy
Takotsubo's cardiomyopathy	Postcardiac arrest shock
Dynamic outflow obstruction	
Advanced valvular disease	

CS = cardiogenic shock; MI = myocardial infarction.

From Cardiogenic Shock. In: Marino PL. *Marino's The ICU Book*. 5th ed. Wolters Kluwer; 2025:257-70. Table 16.1.

made with continuous wave Doppler ultrasound in the apical four-chamber view, which is used to calculate the peak systolic pressure gradient across the subaortic region of the LV (5). Recognition of this condition is important because it is treated differently than other causes of cardiogenic shock: i.e., the goal of management in this case is to slow the heart rate and increase diastolic filling, using nonvasodilating β-blockers (e.g., metoprolol, nadolol).

Cardiac Surgery

Cardiogenic shock is reported in 2-5% of patients who undergo cardiac surgery (6), and this *postcardiotomy shock* can begin in the operating room or in the early postoperative period. Presumed mechanisms include myocardial hibernation ("stunning"), inadequate cardioprotection, and vasodilation (6).

Pregnancy

An idiopathic cardiomyopathy can appear in the later stages of pregnancy or in the early months following delivery, with an incidence of approximately 1 case per 3,000-4,000 pregnancies (7). This cardiomyopathy is characterized by systolic dysfunction and a variable clinical course. Risk factors include age >30 years, multigestational pregnancy, African heritage, and a family history of cardiomyopathy. This condition can progress to cardiogenic shock and even cardiac arrest, and it has a reported mortality rate of 7-20% in the United States (7).

DEFINITION AND CLASSIFICATION

In most guidelines, cardiogenic shock is defined by impaired cardiac output (CO) that causes hypotension (i.e., systolic blood pressure [BP] <90 mm Hg), the need for vasopressors or mechanical support, or evidence of impaired end-organ perfusion (1-2,8-9). Hemodynamic criteria include a cardiac index (CI) ≤2.2 L/min/m^2 and a pulmonary capillary wedge pressure >15 mm Hg (2). In 2019, a classification system was devised, as summarized in Table 17.2 (10).

TABLE 17.2	SCAI Classification Scheme for CS
Stage	Clinical Characteristics
A	No signs or symptoms, but at risk of developing CS due to underlying cardiac pathology
B	Early signs of CS, including tachycardia and hypotension, but without evidence of end-organ hypoperfusion
C	Evidence of end-organ hypoperfusion requiring pharmacological or mechanical support (or both)
D	Deterioration of clinical condition despite initiation of therapy (i.e., decreasing CO, worsening tachycardia and hypotension, lactate elevation)
E	Extremis with refractory shock

CO = cardiac output; CS = cardiogenic shock; SCAI = Society of Cardiovascular Angiography and Interventions.

From Baran DA, Grines CL, Bailey S, et al. SCAI clinical expert consensus statement on the classification of cardiogenic shock. Catheter Cardiovasc Interv 2019;94(1):29-37.

Hemodynamic Changes

The hemodynamic changes in cardiac pump failure are demonstrated in Figure 17.2.

The decrease in CO is accompanied by an increase in cardiac filling pressures (either the central venous pressure or the pulmonary artery wedge pressure, depending on which ventricle has failed) and an increase in systemic vascular resistance (SVR). These changes occur in both heart failure and cardiogenic shock, and *cardiogenic shock is distinguished from heart failure by the presence of tissue hypoperfusion (e.g., hypotension, decreased urine output) and inadequate tissue oxygenation (e.g., elevated plasma lactate levels)*.

Exceptions

The CI in cardiogenic shock is typically <2.2 L/min/m^2 (normal CI = 2.4-4.0 L/min/m^2) (11), but the cardiac filling pressures are not increased in as many as 30% of patients with infarct-related cardiogenic shock (1). In addition, the

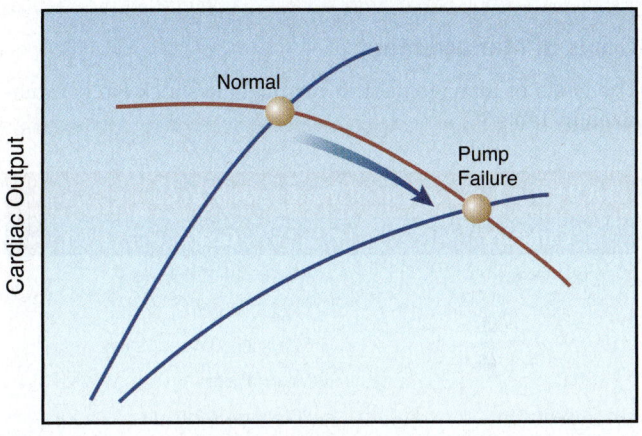

FIGURE 17.2. Graph showing the hemodynamic changes in cardiac pump failure. (From Cardiogenic Shock. In: Marino PL. *Marino's The ICU Book*. 5th ed. Wolters Kluwer; 2025:257-70. Figure 16.2.)

SVR may not be elevated when cardiogenic shock is accompanied by systemic inflammation. Finally, hypotension is absent in about 5% of cases of cardiogenic shock (1). Decreases in capillary perfusion (i.e., *microcirculatory dysfunction*) can persist in cardiogenic shock despite correction of CO and blood pressure (12-13).

Systemic Inflammation

Myocardial necrosis triggers a localized inflammatory response (14), which can progress to a systemic inflammatory response. Signs of systemic inflammation (e.g., fever, leukocytosis) have been reported in 20-40% of patients with cardiogenic shock complicating acute MI, and these patients have a lower SVR (due to the vasodilating effects of nitric oxide) and a higher mortality rate (15).

MANAGEMENT

Goals of Management

The goals of management in cardiogenic shock are summarized in Table 17.3.

TABLE 17.3	Goals of Management in CS
Category	Goals
Hemodynamics	PAWP = 19-20 mm Hg
	CI ≥2.5 L/min/m^2
	SVRI = 25-30 Wood Units[§]
	Mean BP ≥65 mm Hg
Tissue Perfusion	PCO$_2$ gap <6 mm Hg
	Urine output >0.5 mL/kg/h
Tissue Oxygenation	SvO$_2$ >50%
	Plasma lactate <2 mmol/L

CS = cardiogenic shock; PAWP = pulmonary artery wedge pressure; CI = cardiac index; SVRI = systemic vascular resistance index; BP = blood pressure; SvO$_2$ = mixed venous oxygen saturation.

[§]Wood Units = mm Hg/L/min/m^2

From References 2, 17-18.

Monitoring

The management of cardiogenic shock requires a reliable measure of the CO. Doppler echocardiography and pulmonary artery (PA) catheters are the most helpful (see Chapter 7: Bedside Echocardiography and Chapter 9: The Pulmonary Artery Catheter). Echocardiographic measures such as the LV outflow tract velocity-time integral (VTI) and lung ultrasound can be used to monitor stroke volume and pulmonary vascular congestion, respectively (2). The PA catheter provides measurements of the cardiac filling pressures (the central venous and wedge pressures), the SVR, and oxygen transport variables, which makes this device ideal for the management of cardiogenic shock. Many societies, including the American Heart Association, recommend use of the PA catheter in the management of cardiogenic shock because these devices provide continuous data that can inform real-time treatment decisions (2,16-20).

Tissue Perfusion and Oxygenation

Cardiogenic shock can be accompanied by deficits in microcirculatory flow that are independent of the changes in CO and can persist after the CO and blood pressure are normalized (12-13). Although it is not possible to directly monitor tissue O_2 levels, the mixed venous O_2 saturation (SvO_2) can provide information about the balance between O_2 delivery and O_2 consumption, and plasma lactate levels provide an indirect assessment of the adequacy of tissue oxygenation these measures are described in Chapter 15: Approaches to Clinical Shock.

The PCO_2 Gap. Tissue perfusion monitoring can also be assessed using the PCO_2 gap. The venoarterial difference between PCO_2 is normally 2-5 mm Hg (0.3-0.7 kPa), and an increase in the gap to >6 mm Hg (>0.8 kPa) may suggest tissue hypoperfusion (21). Unlike the SvO_2, the PCO_2 is easily obtained and is dependent only on tissue perfusion. The PCO_2 gap *does not provide information about systemic oxygenation and may be elevated in metabolic acidosis* (due to an increase in nonmetabolic CO_2 production).

Optimizing Filling Pressures

The LV filling pressure (i.e., the PA wedge pressure) is not always elevated in cardiogenic shock (1), and when this occurs, volume infusion can be instrumental in augmenting the CO. The target of volume infusion is the highest filling (wedge) pressure that will augment CO without producing pulmonary edema, and this "optimal" pressure is dependent on the colloid osmotic pressure (COP) of plasma. The plasma COP is normally about 28 mm Hg (22), but a lower COP of

20-25 mm Hg is more likely in critically ill patients, who often have a subnormal plasma albumin concentration (the major determinant of plasma COP). Thus, *the optimal LV filling pressure (i.e., wedge pressure) is considered to be 18-20 mm Hg* (23).

Vasopressor Therapy

Vasopressors are used to raise the blood pressure in cardiogenic shock to a systolic BP ≥90 mm Hg or a mean BP ≥65 mm Hg. *The vasopressor of choice in cardiogenic shock is norepinephrine* (2,17-19), a catecholamine that produces systemic vasoconstriction and mild cardiac stimulation. Norepinephrine should be used sparingly, if at all, in cardiogenic shock from dynamic LV outflow obstruction, where a pure vasoconstrictor like phenylephrine (which can trigger a reflex bradycardia) is more appropriate (19).

Dosing

Norepinephrine is given by continuous infusion (without a loading dose) starting at a rate of 0.05 µg/kg/min (or 5 µg/min), titrating upward every 5 min to achieve the desired blood pressure. The usual dose rate in studies of cardiogenic shock is 0.05-0.5 µg/kg/min (or 5-30 µg/min) (24-25).

Inotropic Therapy

Vasopressor therapy does not alleviate the cardiac pump failure and can aggravate it. Inotropic agents used for cardiogenic shock are listed in Table 17.4 (24,26-27). Inotropic therapy is contraindicated in cardiogenic shock from dynamic LV outflow obstruction.

Dobutamine

The most widely used inotropic agent in cardiogenic shock is dobutamine (24,28), a synthetic catecholamine that stimulates β_1 receptors in the heart and increases both CO and heart rate. Dobutamine also has mild vasodilator effects, can increase the heart rate (usually by 5-15 beats/min but can exceed 30 beats/min),

TABLE 17.4	Inotropic Agents for CS
Agent	**Dosing Regimen and Comments**
Dobutamine	1. Start infusion at 3-5 µg/kg/min, and increase in increments of 3-5 µg/kg/min, if needed. Usual dose is 3-20 µg/kg/min. 2. Major disadvantage is an increase in heart rate.

Milrinone	1. Initial dose is 50 µg/kg (over 10 min), followed by an infusion rate of 0.375-0.75 µg/kg/min. Daily dose should not exceed 1.13 mg/kg.
	2. Dose adjustments are advised for renal insufficiency:[5]
	
	   Creatinine Clearance **Infusion Rate**
	   50 mL/min/1.73 m^2 0.43 µg/kg/min
	   40 0.38
	   30 0.33
	   20 0.28
	3. Major disadvantage is the risk of hypotension.

Levosimendan	1. Initial dose is 12 µg/kg (over 10 min), followed by an infusion rate of 0.1 µg/kg/min. After 1 h, infusion rate can be increased to 0.2 µg/kg/min, if needed. 2. Has a long half-life (80 h). 3. Approved for use in about 60 countries, but not in the United States.

CS = cardiogenic shock.
From References 24 and 27.

and can increase in myocardial O_2 consumption (29). These changes are associated with an increase in cardiac work, which is deleterious in the setting of acute MI, and in the failing myocardium, where cardiac work is already increased.

Milrinone

Milrinone is a phosphodiesterase inhibitor that acts as an inotrope by virtue of inhibiting the breakdown of cyclic AMP, which enhances cyclic AMP-mediated calcium influx into cardiac myocytes. It also acts as a vasodilator, which can produce troublesome hypotension (29). The elimination half-life of milrinone (2.5 h) is significantly prolonged in patients with renal insufficiency, and a dosing adjustment is recommended as shown in Table 17.4. The inotropic effects of milrinone are comparable to those of dobutamine, but there is less risk of tachycardia (29). Despite the lower risk of tachycardia, the hypotension associated with milrinone limits its popularity as an inotrope in cardiogenic shock. Milrinone is more appropriate for the management of decompensated heart failure without hypotension.

Levosimendan

Levosimendan has been a popular inotrope in Europe and South America, but it is not approved for use in the United States. Levosimendan increases cardiac contractility by sensitizing cardiac myofilaments to calcium and promotes vasodilation by facilitating potassium influx into vascular smooth muscle (30). This drug is particularly appealing in infarct-related cardiogenic shock because it dilates coronary arteries and does not stimulate myocardial O_2 consumption. Disadvantages associated include hypotension and a long half-life (80 h), so infusions are usually limited to 24 h.

Cardiac Workload

The pharmacological management of cardiogenic shock has the unfortunate consequence of increasing the workload of the heart because vasopressors will increase LV afterload, and inotropes will increase contractility and can increase heart rate. The increase in cardiac work is counterproductive in the failing myocardium, so delays in proceeding to MCS should be avoided if there is no evidence of rapid improvement during pharmacological support (19).

Addressing Underlying Causes

Cardiogenic shock following acute MI is associated with mortality rates of nearly 40% at 30 days and 50% at 1 year (31-32). Current evidence and clinical practice guidelines support immediate revascularization of the infarct-related coronary artery as the primary therapy for cardiogenic shock following acute MI (32). Other causes of cardiogenic shock require specific interventions (e.g., immunosuppression for acute myocarditis, pacing for bradyarrhythmias, surgery for valvular disease) (2). Mixed cardiogenic-septic shock is challenging to manage, and achieving source control is the top priority (2).

Obstructive Shock

The term *obstructive shock* has historically referred to conditions that cause a mechanical impediment to blood flow, leading to inadequate tissue oxygen supply (e.g., *acute pulmonary embolism, pericardial tamponade, tension pneumothorax*) (33). Although debate persists about its categorization and overlap with other types of shock, the hemodynamic consequences are the same as those of cardiogenic shock and management is aimed at correcting the responsible condition.

MECHANICAL CARDIAC SUPPORT

Mechanical cardiac support (MCS) is generally reserved for cases of refractory cardiogenic shock where improvement in cardiac function is an expectation (usually after MI or cardiac surgery), or another intervention is planned (e.g., coronary bypass surgery) (34).

Intra-Aortic Balloon Pump

The intra-aortic balloon pump (IABP) is the oldest form of MCS and continues to be used despite evidence that it does not improve survival (35). Nevertheless, the IABP is the most readily available form of MCS in hospitals other than large, tertiary medical centers, and can be used as a temporary measure, including use for interfacility transports. The IABP reduces cardiac work by unloading the LV while also increasing coronary blood flow and systemic flow. The IABP is contraindicated in patients with aortic valve insufficiency or aortic dissection.

Method

The intra-aortic balloon is an elongated polyurethane balloon that is inserted percutaneously into the femoral artery and advanced up the aorta until the tip lies just below the origin of the left subclavian artery (Figure 17.3).

A pump attached to the balloon uses helium, a low-density gas, to rapidly inflate and deflate the balloon (inflation volume is generally 35-40 mL). Inflation begins at the onset of diastole, just after the aortic valve closes (the R wave on the ECG is a common trigger). The balloon is then deflated at the onset of ventricular systole, just before the aortic valve opens (during isovolumic contraction). This pattern of balloon inflation and deflation produces two changes in the aortic pressure waveform, which are illustrated in Figure 17.3.

1. Inflation of the balloon during diastole increases the peak diastolic pressure, which augments coronary blood flow (which occurs predominantly during diastole), and increases the mean arterial pressure, which augments systemic blood flow.
2. Deflation of the balloon creates a suction effect that reduces pressure in the aorta when the aortic valve opens, decreasing LV afterload and augmenting ventricular stroke output.

Complications

Limb ischemia is the most common serious complication, which can appear while the balloon is in place or shortly after balloon removal. Most cases are the result of in situ

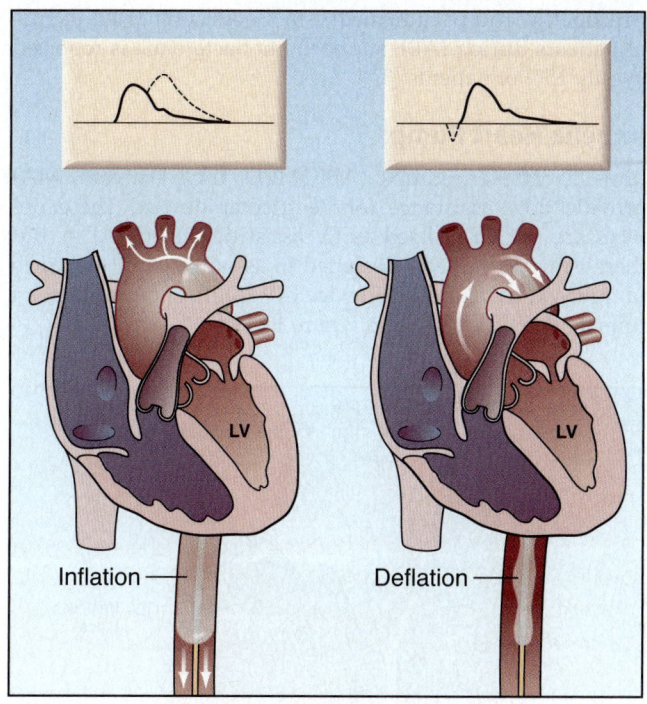

FIGURE 17.3. Intra-aortic balloon counterpulsation, showing balloon inflation in early diastole (on the left), and balloon deflation in late diastole (on the right). The associated changes in the aortic pressure (indicated by the dotted lines) are shown above each maneuver. The arrows show the direction of enhanced flow. (From Cardiogenic Shock. In: Marino PL. *Marino's The ICU Book*. 5th ed. Wolters Kluwer; 2025:257-70. Figure 16.3.)

thrombosis at the catheter insertion site, but aortoiliac injury may also be responsible. Loss of distal pulses alone does not warrant removal of the balloon if sensorimotor function in the legs is intact (36). *Loss of sensorimotor function in the legs should always prompt immediate removal of the device*, and surgical intervention may be required. Other complications of IABP include septicemia, balloon rupture, peripheral neuropathy, and pseudoaneurysm. Fever is reported in 50% of patients during IABP support, but bacteremia is reported in only 15% of patients (37).

Impella Heart Pumps

Impella catheter pumps (ABIOMED, Inc., Danvers, MA) provide flow assistance for ventricular output. These devices are primarily used as LV assist devices (LVADs), but there is also a catheter designed to assist the right ventricle (a right-ventricular assist device [RVAD]). An example of an Impella device is shown in Figure 17.4.

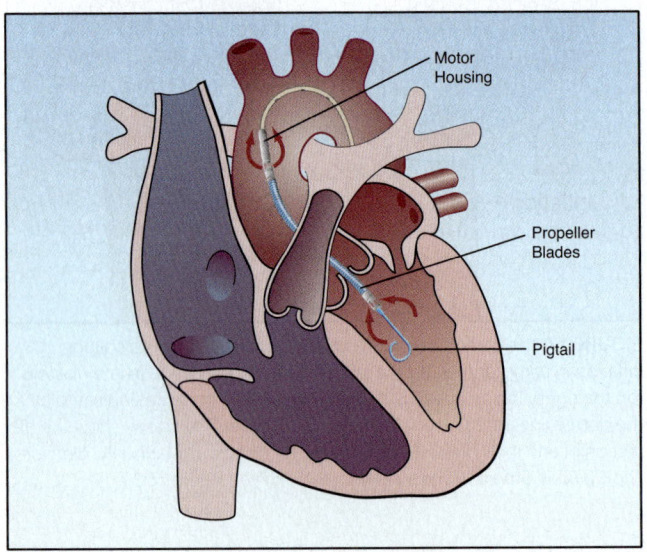

FIGURE 17.4. An Impella catheter, which is equipped with a miniature centrifugal pump. The tip of the catheter is placed in the left ventricle so that the pump's rotational propellers are positioned across the aortic valve. The pump then transfers blood from the ventricle to the proximal aorta (see directional arrows) to unload the ventricle. See text for further explanation. (From Cardiogenic Shock. In: Marino PL. *Marino's The ICU Book*. 5th ed. Wolters Kluwer; 2025:257-70. Figure 16.3.)

The catheter is equipped with a miniature centrifugal pump (i.e., the type of pump that uses rotational "propeller" blades to create nonpulsatile flow), and it is inserted percutaneously into a femoral artery and advanced into the left ventricle. The pump moves blood from the left ventricle to the proximal aorta at flow rates of 2.5-5.5 L/min (flow rates differ with different catheters). The device shown in Figure 17.4 monitors the native CO and automatically adjusts the pump flow to achieve a (preselected) total CO (38).

Hemodynamic Effects

The hemodynamic effects of Impella catheters are similar to the IABP; i.e., they unload the LV and increase CO while also increasing coronary blood flow (39). This similarity also extends to survival value because Impella catheters have not shown a survival advantage over IABP in patients with infarct-related cardiogenic shock (35,40). Impella catheters have an advantage in patients with end-stage LV failure, since they can be implanted for long-term use. These catheters are contraindicated in patients with aortic valve disease or a prosthetic aortic valve and in patients with an LV thrombus.

Complications

The complications of the Impella catheter are similar in type to the IABP, but there is evidence that major bleeding and limb ischemia are more common with Impella catheters (40-41). The incidence of significant hemolysis (5-10%) is also greater with Impella catheters than with other forms of mechanical support (42).

ECMO

Venoarterial extracorporeal membrane oxygenation (VA-ECMO) is an MCS modality that supports both circulatory flow and pulmonary gas exchange to (see Chapter 30: Extracorporeal Membrane Oxygenation). VA-ECMO offers some advantages, including the ability to provide full biventricular support (matched only by combining RV and LV Impella catheters), and the ability to support oxygenation and CO_2 removal, which is advantageous in patients with respiratory failure (a common complication of cardiogenic shock). *VA-ECMO is the preferred method of mechanical support in cases of cardiogenic shock associated with respiratory failure* (43).

Complications

In VA-ECMO, the frequency of complications has been reported as follows (43): major bleeding (41%), sepsis (30%), limb ischemia (17%), lower extremity compartment syndrome (10%), stroke (6%), and lower limb amputation (5%) (see Chapter 30: Extracorporeal Membrane Oxygenation).

LV Afterload. VA-ECMO has a problem that is not shared by the other forms of mechanical support: i.e., the retrograde flow in the aorta increases LV afterload, and this can be severe enough to reduce LV output and cause acute pulmonary edema (43). Efforts to address this problem are discussed in Chapter 30: Extracorporeal Membrane Oxygenation and may include combining an IABP or Impella pump with VA-ECMO to reduce LV afterload or draining blood from the left ventricle to reduce end-diastolic pressure ("venting") (44).

Outcomes

A 42% survival rate to hospital discharge has been reported when VA-ECMO is used for cardiogenic shock (45). A comparison of survival rates with VA-ECMO versus other forms of mechanical support (IABP or LVAD) has had inconsistent results; i.e., survival rates have been better with VA-ECMO in some reports (46) and better with the Impella device in others (47).

Device Selection

The choice of mechanical support device will largely be determined by availability and individual preferences at each institution. VA-ECMO is the method of choice for cardiogenic shock associated with respiratory failure, and there is a trend in favor of VA-ECMO for all mechanical support. However, ECMO is not available in many hospitals, and mechanical support with IABP or an LVAD may be the only options. Patients can then be transferred for ECMO if there is no improvement.

References

1. Clinical Cardiology; Council on Cardiovascular and Stroke Nursing; Council on Quality of Care and Outcomes Research; and Mission: Lifeline. Contemporary management of cardiogenic shock: a scientific statement from the American Heart Association. Circulation 2017;136:e232-68.
2. Alkhunaizi FA, Smith N, Brusca SB, Furfaro D. The management of cardiogenic shock from diagnosis to devices: a narrative review. CHEST Crit Care 2024;2(2):100071.
3. Jentzer JC, Ahmed AM, Vallabhajosyula S, et al. Shock in the cardiac intensive care unit: changes in epidemiology and prognosis over time. Am Heart J 2021;332;94-104.
4. Sobozyk D. Dynamic left ventricular outflow obstruction: underestimated cause of hypotension and hemodynamic instability. J Ultrasonography 2014;4:421-7.
5. Panza JA, Petrone RK, Fananapazir L, Maron BJ. Utility of continuous wave Doppler echocardiography in the noninvasive assessment of left ventricular outflow tract pressure gradient in patients with hypertrophic cardiomyopathy. J Am Coll Cardiol 1992;19:91-6.
6. Masud F, Gheewala G, Giesecke M, et al. Cardiogenic shock in perioperative and intraoperative settings: a team approach. Methodist DeBakey Cardiovasc J 2020;16:e1-e7.
7. Davis MB, Arany Z, McNamara DM, et al. Peripartum cardiomyopathy. JACC state-of-the-art review. J Am Coll Cardiol 2020;75:207-21.
8. Thiele H, Akin I, Sandri M, et al. Strategies in patients with acute myocardial infarction and cardiogenic shock. N Engl J Med 2017; 377(25):2419-32.
9. Heidenreich PA, Bozkurt B, Aguilar D, et al. 2022 AHA/ACC/HFSA guideline for the management of heart failure. J Am Coll Cardiol 2022;79(17):e263-e421.
10. Baran DA, Grines CL, Bailey S, et al. SCAI clinical expert consensus statement on the classification of cardiogenic shock. Catheter Cardiovasc Interv 2019;94(1):29-37.
11. Menon V, White H, LeJemtel T, et al. The clinical profile of patients with suspected cardiogenic shock due to predominant left ventricular failure: a report from the SHOCK Trial Registry: should we emergently revascularize occluded coronaries in cardiogenic shock? J Am Coll Cardiol 2000;36(suppl A):1071-6.

12. Wijntjens GWM, Fengler K, Feurnau G, et al. Prognostic implications of microcirculatory perfusion versus macrocirculatory perfusion in cardiogenic shock: a CULPRIT-SHOCK substudy. Eur Heart J: Acute Cardiovasc Care 2020;9:108-19.
13. Jung C, Fuernau G, de Waha S, et al. Intraaortic balloon counterpulsation and microcirculation in cardiogenic shock complicating myocardial infarction: an IABP-SHOCK II substudy. Clin Res Cardiol 2015;104:679-87.
14. Frangogiannis NG, Smith CW, Entman ML. The inflammatory response in myocardial infarction. Cardiovasc Res 2002;53:31-47.
15. Bertini P, Guarracino F. Pathophysiology of cardiogenic shock. Curr Opin Crit Care 2021;27:409-15.
16. Mathew R, Fernando SM, Hu K, et al. Optimal perfusion targets in cardiogenic shock. JACC Adv 2022;1(2):100034.
17. Lüsebrink E, Binzenhöfer L, Adamo M, et al. Cardiogenic shock. Lancet 2024;404(10466):2006-20.
18. De Luca L, Mistrulli R, Scirpa R, et al. Contemporary management of cardiogenic shock complicating acute myocardial infarction. J Clin Med 2023;12(6):2184.
19. Henry TD, Tomey MI, Tamis-Holland JE, et al. Invasive management of acute myocardial infarction complicated by cardiogenic shock. A scientific statement from the American Heart Association. Circulation 2021;143:e815-e829.
20. Bertaina M, Galluzzo A, Rossello X, et al. Prognostic implications of pulmonary artery catheter monitoring in patients with cardiogenic shock: a systematic review and meta-analysis of observational studies. J Crit Care 2022;69:154024.
21. Scheeren TWL, Wicke JN, Teboul JL. Understanding the carbon dioxide gaps. Curr Opin Crit Care 2018;24(3):181-9.
22. Guyton AC, Hall JE. *Textbook of Medical Physiology*. 10th ed. W.B. Saunders; 2000:169-70.
23. Franciosa JA. Optimal left heart filling pressure during nitroprusside infusion for congestive heart failure. Am J Med 1983;74:457-64.
24. DeBacker D, Ortiz JA, Levy B. The medical treatment of cardiogenic shock: cardiovascular drugs. Curr Opin Crit Care 2021;27:426-32.
25. Rui Q, Jiang Y, Chen M, et al. Dopamine versus norepinephrine in the treatment of cardiogenic shock: a PRISMA-compliant meta-analysis. Medicine 2017;96:e8402.
26. Levy B, Clere-Jehl R, Legras A, et al. Epinephrine versus norepinephrine for cardiogenic shock after acute myocardial infarction. J Am Coll Cardiol 2018;72:173-82.
27. Milrinone Lactate Injection (package insert). Hospira, Inc, Lake Forest, IL, 2021.
28. Desjardin JT, Teerlink JR. Inotropic therapies in heart failure and cardiogenic shock: an educational review. Eur Heart J: Acute Cardiovasc Care 2021;10:676-86.

29. Bayram M, De Luca L, Massie B, Gheorghiade M. Reassessment of dobutamine, dopamine, and milrinone in the management of acute heart failure syndromes. Am J Cardiol 2005;96(suppl):47G-58G.
30. Papp Z, Agostoni P, Alvarez J, et al. Levosimendan efficacy and safety: 20 years of SIMDAX in clinical use. Cardiac Failure Rev 2020;6:e19.
31. Schumann J, Henrich EC, Strobl H, et al. Inotropic agents and vasodilator strategies for cardiogenic shock or low cardiac output syndrome. Cochrane Database Syst Rev 2018;1:CD009669.
32. Samsky MD, Morrow DA, Proudfoot AG, et al. Cardiogenic shock after acute myocardial infarction: a review. JAMA 2021;326(18):1840-50.
33. Zotzmann V, Rottmann FA, Müller-Pelzer K, et al. Obstructive shock, from diagnosis to treatment. Rev Cardiovasc Med 2022;23(7):248.
34. Rob D, Bêlohlávek J. The mechanical support of cardiogenic shock. Curr Opin Crit Care 2021;27:440-6.
35. Thiele H, Zeymer U, Neumann FJ, et al. for the IABP-SHOCK II Trial Investigators. Intraaortic balloon support for myocardial infarction with cardiogenic shock. N Engl J Med 2012;367:1287-96.
36. Baldyga AP. Complications of intra-aortic balloon pump therapy. In: Maccioli GA, ed. *Intra-Aortic Balloon Pump Therapy.* Williams & Wilkins; 1997:127-62.
37. Crystal E, Borer A, Gilad J, et al. Incidence and clinical significance of bacteremia and sepsis among cardiac patients treated with intra-aortic balloon counterpulsation pump. Am J Cardiol 2000;86:1281-4.
38. Impella 5.5 with SmartAssist Instructional Manual. ABIOMED, Inc., 2022.
39. Remmelink M, Sjauw KD, Henriques JP, et al. Effects of left ventricular unloading by Impella recover LP2.5 on coronary hemodynamics. Catheter Cardiovasc Interv 2007;70:532-7.
40. Schrage B, Ibrahim K, Loehn T, et al. Impella support for acute myocardial infarction complicated by cardiogenic shock. Circulation 2019;139:1249-58.
41. Dhruva SS, Ross JS, Mortazavi BJ, et al. Association of use of an intravascular microaxial left ventricular assist device vs intra-aortic balloon pump with in-hospital mortality and major bleeding among patients with acute myocardial infarction complicated by cardiogenic shock. JAMA 2020;323:734-41.
42. Miller PE, Solomon MA, McAreavey D. Advanced percutaneous mechanical circulatory support devices for cardiogenic shock. Crit Care Med 2017;45:1922-9.
43. Combes A, Price S, Slutsky AS, Brodie D. Temporary circulatory support for cardiogenic shock. Lancet 2020;396:199-212.
44. Cevasco M, Takayama H, Ando M, et al. Left ventricular distension and venting strategies for patients on venoarterial extracorporeal membrane oxygenation. J Thorac Dis 2019;11:1676-83.

45. Thiagarajan RR, Barbaro RP, Rycus PT, et al. Extracorporeal Life Support Organization registry international report 2016. ASAIO J 2017;63:60-7.
46. Ouweneel DM, Schotborgh JV, Limpens J, et al. Extracorporeal life support during cardiac arrest and cardiogenic shock: a systematic review and meta-analysis. Intensive Care Med 2016;42:1922-34.
47. Abusnina W, Ismayl M, Al-abdouh A, et al. Impella versus extracorporeal membrane oxygenation in cardiogenic shock: a systematic review and meta-analysis. Shock 2022;58:349-57.

Inflammatory Shock   Chapter 18

Critical to the body's immune system, inflammation is a myriad of the body's biologic responses to injury or infection. These responses are designed to eliminate external threats and heal damaged tissues. Severe or persistent inflammation, e.g., lack of source control in septic shock, can exacerbate tissue damage leading to further activation of inflammation. This process can be self-perpetuating resulting in more harm that causes organ failure, tissue hypoxia, inflammation, and other problems. It is important for the clinician to understand the potential impact of inflammation to all shock syndromes. This chapter discusses the contribution of inflammation in shock states, the systemic inflammatory response syndrome, and two life-threatening conditions where inflammation plays the predominant role: septic shock and anaphylactic shock.

INFLAMMATORY MEDIATORS

Cytokines, eicosanoids, reactive oxygen species (ROS), nitric oxide, platelet activating factor, coagulation factors, and many more have been identified as inflammatory mediators. These mediators may interact to modify cell function, coagulation, regulate the inflammatory response, and initiate responses through a variety of potential pathways (1-4). Clearly, this is the reason there no single therapy for all.

CONSEQUENCES OF ACUTE INFLAMMATION

Edema

Inflammation also promotes endothelial damage from oxidant stress (5), and this leads to increased capillary permeability and edema formation. At the capillary level, edema impairs oxygen delivery to the cells by increasing the distance that oxygen must travel. Pulmonary edema from inflammation, e.g., COVID-19 or acute respiratory distress syndrome (ARDS), fills the alveoli with fluid preventing gas exchange. In the setting of anaphylaxis (discussed in the section that follows), laryngeal edema leads to airway obstruction requiring emergent medical intervention.

Vasoplegia

Vasoplegia is an extreme, uncontrollable vasodilatation resulting in decreased systemic vascular resistance and hypotension with a normal or elevated cardiac output. It was initially described following cardiopulmonary bypass (6-7). The pathophysiology can result from several inflammatory mechanisms including dramatic increases in nitric oxide from inducible nitric oxide synthase (iNOS), endotoxins, endothelins, and other modulators (7-8). A further consequence of vasoplegia is its interference with vascular autoregulation leading to microvascular shunting, which reduces oxygen delivery to the cells and intrapulmonary shunting (physiologic) resulting in poor ventilation/perfusion mismatching.

Cardiac Dysfunction

Cardiac dysfunction can occur from a wide variety of inflammatory mediators (9). Up to 40% of patients with sepsis develop myocardial dysfunction with a mortality rate approaching 70% (10). Sepsis-induced cardiomyopathy (SICM) is described as a global decrease in contractility (biventricular hypokinesis) that is reversible (11-12). Takotsubo cardiomyopathy, also known as "stress cardiomyopathy," can also be seen in severe sepsis/septic shock and manifests as apical "ballooning" (13-14). See Figure 18.1.

Mitochondrial Dysfunction and Cytopathic Hypoxia

The mitochondria, referred to as the "powerhouse of the cell," are responsible for the production of adenosine triphosphate (ATP) through oxidative phosphorylation, with the final step requiring oxygen. (See Chapter 15: Approaches to Clinical Shock.) Mitochondrial dysfunction from inflammation can

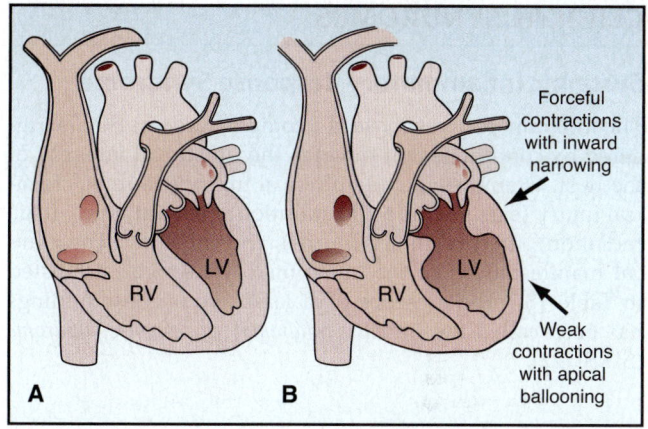

FIGURE 18.1. A. Normal contractility. B. Takotsubo cardiomyopathy with apical "ballooning."

lead to cytotoxic shock where the cells cannot process oxygen despite adequate oxygen delivery. This may manifest as decreased oxygen extraction when increased extraction would be expected. In contrast, hypoxia will cause the release of inflammatory mediators, such as nitric oxide, which damages cells and mitochondrial dysfunction, which impairs oxidative phosphorylation, affecting all organ systems (hypoxia) and contributing to multiple system organ dysfunction and/or failure. This illustrates the self-perpetuating theme (15-17).

Microvascular Thrombosis

Inflammation and coagulation are directly linked with inflammatory mediators stimulating the coagulation cascade and thrombosis and vice versa (18-20). The thrombosis obstructs oxygen delivery to the cells leading to hypoxia, tissue damage, and release of inflammatory mediators further contributing to multiple organ dysfunction syndrome. Microvascular thrombosis plays a major role in the inflammatory response and outcomes in COVID-19 (21).

CLINICAL SYNDROMES

Systemic Inflammatory Response Syndrome

The inflammatory response is a complex process that is triggered by conditions that threaten the functional integrity of the host. Examples include physical injury (trauma), chemical injury (e.g., gastric acid aspiration), oxidant injury (e.g., radiation), thermal injury (burns), and infection. The clinical manifestations of the inflammatory response are listed in Table 18.1; the presence of at least two of these findings has been called the *systemic inflammatory response syndrome* (SIRS) (22).

TABLE 18.1 Systemic Inflammatory Response Syndrome

The diagnosis of SIRS requires at least two of the following:

1. Temperature >38°C or 36°C
2. Heart rate >90 beats/min
3. Respiratory rate >20 breathes/min, or $PaCO_2$ <32 mm Hg (<4.3 kPa)
4. WBC count >12,000/mm^3 or <4000/mm^3, or 10% immature neutrophils (band forms)

SIRS = systemic inflammatory response syndrome.

From Pittet D, Range-Frausto S, Li N, et al. Systemic inflammatory response syndrome, sepsis, severe sepsis, and septic shock: incidence, morbidities and outcomes in surgical ICU patients. Intensive Care Med 1995;21:302-9.

The presence of SIRS does not indicate the presence of infection, i.e., infection is identified in only 25-50% of patients with SIRS (23-24). SIRS may not always indicate inflammation, as conditions like anxiety can cause tachycardia and tachypnea, meeting the criteria for SIRS without an inflammatory response. SIRS is essentially a signal to search for responsible conditions.

Septic Shock

Sepsis is an infection (suspected or confirmed) that is associated with life-threatening organ dysfunction and is the result of a dysregulated host response to infection. Essentially, SIRS is a response to an infection. Septic shock is a subset of sepsis that is characterized by the need for vasopressor support, and by a plasma lactate >2 mmol/L (25). Clearly, a more marked inflammatory response that carries a mortality rate 35-55%, compared with the mortality rate of 10-20% for sepsis (25-27).

Hemodynamic Alterations

Septic shock is characterized by systemic *vasodilation* (vasoplegia) involving both arteries and veins, which reduces ventricular preload (from venodilation) and ventricular afterload (from arterial vasodilation). The vascular changes are attributed to the enhanced production of nitric oxide (inflammatory mediator) in vascular endothelial cells (28). Endothelial injury from neutrophil attachment and degranulation leads to fluid extravasation and hypovolemia (28), further adding to the reduced preload.

Proinflammatory cytokines promote cardiac dysfunction (both systolic and diastolic dysfunction); however, the cardiac output is usually increased early as a result of tachycardia and decreased afterload (29).

Despite the increased cardiac output in early septic shock, splanchnic blood flow is typically reduced in septic shock (28). This can lead to disruption of the intestinal mucosa and "translocation" of enteric pathogens and endotoxins across the mucosa and into the systemic circulation. This can be a source of progressive and unregulated systemic inflammation (which is the source of organ dysfunction in sepsis and septic shock).

In the advanced stages of septic shock, cardiac output begins to decline, eventually resulting in a hemodynamic pattern that resembles cardiogenic shock with high cardiac filling pressures, low cardiac output, and increased systemic vascular resistance (SICM and Takotsubo) (11,13-14).

Mitochondrial Dysfunction and Cytopathic Hypoxia

The decrease in mitochondrial O_2 usage in septic shock is associated with a decrease in O_2 extraction from microcirculation (i.e., a decrease in the arteriovenous O_2 saturation difference). As a result, the central venous O_2 saturation ($ScvO_2$) and mixed venous oxygen saturation (SVO_2) will be inappropriately increased and misleading as a measure of the adequacy of O_2 delivery.

Initial Management

The initial management of septic shock described here is based on the most recent guidelines from the Surviving Sepsis Campaign (30). See Table 18.2.

TABLE 18.2 Initial Management of Septic Shock

Therapy	Recommendations
Volume infusion	• 30 mL/kg (ideal body weight) of a crystalloid fluid, infused within 3 h of presentation
Vasopressor therapy	• Can be initiated through a peripheral vein that is proximal to the antecubital fossa • Begin with norepinephrine and titrate dose to achieve an MAP ≥65 mm Hg. • If the required dose of norepinephrine is 0.25-0.5 μg/kg/min, add vasopressin. • If necessary, add epinephrine as a third vasopressor.
Corticosteroid therapy	• If the norepinephrine dose is >0.25 μg/kg/min, give IV hydrocortisone, 50 mg every 6 h.
Antimicrobial therapy	• Initiate treatment within 1 h of presentation. • Obtain appropriate cultures prior to first dose of antibiotic.

From Evans L, Rhodes A, Alhazzan W, et al. Surviving sepsis campaign: international guidelines for management of sepsis and septic shock, 2021. Intensive Care Med 2021;47:1181-247.

Volume Infusion. The priority in septic shock is preload because cardiac filling (preload) is reduced as a result of vasoplegia and third-spacing from fluid extravasation through "leaky capillaries." Balanced crystalloids are preferred. See Chapter 11: Fluid Management for greater detail.

Vasopressor Therapy. Volume resuscitation does not correct hypotension in septic shock due to vasoplegia, and vasopressor therapy is needed to achieve a mean arterial pressure (MAP) ≥65 mm Hg. Vasopressor options with dosages are shown in Table 18.3 (31-34).

Off-Label Therapy. Methylene blue has evidence to support its use in vasoplegic syndrome from cardiopulmonary bypass (35-36); however, there is some data to support its use in sepsis (37).

Hydroxycobalamin, indicated for cyanide toxicity, is a potent inhibitor of nitric oxide and nitric oxide synthase (6). Similarly, hydroxycobalamin is useful in vasoplegia due to cardiopulmonary bypass, but the current experience regarding septic shock is inconsistent (38-40).

Inotropic Therapy. Although there is no guideline recommendation to initiate inotropic therapy, a cardiac index of <2.2 L/min/m^2 is often cited as a trigger (41). When the ScvO$_2$ is low (<70%), despite correction of the blood pressure with vasopressors and hemoglobin >7.0, then O$_2$ delivery is inadequate, and infusion of the positive inotropic agent is indicated. Inotropic options are shown in Table 18.4. Continuous blood pressure and cardiac output monitoring (invasively or noninvasively) is strongly advised when using inotropes.

Corticosteroids. Corticosteroid therapy is suggested for patients with septic shock who are receiving norepinephrine or epinephrine at a dose ≥0.25 µg/kg/min. The recommended regimen is intravenous (IV) hydrocortisone in a dose of 50 mg every 6 h (200 mg daily) (32). There is no recommendation for the duration of treatment.

TABLE 18.3	Parenteral Vasopressors	
Agent	Dose	Comments
Norepinephrine*	5-40 µg/min	The most widely used vasopressor in clinical shock
Epinephrine	0.1-0.5 µg/kg/min	Drug of choice for anaphylactic shock, and second-line agent for septic shock Promotes lactate production
Dopamine	5-50 µg/kg/min	Once popular, but hampered by undesirable cardiac stimulation
Phenylephrine	0.5-6 µg/kg/min	A pure α agonist used mostly for anesthesia-related hypotension
Vasopressin	0.01-0.04 U/h	A pure α agonist Has no chronic trophic effects
Angiotensin II	*Initial dose:* 20 ng/kg/min via continuous IV infusion *Maintenance dose:* Titrate every 5 min by increments of up to 15 ng/kg/min as needed to achieve or maintain target blood pressure; not to exceed 40 ng/kg/min	Used a second agent in cases of septic shock resistant to norepinephrine

*Preferred vasopressor for septic shock.

Adapted from Approaches to Clinical Shock. In: Marino PL. *Marino's The ICU Book*. 5th ed. Wolters Kluwer; 2025. Table 14.4.

TABLE 18.4	Inotropic Agents		
Agent	Mechanism of Action	Initial Dosing	Comments
Dobutamine	β-1 agonist	5 µg/kg/min	Can cause vasodilatation and hypotension and tachyarrhythmias.
Milrinone	Phosphodiesterase III inhibitor	50 µg/kg over 10 min; followed by 0.5 µg/kg/min	Can cause vasodilatation and hypotension and *tachyarrhythmias*. Preferred for pulmonary hypertension and right heart failure
Levosimendan	Increases myofilament calcium sensitivity	Loading dose: 10 µg/kg over 10 min; followed by 0.1 µg/kg/min	Can cause vasodilatation and hypotension and tachyarrhythmias. Less myocardial oxygen consumption

Antimicrobial Therapy. Delays in initiating appropriate antibiotic therapy can adversely affect outcomes in septic shock, which is the basis for the recommendation that antimicrobial therapy should be started within the first hour after the diagnosis of septic shock (30). Optimally, appropriate cultures should be obtained prior to antibiotic administration to improve pathogen identification (and sensitivities) critical to targeted antibiotic administration.

ANAPHYLACTIC SHOCK

Anaphylaxis is a life-threatening, rapidly progressing allergic reaction produced by the immunogenic release of inflammatory mediators from basophils and mast cells. The characteristic feature is an exaggerated immunoglobulin E (IgE) response to an external antigen, i.e., a hypersensitivity reaction. Common triggers include food, antimicrobial agents, and insect bites. The manifestation of hypotension with evidence of systemic hypoperfusion (e.g., depressed consciousness) defines *anaphylactic shock*.

Clinical Features

Anaphylactic reactions are typically abrupt in onset, appearing within seconds of exposure to the external trigger (42). However, some reactions can appear as late as 72 h after exposure (43). A characteristic feature of anaphylactic reactions is edema and swelling caused by increased vascular permeability and fluid extravasation. The clinical manifestations of anaphylaxis are shown in Table 18.5.

TABLE 18.5 Signs and Symptoms of Anaphylaxis

Manifestation	Frequency of Occurrence
Urticaria and angioedema	60-90%
Upper airway angioedema	50-60%
Flushing	45-55%
Dyspnea, wheezing	45-50%
Hypotension, syncope	30-35%
Abdominal pain, diarrhea	25-30%
Acute coronary syndrome	4-5%

From Lieberman P, Nicklas RA, Randolph, et al. Anaphylaxis—a practice parameter update 2015. Ann Allergy Asthma Immunol 2015;115:341-84.

Management

Anaphylactic shock is an immediate threat to life, with profound hypotension from systemic vasodilation and fluid loss through leaky capillaries. The hemodynamic alterations are similar to those in septic shock but are more pronounced.

Epinephrine

There is no standardized dosing regimen for epinephrine in anaphylactic shock, but the IV regimen (5-15 µg/min), has been cited for its efficacy (43). A bolus dose (5-10 µg) can precede the continuous infusion (44).

Management of Anaphylaxis

Epinephrine is the main treatment for anaphylaxis and has several beneficial effects. A summary of the effects of epinephrine to treat anaphylaxis is shown in Table 18.6.

TABLE 18.6 Summary of Epinephrine Effects on Anaphylaxis

- Blocks the release of inflammatory mediators from sensitized basophils and mast cells
- Vasoconstrictive effects reverse histamine mediated vasodilatation.
- Vasoconstrictive effects reduce laryngospasm by reducing edema.
- Relieves bronchospasm via stimulation of β-2 receptors
- Cardiac stimulant (beta-s receptors) increasing heart rate and contractility

The usual treatment for anaphylactic reactions is 0.3-0.5 mg of epinephrine (0.3-0.5 mL of 1:1,000 epinephrine solution) administered by deep intramuscular (IM) injection in the lateral thigh and repeated every 5 min if necessary (43). Epinephrine can be nebulized for laryngeal edema.

Volume Resuscitation

Aggressive volume resuscitation is essential in anaphylactic shock because *35% of the intravascular volume can be lost through leaky capillaries* (43). The initial volume resuscitation should include 1-2 L of crystalloid fluid (or 20 mL/kg), or 500 mL of 5% albumin, given over 5-10 min (43). Thereafter, the infusion rate of fluids should be tailored to the hemodynamic status of the patient.

Refractory Hypotension

Persistent hypotension despite epinephrine infusion and volume resuscitation can be managed by adding *glucagon* or another vasopressor (e.g., *norepinephrine*).

Glucagon

Epinephrine inhibits degranulation of inflammatory cells by stimulating β-adrenergic receptors, and ongoing therapy with β-receptor antagonists can attenuate or eliminate the response. Glucagon can restore epinephrine responsiveness. The dose of glucagon is 1-5 mg by slow IV injection, followed by a continuous infusion at 5-15 µg/min (45). Glucagon can induce vomiting, and patients with depressed consciousness should be placed on their side to reduce the risk of aspiration.

Adjunctive Treatments

The following drugs are used to treat the consequences of anaphylaxis and will not hasten the resolution of the underlying process.

Antihistamines. Histamine receptor antagonists can be used to relieve pruritus in cutaneous reactions. The histamine-H_1 blocker *diphenhydramine* (25-50 mg PO, IM, or IV) and the histamine-H_2 blocker *ranitidine* (50 mg IV or 150 mg PO) should be given together because they are more effective in combination. The routine use of antihistamines is no longer recommended as initial treatment of anaphylaxis (46).

Bronchodilators. Inhaled β-2 receptor agonists like *albuterol* are used to relieve bronchospasm and are administered by nebulizer (2.5 mL or a 0.5% solution) or by metered-dose inhaler.

Corticosteroids. Despite the popularity of steroids for hypersensitivity reactions, there is no evidence that steroids are effective in reversing, slowing, or preventing recurrences of anaphylactic reactions. As a result, the most recent guideline on treating anaphylaxis does not include a recommendation for steroid therapy (46).

References

1. Akdis M, Aab A, Altunbulakli C, et al. Interleukins (from IL-1 to IL-38), interferons, transforming growth factor β, and TNF-α: receptors, functions, and roles in diseases. J Allergy Clin Immunol 2016;138:984-1010.
2. Eltzschig HK, Carmeliet P. Hypoxia and inflammation. N Engl J Med 2011;364:656-65.
3. Justiz Vaillant AA, Qurie A. Interleukin. [Updated 2022 Aug 22]. In: StatPearls [Internet]. Treasure Island (FL): StatPearls Publishing; 2025 Jan-.
4. Koller GM, Schafer C, Kemp SS, et al. Proinflammatory mediators, IL (interleukin)-1β, TNF (tumor necrosis factor) α, and thrombin directly induce capillary tube regression. Arterioscler Thromb Vasc Biol 2020;40:365-77.
5. Huet O, Obata R, Aubron C, et al. Plasma-induced endothelial oxidative stress is related to the severity of septic shock. Crit Care Med 2007;35:821-6.
6. Busse LW, Barker N, Petersen C. Vasoplegic syndrome following cardiothoracic surgery-review of pathophysiology and update of treatment options. Crit Care 2020;24:36.
7. Ratnani I, Ochani RK, Shaikh A, Jatoi HN. Vasoplegia: a review. Methodist Debakey Cardiovasc J 2023;19:38-47.
8. Levy B, Fritz C, Tahon E, et al. Vasoplegia treatments: The past, the present, and the future. Crit Care 2018;22:52.
9. Reina-Couto M, Pereira-Terra P, Quelhas-Santos J, et al. Inflammation in human heart failure: Major mediators and therapeutic targets. Front Physiol 2021;12:746494.
10. Li Y, Ge S, Peng Y, Chen X. Inflammation and cardiac dysfunction during sepsis, muscular dystrophy, and myocarditis. Burns Trauma 2013;1:109-21.

11. Borkowski P, Borkowski M, Borkowska N, et al. The complexities of sepsis-induced cardiomyopathy: a clinical case and review of inflammatory pathways and potential therapeutic targets. Cureus 2024;16:e75173.
12. Kakihana Y, Ito T, Nakahara M, et al. Sepsis-induced myocardial dysfunction: pathophysiology and management. J Intensive Care 2016;4:22.
13. Sato R, Nasu M. A review of sepsis-induced cardiomyopathy. J Intensive Care 2015;3:48.
14. Zhang H, Liu D. Sepsis-related cardiomyopathy: not an easy task for ICU physicians. J Intensive Med 2022;2:257-9.
15. Bouhamida E, Morciano G, Perrone M, et al. The interplay of hypoxia signaling on mitochondrial dysfunction and inflammation in cardiovascular diseases and cancer: from molecular mechanisms to therapeutic approaches. Biology (Basel) 2022;11.
16. Park DW, Zmijewski JW. Mitochondrial dysfunction and immune cell metabolism in sepsis. Infect Chemother 2017;49:10-21.
17. Staal J, Blanco LP, Perl A. Editorial: mitochondrial dysfunction in inflammation and autoimmunity. Front Immunol 2023;14:1304315.
18. Aksu K, Donmez A, Keser G. Inflammation-induced thrombosis: Mechanisms, disease associations and management. Curr Pharm Des 2012;18:1478-93.
19. Maneta E, Aivalioti E, Tual-Chalot S, et al. Endothelial dysfunction and immunothrombosis in sepsis. Front Immunol 2023;14:1144229.
20. Stark K, Massberg S. Interplay between inflammation and thrombosis in cardiovascular pathology. Nat Rev Cardiol 2021;18:666-82.
21. Wadowski PP, Panzer B, Jozkowicz A, et al. Microvascular thrombosis as a critical factor in severe COVID-19. Int J Mol Sci 2023;24.
22. Bone RC, Sprung CL, Sibbald WJ. Definitions for sepsis and organ failure. Crit Care Med 1992;20:724-6.
23. Pittet D, Rangel-Frausto S, Li N, et al. Systemic inflammatory response syndrome, sepsis, severe sepsis and septic shock: incidence, morbidities and outcomes in surgical ICU patients. Intensive Care Med 1995;21:302-9.
24. Rangel-Frausto MS, Pittet D, Costigan M, et al. The natural history of the systemic inflammatory response syndrome (SIRS). A prospective study. JAMA 1995;273:117-23.
25. Singer M, Deutschman CS, Seymour CW, et al. The third international consensus definitions for sepsis and septic shock (Sepsis-3). JAMA 2016;315:801-10.
26. Kramarow EA. Sepsis-related mortality among adults aged 65 and over: United states, 2019. NCHS Data Brief 2021:1-8.
27. Mahapatra S, Heffner AC. Septic Shock. In: StatPearls. Treasure Island (FL): StatPearls Publishing; 2025.
28. Abraham E, Singer M. Mechanisms of sepsis-induced organ dysfunction. Crit Care Med 2007;35:2408-16.

29. Snell RJ, Parrillo JE. Cardiovascular dysfunction in septic shock. Chest 1991;99:1000-9.
30. Dellinger RP, Levy MM, Rhodes A, et al. Surviving sepsis campaign: international guidelines for management of severe sepsis and septic shock, 2012. Intensive Care Med 2013;39:165-228.
31. Coloretti I, Genovese A, Teixeira JP, et al. Angiotensin II therapy in refractory septic shock: which patient can benefit most? a narrative review. J Anesth Analg Crit Care 2024;4:13.
32. Evans L, Rhodes A, Alhazzani W, et al. Surviving sepsis campaign: international guidelines for management of sepsis and septic shock 2021. Intensive Care Med 2021;47:1181-247.
33. Khanna A, English SW, Wang XS, et al. Angiotensin III for the treatment of vasodilatory shock. N Engl J Med 2017;377:419-30.
34. Sacha GL, Bauer SR. Optimizing vasopressin use and initiation timing in septic shock: a narrative review. Chest 2023;164:1216-27.
35. Kofler O, Simbeck M, Tomasi R, et al. Early use of methylene blue in vasoplegic syndrome: a 10-year propensity score-matched cohort study. J Clin Med 2022;11.
36. Mehaffey JH, Johnston LE, Hawkins RB, et al. Methylene blue for vasoplegic syndrome after cardiac operation: early administration improves survival. Ann Thorac Surg 2017;104:36-41.
37. Naoum EE, Dalia AA, Roberts RJ, et al. Methylene blue for vasodilatory shock in the intensive care unit: a retrospective, observational study. BMC Anesthesiol 2022;22:199.
38. Drug Information Group, Retzkey College of Pharmacy. Is intravenous hydroxocobalamin an effective treatment for vasoplegia-associated shock? Accessed June 28 2025. https://dig.pharmacy.uic.edu/faqs/2024-2/april-2024-faqs/is-intravenous-hydroxocobalamin-an-effective-treatment-for-vasoplegia-associated-shock/
39. Patel JJ, Willoughby R, Peterson J, et al. High-dose IV hydroxocobalamin (vitamin B_{12}) in septic shock: a double-blind, allocation-concealed, placebo-controlled single-center pilot randomized controlled trial (the intravenous hydroxocobalamin in septic shock trial). Chest 2023;163:303-12.
40. Sacco AJ, Cunningham CA, Kosiorek HE, Sen A. Hydroxocobalamin in refractory septic shock: a retrospective case series. Crit Care Explor 2021;3:e0408.
41. Sato R, Hasegawa D, Guo S, et al. Sepsis-induced cardiogenic shock: controversies and evidence gaps in diagnosis and management. J Intensive Care 2025;13:1.
42. Shaker MS, Wallace DV, Golden DBK, et al. Anaphylaxis—a 2020 practice parameter update, systematic review, and Grading of Recommendations, Assessment, Development and Evaluation (GRADE) analysis. J Allergy Clin Immunol 2020;145:1082-123.
43. Lieberman P, Nicklas RA, Oppenheimer J, et al. The diagnosis and management of anaphylaxis practice parameter: 2010 update. J Allergy Clin Immunol 2010;126:477-80.e1-42.

44. Sampson HA, Munoz-Furlong A, Campbell RL, et al. Second symposium on the definition and management of anaphylaxis: summary report—second National Institute of Allergy and Infectious Disease/Food Allergy and Anaphylaxis Network symposium. Ann Emerg Med 2006;47:373-80.
45. Boyce JA, Assa'ad A, Burks AW, et al. Guidelines for the diagnosis and management of food allergy in the United States: report of the NIAID-sponsored expert panel. J Allergy Clin Immunol 2010;126:S1-58.
46. Dodd A, Hughes A, Sargant N, et al. Evidence update for the treatment of anaphylaxis. Resuscitation 2021;163:86-96.

CARDIAC DISORDERS
SECTION V

Acute Heart Failure(s)
Chapter 19

This chapter describes the diagnosis and management of acute heart failure. Heart failure is becoming increasingly prevalent in the United States, with over 6.7 million adults with heart failure and 50% more deaths attributed to heart failure in 2020 as compared to 2010 (1).

TYPES OF HEART FAILURE

Heart failure can be the result of a decrease in contractile strength (systolic dysfunction) or impaired cardiac filling (diastolic dysfunction). The end-diastolic volume (EDV) can distinguish between systolic and diastolic dysfunction in patients with heart failure. An EDV >97 mL/m^2 indicates systolic dysfunction and an EDV <97 mL/m^2 indicates diastolic dysfunction (2).

Systolic Dysfunction

The ejection fraction (EF) is a measurement of the blood volume ejected during systole and is most often assessed with echocardiography. An EF >55% is considered normal, but in patients with heart failure, a lower value (>50%) is used because increases in afterload can reduce the EF by 5-10% (3). The left ventricular EF (LVEF) is used to classify heart failure as shown in Table 19.1.

Diastolic Dysfunction

Diastolic dysfunction is defined by a decrease in ventricular distensibility with impairment of ventricular filling during diastole. Diastolic dysfunction is recognized as a cause of heart failure in at least 50% of cases (3). In diastolic dysfunction, the

EF is preserved Heart Failure with preserved ejection fraction (HFpEF), but the stroke volume is decreased due to a decrease in EDV. Common causes of heart failure with HFpEF are ventricular hypertrophy, myocardial ischemia, restrictive (fibrotic) cardiomyopathy, and pericardial tamponade. High intrathoracic pressures during mechanical ventilation can also impair ventricular filling and aggravate HFpEF (4).

TABLE 19.1 Classification of Heart Failure Based on Left Ventricular Ejection Fraction (LVEF)

Category	LVEF	Problem
Heart Failure with preserved ejection fraction (HFpEF)	≥50%	Diastolic Dysfunction
Heart Failure with mildly reduced ejection fraction (HFmrEF)	41-49%	Systolic Dysfunction (mild)
Heart Failure with reduced ejection fraction (HFrEF)	≤40%	Systolic Dysfunction (moderate/severe)

From Bozkurt B, Coats AJ, Tsutsui H, et al. Universal definition and classification of heart failure: a report of the Heart Failure Society of America, Heart Failure Association of the European Society of Cardiology, Japanese Heart Failure Society and Writing Committee of the Universal Definition of Heart Failure. J Card Fail 2021;27:387-413.

Right Heart Failure

Right heart failure (RHF) is defined as the inability of the right ventricle to maintain optimal circulation in the presence of adequate preload (5). RHF is distinguished from structural right ventricular (RV) dysfunction using signs and symptoms that define RHF as a clinical syndrome (5). Common causes of acute RHF are listed in Table 19.2 and include disease processes that decrease RV contractility and conditions associated with RV volume or pressure overload.

TABLE 19.2 Causes of Acute RHF

Decreased RV Contractility	RV Volume Overload	RV Pressure Overload
Sepsis	Sepsis	Acidosis
LVAD support	LVAD support	Hypoxia
Right ventricular myocardial infarction	Excessive transfusions	Pulmonary embolism
Myocarditis	Excessive crystalloid / colloid infusions	ARDS
Perioperative injury / ischemia (postcardiotomy)		Positive pressure ventilation

ARDS = acute respiratory distress syndrome (see Chapter 25); LVAD = left ventricular assist device; RHF = right heart failure; RV = right ventricular.

From Konstam MA, Kiernan MS, Bernstein D, et al. Evaluation and management of right-sided heart failure: a scientific statement from the American Heart Association. Circulation 2018;137(20):e578-e622.

Under normal physiological conditions, the RV pumps blood into a highly compliant low resistance pulmonary circulation (5). *Hence, the RV is highly sensitive to afterload, and minor increases in pulmonary artery pressures can lead to significant decreases in stroke volume.* Normal and abnormal RV anatomy is demonstrated in Figure 19.1.

Echocardiography

Transthoracic echocardiography is the standard for assessing right heart function (see Chapter 7: Bedside Echocardiography) (6). In Figure 19.2, the pathophysiological consequences associated with RV dilation are shown.

Cardiac Filling Pressures

When data from a pulmonary artery catheter is available, RHF is likely when the central venous pressure (CVP) is equal to, or greater than, the pulmonary artery wedge pressure

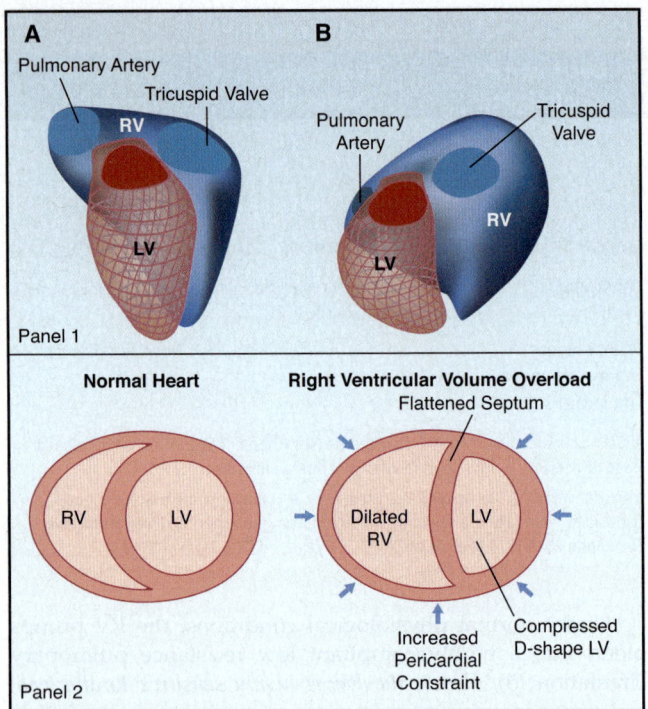

FIGURE 19.1. A. Normal right ventricle (RV). Note the hemi-ellipsoid shape that partially surrounds the left ventricle (LV). In cross section (panel 2), the RV approximates 2/3 of the LV volume. B. RV failure. The RV is distended and the shape distorted. In panel 2, the distended RV causes a leftward shift of the interventricular septum towards the LV. As a result of these changes, cardiac output is decreased. (Derived from Konstam MA, Kiernan MS, Bernstein D, et al. Evaluation and management of right-sided heart failure: a scientific statement from the American Heart Association. Circulation 2018;137[20]:e578-e622.)

(PAWP) (7). CVP and PAWP equalization is also possible in pericardial tamponade; thus, echocardiography is required to distinguish tamponade from RHF.

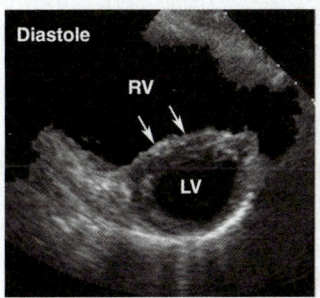 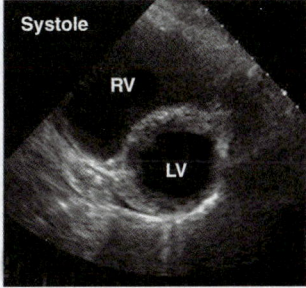

FIGURE 19.2. Transthoracic ultrasound image in the parasternal short-axis view showing RV enlargement, where the RV cavity is larger than the LV cavity. Note also that the interventricular septum is flattened during diastole (indicated by the arrows) which is a sign of RV volume overload. (Image retouched from Rudski LG, Lai WW, Afilalo J, et al. Guidelines for the echocardiographic assessment of the right heart in adults: a report from the American Society of Echocardiography endorsed by the European Association of Echocardiography, a registered branch of the European Society of Cardiology, and the Canadian Society of Echocardiography. J Am Soc Echocardiogr 2010;23[7]:685-788.)

CARDIOVASCULAR CONSEQUENCES

The pathophysiological consequences of heart failure are the result of venous congestion and a reduction of forward blood flow.

Stages and Classes of Heart Failure

Progressive changes in cardiac performance and symptoms (i.e., New York Heart Association Classification) occur as heart failure worsens, as listed in Table 19.3 (8).

Neurohumoral Responses

As the EDV increases, atrial and ventricular wall tension increases, resulting in the release of natriuretic peptides from cardiac myocytes. Concentrations of brain-type (B-type) natriuretic peptide (BNP) and other natriuretic proteins can be assessed with blood tests (9). Assays include BNP, pro-BNP (a prohormone), and N-terminal (NT)-proBNP (a byproduct of pro-BNP cleavage). Heart failure is unlikely if BNP levels are <100 picograms/mL or if NT-pro-BNP levels are <300 picograms/mL (10-12). There are several conditions, aside from heart failure, that elevate natriuretic proteins, as listed in Table 19.4.

TABLE 19.3 Progressive Physiological Stages of Heart Failure and Corresponding NYHA Heart Failure Classes

Physiological Changes	NYHA Class[†]
• Increased end-diastolic filling pressure (pulmonary capillary wedge pressure) • Stroke volume is maintained	I - No limitation of physical activity. Ordinary physical activity does not cause undue fatigue, palpitation or shortness of breath.
• Venous congestion, dyspnea	II - Slight limitation of physical activity. Comfortable at rest. Ordinary physical activity results in fatigue, palpitations, shortness of breath or chest pain.
• Decreased stroke volume • Increased heart rate (to offset the decreased stroke volume)	III - Marked limitation of physical activity. Comfortable at rest. Less than ordinary activity causes fatigue, palpitations, shortness of breath or chest pain.
• Decreased cardiac output (signifies the transition from compensated to decompensated heart failure) • Further increase in end-diastolic filling pressure	IV - Symptoms of heart failure at rest. Any physical activity causes further discomfort.

NYHA = New York Heart Association.

[†]NHYA class symptoms may vary between physiological stages, depending on the level of compensation.

From Dolgin M. *Nomenclature and Criteria for Diagnosis of Diseases of the Heart and Great Vessels*. 9th ed. Little Brown & Co; 1994.

TABLE 19.4 Causes of Elevated Natriuretic Peptide Levels

Cardiac	Noncardiac
Heart failure (R and L)	Advanced Age
Myocarditis	Renal Failure
Ventricular Hypertrophy	Anemia
Acute Coronary Syndromes	Pulmonary Embolism
Pericardial Disease	Pulmonary Hypertension
Atrial Fibrillation	Bacterial Sepsis
Cardioversion	Critical Illness
Cardiac Surgery	

From Heidenreich PA, Bozkurt B, Aguilar D, et al. 2022 AHA/ACC/HFSA guideline for the management of heart failure: executive summary: a report of the American College of Cardiology/American Heart Association Joint Committee on clinical practice guidelines. J Am Coll Cardiol 2022;79(17):1757-80.

Because of the nonspecific nature of elevated peptide levels in critically ill patients, these assays are best suited to *rule out* acute heart failure (10).

Sympathetic Nervous System

Baroreceptors in the carotid and pulmonary arteries detect decreases in stroke volume, activating positive inotropic and chronotropic effects in the heart. Peripheral vasoconstriction also occurs as a sympathetic response aimed at maintaining blood flow to the vital organs.

Renin-Angiotensin-Aldosterone System

Renin is released from cells in the renal arterioles in response to renal hypoperfusion and adrenergic β-receptor activation. Renin stimulates the formation of angiotensin II, production of aldosterone in the adrenal cortex, and the release of arginine vasopressin from the posterior pituitary. *Angiotensin* produces systemic vasoconstriction, *aldosterone* promotes renal sodium and water retention, and *vasopressin* promotes both vasoconstriction and renal water retention (13). In advanced stages of heart failure, these changes can be deleterious because vasoconstriction can increase afterload, impeding systemic blood flow, and the retention of sodium and water can promote edema.

Venous Congestion

The principal manifestations of acute, decompensated heart failure are related to venous congestion (14). Pulmonary edema (as shown in Figure 19.3) and pleural effusions are common and will manifest as dyspnea and the presence of basilar crackles on lung auscultation.

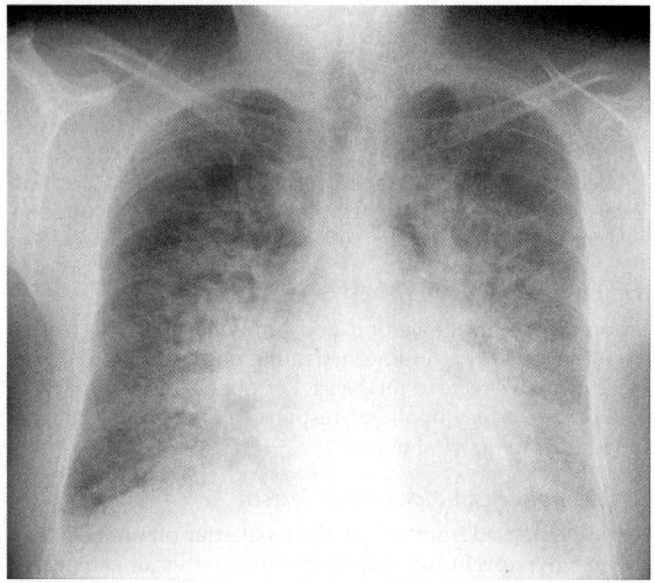

FIGURE 19.3. Portable chest x-ray in a patient with acute heart failure and pulmonary edema. Note that the infiltrates radiate out from the hilar regions, which is a feature that distinguishes cardiogenic from noncardiogenic pulmonary edema. (From Acute Heart Failure[s]. In: Marino PL. *Marino's The ICU Book*. 5th ed. Wolters Kluwer; 2025:291-306. Figure 18.4.)

Cardiorenal Syndrome. Heart failure is frequently accompanied by renal dysfunction (15). The renal dysfunction in acute heart failure is likely due to increased venous pressure rather than a reduction in cardiac output, though in cases with a low cardiac output, severe hypotension (i.e., cardiogenic shock) may also be contributory.

MANAGEMENT STRATEGIES

The management strategies discussed here pertain to acute left-sided systolic and diastolic heart failure.

High Blood Pressure

Vasodilators

Hypertension is common in heart failure and is often a secondary phenomenon caused by hypoxemia or agitation. Occasionally, hypertension is the primary problem (e.g., hypertensive emergency). Management begins with an infusion of a vasodilator, as listed in Table 19.5 (16-19).

Diuretics

Diuretics are administered after the blood pressure has been normalized because furosemide, the most popular diuretic used in heart failure, may produce an acute *arteriolar* vasoconstrictor response (20). Diuretics are discussed in more detail in the section that follows.

Normal Blood Pressure

In acute heart failure with a normal blood pressure, intravenous diuretics are indicated as an initial intervention. There are three concerns about intravenous diuretics that must be considered in acute heart failure with normal blood pressure:

1. Diuretics may cause a decrease in cardiac output in acute heart failure as the result of a decrease in venous return; the degree of this response depends on a patient's

TABLE 19.5 Vasodilator Infusions for Acute Heart Failure in Patients with High Blood Pressure

Agent	Mechanism of Action	Dosing Recommendations
Nitroglycerin	1. Nitroglycerin is converted to nitric oxide. 2. Nitric oxide activates guanylyl cyclase. 3. cGMP is generated, activating protein kinases that cause smooth muscle relaxation. 4. The primary action is *venodilation*.	1. Start infusion at 5 μg/min, and increase by 5 μg/min every 5 min to achieve the desired effect. The effective dose is 5-100 μg/min in most cases and doses above 200 μg/min are not advised. 2. The drug binds (up to 80%) to plastics such as polyvinylchloride, so glass bottles and polyethylene tubes must be used. 3. Tachyphylaxis is common after 24 h of continuous use. 4. Propylene glycol toxicity is a risk with prolonged infusions. 5. High doses can produce methemoglobinemia.
Nitroprusside	1. Acts as a prodrug 2. Reacts with sulfhydryl groups on erythrocytes and proteins (albumin) 3. Produces nitric oxide 4. The primary action is both *arteriolar* and *venodilation*.	1. Start infusion at 0.2 μg/kg/min and titrate upward every 5 min to achieve the desired effect. The effective dose is 2-5 μg/kg/min in most cases and the maximum dose allowed is 10 μg/kg/min. 2. Cyanide toxicity is possible as the agent contains 5 cyanide atoms; to reduce the risk of toxicity, avoid prolonged infusions >3 μg/kg/min (thiosulfate [500 mg] can be added to the infusate to bind the cyanide). 3. Since the liver and kidneys participate in cyanide clearance, the drug should not be used in patients with renal or hepatic insufficiency. 4. Not recommended for heart failure associated with coronary ischemia (can produce coronary steal syndrome).

cGMP = cyclic guanosine monophosphate.

From References 9, 16-19.

sodium status and degree of renin-angiotensin system activation (21).
2. Diuretics should be used cautiously in acute heart failure with preserved ejection fraction (HFpEF) because there is decreased cardiac filling in this form of heart failure (i.e., exacerbated by diuretics).
3. The presence of pulmonary edema may be due to myocardial stunning during ischemia (i.e., "flash" pulmonary edema). Diuretics should be used cautiously in this situation.

Table 19.6 lists dosing regimens for diuretics used in acute heart failure.

TABLE 19.6	Diuretic Therapy for Acute Heart Failure
Agent	Dosing Recommendations
Furosemide	1. For patients who are furosemide-naïve, start with an IV dose of 40 mg (for normal renal function) or 60-80 mg (for renal impairment).
	2. For patients already receiving furosemide, start with an IV dose equal to the total daily furosemide dose.
	3. If response not satisfactory after 2 h, double the dose, and continue this, if necessary, to a maximum dose of 200 mg.
	4. The effective IV dose is then given twice daily.
Bumetanide Torsemide	1. These loop diuretics have a greater bioavailability than furosemide and can be effective in cases of furosemide resistance.
	2. Dose equivalence: 40 mg furosemide = 1 mg bumetanide = 20 mg torsemide
Metolazone	1. A thiazide diuretic that can augment the effect of loop diuretics.
	2. Dose is 2.5-10 mg PO daily and should be given a few hours prior to the loop diuretic.
	3. Combination therapy increases the risk of hypokalemia.

From Heidenreich PA, Bozkurt B, Aguilar D, et al. 2022 AHA/ACC/HFSA guideline for the management of heart failure: executive summary: a report of the American College of Cardiology/American Heart Association Joint Committee on clinical practice guidelines. J Am Coll Cardiol 2022;79(17):1757-80.

Furosemide

Diuresis with furosemide should begin within 5 min and peak by 20-60 min. Higher doses are suggested (see Table 19.6) for patients with renal insufficiency (22-23). Prior to the diuretic effect, patients with pulmonary edema may report immediate relief of symptoms, possibly due to synthesis of prostaglandins, decreased pulmonary resistance, and improved gas exchange (23). When venous congestion has improved, furosemide can be given orally, but only 50% of an oral dose is absorbed, so doses may need to be adjusted upwards (22-23). In patients with hypoalbuminemia, some patients may have a poor response because furosemide is highly protein-bound. In cases of furosemide resistance, alternative loop diuretics should be considered, or thiazides such as metolazone may be added (see Table 19.6).

Continuous Furosemide Infusion. Compared to intermittent dosing, a continuous infusion of furosemide may be theoretically advantageous for patients who are massively volume-overloaded (24). Although continuous infusions are not consistently associated with improved outcomes such as decreased mortality or length of hospital stay, greater body weight reduction has been observed in some studies without any difference in adverse effects (24-25). A dosing regimen for continuous-infusion furosemide is provided in Figure 19.4 (26).

Management of Right Heart Failure

Volume Management

Volume management in acute RHF is a critical consideration because the myocardium of the RV is thinner and is incapable of generating as much pressure as the LV. Hence, *due to its highly compliant nature, the RV is more susceptible to volume overload*. In some cases, a small fluid bolus may be reasonable to prevent precipitous drops in preload, but more often diuresis is indicated to attenuate RV dilation, tricuspid regurgitation, increased RV afterload, and worsening myocardial tension (5). Diuretics, as described previously in this chapter, should not be held in most cases, including hypotensive patients who are volume overloaded on clinical exam (5).

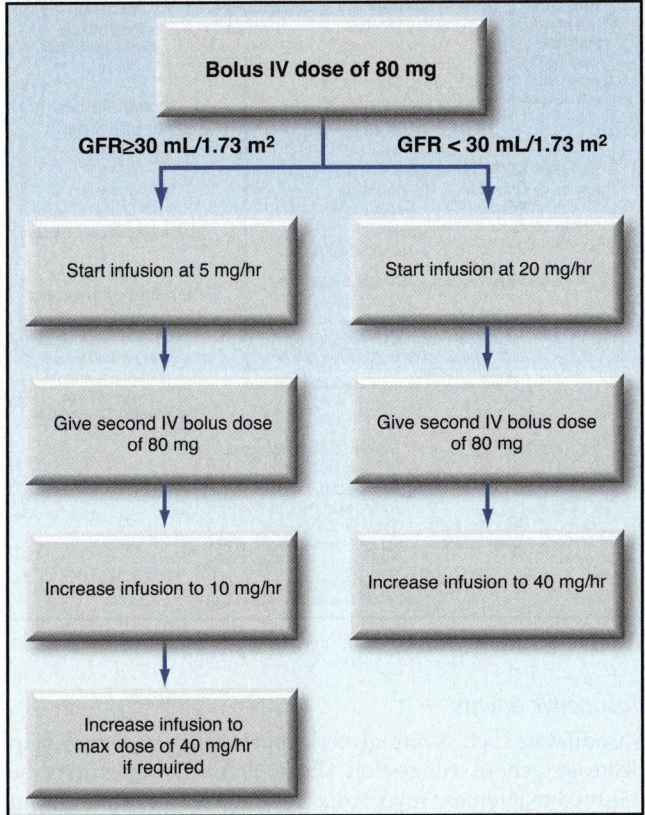

FIGURE 19.4. Dosing regimen for diuresis with continuous infusion furosemide. GFR = glomerular filtration rate. (From Ellison DH, Felker GM. Diuretic treatment in heart failure. N Engl J Med 2017;377[20]:1964-75.)

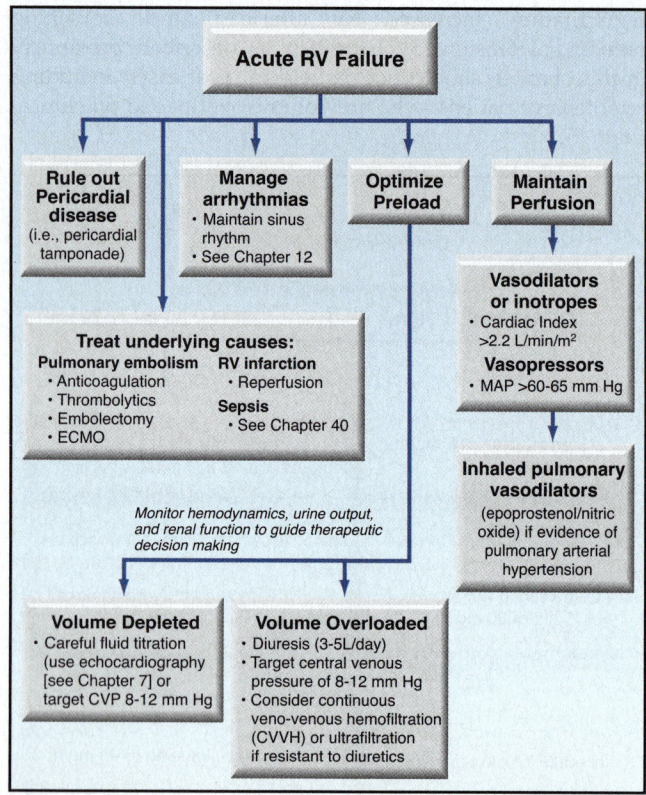

FIGURE 19.5. Management of right heart failure. (From Reference 5.)

Vasoactive Agents

Vasodilators such as nitroglycerin and nitroprusside may help decrease venous congestion (Table 19.5). Inotropes may be required to augment myocardial contractility if cardiac output and blood pressure are inadequate (5). Similar clinical outcomes have been observed with milrinone and dobutamine, though milrinone may have more potent pulmonary vasodilation properties and may be less likely to cause tachycardia (5).

In cases where hypotension persists, malperfusion and ischemia of the RV is possible and vasopressors such as dopamine, vasopressin, or norepinephrine may be needed. Vasopressin has been reported to have less pulmonary vasoconstrictive effects compared to other vasopressors and may also support glomerular filtration through its action as a selective efferent arteriolar constrictor (5). Figure 19.5 shows an overview of the management of RHF (5).

References

1. Tsao CW, Aday AW, Almarzooq ZI, et al. Heart disease and stroke statistics-2023 update: a report from the American Heart Association. Circulation 2023;147(8):e622.
2. Paulus WJ, Tschöpe C, Sanderson JE, et al. How to diagnose diastolic heart failure: a consensus statement on the diagnosis of heart failure with normal left ventricular ejection fraction by the Heart Failure and Echocardiography Associations of the European Society of Cardiology. Eur Heart J 2007;28(20):2539-50.
3. Bozkurt B, Coats AJ, Tsutsui H, et al. Universal definition and classification of heart failure: a report of the Heart Failure Society of America, Heart Failure Association of the European Society of Cardiology, Japanese Heart Failure Society and Writing Committee of the Universal Definition of Heart Failure. J Card Fail 2021;27:387-413.
4. Mahmood SS, Pinsky MR. Heart-lung interactions during mechanical ventilation: the basics. Ann Transl Med 2018;6(18):349.
5. Konstam MA, Kiernan MS, Bernstein D, et al. Evaluation and management of right-sided heart failure: a scientific statement from the American Heart Association. Circulation 2018;137(20):e578-e622.
6. Rudski LG, Lai WW, Afilalo J, et al. Guidelines for the echocardiographic assessment of the right heart in adults: a report from the American Society of Echocardiography endorsed by the European Association of Echocardiography, a registered branch of the European Society of Cardiology, and the Canadian Society of Echocardiography. J Am Soc Echocardiogr 2010;23(7):685-788.
7. Lopez-Sendon J, Coma-Canella I, Gamallo C. Sensitivity and specificity of hemodynamic criteria in the diagnosis of acute right ventricular infarction. Circulation 1981;64(3):515-25.
8. Dolgin M, Association NYH, Fox AC, Gorlin R, Levin RI, *New York Heart Association. Criteria Committee. Nomenclature and criteria for diagnosis of diseases of the heart and great vessels*. 9th ed. Little Brown & Co; 1994.

9. Heidenreich PA, Bozkurt B, Aguilar D, et al. 2022 AHA/ACC/HFSA guideline for the management of heart failure: executive summary: a report of the American College of Cardiology/American Heart Association Joint Committee on clinical practice guidelines. J Am Coll Cardiol 2022;79(17):1757-80.
10. Maisel AS, Krishnaswamy P, Nowak RM, et al. Rapid measurement of B-type natriuretic peptide in the emergency diagnosis of heart failure. N Engl J Med 2002;347(3):161-7.
11. Januzzi JL, van Kimmenade R, Lainchbury J, et al. NT-proBNP testing for diagnosis and short-term prognosis in acute destabilized heart failure: an international pooled analysis of 1256 patients: the International Collaborative of NT-proBNP Study. Eur Heart J 2006;27(3):330-7.
12. Maisel AS, McCord J, Nowak RM, et al. Bedside B-Type natriuretic peptide in the emergency diagnosis of heart failure with reduced or preserved ejection fraction. Results from the Breathing Not Properly Multinational Study. J Am Coll Cardiol 2003;41(11):2010-7.
13. Maryam, Varghese TP, B T. Unraveling the complex pathophysiology of heart failure: insights into the role of renin-angiotensin-aldosterone system (RAAS) and sympathetic nervous system (SNS). Curr Probl Cardiol 2024;49(4):102411.
14. Gheorghiade M, Pang PS. Acute heart failure syndromes. J Am Coll Cardiol 2009;53(7):557-73.
15. Heywood JT, Fonarow GC, Costanzo MR, et al. for the ADHERE Scientific Advisory Committee and Investigators. High prevalence of renal dysfunction and its impact on outcome in 118,465 patients hospitalized with acute decompensated heart failure: a report from the ADHERE database. J Card Fail 2007;13(6):422-30.
16. Demey HE, Daelemans RA, Verpooten GA, et al. Propylene glycol-induced side effects during intravenous nitroglycerin therapy. Intensive Care Med 1988;14(3):221-6.
17. Curry SC, Arnold-Capell P. Toxic effects of drugs used in the ICU. Nitroprusside, nitroglycerin, and angiotensin-converting enzyme inhibitors [published correction appears in Crit Care Clin 1994 Oct;10(4):xi]. Crit Care Clin 1991;7(3):555-81.
18. Hall VA, Guest JM. Sodium nitroprusside-induced cyanide intoxication and prevention with sodium thiosulfate prophylaxis. Am J Crit Care 1992;1(2):19-27.
19. Mann T, Cohn PF, Holman LB, et al. Effect of nitroprusside on regional myocardial blood flow in coronary artery disease. Results in 25 patients and comparison with nitroglycerin. Circulation 1978;57(4):732-8.
20. Francis GS, Siegel RM, Goldsmith SR, et al. Acute vasoconstrictor response to intravenous furosemide in patients with chronic congestive heart failure. Activation of the neurohumoral axis. Ann Intern Med 1985;103(1):1-6.

21. Jhund PS, McMurray JJ, Davie AP. The acute vascular effects of frusemide in heart failure. Br J Clin Pharmacol 2000;50(1):9-13.
22. Brater DC. Diuretic therapy. N Engl J Med 1998;339(6):387-95.
23. Huang X, Dorhout Mees E, Vos P, et al. Everything we always wanted to know about furosemide but were afraid to ask. Am J Physiol Renal Physiol 2016;310(10):F958-71.
24. Kuriyama A, Urushidani S. Continuous versus intermittent administration of furosemide in acute decompensated heart failure: a systematic review and meta-analysis. Heart Fail Rev 2019;24(1):31-9.
25. Fudim M, Spates T, Sun JL, et al. Early diuretic strategies and the association with in-hospital and post-discharge outcomes in acute heart failure. Am Heart J 2021;239:110-9.
26. Ellison DH, Felker GM. Diuretic treatment in heart failure. N Engl J Med 2017;377(20):1964-75.

Dysrhythmias — Chapter 20

This chapter describes tachyarrhythmias and bradyarrhythmias that require prompt evaluation and management in the ICU.

TACHYARRHYTHMIAS

There are three fundamental electrocardiograph (ECG) findings to consider when diagnosing a tachyarrhythmia: the duration of the QRS complex, the uniformity of the RR intervals, and the characteristics of the atrial activity. Figure 20.1 summarizes an approach for the evaluation of tachyarrhythmias based on these criteria.

Narrow Complex Tachycardias

A narrow QRS complex is defined as <0.12 s (1). Narrow complex tachyarrhythmias originate from a site above the atrioventricular (AV) conduction system and include sinus tachycardia, atrial tachycardia, AV nodal reentrant tachycardia (i.e., paroxysmal supraventricular tachycardia [PSVT]), atrial flutter, and atrial fibrillation (AF). The RR interval and characteristics of the atrial activity are used to identify the tachyarrhythmia (2).

Regular Rhythm

Tachyarrhythmias with a uniform RR interval include sinus tachycardia, AV nodal reentrant tachycardia (AVNRT), and atrial flutter with a fixed (i.e., 2:1, 3:1) AV block.

- *Uniform P waves and PR intervals are consistent with sinus tachycardia.*
- *The absence of P waves suggests an AVNRT (Figure 20.2).*
- *Sawtooth waves are evidence of atrial flutter.*

CHAPTER 20 ■ Dysrhythmias

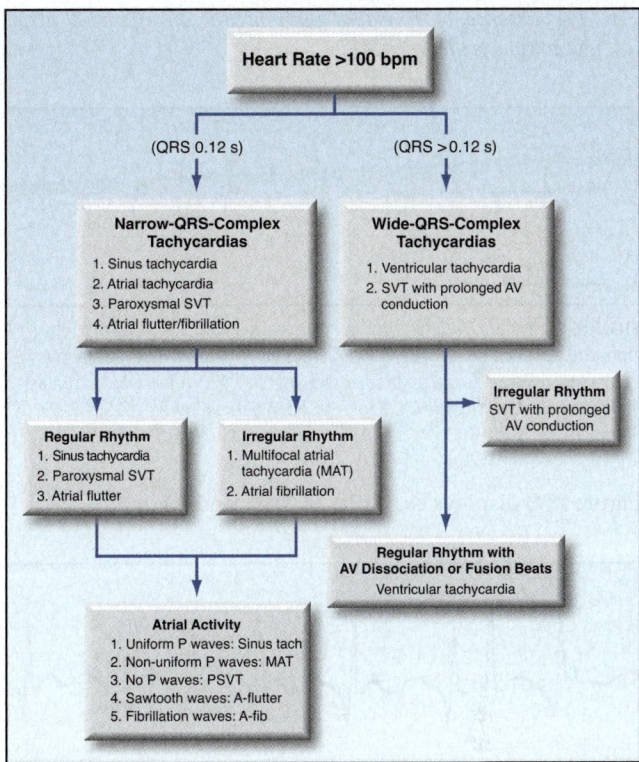

FIGURE 20.1. Flow diagram for the evaluation of tachycardias. SVT = supraventricular tachycardia. (From Tachyarrhythmias. In: Marino PL. *Marino's The ICU Book*. 5th ed. Wolters Kluwer; 2025:307-25. Figure 19.1.)

Irregular Rhythm

If the RR intervals are not uniform in length (i.e., an *irregularly irregular* tachycardia), the likely tachyarrhythmias are multifocal atrial tachycardia (MAT) or AF.

- *Multiple P wave morphologies and variable PR intervals are evidence of MAT.*

- The absence of P waves with highly disorganized atrial activity is evidence of AF.

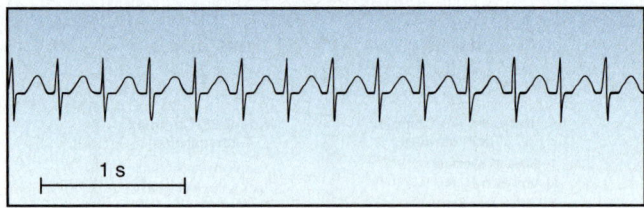

FIGURE 20.2. Narrow-QRS-complex tachycardia with a regular rhythm. Note the absence of visible P waves. This is an AV nodal reentrant tachycardia (paroxysmal supraventricular tachycardia). (From Tachyarrhythmias. In: Marino PL. *Marino's The ICU Book*. 5th ed. Wolters Kluwer; 2025:307-25. Figure 19.2.)

Figure 20.3 displays examples of MAT and AF.

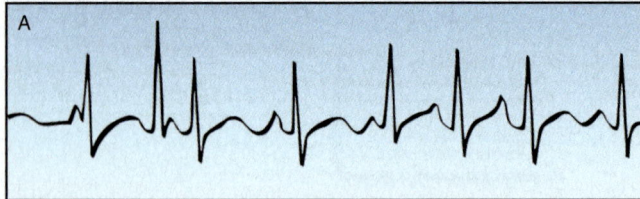

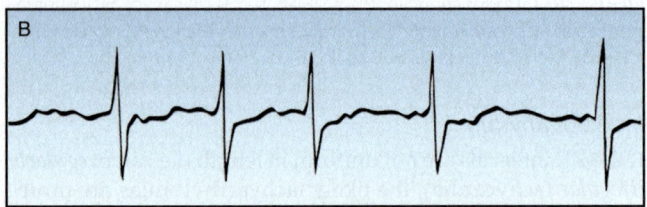

FIGURE 20.3. Panel A shows MAT, identified by multiple P wave morphologies and variable PR intervals. Panel B shows AF, identified by the absence of P waves with highly disorganized atrial activity (fibrillation waves). (From Tachyarrhythmias. In: Marino PL. *Marino's The ICU Book*. 5th ed. Wolters Kluwer; 2025:307-25. Figure 19.3.)

Wide Complex Tachycardias

Tachycardias with a QRS complex >0.12 s originate from a site below the AV conduction system or represent a supraventricular tachycardia (SVT) with prolonged AV conduction. Monomorphic (i.e., showing little variation in ECG form) ventricular tachycardia (VT) can be difficult to distinguish from SVT. The difference between the two tachyarrhythmias is often only evident after the arrhythmia is terminated, as demonstrated in Figure 20.4.

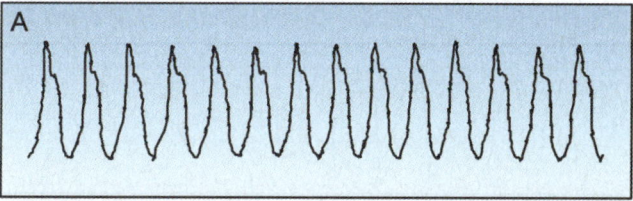

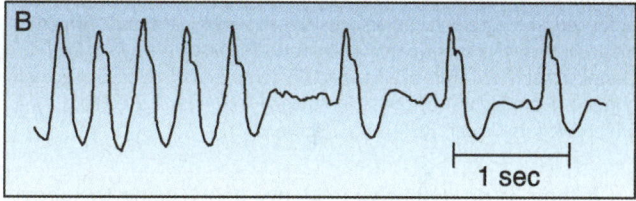

FIGURE 20.4. Differentiating VT from an SVT with prolonged AV conduction. The upper panel shows a wide-QRS-complex tachycardia that looks like monomorphic VT. In the lower panel, when the arrhythmia is terminated, an underlying bundle branch block is revealed, indicating that the rhythm in the upper panel is an SVT with a preexisting bundle branch block. (Tracings courtesy of Richard M. Greenberg, MD.)

Additional Clues to Identify VT

There are ECG abnormalities that may help identify VT as the cause of a wide-QRS-complex tachycardia.

- *The atria and ventricles beat independently in VT, resulting in AV dissociation (i.e., no fixed relationship between P waves*

and QRS complexes). The inferior and anterior precordial leads are best for identifying the P waves that may indicate dissociation.
- *Fusion beats (Figure 20.5) are indirect evidence of VT. A hybrid QRS complex that is a mixture of the normal QRS complex, and the ventricular ectopic impulse, is highly suggestive of VT.*
- *There are several scoring systems, including the Brugada criteria, that may help establish the diagnosis of VT as the cause of a wide complex tachydysrhythmia, though no set of criteria provides perfect diagnostic accuracy (3-4).*

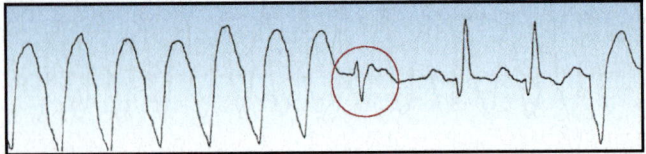

FIGURE 20.5. An example of a fusion beat (circled in red). A fusion beat is produced by the retrograde transmission of a ventricular ectopic impulse that collides with a supraventricular impulse. The result is a hybrid QRS complex that is a mixture of a normal QRS complex and ventricular ectopic impulse. (From Tachyarrhythmias. In: Marino PL. *Marino's The ICU Book*. 5th ed. Wolters Kluwer; 2025:307-25. Figure 19.7.)

If there is no definitive evidence of VT using the abovementioned ECG abnormalities, a wide-QRS-complex tachyarrhythmia in a patient with known underlying heart disease should be treated as *probable VT*, because VT is the cause of 95% of wide-QRS-complex tachycardias in patients with heart disease (5-6).

Atrial Fibrillation

Prevalence

AF is the most common tachyarrhythmia encountered clinically worldwide (6-7). The prevalence of AF increases with age, and the incidence of AF in the ICU varies widely, depending on age, gender, and disease state (i.e., coronary disease, sepsis, shock, respiratory failure) (6).

Adverse Consequences

AF can impair cardiac performance and increase the risk for stroke. Since atrial contraction is responsible for approximately 25% of the ventricular end diastolic volume, loss of atrial contraction in AF can lead to inadequate cardiac output (i.e., a pulse deficit) (8). This effect is most pronounced in conditions that decrease diastolic filling, such as mitral stenosis or ventricular hypertrophy. AF predisposes to thrombus formation in the left atrium and left atrial appendage, and the presence of AF increases the risk for stroke 5-fold (7).

Treatment

Heart Rate Control. Heart rate control is recommended as the initial management strategy for ICU patients with AF who are hemodynamically stable (7,9). Drugs available for this purpose are listed in Table 20.1.

A heart rate goal of <110 bpm is recommended (7,9). Elimination of the pulse deficit (Figure 20.6), or resolution of the variable systolic pressure in rapid AF, may be a more physiological goal.

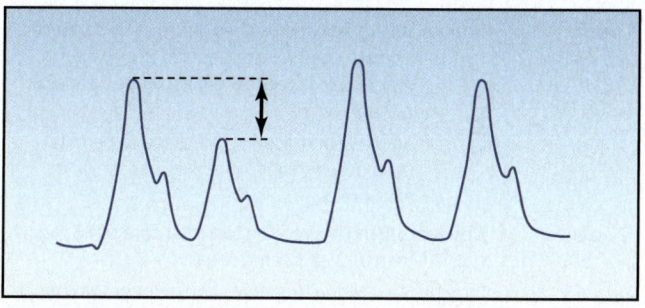

FIGURE 20.6. Arterial pressure tracing in AF. Note that there is a decrease in systolic pressure when two heartbeats occur in rapid succession. This effect can produce a "pulse deficit," where apical impulses are not always transmitted to the periphery. (From Tachyarrhythmias. In: Marino PL. *Marino's The ICU Book.* 5th ed. Wolters Kluwer; 2025:307-25. Figure 19.4.)

In patients with preserved left ventricular ejection fraction (LVEF) (>40%), β-blockers, diltiazem, verapamil, or digoxin

TABLE 20.1 Drug Regimens for Acute Rate Control in Atrial Fibrillation

Drug	Dosing Regimens and Comments
Diltiazem	**Dosing:** 0.25 mg/kg IV over 2 min, then infuse at 5-15 mg/h **Comment:** A popular agent for acute rate control, but use is limited by the risk of hypotension (20-30% of cases), and by negative inotropic effects
Amiodarone	**Dosing:** 150 mg IV over 10 min, and repeat if needed, then infuse at 1 mg/min for 6 h and 0.5 mg/min for 18 h; total dose should not exceed 2.2 g in 24 h. **Comment:** An effective alternative to diltiazem and beta blockers, and may be preferred in HFrEF; can occasionally promote conversion to sinus rhythm
Metoprolol	**Dosing:** 2.5-5 mg IV over 2 min, and repeat every 5-10 min if needed to a total of 3 doses **Comment:** Most effective in AF associated with hyper-adrenergic states; similar to diltiazem in risk of hypotension and negative inotropic effects
Esmolol	**Dosing:** 500 µg/kg IV bolus, then infuse at 50 µg/kg/min; increase dose in increments of 25 µg/kg/min every 5 min if needed to a maximum rate of 200 µg/kg/min. **Comment:** An ultra-short-acting β blocker that permits rapid dose titration; other features similar to metoprolol
Digoxin	**Dosing:** 0.25 mg IV every 2 h to a total dose of 1.5 mg, then 0.125-0.375 mg IV daily **Comment:** Slow-acting drug that should not be used alone for acute rate control; used primarily for long-term rate control in patients with HFrEF.

HFrEF = heart failure with reduced ejection fraction.

From Tachyarrhythmias. In: Marino PL. *Marino's The ICU Book*. 5th ed. Wolters Kluwer; 2025:307-25. Table 19.1.

are recommended as first choice rate control agents (7,9). β-blockers and/or digoxin are recommended in patients with AF and a LVEF (<40%) (7). Digoxin has a limited role in the *acute* management of AF because of a delayed onset of action. Intravenous magnesium sulfate may also be considered; doses of 3-10 mg IV given over 1 h have been shown to be effective when combined with other standard-of-care drugs (10).

Cardioversion. Synchronized, direct-current cardioversion is indicated for hemodynamically unstable patients (i.e., *patients with hypotension, altered mental status, cardiac ischemia, or evidence of heart failure*) (11). Biphasic waveforms, high-energy shocks (>200 J) and manual pressure have been shown to increase the success of electrical cardioversion for AF (12). Time permitting, transesophageal echocardiography (TEE) should be performed to rule out the presence of an atrial thrombus. Anticoagulation is started as soon as possible prior to or immediately after the procedure unless the AF is new onset, defined as a duration of <48 h.

Transition to Oral Therapy. The transition from IV to oral amiodarone begins with an oral dose of 400 mg, which is given 4-5 h before discontinuing the infusion. The initial oral regimen is 400 mg twice daily, which is continued until the total loading dose (IV and PO) reaches 10 g (13). Digoxin may also be considered for long-term rate control in patients with AF and heart failure with reduced ejection fraction (HFrEF), although it should be noted that digoxin is associated with a moderately increased risk of all-cause and cardiovascular mortality in AF patients regardless of the presence of heart failure (14).

Stroke Prevention

Risk factors for thromboembolic stroke in AF can be assessed with the CHA_2DS_2-VASc score (Table 20.2). The CHA_2DS_2-VASc score does not apply to AF associated with mitral stenosis or a prosthetic valve because these conditions always require anticoagulation (7,9).

TABLE 20.2 Risk Assessment for Oral Anticoagulation in Atrial Fibrillation

CHA_2DS_2-VASc Scoring		Indications for Anticoagulation
Condition	**Points**	
(C) CHF	1	<u>Definite</u> Males: ≥2 points Females: ≥3 points <u>Consider</u> Males: 1 point Females: 2 points
(H) Hypertension	1	
(A) Age >75 yrs	2	
(D) Diabetes	1	
(S) Stroke/TIA/VTE	2	
(V) Vascular Disease	1	
(A) Age 65-74 yrs	1	
(Sc) Sex Category (♀)	1	

CHF = congestive heart failure; TIA = transient ischemic attack; VTE = venous thromboembolism.

From References 6-7, 9.

Oral anticoagulants used for stroke prevention in AF are listed in Table 20.3.

Direct-acting oral anticoagulants (DOACs) include direct thrombin inhibitors (e.g., dabigatran) and drugs that inhibit factor Xa (e.g., rivaroxaban, apixaban, and edoxaban). DOACs have a more predictable anticoagulant effect, do not require frequent monitoring (Factor Xa levels are used to assess adequacy of anticoagulation), and are as effective as warfarin for reducing stroke. For these reasons, *DOACs are preferred to warfarin in nonvalvular AF* (7,9). Warfarin is the drug of choice for patients with significant mitral stenosis or a prosthetic valve (7,9).

Wolff-Parkinson-White Syndrome and AF

The Wolff-Parkinson-White (WPW) syndrome is diagnosed by a short PR interval (<120 ms) and a delta wave (i.e., a slurred

QRS upstroke) on ECG. This arrhythmia should be suspected when a patient in the ICU develops a paroxysmal tachyarrhythmia with a delta wave. When AF occurs in a patient with the WPW syndrome, drugs that block conduction in the AV node (e.g., calcium channel blockers, β-blockers, digoxin, amiodarone) are unlikely to slow the ventricular rate because the accessory pathway is not blocked. Moreover, selective block of the AV node can precipitate ventricular fibrillation. Therefore, drugs that block the AV node should not be used when AF is associated with the WPW syndrome. Electrical cardioversion is indicated in hemodynamically unstable patients. In patients who are hemodynamically stable, procainamide or ibutilide are recommended due to each agent's lack of AV nodal blocking properties (15-16).

TABLE 20.3   Oral Anticoagulants for Atrial Fibrillation

Drug	Dosing Recommendations
Dabigatran (Pradaxa)	Standard dose: 50 mg BID Reduced dose: 110 mg BID for age ≥80 yrs or CrCL <30 mL/min
Rivaroxaban (Xarelto)	Standard dose: 20 mg once daily Reduced dose: 15 mg once daily for CrCL <30 mL/min
Apixaban (Eliquis)	Standard dose: 5 mg BID. Reduced dose: 2.5 mg BID for two of the following: age ≥80 yrs, weight ≤60 kg, serum creatinine ≥1.5 mg/dL
Edoxaban (Lixiana)	Standard dose: 60 mg once daily. Reduced dose: 30 mg once daily for CrCL <30 mL/min, weight ≤60 kg, or therapy with erythromycin or ketoconazole.
Warfarin (Coumadin)	Starting dose is usually 5 mg once daily, which is adjusted to achieve an INR of 2-3.

From References 7, 9.

Multifocal Atrial Tachycardia

Etiology and Diagnosis

MAT is a tachyarrhythmia that occurs predominantly in the elderly and in those with lung disease (over 60% of cases) (17). MAT may also be associated with hypomagnesemia, hypokalemia, and coronary artery disease. The diagnosis of MAT requires the presence of tachycardia (heart rate >100 bpm), P waves with at least three different morphologies, P waves that return to the baseline and are separated by isoelectric intervals, and variable PP intervals, PR duration, and RR intervals (17).

Treatment

MAT is often a stubborn tachyarrhythmia that is difficult to treat if the underlying disease process is not managed adequately (15,17). The following steps are recommended for treatment (15,17):

1. *Electrolyte repletion.* Hypomagnesemia and hypokalemia should be corrected.
2. *Empiric magnesium.* Even if serum magnesium levels are normal, total body magnesium is often depleted. IV magnesium can be given empirically with *2 g magnesium sulfate over 15 min followed by a 6 g infusion over 6 h.*
3. *Metoprolol.* If chronic obstructive pulmonary disease (COPD) is not the cause and the prior measures fail, metoprolol can be given using the doses listed in Table 20.1.
4. *Verapamil.* If metoprolol is contraindicated, verapamil can be used. MAT may not convert to a sinus rhythm, but the ventricular rate may be slowed. A dose of *0.25-5 mg IV over 2 min can be given and repeated every 15-30 min if necessary to a total dose of 20 mg* (17). Verapamil is not recommended for patients with HFrEF as this agent is a potent negative inotrope.

Paroxysmal Supraventricular Tachycardias

Prevalence

PSVT are narrow-QRS-complex tachycardias that are second only to AF as the most prevalent rhythm disturbances in the general population (15,18). AVNRT accounts for 50-60% of all PSVT cases. AVNRT occurs more frequently in woman than men and in patients *without* a history of heart disease.

Diagnosis

The ECG shows a narrow-QRS-complex tachycardia with a regular rhythm and a heart rate between 140 and 250 bpm (15,19). There are often no discernible P waves on the 12-lead ECG.

Treatment

Maneuvers. Maneuvers that increase vagal tone are recommended as an initial intervention to terminate PSVT. These maneuvers include carotid sinus massage (only when there are no carotid bruits), the Valsalva maneuver (maximal expiratory effort with a closed glottis), induced gag reflex (stimulating the posterior oropharynx with a tongue depressor), and application of an ice-cold, wet towel to the face (15). Vagal maneuvers have limited success in terminating PSVTs, including AVNRTs (20).

Adenosine. When vagal maneuvers fail, adenosine is the drug of choice for terminating PSVT (15,19). Adenosine is an endogenous nucleotide that relaxes smooth muscle and slows conduction in the AV node. Adenosine has a quick onset of action (<30 s) and short duration of action (1-2 min). The dosing regimen, drug interactions, adverse effects, and contraindications for adenosine are listed in Table 20.4.

Other Therapies. When PSVT does not respond to adenosine, calcium channel blockers (diltiazem) can be effective (see

Table 20.1). For PSVT that is resistant to drugs or associated with hemodynamic instability, synchronized electrical cardioversion is indicated. Energy levels >100 J may be necessary (11,15,19).

TABLE 20.4	Intravenous Adenosine for Paroxysmal SVT
Feature	Recommendations
Dosing regimen	1. Deliver through a peripheral vein. 2. Give 6 mg by rapid IV injection and flush catheter with saline. 3. If response is inadequate after 2 min, give 12 mg by rapid IV injection and flush catheter with saline. 4. If response is still inadequate after 2 min, another 12 mg can be given by rapid IV injection.
Dose adjustments	Decrease dose by 50% for the following: • Drug delivery into the superior vena cava • Patient receiving calcium channel blocker, β-blocker, or dipyridamole
Drug interactions	• Dipyridamole (blocks adenosine uptake) • Theophylline (blocks adenosine receptors)
Adverse effects	• Bradycardia, AV block (50%) • Facial flushing (20%) • Dyspnea (12%) • Chest pressure (7%)
Contraindications	• Asthma • 2nd or 3rd degree AV block • Sick sinus syndrome

From References 11, 15, 19.

Ventricular Tachycardia

Diagnosis

VT is a wide-QRS-complex tachycardia that has an abrupt onset, regular rhythm, and a rate that is typically 140-200 bpm. As discussed previously in this chapter, distinguishing between VT and supraventricular arrhythmias on ECG can be difficult. VT can also present as an irregular broad complex tachyarrhythmia, so an irregular rhythm does not exclude it as a diagnosis (21). Most VT occurs in patients with underlying heart disease, but up to 10% of cases occur in patients with structurally normal hearts (21).

Treatment

The management of VT is shown in Figure 20.7.

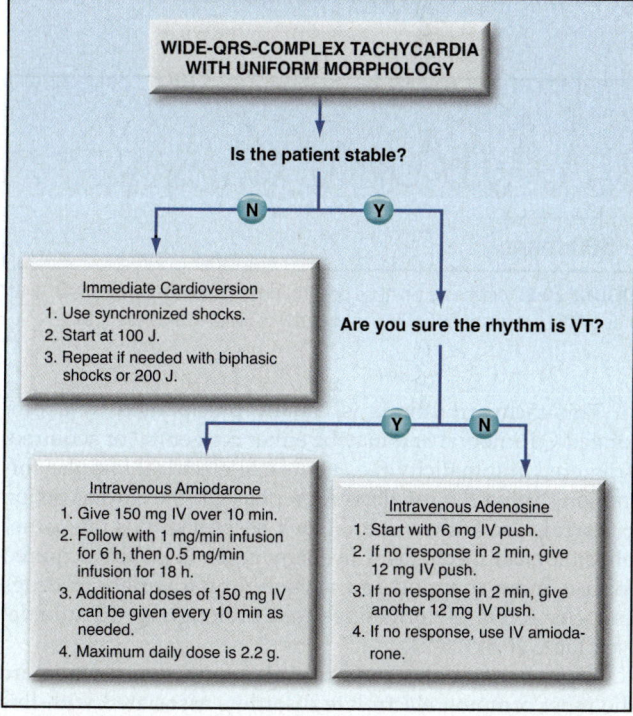

FIGURE 20.7. Flow diagram for the acute management of patients with wide-QRS-complex tachycardia. (Based on recommendations in Reference 11.)

Electrical cardioversion is the treatment of choice if there is evidence of hemodynamic compromise. Shocks should be synchronized (timed with the QRS complex) and 100 J may be used initially (11,22). If the QRS complex is wide and bizarre or if the VT is polymorphic, nonsynchronized defibrillation should be performed using 200 J for a biphasic device, to avoid the delivery of electricity during a T wave, which could provoke ventricular fibrillation.

Torsade de Pointes

Torsade de pointes (French for "twisting around the points") is a polymorphic VT, as shown in Figure 20.8.

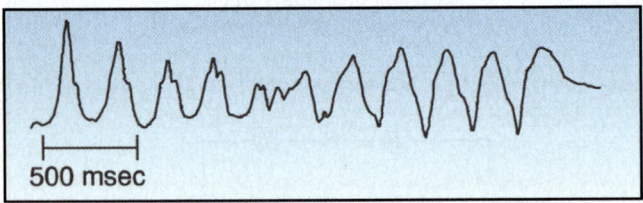

FIGURE 20.8. Torsade de points, a polymorphic VT. The QRS appears to "twist" around the isoelectric line. (Tracing courtesy of Richard Greenberg, MD.)

This tachyarrhythmia is usually precipitated by a prolonged QT interval and may be either congenital or acquired. Triggered automaticity (i.e., abnormal electrical impulse formation during the repolarization phase of the cardiac action potential, also known as an *R on T phenomenon*) is the pathophysiological mechanism in many cases (24). The acquired form is more common and is caused by a variety of drugs and electrolyte abnormalities that prolong the QT interval (see Table 20.5) (23-24).

Hypomagnesemia, hypokalemia, and hypocalcemia are the most common electrolyte disorders associated with this arrhythmia.

QT Interval Measurement. The QT interval represents ventricular depolarization and repolarization. This interval is measured from the onset of the QRS complex to the end of the T wave and is best measured in leads V3 and V4. The QT interval varies inversely with heart rate, and a rate-correction (QTc) is required in tachycardia. The method for determining the QTc is shown in Equation 20.1:

$$QTc = \frac{QT}{\sqrt{RR}} \qquad (20.1)$$

A normal QTc is 350-450 ms for adult men and 360-460 ms for adult women, but 10-20% of healthy adults may have intervals outside of these ranges (25). A QTc >0.5 represents a risk for torsade de pointes (25-26).

TABLE 20.5 Drugs that can Induce Torsade de Pointes

Antiarrhythmics	Antimicrobials	Neuroleptics	Others
IA: Quinidine, Disopyramide, Procainamide	Clarithromycin, Erythromycin, Pentamidine	Chlorpromazine, Tioridazine, Droperidol, Haloperidol	Cisapride, Methadone
III: Ibutilide, Sotalol			

From www.torsades.org and References 23 and 24.
IA and III refer to the Vaughan Williams classification for antiarrhythmics.

Treatment. Sustained polymorphic VT requires cardioversion. Intravenous magnesium is popular for terminating torsade de pointes and can be combined with electrical cardioversion at a dose of 1-2 grams magnesium sulfate IV over 15 min (11,27). For polymorphic VT with a normal QT interval, amiodarone or β-blockers can help prevent recurrences (27). Other measures for preventing torsade de pointes include correcting electrolyte disorders and discontinuing high-risk drugs (see Table 20.5).

BRADYARRHYTHMIAS

Definition and Causes

Bradyarrhythmias have been associated with sudden cardiac arrest in 20-40% of hospitalized patients (28). In this section, common bradyarrhythmias in the ICU are reviewed, to include management options, such as physiological pacing.

Sinus Bradycardia

Sinus bradycardia is a disorder of cardiac electrical *impulse generation* and is defined as a heart rate <50 bpm (28). Typical causes for sinus bradycardia include drugs, including β-blockers, calcium channel blockers, and sedatives. Sinus bradycardia may be the initial presenting rhythm in up to 25% of acute myocardial infarctions, especially if the right coronary artery is affected, because this artery supplies the sinoatrial node in 60% of patients (28).

Atrioventricular Block

AV blocks represent a disorder of *impulse propagation*, and are caused by medications, electrolyte disorders (e.g., hyperkalemia), ischemia, infections (e.g., Lyme disease), inflammation, or other disorders (28). First-degree AV block is a risk factor for the development of AF (29). AV blocks encountered after cardiac surgical procedures may be due to trauma, localized inflammation, or direct mechanical compression (28).

Intraventricular Conduction Disturbances

Intraventricular conduction disturbances involve conduction disorders at the level of the left bundle branch (including anterior and posterior fascicles), the right bundle branch, or septal fascicle. Bundle branch blocks are associated with an increased risk for complete heart block and sudden cardiac death, especially when a first-degree

AV block is also present (30). Ischemia should strongly be considered when new onset intraventricular bundle branch blocks are encountered in the ICU.

Treatment

Atropine

Atropine is a parasympathetic blocking agent that works by inhibiting the muscarinic actions of acetylcholine. Atropine is a first-line agent for symptomatic bradycardia and can be given in doses of 0.5 mg IV every 3-5 min to a total dose of 3 mg (Figure 20.9) (11,28). Atropine is ineffective in heart transplant patients due to the absence of vagal innervation; aminophylline or isoproterenol may be considered as alternative pharmacological treatments.

Second-Line Agents

For bradycardia that is refractory to atropine and associated with hemodynamic compromise, epinephrine can be given at a dose of 2-10 µg/min (0.025-0.125 µg/kg/min) (11,28). Dopamine (2-20 µg/kg/min) is another option. Isoproterenol is a non-selective beta agonist that may be effective in cases of sinus node dysfunction, but this agent cannot be used during myocardial ischemia since experimental models have shown that isoproterenol can induce or exacerbate myocardial damage (31-32).

Management of Drug Culprits

If drug toxicity is suspected as the cause of hemodynamically significant bradycardia, antidotes should be considered. β-blocker overdoses should be treated with glucagon (5 mg IV over 60 s), which increases intracellular cyclic adenosine monophosphate through a non-beta-adrenergic receptor pathway (28). IV calcium (10-20 mL of 10% calcium chloride [30-60 mL if calcium gluconate is used]) can be given every 10-20 min for 3-4 doses until a clinical response is achieved (33). Calcium should be given over 5 min to avoid

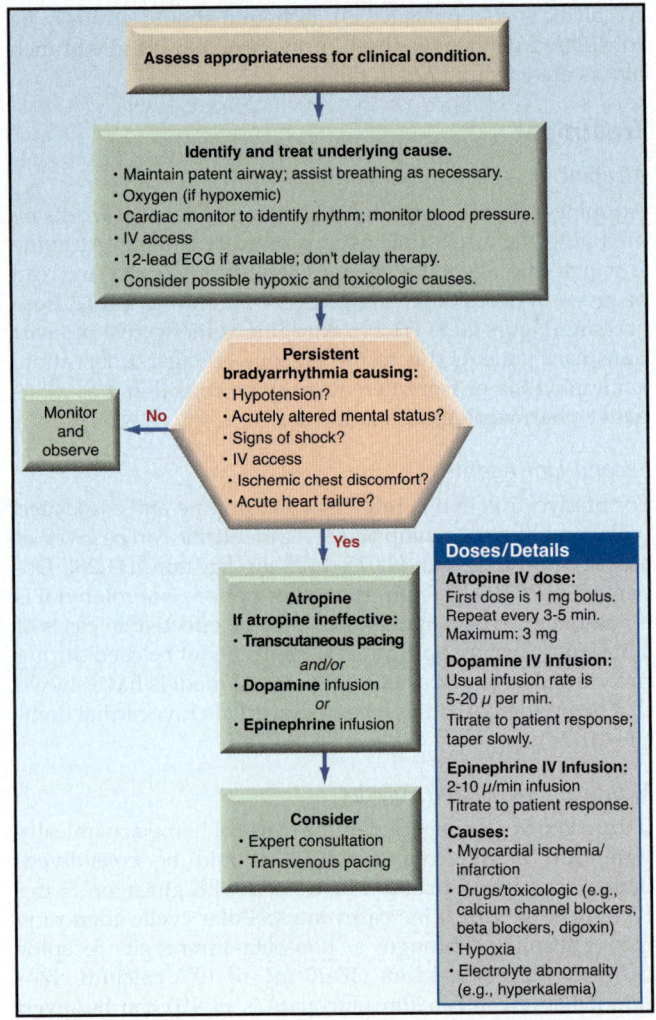

FIGURE 20.9. Flow diagram for the management of symptomatic bradycardia. See text for details. (© 2020 American Heart Association.)

TABLE 20.6 Indications and Guidelines for Initial Temporary Pacemaker Settings

- Acute MI (especially anterior MI or alternating RBBB and LBBB or RBBB with alternating LAHB or LPHB)
- Drug overdose (digoxin, beta blockers, calcium channel blockers)
- Hyperkalemia
- AV node or His-Purkinje system damage after cardiac surgery
- Infectious diseases (Lyme disease, Chagas)
- Catheter-induced injury to the right bundle branch in a patient with a left bundle branch block
- Subacute bacterial endocarditis or myocarditis
- Direct cardiac trauma

Transcutaneous Pacing

1. **Pad placement**: Pads should be preferably placed in an anterior-posterior configuration but not over an AICD or transdermal drug patches.
2. **Rate**: Set to desired heart rate (60-80 bpm or 30 bpm above the patient's intrinsic rhythm).
3. **Output**: Start at 70 mA and increase in 5-10 mA increments until capture is achieved.
4. A wide-complex-QRS that follows each pacer spike indicates capture.
5. Once capture is confirmed, increase current by 5-10 mA to prevent loss of capture.
6. If capture is not achieved at a current above 120 mA, the pads should be repositioned and the process is repeated.

Transvenous Pacing

1. The preferred sites for insertion of a 6 Fr cordis catheter are either the right internal jugular or left subclavian vein (see Chapter 2: Airway Management).
2. Attach sheath to pacer wire before inserting it into the cordis.
3. Insert the pacer wire to approximately 15 cm through the cordis.
4. Inflate the balloon with 1.5 mL of air and lock in the inflated position.
5. Turn on pacemaker.
   a. **Rate**: 80 bpm
   b. **Output**: 10 mA (A and V)
   c. **Mode**: DDD
6. Advance pacemaker wire with balloon inflated.
7. Assess for capture.
8. Once capture is achieved, hold pacemaker wire in place and deflate balloon
   a. The tip of the wire should be in the apex of the right ventricle
   b. Tip placement can be assessed with echocardiography (subcostal view).
9. Turn output down to point when capture is lost. From this minimum threshold, increase output to 2.5 times the minimal output to prevent loss of capture.

AICD = automated implantable cardioverter defibrillator; DDD = refers to pacing nomenclature, where both atrium and ventricle are paced, both atrium and ventricle are sensed, and the device can trigger or inhibit sensed events; LAHB = left anterior hemiblock; LBBB = left bundle branch block; LPHB = left posterior hemiblock; MI = myocardial infarction; RBBB = right bundle branch block.

From References 28, 35-37.

hypotension and preferably via a central line to avoid the risk of extravasation and skin necrosis. An infusion of calcium chloride may be considered at a rate of 0.2-0.4 mL/kg/h, with close monitoring of calcium levels (after first 30 min then every 2 h during the infusion) (34). Digitalis toxicity should be treated with digitalis-specific antibody fragments; consultation with a local toxicology center or pharmacist is recommended for dosing adjustments (28,35).

Pacing

The indications for temporary pacing in the ICU are when permanent pacing is indicated but not appropriate (i.e., presence of an active bloodstream infection), or when a symptomatic bradyarrhythmia is temporary or reversible (28,35-37). Table 20.6 lists indications for pacing with guidelines for initial transcutaneous and transvenous pacemaker settings.

References

1. Ganz LI, Friedman PL. Supraventricular tachycardia. N Engl J Med 1995;332(3):162-73.
2. Katritsis DG, Josephson ME. Differential diagnosis of regular, narrow-QRS tachycardias. Heart Rhythm 2015;12(7):1667-76.
3. Lau EW, Pathamanathan RK, Ng GA, et al. The Bayesian approach improves the electrocardiographic diagnosis of broad complex tachycardia. Pacing Clin Electrophysiol 2000;23(10 Pt 1):1519-26.
4. Vereckei A, Duray G, Szénási G, et al. Application of a new algorithm in the differential diagnosis of wide QRS complex tachycardia. Eur Heart J 2007;28(5):589-600.
5. Akhtar M, Shenasa M, Jazayeri M, et al. Wide QRS complex tachycardia. Reappraisal of a common clinical problem. Ann Intern Med 1988;109(11):905-12.
6. Wetterslev M, Haase N, Hassager C, et al. New-onset atrial fibrillation in adult critically ill patients: a scoping review. Intensive Care Med 2019;45(7):928-38.
7. Van Gelder IC, Rienstra M, Bunting KV, et al. 2024 ESC guidelines for the management of atrial fibrillation developed in collaboration with the European Association for Cardio-Thoracic Surgery (EACTS). Eur Heart J 2024;30:ehae176.
8. Guyton AC. The relationship of cardiac output and arterial pressure control. Circulation 1981;64:1079-88.

9. Joglar JA, Chung MK, et al. 2023 ACC/AHA/ACCP/HRS guideline for the diagnosis and management of atrial fibrillation: a report of the American College of Cardiology/American Heart Association joint committee on clinical practice guidelines. J Am Coll Cardiol 2024;83(9):959.
10. Ramesh T, Lee PYK, Mitta M, Allencherril J. Intravenous magnesium in the management of rapid atrial fibrillation: a systematic review and meta-analysis. J Cardiol 2021;78(5):375-81.
11. Panchal AR, Bsartos JA, Cabañas JG, et al. Part 3: adult basic and advanced life support: 2020 American Heart Association guidelines for cardiopulmonary resuscitation and emergency cardiovascular care Circulation 2020;142(16 Suppl 2):S366-S468.
12. Nguyen ST, Belley-Côté EP, Ibrahim O, et al. Techniques improving electrical cardioversion success for patients with atrial fibrillation: a systematic review and meta-analysis. Europace 2023;25(2):318-30.
13. Amiodarone injection. Prescribing information. Fresenius Kabi; 2020.
14. Gazzaniga G, Menichelli D, Scaglione F, et al. Effect of digoxin on all-cause and cardiovascular mortality in patients with atrial fibrillation with and without heart failure: an umbrella review of systematic reviews and 12 meta-analyses. Eur J Clin Pharmacol 2023;79(4):473-83.
15. Page RL, Joglar JA, Caldwell MA, et al. 2015 ACC/AHA/HRS guideline for the management of adult patients with supraventricular tachycardia: a report of the American College of Cardiology/American Heart Association Task Force on clinical practice guidelines and the Heart Rhythm Society. Circulation 2016;134(11):e234-5.
16. January CT, Wann LS, Alpert JS, et al. 2014 AHA/ACC/HRS guideline for the management of patients with atrial fibrillation: executive summary: a report of the American College of Cardiology/American Heart Association Task Force on practice guidelines and the Heart Rhythm Society. Circulation 2014;130(23):2071-104.
17. Kastor JA. Multifocal atrial tachycardia. N Engl J Med 1990;322(24):1713-17.
18. Rehorn M, Sacks NC, Emden MR, et al. Prevalence and incidence of patients with paroxysmal supraventricular tachycardia in the United States. J Cardiovasc Electrophysiol 2021;32(8):2199-206.
19. Trohman RG. Supraventricular tachycardia: implications for the intensivist. Crit Care Med 2000;28(10 Suppl):N129-N135.
20. Ceylan E, Ozpolat C, Onur O, et al. Initial and sustained response effects of 3 Vagal maneuvers in supraventricular tachycardia: a randomized, Clinical Trial. J Emerg Med 2019;57(3):299-305.
21. Whitaker J, Wright MJ, Tedrow U. Diagnosis and management of ventricular tachycardia. Clin Med (Lond) 2023;23(5):442-8.

22. Link MS, Atkins DL, Passman RS, et al. Part 6: electrical therapies: automated external defibrillators, defibrillation, cardioversion, and pacing: 2010 American Heart Association guidelines for cardiopulmonary resuscitation and emergency cardiovascular care. Circulation 2010;122(18 Suppl 3):S706-19.
23. Gupta A, Lawrence AT, Krishnan K, et al. Current concepts in the mechanisms and management of drug-induced QT prolongation and torsade de pointes. Am Heart J 2007;153(6):891-9.
24. Antzelevitch C, Burashnikov A. Overview of basic mechanisms of cardiac arrhythmia. Card Electrophysiol Clin 2011;3(1):23-45.
25. Rezuş C, Moga VD, Ouatu A, Floria M. QT interval variations and mortality risk: is there any relationship? Anatol J Cardiol 2015;15(3):255-8.
26. Al-Khatib SM, LaPointe NM, Kramer JM, Califf RM. What clinicians should know about the QT interval. JAMA 2003;289(16):2120-7.
27. Al-Khatib SM, Stevenson WG, Ackerman MJ, et al. 2017 AHA/ACC/HRS guideline for management of patients with ventricular arrhythmias and the prevention of sudden cardiac death: executive summary: a report of the American College of Cardiology/American Heart Association Task Force on clinical practice guidelines and the Heart Rhythm Society. Heart Rhythm 2018;15(10):e190-e252.
28. Lattell J, Upadhyay GA. Bradyarrhythmias and physiologic pacing in the ICU. J Intensive Care Med 2022;37(5):595-610.
29. Cheng S, Keyes MJ, Larson MG, et al. Long-term outcomes in individuals with prolonged PR interval or first-degree atrioventricular block. JAMA 2009;301(24):2571-7.
30. Maddali M. Cardiac pacing in left bundle branch/bifascicular block patients. Ann Card Anaesth 2010;13(1):7-15.
31. Overgaard CB, Dzavík V. Inotropes and vasopressors: review of physiology and clinical use in cardiovascular disease. Circulation 2008;118(10):1047-56.
32. Ma S, Ma J, Tu Q, et al. Isoproterenol increases left atrial fibrosis and susceptibility to atrial fibrillation by inducing atrial ischemic infarction in rats. Front Pharmacol 2020;11:493.
33. Carlon GC, Howland WS, Goldiner PL, et al. Adverse effects of calcium administration. Report of two cases. Arch Surg 1978;113(7):882-5.
34. Chin RL, Garmel GM, Harter PM. Development of ventricular fibrillation after intravenous calcium chloride administration in a patient with supraventricular tachycardia. Ann Emerg Med 1995;25(3):416-9.
35. Glikson M, Nielsen JC, Kronborg MB, et al. 2021 ESC guidelines on cardiac pacing and cardiac resynchronization therapy. Eur Heart J 2021;42(35):3427-3520.
36. Kusumoto FM, Schoenfeld MH, Barrett C, et al. 2018 ACC/AHA/HRS guideline on the evaluation and management of patients with

bradycardia and cardiac conduction delay: executive summary: a report of the American College of Cardiology/American Heart Association Task Force on clinical practice guidelines, and the Heart Rhythm Society. Circulation 2019;140(8):e333-e381.
37. Roberts, JR, Hedges, JR. *Ch 15 Emergency Cardiac Pacing in Clinical Procedures in Emergency Medicine*, 5th ed. Elsevier; 2010.

Acute Coronary Syndromes — Chapter 21

This chapter describes the diagnosis and early management of acute myocardial infarction and unstable angina (i.e., *acute coronary syndromes* [ACS]). While advances in reperfusion therapy have contributed to a 20% decline in the annual mortality rate, coronary disease continues to be the leading cause of death in leading cause of death worldwide (1-2). This chapter emphasizes management within the first 24-36 h after presentation. Acute aortic dissection is also discussed because the clinical presentation of this disease process may be confused with ACS.

PATHOGENESIS

Coronary Thrombosis

Acute myocardial infarction is the result of an occlusive thrombus in one or more coronary arteries. The trigger for thrombus generation is rupture of an atherosclerotic plaque, which releases thrombogenic lipids (Figure 21.1). Plaque disruption is also related to inflammation and hydraulic shear stress (3-4).

CLINICAL SYNDROMES

Acute coronary thrombosis produces three distinct clinical syndromes which are described as *ACS* (5). ACS are classified according to Electrocardiogram (ECG) findings:

1. ST-elevation myocardial infarction (STEMI), which is a transmural infarction caused by complete occlusion of the infarct-related artery.
2. Non-ST-elevation myocardial infarction (NSTEMI), which is the result of incomplete or partial occlusion of the infarct-related artery.

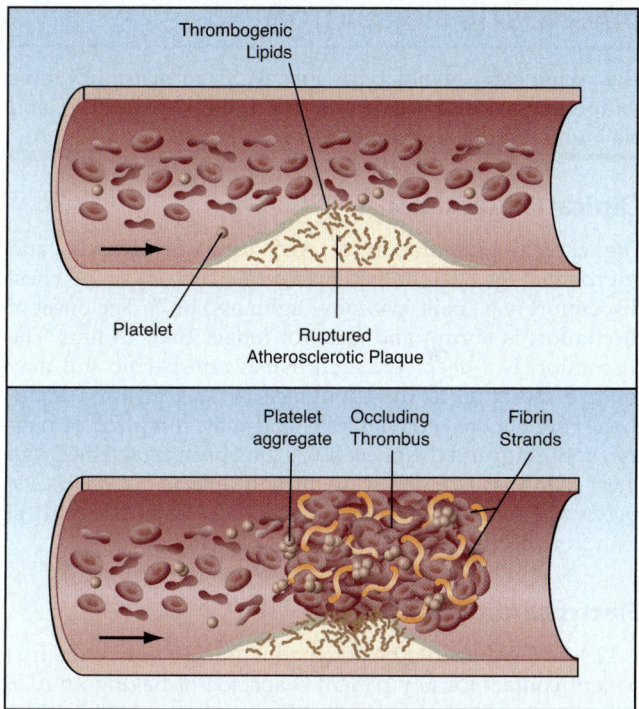

FIGURE 21.1. Pathogenesis of acute coronary syndromes. Rupture of an atherosclerotic plaque releases thrombogenic lipids that activate platelets and clotting factors (upper panel), resulting in the formation of an occlusive thrombus. (From Acute Coronary Syndromes. In: Marino PL. *Marino's The ICU Book*. 5th ed. Wolters Kluwer; 2025:326-42. Figure 20.1.)

3. Unstable angina (UA), which is not associated with ST-elevation on the ECG and is the result of *intermittent* episodes of coronary occlusion.

Newer nomenclature has been proposed to distinguish *acute myocardial ischemic syndromes* (AMIS) caused by plaque rupture or infarction versus *non-acute* myocardial ischemic syndromes (i.e., epicardial coronary stenosis, ischemia with non-obstructive coronary arteries) (5).

DIAGNOSTIC EVALUATION

The diagnostic evaluation for ACS consists of three components: the clinical presentation, the 12-lead ECG, and the high-sensitivity troponin assay.

Clinical Presentation

The clinical presentation of ACS can vary widely, and approximately 80% of patients have some type of chest discomfort (e.g., pain, pressure, tightness) (6-7). The onset of discomfort is abrupt and lasts for longer than 15 min. The discomfort is a deep sensation that is nonspecific and may involve radiation to the shoulders, neck, arms, and abdomen. Patients are often anxious and may complain of nausea, vomiting, and dyspnea. It has long been established that chest pain that is relieved by nitroglycerin is *not evidence of myocardial ischemia*, since nitroglycerin can also relieve chest pain from esophageal spasm (8).

Electrocardiogram

A 12-lead ECG should be obtained within 10 min of the first patient contact for any patient suspected of having an ACS (6-7). Typical ECG changes in ACS are shown in Table 21.1 (9).

ECG evidence of STEMI merits emergency reperfusion therapy. NSTEMI and UA may be characterized by ST depressions or T-wave inversions, but the ECG can also be normal in these conditions. Bundle branch blocks or paced rhythms can mask ischemic ECG changes.

Troponin Assay

Plasma levels of cardiac troponin (cTn) are used to detect the presence of myocardial cell injury. A high-sensitivity cardiac troponin (hs-cTn) assay can detect elevations of cTn as early as 3 h after the onset of symptoms (10). Reference values differ for various commercial cTn assays. The following protocol is recommended for interpreting hs-cTn in suspected ACS (6-7,10-11):

1. Plasma levels of hs-cTn should be measured at the time of presentation and again 1 h later.
2. If the hs-cTn level is elevated above the 99th percentile upper reference level for the assay, and at least 3 h have transpired since the onset of symptoms, myocardial necrosis is likely. Conditions other than ischemia can cause myocardial injury, so hs-cTn should be repeated at 1 h.

TABLE 21.1 ECG Changes in Acute Coronary Syndromes

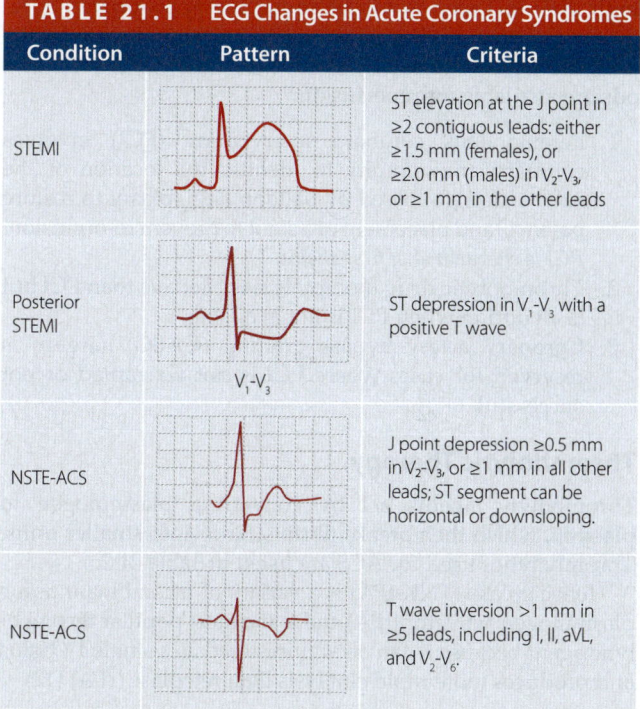

Condition	Pattern	Criteria
STEMI		ST elevation at the J point in ≥2 contiguous leads: either ≥1.5 mm (females), or ≥2.0 mm (males) in V_2-V_3, or ≥1 mm in the other leads
Posterior STEMI	V_1-V_3	ST depression in V_1-V_3 with a positive T wave
NSTE-ACS		J point depression ≥0.5 mm in V_2-V_3, or ≥1 mm in all other leads; ST segment can be horizontal or downsloping.
NSTE-ACS		T wave inversion >1 mm in ≥5 leads, including I, II, aVL, and V_2-V_6.

From Amsterdam EA, Wenger NK, Brindis RG, et al. 2014 AHA/ACC guideline for the management of patients with non-ST-elevation acute coronary syndromes: a report of the American College of Cardiology/American Heart Association task force on practice guidelines. J Am Coll Cardiol 2014;64(24):2713-4.

3. A significant change (usually >10%) in the second hs-cTn level is evidence of acute myocardial infarction.

There are several non-ischemic causes of elevated hs-cTN, such as heart failure, sustained tachycardia, pulmonary hypertension, and sepsis, but these conditions should not cause an acute change in hs-cTN levels (6,10).

REPERFUSION STRATEGIES

When the likelihood of an acute coronary occlusion is very high, the next step is to determine the appropriate strategy for reperfusion. Reperfusion strategies are based on the presence or absence of ST-elevation on the ECG. Three methods are available for reperfusion:

1. Percutaneous coronary intervention (PCI) involves coronary angiography to identify the location of the obstruction, followed by balloon angioplasty to restore patency, and placement of a stent to prevent re-occlusion. *PCI is the method of first choice*.
2. Thrombolytic drug therapy is less effective than PCI but is an option when PCI is not available.
3. Coronary artery bypass grafting (CABG) surgery is reserved for cases where PCI is not warranted or not successful.

Thrombolytic Therapy

Thrombolytic agents act by converting plasminogen to plasmin, which then breaks fibrin strands into smaller units. Thrombolytics used for ACS are listed in Table 21.2.

Tenecteplase (TNK-tPA) is a variant of recombinant tissue plasminogen activator (tPA) and is the most popular thrombolytic agent because it can be administered as a single IV bolus and produces more rapid clot lysis than reteplase (rPA) (12).

Bleeding Attributed to Thrombolytics

Thrombolytic therapy for ACS is complicated by significant bleeding—defined as the requirement for a blood transfusion—

TABLE 21.2 Thrombolytic Therapy for Acute Coronary Occlusion

Agent	Dosing Regimen	Patency Rate at 90 min
Alteplase (tPA)	15 mg IV bolus, then 0.75 mg/kg (not >50 mg) over 30 min, then 0.5 mg/kg (not >35 mg) over 60 min. Max dose: 100 mg over 90 min	73-84%
Reteplase (rPA)	10 Units as IV bolus and repeat in 30 min	84%
Tenecteplase (TNK-tPA)	Single IV bolus: 30 mg for wt. <60 kg, 35 mg for 60-69 kg, 40 mg for 70-79 kg, 45 mg for 80-89 kg, and 50 mg for ≥90 kg	85%

From O'Gara PT, Kushner FG, Ascheim DD, et al. 2013 ACCF/AHA guideline for the management of ST-elevation myocardial infarction: executive summary: a report of the American College of Cardiology Foundation/American Heart Association task force on practice guidelines. J Am Coll Cardiol 2013;61(4):485-510.

in approximately 10% of cases (13). Thrombolytic-associated bleeding is more likely in older patients and women, and in patients with diabetes, hypertension, anemia, renal dysfunction, high-risk ACS, and those undergoing invasive procedures (14). Major bleeding is associated with a 60% increased risk of in-hospital death, and a fivefold increase in one-year mortality and reinfarction (14). When associated with low fibrinogen levels (<100 mg/dL), fibrinogen concentrates or cryoprecipitate can be given (see Chapter 13: Platelets and Plasma). The use of antifibrinolytic agents such as tranexamic acid or aminocaproic acid is discouraged because of the risk of re-thrombosis but may be used as a last resort if bleeding is severe (15-16).

ST-Elevation Myocardial Infarction

The optimal management of STEMI is PCI, ideally performed within 90-120 min of hospital arrival (i.e., "door to balloon" time); *PCI less than 90 min* from time of initial presentation is ideal (17-19). If PCI is unavailable, patients should be transferred to a PCI-capable center, but if the transfer time exceeds 120 min, thrombolytic therapy should be administered within 30 min of initial hospital arrival (20). CABG is reserved for patients with multi-vessel coronary artery disease, complex anatomy, or when PCI is ineffective.

Non-ST-Elevation Myocardial Infarction

Urgent PCI is advised for cases of NSTEMI that are complicated by hemodynamic instability, cardiogenic shock, acute heart failure, or persistent chest pain (6-7,9). In NSTEMI, thrombolytic therapy has no benefit and is not used as an alternative to PCI. Patients with UA who are not hemodynamically stable and devoid of pain may not require PCI during hospitalization.

CARDIOPROTECTIVE MEASURES

A summary of measures used to improve the balance between myocardial O_2 supply and O_2 demand are summarized in Table 21.3.

Oxygen

Although used for over a century in the management of patients with acute myocardial infarction, supplemental O_2 provides *no benefit* in normoxemic patients (SpO_2 >90%) (21-22). Hence, supplemental oxygen is only recommended in patients who are hypoxemic (i.e., SpO_2 <90%) (6,9,17,20).

Nitroglycerin

The mechanism of pain relief with nitroglycerin is unclear; vasodilation has been considered as the primary mechanism, but other vasodilators do not relieve pain in ACS. Nitroglycerin reduces both preload and afterload, particularly in the coronary arteries, and this dual action is thought to confer a mortality benefit, although most studies showing such a benefit used IV rather than sublingual preparations (23-24).

Morphine

Morphine is the drug of choice for treating chest pain that is refractory to nitroglycerin. Morphine may impair the antiplatelet effects of P2Y12 inhibitors, although the clinical significance of this effect is unproven (6,25). Use of morphine in ACS has been associated with an increased risk of in-hospital mortality in one systematic review, although the review identified a high risk of bias, and therefore low confidence in this finding (25).

TABLE 21.3 Cardioprotective Measures

Agent	Dosing Regimens and Comments
Oxygen	Dosing: Whatever is needed to maintain an SpO_2 ≥90%. Comment: Use supplemental O_2 judiciously, because it promotes coronary artery vasoconstriction.
Nitroglycerin	Dosing: For chest pain: 0.4 mg sublingual or by mouth spray every 5 min × 3, as needed. For recurrent pain, high BP or CHF: infuse at 5 µg/min initially, then titrate upward to desired end-point. Comment: Avoid in RV infarction, aortic stenosis, and for 24-48 h after a dose of phosphodiesterase inhibitors. Tachyphylaxis is common with prolonged (>24 h) infusions.
Morphine	Dosing: 4-8 mg IV, and follow with 2-8 mg IV every 5-15 min as needed. Comment: Reduces antiplatelet effect of P2Y12 inhibitors, but clinical significance is uncertain
Metoprolol	Dosing: 5 mg IV, repeated every 5 min for up to 3 doses as needed based on heart rate and blood pressure, up to 15 mg maximum total dose. Comment: Avoid early use of β-blockers in acute heart failure, but not after the condition stabilizes. β-blockers contraindicated in cocaine-related ischemia.

From Acute Coronary Syndromes. In: Marino PL. *Marino's The ICU Book*. 5th ed. Wolters Kluwer; 2025:326-42. Table 20.3.

β-Blockers

β-receptor antagonists (blockers) are usually started within the first 24 h after diagnosis of ACS and may be helpful for patients with tachycardia and hypertension. In addition to the contraindications listed in Table 21.3, β-blockers should be avoided when the systolic BP is <120 mm Hg, due to an increased risk for cardiogenic shock (26-27).

ANTITHROMBOTIC MEASURES

Antiplatelet Agents

Antiplatelet therapy has an important role in ACS. The antiplatelet agents and recommended dosing regimens for ACS are listed in Table 21.4.

TABLE 21.4	Antiplatelet Measures for Acute Coronary Thrombosis
Agent	**Dosing Regimen**
Aspirin	162-325 mg (in chewable form) at first patient contact, then daily dose of 81 mg (for dual anti-platelet R_x) or 325 mg
	If aspirin allergy, use clopidogrel.
P2Y12 Inhibitors	
Clopidogrel (Plavix)	PO: 300-600 mg initially, then 75 mg daily
Ticagrelor (Brilinta)	PO: 180 mg initially, then 90 mg twice daily
Prasugrel (Effient)	PO: 60 mg initially, then 10 mg daily
GP IIb-IIIa Inhibitors	
Eptifibatide (Integrilin)	4-8 mg IV, and follow with 2-8 mg IV every 5-15 min as needed
Tirofiban (Aggrastat)	Reduces antiplatelet effect of P2Y12 inhibitors, but clinical significance is uncertain.

From References 6, 9, 20.

Anticoagulant Therapy

Anticoagulation with heparin is recommended for all patients with ACS and is started at the time of diagnosis. Anticoagulation options are described in Table 21.5 (6,11,28-29).

LONG-TERM THERAPIES

Once a patient is clinically stable, several agents are recommended. A high-intensity statin (i.e., atorvastatin, 80 mg daily) is recommended for all patients with ACS (6,9,17-18,20). Inhibition of the renin-angiotensin-aldosterone (RAA) system is recommended for all patients with ACS, especially for patients with hypertension, anterior STEMI, or heart failure associated with reduced ejection fraction (6,9,20). Sacubitril/valsartan (Entresto) is a combination drug with an angiotensin receptor antagonist and a drug (sacubitril) that inhibits neprilysin, an enzyme that degrades natriuretic peptides (30). RAA inhibitors are contraindicated in patients with a history of angioedema and should be used cautiously in patients with renal impairment due to the risk of hyperkalemia. *Long-term* treatment with β-blockers is recommended for all patients with ACS, especially in cases of heart failure associated with reduced ejection fraction (see Chapter 18: Inflammatory Shock).

ACUTE AORTIC DISSECTION

Acute aortic dissection can mimic or include ACS. This condition is a surgical emergency with a mortality rate of >60% without prompt surgical intervention (31).

Pathophysiology

Aortic dissection occurs when a tear in the aortic intima allows blood to dissect between the intimal and medial layers of the aortic wall, creating a false lumen. This process can be the result of atherosclerotic disease or degradation of the aortic wall from a genetic disorder (e.g., Marfan's syndrome).

TABLE 21.5 Anticoagulant Therapy for Acute Coronary Syndromes

Agent	Dosing	Monitoring	Comment
Unfractionated heparin	60 U IV bolus then an infusion of 12 U/kg/h (maximum dose, 1,000 U/h)	aPTT 1.5-2 times control	• Preferred agent for patients receiving PCI • Usually continued for 24-48 h
Low-molecular-weight heparin	30 mg IV bolus followed in 15 min by 1 mg/kg subcutaneously every 12 h	Anti-Xa level 0.6-1.8 IU mL^{-1}	• Used when PCI is non-emergent or deferred • Bolus dosing is not recommended for patients older than 75 years. • 50% dose reduction is recommended when the creatinine clearance is <30 mL/min.
Bivalirudin (direct thrombin inhibitor)	0.75 mg/kg IV bolus followed by an infusion of 1.75 mg/kg/h.	aPTT 1.5-2.5 times control	• Alternative agent for patients with HIT (Chapter 12: Erytrocyte Transfusions) band requiring PCI • Reduce infusion rate to 1 mg/kg/h for creatinine clearance <30 mL/min.
Fondaparinux (factor Xa inhibitor)	2.5 mg IV bolus then 24 h later start 2.5 mg subcutaneous injections daily until catheterization complete	Does not require routine monitoring.*	• Contraindicated if creatinine clearance <30 mL/min.

*May consider dedicated anti-Xa assays in high-risk patient populations (i.e., renal insufficiency, bodyweight <50 kg).

From References 6, 11, 28-29.

The dissection can originate in the ascending or descending aorta. A *Type A* dissection involves the ascending aorta, between the aortic valve and the brachiocephalic artery, and a *Type B* dissection involves the descending aorta, distal to the brachiocephalic artery. Retrograde progression of an aortic dissection can cause aortic valve insufficiency, coronary artery occlusion, and pericardial tamponade, whereas antegrade propagation can lead to neurologic deficits from occlusion of the aortic arch vessels.

Clinical Presentation

Acute aortic dissection presents with a range of symptoms, including considerable overlap with ACS. The hallmark presentation of acute aortic dissection is abrupt "ripping" or "tearing" chest pain which may be substernal (Type A) or in the back (Type B) (32). Only 5% of patients do not have pain (32-33). Chest pain can subside for hours to days and the return of chest pain is often a sign of impending aortic rupture (32-34). *The spontaneous resolution of chest pain is an important symptom that if overlooked, could result in a missed diagnosis* (34). Hypertension is present in >50% of patients but the "classic" sign of unequal pulses in the upper extremities (from obstruction of the left subclavian artery) is only present in 15% of cases (33). The ECG may show ischemic changes in 15% and the chest x-ray can show a widened mediastinum in 60% of cases (33).

Diagnostic Imaging

Because of the limited sensitivity of clinical findings, one of four imaging modalities is required to establish the diagnosis: MRI, transesophageal echocardiography (TEE), contrast enhanced CT, or aortography (35-36). CT is often chosen as the initial study in hemodynamically stable patients due to availability and access. In hemodynamically *unstable* patients, TEE is frequently used as an initial modality to obtain information more rapidly. MRI is the most sensitive and specific test, but multiple tests are frequently required to appropriately guide definitive management (37). Figure 21.2 shows a dissection of the ascending aorta with contrast-enhanced CT.

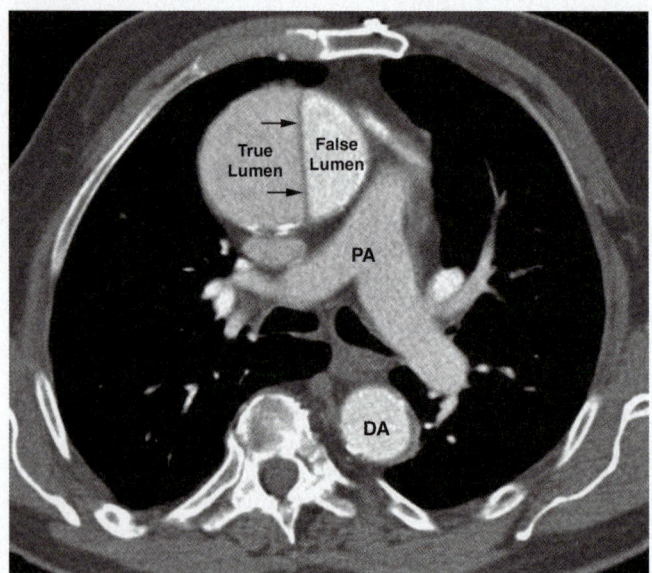

FIGURE 21.2. Contrast-enhanced CT image showing an acute dissection in the ascending aorta. The intimal flap that separates the true and false lumens (indicated by the small arrows) distinguishes an aortic dissection from a saccular aneurysm. PA = pulmonary artery, DA = descending aorta. (From Acute Coronary Syndromes. In: Marino PL. *Marino's The ICU Book*. 5th ed. Wolters Kluwer; 2025:326-42. Figure 20.4.)

Management

The phases of management and hemodynamic goals for aortic dissections are presented in Figure 21.3 (31,38-39).

Table 21.6 lists antihypertensive agents used in acute aortic dissection.

Antihypertensive therapy for aortic dissection *should not be accompanied by tachycardia or an increase in the cardiac output, as these conditions will augment the shear forces*

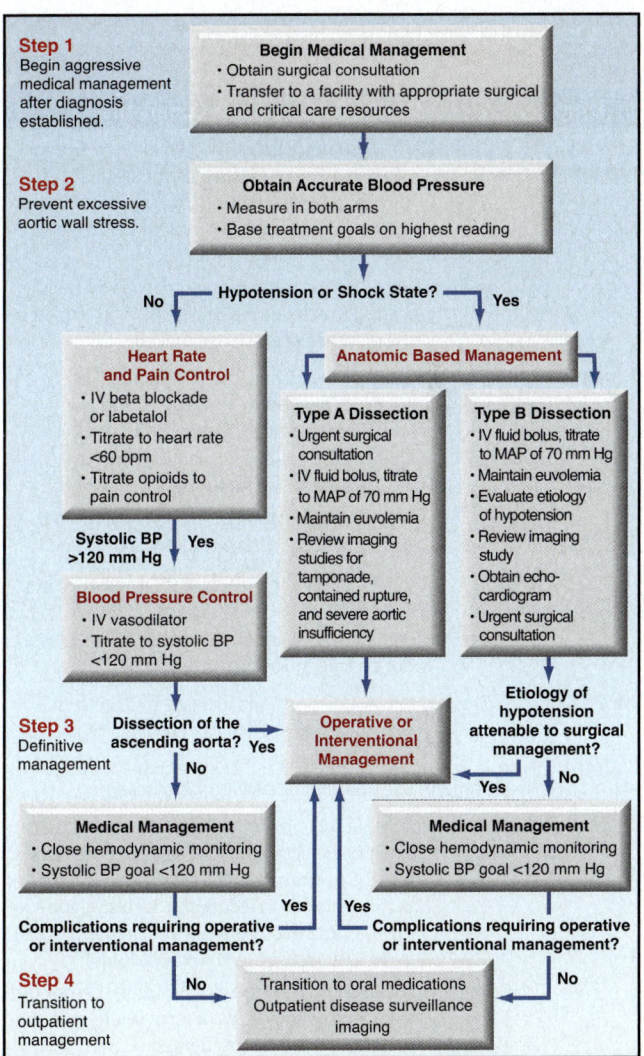

FIGURE 21.3. Acute aortic dissection management. (From References 31, 38-39.)

TABLE 21.6 Antihypertensive Therapy for Acute Aortic Dissection*

Drug	Dosing Regimens and Comments
Esmolol	Dosing: 500 µg/kg as IV bolus, then infuse at 50 µg/kg/min and increase rate in increments of 25 µg/kg/min to desired BP, or to maximum of 200 µg/kg/min. Give a repeat bolus dose before each increment in infusion rate. Comment: Ultra rapid-acting β-blocker that can be rapidly titrated to achieve the desired BP. Not advised in the presence of acute heart failure.
Labetalol	Dosing: 20 mg IV over 2 min, then 20-40 mg IV every 10 min as needed, or infuse at 1-2 mg/min and titrate to desired BP. Max. cumulative dose is 300 mg. Comment: A combined α- and β-blocker that is used as monotherapy. Avoid use in acute heart failure.
Metoprolol	Dosing: 5 mg as IV bolus and repeat in 5 min × 2, if needed. Continue with 5-10 mg IV every 4-6 h, as needed. Comment: Reduces antiplatelet effect of P2Y12 inhibitors, but clinical significance is uncertain.
Nicardipine	Dosing: Infuse at 5 mg/h, and increase by 2.5 mg/h every 5 min as needed to maximum infusion of 15 mg/h. Comment: Use in combination with a β-blocker.
Nitroprusside	Dosing: Infuse at 0.2 µg/kg/min and titrate upward every 5 min to the desired effect. Effective dose is typically 2-5 µg/kg/min, but avoid prolonged infusions at >3 µg/kg/min to reduce the risk of cyanide toxicity. Can add thiosulfate (500 mg) to the infusate (binds cyanide released by nitroprusside). Comment: Use in combination with a β-blocker. Do not use in patients with hepatic or renal failure, or in the presence of coronary ischemia.

*Dosing regimens are manufacturer's recommendations.

From Acute Coronary Syndromes. In: Marino PL. *Marino's The ICU Book*. 5th ed. Wolters Kluwer; 2025:326-42. Table 20.5.

that promote dissection. Titratable β-blockers such as esmolol are co-administered when other antihypertensives are used. Equally important is pain management, because increases in heart rate, cardiac output, and blood pressure are induced by pain. Prompt surgical intervention is required because the mortality rate for acute, Type A dissections increases 1-2% per hour after the onset of symptoms (38).

References

1. Leading Causes of Death. Centers for Disease Control and Prevention. Updated May 2, 2024. Accessed November 2, 2024. https://www.cdc.gov/nchs/fastats/leading-causes-of-death.htm
2. Martin SS, Aday AW, Almarzooq ZI, et al. 2024 heart disease and stroke statistics: a report of US and global data from the American Heart Association. Circulation 2024;149(8):e347-e913.
3. van der Wal AC, Becker AE, van der Loos CM, Das PK. Site of intimal rupture or erosion of thrombosed coronary atherosclerotic plaques is characterized by an inflammatory process irrespective of the dominant plaque morphology. Circulation 1994;89(1):36-44.
4. Malek AM, Alper SL, Izumo S. Hemodynamic shear stress and its role in atherosclerosis. JAMA 1999;282(21):2035-42.
5. Boden WE, De Caterina R, Kaski JC, et al. Myocardial ischaemic syndromes: a new nomenclature to harmonize evolving international clinical practice guidelines. Eur Heart J 2024;45(36):3701-6.
6. Byrne RA, Rossello X, Coughlan JJ, et al. 2023 ESC guidelines for the management of acute coronary syndromes. Eur Heart J Acute Cardiovasc Care 2024;13(1):55-161.
7. Gulati M, Levy PD, Mukherjee D, et al. 2021 AHA/ACC/ASE/CHEST/SAEM/SCCT/SCMR guideline for the evaluation and diagnosis of chest pain: a report of the American College of Cardiology/American Heart Association joint committee on clinical practice. Circulation 2021;144(22):e368-e454.
8. Swamy N. Esophageal spasm: clinical and manometric response to nitroglycerine and long-acting nitrites. Gastroenterology 1977;72(1):23-7.
9. Amsterdam EA, Wenger NK, Brindis RG, et al. 2014 AHA/ACC guideline for the management of patients with non-ST-elevation acute coronary syndromes: a report of the American College of Cardiology/American Heart Association task force on practice guidelines. J Am Coll Cardiol 2014;64(24):2713-4.
10. Thygesen K, Mair J, Giannitsis E, et al. How to use high-sensitivity cardiac troponins in acute cardiac care. Eur Heart J 2012;33(18):2252-7.

11. Lawton JS, Tamis-Holland JE, Bangalore S, et al; Writing Committee Members. 2021 ACC/AHA/SCAI guideline for coronary artery revascularization: a report of the American College of Cardiology/American Heart Association joint committee on clinical practice guidelines J Am Coll Cardiol 2022;79(15):1547.
12. Llevadot J, Giugliano RP, Antman EM. Bolus fibrinolytic therapy in acute myocardial infarction. JAMA 2001;286(4):442-449.
13. Berkowitz SD, Granger CB, Pieper KS, et al. Incidence and predictors of bleeding after contemporary thrombolytic therapy for myocardial infarction. The Global Utilization of Streptokinase and Tissue Plasminogen activator for Occluded coronary arteries (GUSTO) I Investigators. Circulation 1997;95(11):2508-16.
14. Fitchett D. The impact of bleeding in patients with acute coronary syndromes: how to optimize the benefits of treatment and minimize the risk. Can J Cardiol 2007;23(8):663-71.
15. Young GP, Hoffman JR. Thrombolytic therapy. Emerg Med Clin North Am 1995;13(4):735-58.
16. Rinaldi R, Ruberti A, Brugaletta S. Antithrombotic Therapy in acute coronary syndrome. Interv Cardiol Clin 2024;13(4):507-16.
17. O'Connor RE, Brady W, Brooks SC, et al. Part 10: acute coronary syndromes: 2010 American Heart Association guidelines for cardiopulmonary resuscitation and emergency cardiovascular care. Circulation 2010;122(18 Suppl 3):S787-S817.
18. Damluji AA, Forman DE, Wang TY, et al. Management of acute coronary syndrome in the older adult population: a scientific statement from the American Heart Association. Circulation 2023;147(3):e32-e62.
19. Levine GN, Bates ER, Blankenship JC, et al. 2015 ACC/AHA/SCAI focused update on primary percutaneous coronary intervention for patients with ST-elevation myocardial infarction: an update of the 2011 ACCF/AHA/SCAI guideline for percutaneous coronary intervention and the 2013 ACCF/AHA guideline for the management of ST-Elevation myocardial infarction: a report of the American College of Cardiology/American Heart Association Task Force on clinical practice guidelines and the Society for Cardiovascular Angiography and Interventions. Circulation 2016;133(11):1135-47.
20. O'Gara PT, Kushner FG, Ascheim DD, et al. 2013 ACCF/AHA guideline for the management of ST-elevation myocardial infarction: executive summary: a report of the American College of Cardiology Foundation/American Heart Association task force on practice guidelines. J Am Coll Cardiol 2013;61(4):485-510.
21. Sepehrvand N, James SK, Stub D, et al. Effects of supplemental oxygen therapy in patients with suspected acute myocardial infarction: a meta-analysis of randomised clinical trials. Heart 2018;104(20):1691-8.
22. Hofmann R, Svensson L, James SK. Oxygen therapy in suspected acute myocardial infarction. N Engl J Med. 2018;378(2):201-2.

23. Perez MI, Musini VM, Wright JM. Effect of early treatment with anti-hypertensive drugs on short and long-term mortality in patients with an acute cardiovascular event. Cochrane Database Syst Rev 2009;(4):CD006743.
24. Twiner MJ, Hennessy J, Wein R, Levy PD. Nitroglycerin use in the emergency department: current perspectives. Open Access Emerg Med 2022;14:327-33.
25. Duarte GS, Nunes-Ferreira A, Rodrigues FB, et al. Morphine in acute coronary syndrome: systematic review and meta-analysis. BMJ Open 2019;9(3):e025232.
26. Chen ZM, Pan HC, Chen YP, et al. Early intravenous then oral metoprolol in 45,852 patients with acute myocardial infarction: randomised placebo-controlled trial. Lancet 2005;366(9497):1622-32.
27. McCord J, Jneid H, Hollander JE, et al. Management of cocaine-associated chest pain and myocardial infarction: a scientific statement from the American Heart Association acute cardiac care committee of the council on clinical cardiology. Circulation 2008;117(14):1897-907.
28. Sanchez-Pena P, Hulot JS, Urien S, et al. Anti-factor Xa kinetics after intravenous enoxaparin in patients undergoing percutaneous coronary intervention: a population model analysis. Br J Clin Pharmacol 2005;60(4):364-73.
29. Khan MY, Ponde CK, Kumar V, Gaurav K. Fondaparinux: a cornerstone drug in acute coronary syndromes. World J Cardiol 2022;14(1):40-53.
30. Velazquez EJ, Morrow DA, DeVore AD, et al. Angiotensin-neprilysin inhibition in acute decompensated heart failure. N Engl J Med 2019;380(6):539-48.
31. Isselbacher EM, Preventza O, Hamilton Black J 3rd, et al. 2022 ACC/AHA guideline for the diagnosis and management of aortic disease: a report of the American Heart Association/American College of Cardiology joint committee on clinical practice guidelines. Circulation 2022;146(24):e334-e482.
32. Tsai TT, Nienaber CA, Eagle KA. Acute aortic syndromes. Circulation 2005;112(24):3802-13.
33. Knaut AL, Cleveland JC Jr. Aortic emergencies. Emerg Med Clin North Am 2003;21(4):817-45.
34. Lovatt S, Wong CW, Schwarz K, et al. Misdiagnosis of aortic dissection: a systematic review of the literature. Am J Emerg Med 2022;53:16-22.
35. Isselbacher EM, Preventza O, et al. 2022 ACC/AHA guideline for the diagnosis and management of aortic disease: a report of the American Heart Association/American College of Cardiology Joint Committee on clinical practice guidelines. J Thorac Cardiovasc Surg 2023;166(5):e182-e331.

36. Kienzl D, Prosch H, Töpker M, Herold C. Imaging of non-cardiac, non-traumatic causes of acute chest pain. Eur J Radiol 2012;81(12):3669-74.
37. Evangelista A, Isselbacher EM, Bossone E, et al. Insights from the International Registry of Acute Aortic Dissection: a 20-year experience of collaborative clinical research. Circulation 2018;137(17):1846-60.
38. Malaisrie SC, Szeto WY, Halas M, et al. 2021 The American Association for Thoracic Surgery expert consensus document: surgical treatment of acute type A aortic dissection. J Thorac Cardiovasc Surg 2021;162(3):735-8.
39. Hiratzka LF, Bakris GL, Beckman JA, et al. 2010 ACCF/AHA/AATS/ACR/ASA/SCA/SCAI/SIR/STS/SVM guidelines for the diagnosis and management of patients with thoracic aortic disease. A report of the American College of Cardiology Foundation/American Heart Association Task Force on practice guidelines, American Association for Thoracic Surgery, American College of Radiology, American Stroke Association, Society of Cardiovascular Anesthesiologists, Society for Cardiovascular Angiography and Interventions, Society of Interventional Radiology, Society of Thoracic Surgeons, and Society for Vascular Medicine J Am Coll Cardiol 2010;55(14):e27-e129.

Cardiac Arrest

Chapter 22

This chapter describes the practical aspects of cardiopulmonary resuscitation (CPR) and the management that ensues after a successful resuscitation effort. The recommendations in this chapter are taken from the most recent and most relevant consensus guidelines and instruction manuals on CPR (1-4).

BASIC LIFE SUPPORT

Time Dependence

The heart is an exceptionally resilient organ, beating over 2-3 billion times during the average human lifespan. Hence, *cardiac arrest represents an extreme physiological event*, and the success of CPR depends on the rapid restoration of blood flow to prevent irreversible cell death. The total O_2 content of the adult human body is about 1 L, with a normal O_2 consumption of approximately 250 mL/min at rest. Thus, *following the cessation of blood flow from a cardiac arrest, anoxic cell death is expected in just 4-5 min*. This emphasizes the need to perform CPR as soon as possible because "time is tissue."

The trigger for CPR is the absence of pulses in an unresponsive patient who has minimal or no spontaneous breathing efforts (i.e., a pulseless and apneic patient). Chest compressions should begin within 10 s, using the depth and frequency of compressions shown in Table 22.1. Two lung inflations should be delivered with a bag-mask device after every 30 chest compressions (1-6). After an endotracheal tube is placed, lung inflations are delivered at 6-s intervals (10/min) without interrupting chest compressions. An ECG monitor/defibrillator should be attached to the patient as soon as possible.

TABLE 22.1 Essential Elements of Basic Life Support

1. Chest compressions should begin within 10 s of detecting the absence of pulses.
2. Each chest compression should depress the lower third of the sternum by 2-2.5 inches (5-6 cm), and the chest should be allowed to recoil completely before the next compression.
3. The rate of compressions should be 100-120/min.
4. After 30 chest compressions, 2 lung inflations are delivered (with a bag-mask device) without interrupting the compressions, and this (30:2) cycle is repeated until the patient is intubated.
5. Following intubation, lung inflations are delivered every 6 s (10/min) without interrupting chest compressions.
6. Chest compressions should be continued without interruption until a defibrillator is attached to the patient.
7. Each person performing chest compressions should be relieved after 2 min, if possible.

From References 1-4.

Chest Compressions

The foundation of Basic Life Support (BLS) is high-quality chest compressions with minimal interruptions, because interruptions contribute to poor outcomes (5). High-quality chest compressions are defined as having a rate of 100-120/min, a depth of 2-2.5 inches (5-6 cm), and allowance for full chest recoil between compressions (1-4). Fatigue during CPR is common, and each person performing compressions should be replaced after 2 min (3-4).

Lung Inflations

The recommended volume for each lung inflation when using a self-inflating bag is 500-600 mL (3-4). The volume capacity of most adult ventilation bags is 1-2 L; thus, large inflation volumes are common during CPR (6). To prevent excessive inflation volumes, breaths should be delivered until the chest wall visibly rises. Rapid lung inflations are also common during CPR and should be avoided so the lungs have sufficient time to empty. Rapid breathing leads to progressive hyperinflation and positive end-expiratory pressure (PEEP), reducing venous return (preload) to the heart and reducing coronary perfusion pressure (7). Accordingly, hyperventilation should be avoided by administering breaths at a frequency of 10 per min (i.e., every 6 s) during CPR.

ADVANCED LIFE SUPPORT

Advanced Cardiovascular Life Support (ACLS) includes electrical therapies (i.e., cardioversion or defibrillation) and the use of drugs to support the resuscitation attempt (2,4). The ACLS management algorithm is shown in Figure 22.1. The main features are summarized here:

1. If the rhythm is shockable (i.e., ventricular fibrillation [VF]/ventricular tachycardia [VT]), immediate defibrillation is recommended. The initial shock is 120-200 J for biphasic shocks (unless otherwise specified by the manufacturer). If not successful, a higher energy level can be used for subsequent shocks, if allowed by the defibrillator.
2. Chest compressions are paused when the defibrillation shock is delivered and are resumed immediately thereafter. At least 2 min of high-quality chest compressions are recommended after each defibrillation before checking the post-shock rhythm.
3. If a second defibrillation is required, 1 mg of *epinephrine* is administered (IV or intraosseous [IO]) every 3-5 min throughout the resuscitation attempt.
4. If a third defibrillation is needed, *amiodarone* is given as a bolus dose of 300 mg (IV or IO) and followed by a second dose of 150 mg if needed. If amiodarone is not available, *lidocaine* can be given in an initial dose of 1-1.5 mg/kg (IV or IO), followed by 0.5-0.75 mg/kg every 5-10 min as needed, to a maximum dose of 3 mg/kg (2,4).

Adult Cardiac Arrest Algorithm.

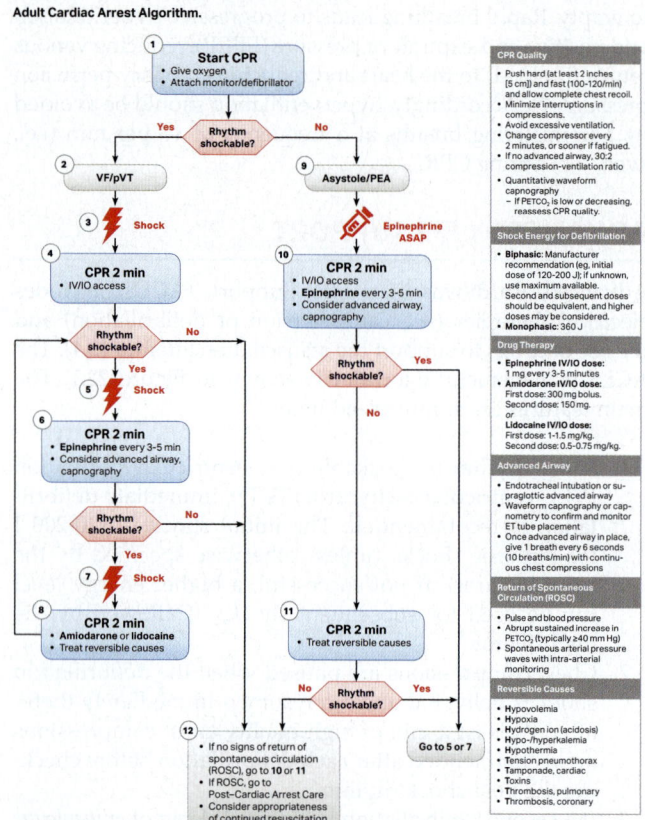

FIGURE 22.1. The American Heart Association algorithm for ACLS. (Reprinted from American Heart Association. *Advanced Cardiovascular Life Support Provider Manual*. American Heart Association; 2020.)

Reversible causes of cardiac arrest should be considered throughout the resuscitation effort and are described by the "H's" and "T's," as listed in Table 22.2. Point-of-care ultrasound is a valuable aid for identifying many of these conditions (see Chapter 7: Bedside Echocardiography).

TABLE 22.2 Reversible Causes of Cardiac Arrest (i.e., the "H's" and "T's")

"H's"	"'Ts"
Hypovolemia	Tension pneumothorax
Hypoxemia	Tamponade (pericardial)
Hydrogen ions (i.e., acidosis)	Thromboembolism (i.e., pulmonary embolism)
Hypo- or Hyperkalemia	
Hypothermia Toxins	Thrombosis (i.e., coronary artery thrombosis)
	Toxins

From American Heart Association. *Advanced Cardiovascular Life Support Provider Manual*. American Heart Association; 2020.

Defibrillation

The delivery of asynchronous electrical shocks (i.e., not timed to the QRS complex) is called *defibrillation*. The survival benefit for defibrillation is one of only a few interventions that has been shown to improve survival in cardiac arrest victims, but the survival benefit is time dependent. In one study that studied the relationship between survival and time from collapse from cardiac arrest, 40% of patients survived when the first shock was delivered within 5 min whereas fewer than 10% of patients survived when defibrillation was delayed until 20 min after the arrest (8-9).

Impulse Energy

Contemporary defibrillators deliver biphasic shocks, with an energy level that varies from as low as 100 J to as high as 360 J (10). Biphasic shocks can convert VF and VT at lower energy than monophasic shocks. Automatic external defibrillators (AEDs) deliver fixed-energy shocks. Double sequential external defibrillation (DSED, also termed *double defibrillation*), is the administration of shocks from two defibrillators with defibrillation pads placed in two different planes (anterior–lateral and anterior–posterior) (10). Although this technique has been shown to be effective for refractory VF in some studies, others have not demonstrated a benefit (11-12).

Ventricular Fibrillation and Pulseless Ventricular Tachycardia

The principal intervention for VF and pulseless VT is defibrillation. When three defibrillation attempts (see Figure 22.1) fail to convert VF or VT, the prognosis is very poor, with only 5% of cases resulting in a satisfactory outcome (13). In cases of shock-resistant VF/VT, management with veno-arterial extracorporeal membrane oxygenation (VA ECMO) has been used with neurologically favorable survival rates approaching 30% (14). This approach is termed *extracorporeal cardiopulmonary resuscitation* (ECPR) (15). A list of potential indications for ECPR is presented in Table 22.3.

TABLE 22.3 Indications for Extracorporeal Cardiopulmonary Resuscitation

- Age <70 years
- Witnessed arrest
- Arrest to first CPR (i.e., "no-flow interval") <5 min
- Initial cardiac rhythm of VF/VT/PEA
- Arrest to ECMO flow time of <60 min (i.e., "low flow interval")
- $ETCO_2$ >10 mm Hg (1.3 kPa) during CPR prior to cannulation for ECMO
- Intermittent ROSC and/or recurrent VF
- Signs of life during conventional CPR (i.e., breathing, spontaneous movements, gagging, intermittent ROSC)
- Absence of life-limiting medical conditions (e.g., end stage heart failure, chronic obstructive pulmonary disease, end stage renal failure, liver failure)
- No known aortic valve incompetence

CPR = cardiopulmonary resuscitation; ECMO = extracorporeal membrane oxygenation; PEA = pulseless electrical activity; ROSC = return of spontaneous circulation, VF = ventricular fibrillation; VT = ventricular tachycardia.

From Reference 15.

Asystole and Pulseless Electrical Activity

The management of asystole and pulseless electrical activity (PEA) is described on the right side of Figure 22.1. Aside from high-quality CPR and attempts to reverse the underlying etiology, the major intervention for asystole and PEA is vasopressor therapy with *epinephrine*. Defibrillation is not indicated unless the rhythm changes to VF and pulseless VT.

Epinephrine

Although epinephrine has been shown to increase the rate of return of spontaneous circulation (ROSC), the impact on survival is uncertain (16). Use of standard-dose epinephrine has been shown to increase ROSC and survival to hospital admission but may not improve survival to discharge or functional outcome (17). Moreover, the survival benefit may be more pronounced among patients with a non-shockable rhythm but not those with a shockable rhythm (17).

Epinephrine, Vasopressin and Steroids

Epinephrine, when given in combination with vasopressin (i.e., 20 IU every CPR cycle for a maximum of 4 or 5 doses) and steroids (i.e., 40 mg methylprednisolone or 240-300 mg hydrocortisone), have been shown to be associated with significant increases in ROSC, survival to hospital discharge, favorable neurological outcomes, higher blood pressure, and fewer organ failures (18). The effect of this combination seems to be most pronounced with in-hospital cardiac arrest.

RESUSCITATION MONITORING

End-Tidal PCO_2

Monitoring for ROSC has been traditionally limited to manual pulse checks, although this practice has low sensitivity (19). The PCO_2 in exhaled gas at the end of expiration is known as the end-tidal CO_2 ($ETCO_2$). The $ETCO_2$ provides physiological insight regarding the balance between ventilation and perfusion because when alveolar ventilation is constant, changes in $ETCO_2$ reflect proportional changes in cardiac output (i.e., a 30% decrease in $ETCO_2$ indicates a 30% decrease in cardiac output). $ETCO_2$ measurements can be used to identify the likelihood of ROSC. Figure 22.2 shows the relationship between ROSC and serial changes in $ETCO_2$ (20).

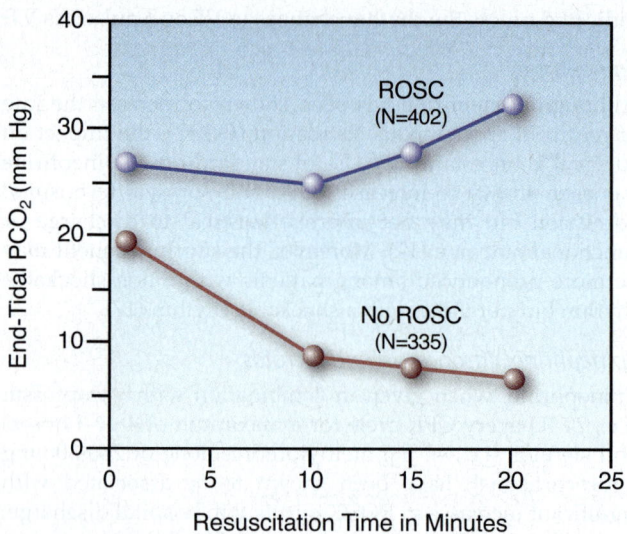

FIGURE 22.2. Serial changes in end tidal PCO_2 during CPR in relation to return of spontaneous circulation (ROSC) in 737 cases of out-of-hospital cardiac arrest. N indicates the number of patients in each group and data points represent mean values. CPR = cardiopulmonary resuscitation. (From Rolston DM. Time is running out for manual pulse checks, as ultrasound races past. Resuscitation 2022;179:59-60.)

The majority of evidence indicates that a successful resuscitation is unlikely if the $ETCO_2$ is not higher than 10-15 mm Hg after 20 min of CPR (i.e., an $ETCO_2$ <10 mm Hg after 20 min of CPR is associated with a 0.5% likelihood of ROSC) (21). The reader is referred to an excellent online reference for clinical capnography, which includes $ETCO_2$ tracings during cardiac arrest (https://www.capnography.com/).

Ultrasound

Point-of-care ultrasound is invaluable for the detection of potentially reversible causes of cardiac arrest, including tension pneumothorax or pericardial tamponade (see Chapter 7: Bedside Echocardiography). The classic echocardiographic signs of pericardial tamponade (i.e., diastolic collapse of the right ventricle) are unreliable during a cardiac arrest due to low intracardiac pressures, so the presence of any pericardial effusion during an arrest should prompt immediate pericardiocentesis (Figure 22.3).

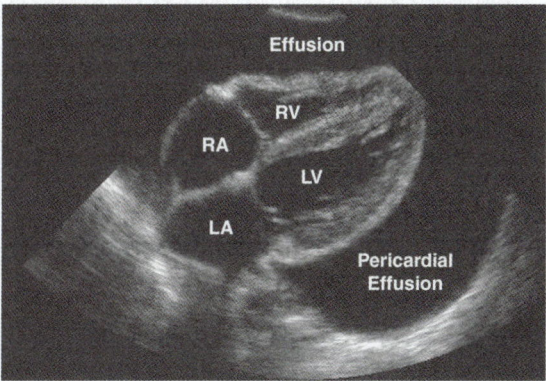

FIGURE 22.3. Ultrasound image (subcostal view) showing a large pericardial effusion which appears as a broad anechoic band surrounding the heart. RA = right atrium; RV = right ventricle; LA = left atrium; LV = left ventricle.

POST-RESUSCITATION PERIOD

The immediate goal of CPR is ROSC, but this does not guarantee a satisfactory outcome. Approximately 70% of patients who survive resuscitation following cardiac arrest do not survive the hospitalization (23). This section describes the common problems encountered following a successful resuscitation of cardiac arrest.

Post-Cardiac Arrest Syndrome

The *post-cardiac arrest syndrome* refers to dysfunction in one or more major organs. The principal features of this syndrome are as follows:

1. Brain injury is the most common manifestation of the post-cardiac arrest syndrome and is responsible for 23-68% of deaths following cardiac arrest (24). Clinical manifestations include persistent coma, myoclonus, and generalized seizures.
2. Post-arrest cardiac dysfunction is a combination of systolic and diastolic heart failure that can progress to cardiogenic shock (see Chapters 16: Hemorrhagic Shock and 18: Inflammatory Shock). Myocardial "stunning," a type of reperfusion injury, is the usual cause and normally resolves within 72 h (24).
3. A systemic inflammatory response (i.e., fever, leukocytosis) is almost universally present after cardiac arrest (see Chapter 17: Cardiogenic Shock).

Temperature Control

Elevated body temperature is well-known for its ability to aggravate ischemic brain injury (25). *The goal of temperature control is to prevent fever (i.e., a target body temperature of <37.5° C [<99.5° F]) in comatose survivors of cardiac arrest.* The elements of temperature control are described in Table 22.4.

Candidates for temperature control include all patients who do not regain consciousness after ROSC (1). Temperature-controlled cooling devices are only used if the body temperature rises above 37.7° C (99.9° F), and surface cooling is usually sufficient, with a target temperature set at 37.5° C.

Additional Management Goals

In the early post-arrest period, there are additional critical care management concerns, as summarized in Table 22.5.

TABLE 22.4	Temperature Control
Feature	Recommendations†
Indication	Patients who do not regain consciousness after ROSC
Goal	Body temperature ≤37.5° C (≤99.5° F) for 72 h
Monitoring	Continuous monitoring of core body temperature; e.g., with a thermistor-equipped bladder catheter
Treatment Plan	1. Patients with mild hypothermia (32°-36° C) after ROSC should not be actively rewarmed. 2. Maintain body temperature at ≤37.5° C with acetaminophen and reduced room temperature, if needed. 3. If body temperature rises >37.7° C (>99.9° F), start active cooling, and set target temperature at 37.5° C (99.5° F). 4. Surface cooling is acceptable. 5. Body temperature is kept at ≤37.5° C for 72 h, unless the patient awakens.

From Reference 1.

TABLE 22.5	Additional Management Concerns Following Resuscitation from Cardiac Arrest
Intervention	Comment
Oxygen therapy	Hyperoxia aggravates neurologic injury after cardiac arrest so O_2 inhalation should be used only to correct hypoxemia (SpO_2 <90%).
Vasopressor	Targeting a MAP >75 mm Hg may be beneficial for neurologic recovery. Norepinephrine is preferred to epinephrine.
Glycemic control	*Hyper*glycemia aggravates neurologic injury after cardiac arrest, as does *hypo*glycemia. Hence, "tight" glycemic control is avoided due to the risk of *hypo*glycemia. A blood glucose goal in the range of 145-180 mg/dL is considered a reasonable range post-arrest.

MAP = mean arterial pressure.

From References 1, 23-24, 28.

Although a standard recommendation for hypotension is to maintain a mean arterial pressure (MAP) >65 mm Hg, observational studies have shown that patients with higher blood pressure have better neurologic outcomes (26-27). The preferred vasopressor in post-cardiac arrest shock has not been established with robust clinical outcomes data, although norepinephrine has been shown to be advantageous in a few studies (28-29).

Predicting Neurologic Recovery

The predictors of a poor neurologic outcome after cardiac arrest are listed in Table 22.6 (30).

TABLE 22.6 Predictors of a Poor Neurologic Outcome After Cardiac Arrest

1. Absence of pupillary light reflexes bilaterally on day 4 after ROSC.
2. Absence of corneal reflexes bilaterally on day 4 after ROSC.
3. Absence of oculocephalic or gag reflexes on day 2 after ROSC.
4. Myoclonic status at any time after ROSC.
5. Bilateral absence of the N20 peak on somatosensory evoked potentials.
6. An EEG that shows nonconvulsive status epilepticus or background suppression with periodic discharges.
7. A CT scan that shows diffuse cerebral edema.

CT = computed tomography; EEG = electroencephalogram; ROSC = return of spontaneous circulation.

From Sandroni CD, Arrigo S, Cacciola S, et al. Prediction of poor neurologic outcome in comatose survivors of cardiac arrest: a systematic review. Intensive Care Med 2020;46:1803-51.

Approximately 80-95% of patients who regain consciousness after ROSC awaken after 72 h, but it may take 5 days or even longer, especially if patients are subjected to hypothermia (i.e., target temperatures of 32-34° C) (31-32).

References

1. Wyckoff MH, Greif R, Morley PT, et al. 2022 International consensus on cardiopulmonary resuscitation and emergency cardiovascular care science with treatment recommendations: summary from the Basic Life Support; Advanced Life Support; Pediatric Life Support; Neonatal Life Support; Education, Implementation and Teams; and First Aid Task Forces. Resuscitation 2022;208-88.
2. Panchal AR, Bartos JA, Cabañas JG, et al. Part 3: Adult basic and advanced life support: 2020 American Heart Association guidelines for cardiopulmonary resuscitation and emergency cardiovascular care. Circulation 2020;142(Suppl 2):S366-S468.
3. American Heart Association. *Basic Life Support Provider Manual*. American Heart Association; 2016.
4. American Heart Association. *Advanced Cardiovascular Life Support Provider Manual*. American Heart Association; 2020.
5. Wit L, Kramer-Johansen J, Mykelbust H, et al. Quality of cardiopulmonary resuscitation during out-of-hospital cardiac arrest. JAMA 2005;293:299-304.
6. Berg RA, Hemphill R, Abella BS, et al. Part 5: Adult basic life support: 2010 American Heart Association guidelines for cardiopulmonary resuscitation and emergency cardiovascular care. Circulation 2010;122(Suppl 3):S685-S705.
7. Aufderheide TP, Lurie KG. Death by hyperventilation: a common and life-threatening problem during cardiopulmonary resuscitation. Crit Care Med 2004;32(Suppl):S345-51.
8. Larsen MP, Eisenberg M, Cummins RO, Hallstrom AP. Predicting survival from out of hospital cardiac arrest: a graphic model. Ann Emerg Med 1993;22:1652-8.
9. Koster RW, Walker RG, Chapman FW. Recurrent ventricular fibrillation during advanced life support care of patients with prehospital cardiac arrest. Resuscitation 2008;78:252-7.
10. Hoch DH, Batsford WP, Greenberg SM, et al. Double sequential external shocks for refractory ventricular fibrillation. J Am Coll Cardiol 1994;23(5):1141-5.
11. Yu J, Yu Y, Liang H, et al. Defibrillation strategies for patients with refractory ventricular fibrillation: a systematic review and meta-analysis. Am J Emerg Med 2024;84:149-57.
12. Cheskes S, Verbeek PR, Drennan IR, et al. Defibrillation strategies for refractory ventricular fibrillation. N Engl J Med 2022;387(21):1947-56.
13. Sakai T, Iwami T, Tasaki O, et al. Incidence and outcomes of out-of-hospital cardiac arrest with shock-resistant ventricular fibrillation: data from a large population-based cohort. Resuscitation 2010;81:956-61.

14. Fernando SM, Mathew R, Sadeghirad B, et al. Epinephrine in out-of-hospital cardiac arrest: a network meta-analysis and subgroup analyses of shockable and nonshockable rhythms. Chest 2023;164(2):381-93.
15. Richardson ASC, Tonna JE, Nanjayya V, et al. Extracorporeal cardiopulmonary resuscitation in adults. Interim guideline consensus statement from the Extracorporeal Life Support Organization. ASAIO J 2021;67(3):221-8.
16. Perkins GD, Ji C, Deakin CD, et al; for the PARAMEDIC2 Collaborators. A randomized trial of epinephrine in out-of-hospital cardiac arrest. N Engl J Med 2018;379:711-21.
17. Fernando SM, Mathew R, Sadeghirad B, et al. Epinephrine in out-of-hospital cardiac arrest: a network meta-analysis and subgroup analyses of shockable and nonshockable rhythms. Chest 2023;164(2):381-93.
18. Ho JK, Tam HL, Leung LY. Effectiveness of vasopressin against cardiac arrest: a systematic review of systematic reviews. Cardiovasc Drugs Ther 2024; Online ahead of print.
19. Rolston DM. Time is running out for manual pulse checks, as ultrasound races past. Resuscitation 2022;179:59-60.
20. Kolar M, Krizmaric M, Klemen P, Grmec S. Partial pressure of end-tidal carbon dioxide predicts successful cardiopulmonary resuscitation in the field: a prospective observational study. Crit Care 2008;12:R115.
21. Paiva EF, Paxton JH, O'Neil BJ. The use of end-tidal carbon dioxide (ETCO2) measurement to guide management of cardiac arrest: a systematic review. Resuscitation 2018;123:1-7.
22. Medical Education Curriculum in Radiology. Stritch School of Medicine. Accessed November 18, 2024. https://www.luc.edu/stritch/
23. Nolan JP, Neumar RW, Adrie C, et al. Post-cardiac arrest syndrome: epidemiology, pathophysiology, and prognostication. A scientific statement from the International Liaison Committee on Resuscitation; the American Heart Association Emergency Cardovascular Care Committee; the Council on Cardiovascular Surgery and Anesthesia; the Council on Cardiopulmonary, Perioperative, and Critical Care; the Council on Clinical Cardiology; the Council on Stroke. Resuscitation 2008;79:350-79.
24. Huet O, Dupic L, Batteux F, et al. Post-resuscitation syndrome: potential role of hydroxyl radical-induced endothelial cell damage. Crit Care Med 2011;39:1712-20.
25. Zeiner A, Holzer M, Sterz F, et al. Hyperthermia after cardiac arrest is associated with an unfavorable neurologic outcome. Arch Intern Med 2001;161:2007-12.
26. Müllner M, Sterz F, Binder M, et al. Arterial blood pressure after human cardiac arrest and neurologic recovery. Stroke 1996;27:59-62.

27. Kilgannon JH, Roberts BW, Jones AE, et al. Arterial blood pressure and neurologic outcome after resuscitation from cardiac arrest. Crit Care Med 2014;42:2083-91.
28. Lawson CK, Faine BA, Rech MA, et al. Norepinephrine versus epinephrine for hemodynamic support in post-cardiac arrest shock: a systematic review. Am J Emerg Med 2024;77:158-63.
29. Bougouin W, Slimani K, Renaudier M, et al; for the Sudden Death Expertise Center Investigators. Epinephrine versus norepinephrine in cardiac arrest patients with post-resuscitation shock. Intensive Care Med 2022;48(3):300-10.
30. Sandroni CD, Arrigo S, Cacciola S, et al. Prediction of poor neurologic outcome in comatose survivors of cardiac arrest: a systematic review. Intensive Care Med 2020;46:1803-51.
31. Wijdicks EFM. Brain injury after cardiac arrest: refining prognosis. Neurol Clin 2025;43(1):79-90.
32. Lybeck A, Cronberg T, Aneman A, et al. Time to awakening after cardiac arrest and the association of targeted temperature management. Resuscitation 2018;126:166-71.

RESPIRATORY DISORDERS — SECTION VI

Pulmonary Embolism — Chapter 23

CLINICAL EVALUATION

Clinical Presentation

The typical clinical presentation of acute pulmonary embolism (PE) is dyspnea, tachycardia, and hypoxemia. Unfortunately, these are also common signs of many acute cardiopulmonary diseases. Overall, *the diagnosis of PE is confirmed in only 10% of suspected cases* (1), which reflects the nonspecific clinical presentation of PE. Table 23.1 demonstrates the predictive value of clinical findings in suspected PE (2).

Note that none of the findings are reliable for confirming or excluding the presence of PE. In particular, hypoxemia has only a 70% negative predictive value, which means 30% of patients with acute PE have a normal arterial PO_2! Except for extremity swelling which may represent deep venous thrombosis (DVT) and indirectly implicate PE, there are no specific physical exam findings diagnostic of PE. A detailed physical examination, however, may elucidate another cardiopulmonary process to explain a patient's presentation, e.g., pneumothorax, heart failure, pneumonia. Considering the lack of specificity of the physical exam, clinical signs and symptoms, diagnostic testing is required.

Diagnostic Studies

Laboratories

- *D-dimer* is a product of clot breakdown and is elevated in the presence of acute thrombosis. In practicality, its utility is limited to screening in outpatient or emergency department settings as it has high sensitivity but low

specificity (3-4). D-dimer is also elevated in other conditions such as sepsis, inflammatory conditions, heart failure, renal failure, pregnancy, and advanced age (3), and is therefore not considered a useful diagnostic *or screening* test for acute PE in the ICU setting.
- *B-Type Natriuretic Peptide (BNP)* is a cardiovascular hormone that is released from the heart in response to ventricular dilatation. Right ventricular overload due to acute PE will result in elevated BNP (5). Other cardiac disorders will cause increased BNP level limiting its use as a diagnostic tool, however, elevated BNP in acute PE is associated with a worse outcome (6-8).
- *Troponins* are cardiac proteins that regulate myocardial contraction and are elevated in cardiac injury (9). Not specific to PE, the elevation is a marker of myocardial

TABLE 23.1 Predictive Value of Clinical Findings for Diagnosis of Pulmonary Embolism

Findings	Positive Predictive Value[†]	Negative Predictive Value[‡]
Dyspnea	37%	75%
Tachycardia	47%	86%
Tachypnea	48%	75%
Pleuritic chest pain	39%	71%
Hemoptysis	32%	67%
Pulmonary infiltrate	33%	71%
Pleural effusion	40%	69%
Hypoxemia	34%	70%

[†]Positive predictive value is the percentage of patients with the finding who have a pulmonary embolus.

[‡]Negative predictive value is the percentage of patients without the finding who do not have a pulmonary embolus.

From Hoellerich VL, Wigton RS. Diagnosing pulmonary embolism using clinical findings. Arch Intern Med 1986;146:1699-704.

stress (e.g., right ventricular dilatation) and is also associated with increased mortality (8,10).

Chest X-Ray

There are several eponymous chest x-ray findings that are "suggestive" of PE (i.e., Westermark sign, Hampton's hump, Fleischner's sign, the Knuckle sign, and others), however, none are diagnostic. The value of a plain film chest x-ray is the ability to identify other potential causes of the patient's symptomatology and presentation, *potentially* negating the need for computed tomographic angiography (CTA).

Venous Duplex Ultrasonography

Since most PE originate from DVT in proximal lower extremity veins (5), venous duplex ultrasonography (VDUS) looking for lower extremity DVT seems like a rational approach to suspected PE. Duplex ultrasonography has numerous advantages: noninvasive, no radiation, does not require radiocontrast dye, and it can be done at the bedside. Color-flow doppler can be added to show speed and direction of flow. Unfortunately, DVT is identified on VDUS in <50% of PE, as thrombi have already embolized to the lung (11). The utility of VDUS in venous thromboembolism as a whole is its ability to diagnose and treat DVT to *prevent* PE (12). An example of positive color-flow VDUS is shown in Figure 23.1.

Bedside Echocardiography

Unfortunately, there are no well-defined parameters for the diagnosis of PE using echocardiography (ECHO), and smaller PE may not result in cardiac changes. Even the "classic" McConnell's sign is only *suggestive* of PE (5). Bedside echocardiography may also elucidate other cardiac causes of the clinical presentation but clearly also has a role in risk stratification in patients who do demonstrate cardiac dysfunction (13). In hemodynamically unstable patients with high suspicion for PE and clear ECHO findings of right heart dysfunction, immediate pulmonary reperfusion efforts should proceed without further testing (5,14).

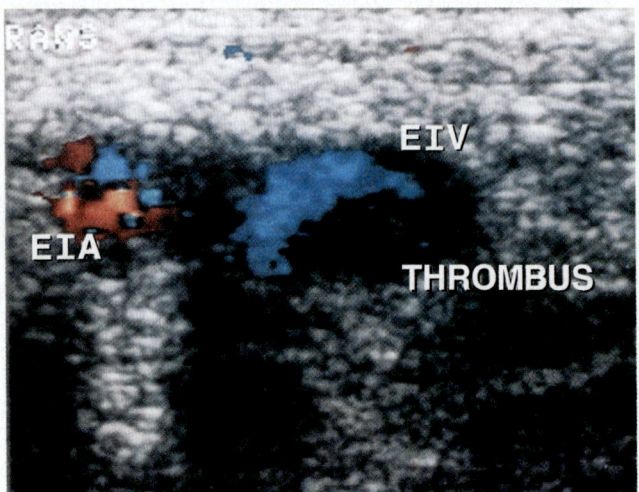

FIGURE 23.1. Color-flow venous doppler ultrasound of external iliac deep venous thrombosis. EIA = external iliac artery; EIV = external iliac vein.

Computed Tomographic Angiography

CTA is the imaging modality of choice for the diagnosis of PE (5,15-16). CTA's value is not limited to the diagnosis of PE (diagnostic as far out as the segmental pulmonary artery branches); it also provides information regarding clot *burden, and potential* right heart strain (15) not to mention the ability to identify other cardiopulmonary pathology (e.g., pneumonia, atelectasis, pleural effusions, pneumothoraces, pericardial effusion). Current technological advances in computed tomography have improved the sensitivity and specificity of CTA for the diagnosis of PE to 94% and 98% respectively (16). Examples of CTA diagnoses of PE are shown in Figure 23.2.

Ventilation-Perfusion Lung Scan

A ventilation-perfusion lung (V/Q) scan is a radionucleotide imaging study that has limited utility in the ICU patient. The presence of lung disease (essentially ubiquitous in the ICU patient) significantly impacts V/Q scan interpretation. The classic indications for V/Q scans are for those patients that have contraindication to CTA (which requires a significant radiation exposure and iodinated contrast). Contraindications include pregnancy, renal insufficiency, chronic kidney disease stage 4 or greater, or severe contrast allergy (17). These contraindications for CTA are debatable when the need for a clear diagnosis is essential, the pitfalls of V/Q scans are considered, and there are interventions to mitigate complications. An individualized risk-to-benefit analysis for each case is necessary i.e., weighing the risks of contrast exposure in the face of renal insufficiency, radiation during pregnancy, and anaphylaxis with severe allergies. Regarding pregnancy, current CT scanning technology delivers less radiation, and diagnostic accuracy is better, making CTA the test of choice in pregnancy over V/Q scanning (18). Furthermore, pregnant patients can have the additional protective lead apron coverage of the abdomen and pelvis during scanning. Severe contrast allergies can be addressed with desensitization protocols (19-21). Finally, V/Q scanning requires pharmacy preparation of the nucleotides, so along with the scan it takes a minimum of 3 h to perform.

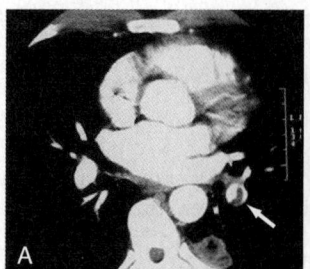 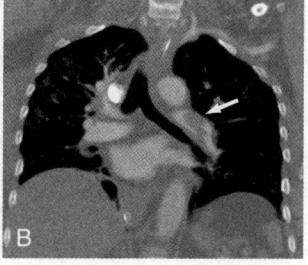

FIGURE 23.2. CTA diagnoses of pulmonary emboli. (A) Axial image of pulmonary embolism (*arrow*). (B) Coronal image of pulmonary embolism (*arrow*).

Magnetic Resonance Angiography

Although a promising radiation-free technology, magnetic resonance angiography (MRA) for diagnosing PE currently has low sensitivity (5). Time for image acquisition and other logistical limitations of magnetic resonance scans contraindicate this modality in unstable patients (22).

Pulmonary Angiography

Once the "gold standard" method for the diagnosis of PE, CTA has supplanted pulmonary angiography for the diagnosis of PE. Its only role now is as a road map for therapeutic interventions such as catheter-directed thrombolysis.

MANAGEMENT

Multiple scoring systems are available for predicting the probability of PE; however, the value of clinical judgment has also been validated. Expectations are that the proportion of confirmed PE would be expected to be <10% (low-probability); 30% (intermediate-probability); and 65% (high-probability) (5). Anticoagulation should be initiated for high- and intermediate-probability patients during the diagnostic phase (*prior to diagnosis!*) unless there is high bleeding risk, e.g., recent major surgery (5,23).

Risk stratification can guide therapy. The American Heart Association and the European Society of Cardiology PE severity and risk classification is shown in Table 23.2.

Anticoagulation

The initial management of VTE that is not immediately life-threatening is anticoagulation with heparin.

Low-Molecular-Weight Heparin

Low-molecular-weight heparin (LMWH) is preferred in hemodynamically stable patients due to simplicity and less bleeding complications, reduced VTE recurrence, and a lower incidence of heparin-induced thrombocytopenia compared with unfractionated heparin (5,24-25).

Enoxaparin is favored because it is the LMWH studied most extensively in acute PE. The dosing and monitoring of enoxaparin are shown in Figure 23.3 (26-27).

Unfractionated Heparin

Intravenous heparin (bolus, then infusion) has been preferred for the initial management of intermediate and high-risk patients because it achieves rapid anticoagulation and off-set monitoring is easily available to ensure therapeutic anticoagulation is achieved.

It is recommended that heparin dosing be based on *total* body weight (27-28). Dosing and monitoring are outlined in Figure 23.4 (26-28).

TABLE 23.2 AHA/ESC Pulmonary Embolism Classification

Classification	Characteristics	Percentage of PE's	30-Day Mortality Rate
Massive/ High-risk	• Presence of hypotension, systolic BP <90 mm Hg, or drop of ≥40 mm Hg for at least 15 min • Requirement of vasopressor support	5%	~65%
Submassive/ Intermediate risk	• Presence of RV strain, dilation or dysfunction • Intermediate-to-high: RV dysfunction or RV injury • Intermediate-to-low: if only one or neither	40%	5-25%
Low risk	• Do not meet criteria for submassive or intermediate risk	40-60%	~1%

AHA/ESC = American Heart Association/ European Society of Cardiology; BP = blood pressure; PE = pulmonary embolism; RV = right ventricular.

From Russell C, Keshavamurthy S, Saha S. Classification and stratification of pulmonary embolisms. Int J Angiol 2022;31(3):162-5. Table 1.

Enoxaparin Dosing   Anti-Xa Level Target*

1. 1 mg/kg SQ twice daily   0.5-1 units/mL
2. 1.5 mg/kg SQ once daily   1-2 units/mL

*The pharmacokinetics of enoxaparin are predictable and the use of anti-Xa levels is typically not necessary. Levels may be useful in patients with extremes of weight (<50 kg or >150 kg), pregnancy, or renal insufficiency (serum creatinine clearance <39 mL/min). Consider use of unfractionated heparin in these populations.

FIGURE 23.3. Dosing and monitoring for enoxaparin. (From References 26-27.)

Unfractionated Heparin Dosing
Bolus: 80 units/kg
Infusion: 18 units/kg/h

Unfractionated Heparin Monitoring*
aPTT	1.5-2.5 times control (in seconds)
Anti-Xa	0.3-0.7 units/mL

*Levels should be drawn every 6 h until two consecutive therapeutic levels then interval can expand to once daily.

FIGURE 23.4. Dosing and monitoring for unfractionated heparin. aPTT = activated partial thromboplastin time; Anti-Xa = anti-Factor Xa level. (From References 26 and 28.)

Thrombolytic Therapy

Systemic Thrombolysis

National and international guidelines recommend systemic thrombolysis for massive/high-risk pulmonary emboli (5,14,

25,29). The recommended drug regimen is a 2-h infusion of alteplase (recombinant tissue plasminogen activator) (14). An accelerated regimen (0.6 mg/kg over 15 min to a maximum dose of 50 mg) has not been officially approved but may be considered in impending cardiovascular collapse (5,14).

Continuous-infusion heparin is used in conjunction with thrombolytic therapy. Heparin is particularly advantageous after thrombolysis because clot dissolution releases thrombin, which can lead to thrombotic re-occlusion of the involved vessel.

Contraindications to thrombolytic therapy include the following:

- Active bleeding
- Prior hemorrhagic stroke
- Ischemic stroke within the past 6 months
- Central nervous system neoplasm
- Major trauma, surgery, or head injury in the past 3 weeks (5)

Catheter-Directed Therapies

Although there is limited data, the use of catheter-directed therapies (CDT) has increased (30). Ongoing innovations in catheter-based therapies not only include catheter-directed thrombolysis but mechanical fragmentation and embolectomy with or without pharmacologic thrombolysis. Considerations include not only local expertise but carefully selected patients (rapidly deteriorating or severely compromised patients) or those who have failed systemic thrombolysis (14,30-31).

Surgical Embolectomy

If local expertise is available, surgical embolectomy can be considered for life-threatening PE. Indications include contraindication to systemic thrombolytic therapy, failure of thrombolysis, and free-floating right atrial thrombus (32). Survival rates of 87% have been reported with emergency surgical embolectomy (33). A specimen from a surgical embolectomy is shown in Figure 23.5.

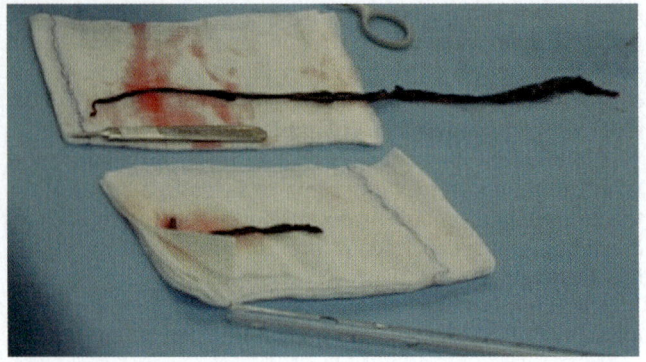

FIGURE 23.5. Specimen from a surgical embolectomy.

Extracorporeal Membrane Oxygenation

Not typically available outside of major medical centers, extracorporeal membrane oxygenation (ECMO) is generally used as a bridge to or supportive care during catheter-based thrombectomy/thrombolysis or surgical embolectomy in cardiogenic (obstructive) shock due to acute massive PE (33-35).

Vena Cava Filter

Filters can be placed (percutaneously) in the inferior vena cava to trap thrombi that break loose from leg veins and prevent them from embolizing to the lungs (36). An image of a trapped thrombus in a vena cava filter can be seen in Figure 4.2, Chapter 4: Prophylaxis for VTE.

Indications for a vena cava filter include the following:

- Acute PE despite therapeutic anticoagulation
- Evidence of VTE with an absolute contraindication to anticoagulation
- Proximal DVT in the legs, with a free-floating thrombus (i.e., the leading edge of the thrombus is not adherent to the vessel wall), or with limited cardiopulmonary reserve (i.e., unlikely to tolerate a pulmonary embolus)

- In selected patients undergoing catheter-based interventions (37)

References

1. Kabrhel C, Camargo CA Jr., Goldhaber SZ. Clinical gestalt and the diagnosis of pulmonary embolism: does experience matter? Chest 2005;127:1627-30.
2. Hoellerich VL, Wigton RS. Diagnosing pulmonary embolism using clinical findings. Arch Intern Med 1986;146:1699-704.
3. Bounds EJ, Kok SJ. D Dimer. In: StatPearls. Treasure Island (FL): StatPearls Publishing; 2025.
4. Kearon C, de Wit K, Parpia S, et al. Diagnosis of pulmonary embolism with d-dimer adjusted to clinical probability. N Engl J Med 2019;381:2125-34.
5. Konstantinides SV, Meyer G, Becattini C, et al. 2019 ESC Guidelines for the diagnosis and management of acute pulmonary embolism developed in collaboration with the European Respiratory Society (ERS). Eur Heart J 2020;41:543-603.
6. Coutance G, Le Page O, Lo T, Hamon M. Prognostic value of brain natriuretic peptide in acute pulmonary embolism. Crit Care 2008;12:R109.
7. Kucher N, Printzen G, Goldhaber SZ. Prognostic role of brain natriuretic peptide in acute pulmonary embolism. Circulation 2003;107:2545-7.
8. Lega JC, Lacasse Y, Lakhal L, Provencher S. Natriuretic peptides and troponins in pulmonary embolism: a meta-analysis. Thorax 2009;64:869-75.
9. Potter JM, Hickman PE, Cullen L. Troponins in myocardial infarction and injury. Aust Prescr 2022;45:53-7.
10. Sonne-Holm E, Winther-Jensen M, Bang LE, et al. Troponin dependent 30-day mortality in patients with acute pulmonary embolism. J Thromb Thrombolysis 2023;56:485-94.
11. Gornik HL, Sharma AM. Duplex ultrasound in the diagnosis of lower-extremity deep venous thrombosis. Circulation 2014;129:917-21.
12. Kay AB, Morris DS, Woller SC, et al. Trauma patients at risk for venous thromboembolism who undergo routine duplex ultrasound screening experience fewer pulmonary emboli: a prospective randomized trial. J Trauma Acute Care Surg 2021;90:787-96.
13. Nasser MF, Jabri A, Limaye S, et al. Echocardiographic evaluation of pulmonary embolism: a review. J Am Soc Echocardiogr 2023;36:906-12.
14. Chopard R, Behr J, Vidoni C, et al. An update on the management of acute high-risk pulmonary embolism. J Clin Med 2022;11(16):4807.

15. Albrecht MH, Bickford MW, Nance JW Jr, et al. State-of-the-art pulmonary CT angiography for acute pulmonary embolism. AJR Am J Roentgenol 2017;208:495-504.
16. Patel P, Patel P, Bhatt M, et al. Systematic review and meta-analysis of test accuracy for the diagnosis of suspected pulmonary embolism. Blood Adv 2020;4:4296-311.
17. Mirza H, Hashmi MF. Lung Ventilation Perfusion Scan (VQ Scan). In: StatPearls. Treasure Island (FL): StatPearls Publishing; 2025.
18. Simcox LE, Ormesher L, Tower C, Greer IA. Pulmonary thrombo-embolism in pregnancy: diagnosis and management. Breathe (Sheff) 2015;11:282-9.
19. Gandhi S, Litt D, Chandy M, Nguyen BM, et al. Successful rapid intravenous desensitization for radioiodine contrast allergy in a patient requiring urgent coronary angiography. J Allergy Clin Immunol Pract 2014;2:101-2.
20. Sanan N, Rowane M, Hostoffer R. Radiologic contrast media desensitization for delayed cardiac catheterization. Allergy Rhinol (Providence) 2019;10:2152656719892844.
21. The University of Texas MD Anderson Cancer Center. Management of Contrast Media Reactions–Adult 2023. Available from: https://www.mdanderson.org/documents/for-physicians/algorithms/clinical-management/clin-management-contrast-reactions-adult-web-algorithm.pdf.
22. Tsuchiya N, van Beek EJ, Ohno Y, et al. Magnetic resonance angiography for the primary diagnosis of pulmonary embolism: a review from the international workshop for pulmonary functional imaging. World J Radiol 2018;10:52-64.
23. Moreland S, Mukherjee D, Nickel NP. Contemporary treatment of pulmonary embolism: medical treatment and management. Int J Angiol 2022;31:155-61.
24. Maughan BC, Kabrhel C, Jarman AF. Evidence-based anticoagulation choice for acute pulmonary embolism. JAMA Netw Open 2025;8:e2452850.
25. Stevens SM, Woller SC, Kreuziger LB, et al. Antithrombotic Therapy for VTE Disease: second update of the CHEST Guideline and Expert Panel Report. Chest 2021;160:e545-e608.
26. Centers for Medicare & Medicaid Services. Enoxaparin: U.S. Food and Drug Administration-Approved Indications, Dosages, and Treatment Durations Available from: https://www.cms.gov/medicare-medicaid-coordination/fraud-prevention/medicaid-integrity-education/pharmacy-education-materials/downloads/enox-dosingchart11-14.pdf.
27. Smythe MA, Priziola J, Dobesh PP, et al. Guidance for the practical management of the heparin anticoagulants in the treatment of venous thromboembolism. J Thromb Thrombolysis 2016;41:165-86.

28. Samimi MN, Hale A, Schults J, et al. Clinical guidance for unfractionated heparin dosing and monitoring in critically ill patients. Expert Opin Pharmacother 2024;25:985-97.
29. Ortel TL, Neumann I, Ageno W, et al. American Society of Hematology 2020 guidelines for management of venous thromboembolism: treatment of deep vein thrombosis and pulmonary embolism. Blood Adv 2020;4:4693-738.
30. Carroll BJ, Larnard EA, Pinto DS, Giri J, Secemsky EA. Percutaneous management of high-risk pulmonary embolism. Circ Cardiovasc Interv 2023;16:e012166.
31. Kuo WT, Sista AK, Faintuch S, et al. Society of Interventional Radiology Position statement on catheter-directed therapy for acute pulmonary embolism. J Vasc Interv Radiol 2018;29:293-7.
32. Saxena P, Smail H, McGiffin DC. Surgical techniques of pulmonary embolectomy for acute pulmonary embolism. Oper Tech Thorac Cardiovasc Surg 2016;21:80-8.
33. Iaccarino A, Frati G, Schirone L, et al. Surgical embolectomy for acute massive pulmonary embolism: state of the art. J Thorac Dis 2018;10:5154-61.
34. Davies MG, Hart JP. Current status of ECMO for massive pulmonary embolism. Front Cardiovasc Med 2023;10:1298686.
35. George TJ, Sheasby J, Sawhney R, et al. Extracorporeal membrane oxygenation for large pulmonary emboli. Proc (Bayl Univ Med Cent.) 2023;36:314-7.
36. Fairfax LM, Sing RF. Vena cava interruption. Crit Care Clin 2011;27:781-804, v.
37. Kaufman JA, Barnes GD, Chaer RA, et al. Society of Interventional Radiology clinical practice guideline for inferior vena cava filters in the treatment of patients with venous thromboembolic disease: developed in collaboration with the American College of Cardiology, American College of Chest Physicians, American College of Surgeons Committee on Trauma, American Heart Association, Society for Vascular Surgery, and Society for Vascular Medicine. J Vasc Interv Radiol 2020;31:1529-44.

Severe Asthma and COPD in the ICU

Chapter 24

Respiratory failure for acute exacerbations of both asthma and chronic obstructive pulmonary disease (COPD) is a risk factor for mortality (1-2). In addition, asthma and COPD as a comorbidity in critically ill patients is associated with poorer prognosis (3-4). Although they have a number of etiologic differences, they have similar clinical presentations and treatment strategies. This chapter describes the management of acute exacerbations of asthma and COPD.

ACUTE ASTHMA EXACERBATION

Acute asthma exacerbations are clinically characterized by wheezing, cough, and dyspnea.

Pathophysiology

Asthma is a chronic inflammatory condition, the hallmark being hyperactive airways. Environmental triggers, whether intrinsic or extrinsic (e.g., allergies) activate a cascade of inflammatory responses resulting in bronchospasm, airway obstruction, dynamic hyperinflation, and mucous plugging (4-5).

Bronchospasm

Contraction or "spasm" of the smooth muscles of the airway leads to airway resistance and clinical wheezing. The absence of wheezing, i.e., a "silent chest," denotes severe airway obstruction (6).

- Bronchospasm narrows the airways, limiting expiratory flow, impairing alveolar emptying which leads to increased obstruction and decreased expiratory airflow. The impact on expiratory flow can be visualized in mechanically ventilated patients following the *Flow-Time* graphics on the ventilator (Figure 24.1).

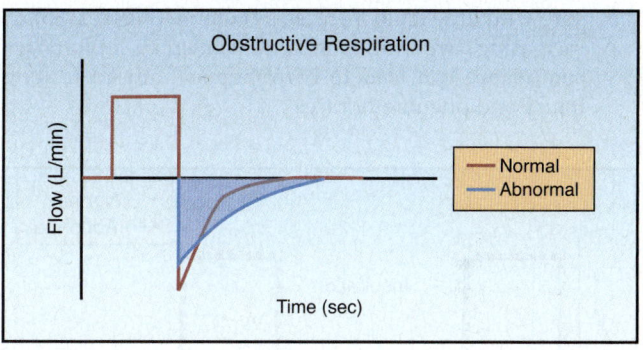

FIGURE 24.1. Flow-Time graphics diagram demonstrating bronchospasm resulting in obstruction of air flow.

Airway Obstruction and Air Trapping

- The increase in expiratory flow resistance results in air trapping, also known as "stacking breaths." This occurs with an incomplete tidal volume expiration compared with inspiratory tidal volume, resulting in hyperinflation of the lung.
- Air trapping, also known as "auto-PEEP," can also be seen on the *Flow-Time* graphic of the mechanical ventilator (Figure 24.2).

Dynamic Hyperinflation

- As air trapping continues, end-expiratory lung volume increases, leading to "dynamic hyperinflation." Lungs becomes stiffer and less compliant as the increased end-expiratory volume overcomes the elasticity limit of the lung. This results in decreased gas exchange, with an increased work of breathing and fatigue.
- Increases in end-expiratory lung volumes cannot be determined even by ventilator *graphics* as only the inhaled tidal volume and exhaled tidal volumes are

measured. However, as the hyperinflation increases, this "overdistention" can be inferred by examining the *Volume-Pressure* loop which shows an increase in pressure with little to no increase in volume (Figure 24.3).
- Increasing hyperinflation and worsening pulmonary compliance can lead to barotrauma (both acute lung injury and pneumothoraces).

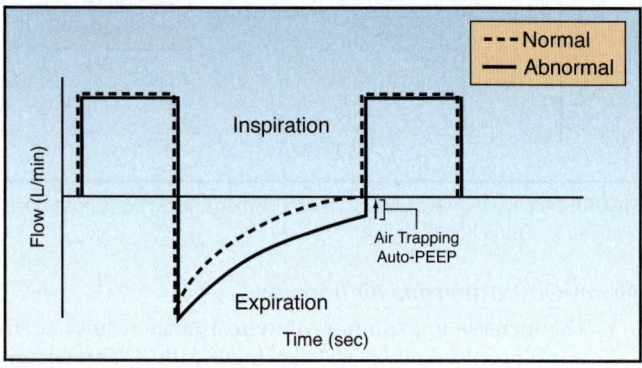

FIGURE 24.2. Flow-Time graphics demonstrating air trapping.

Mucous Plugging

The chronic inflammation leads to increased goblet cell hyperplasia in the airways and acute inflammation (exacerbation) leads to hypersecretion (5,7).

Management of Acute Exacerbation

Figure 24.4 shows the recommendations of the National Asthma Education Program for the initial management of adults with acute exacerbations of asthma (8). This protocol uses objective measures of airway obstruction (Forced expiratory volume in one second [FEV_1] and peak expiratory flow rate) to determine disease severity, but these measures are difficult to obtain in acutely ill patients, so clinical assessment of disease severity is used to guide management (8).

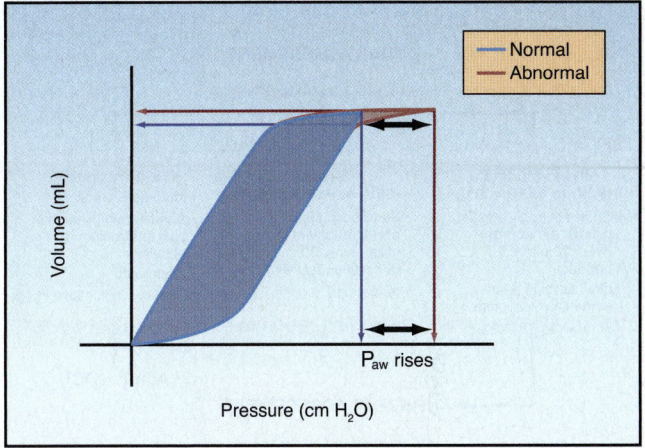

FIGURE 24.3. Volume-Pressure loop showing overdistention/hyperinflation. At end inspiration there is little to no increase in tidal volume with increases in airway pressure.

Inhaled Bronchodilators

Short-Acting β_2 Agonists (SABA). SABAs are the foundation of day-to-day maintenance and the treatment of acute asthma exacerbations. They are the preferred bronchodilators for acute exacerbations of asthma, and are given as an inhaled aerosol, which is more effective than parenteral drug therapy, and has fewer side effects (9). Bronchodilator effects are usually apparent in 2-3 min, reach a peak at 30 min, and last for 2-5 h (10).

1. The most widely used drug in this class is *albuterol*, which is a racemic mixture of two isomers, only one being active. *Levalbuterol* is the active isomer in albuterol and was introduced as a more powerful bronchodilator than albuterol. However, clinical studies have shown no advantages with levalbuterol in acute asthma (11).
2. The dosing regimens for albuterol in asthma are shown in Table 24.1. Treatment usually begins with a series of

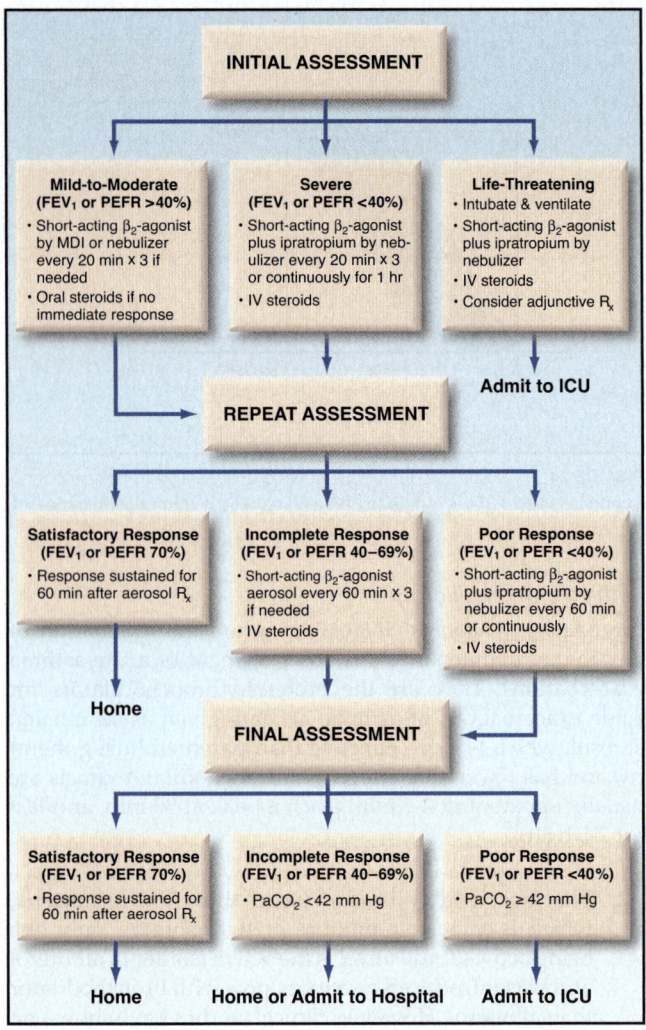

FIGURE 24.4. The management of acute exacerbations of asthma. FEV_1 = forced expiratory volume in one second; PEFR = peak expiratory flow rate. (From Reference 8.)

3 consecutive aerosol treatments at 20-min intervals, and nebulizers are preferred to metered dose inhalers (MDIs) for moderate-to-severe airflow obstruction (8).
3. Albuterol can also be given as a continuous aerosol using a large-volume nebulizer and a dose of 10-15 mg for the first hour (8). This method has become popular and is more effective than intermittent aerosol therapy for severe airflow obstruction (12).
4. When the acute episode begins to resolve, albuterol is given by intermittent aerosol treatments every 4-6 h for the duration of the hospital stay.
5. Adverse effects of high-dose aerosol therapy with β_2-agonists include tachycardia, fine tremors, hyperglycemia, and electrolyte "hypo's" (i.e., hypokalemia, hypomagnesemia, and hypophosphatemia) (13-14). Albuterol may also be responsible for the increase in serum lactate levels that are observed during acute exacerbations of asthma (15).

Anticholinergic Aerosols

1. The only anticholinergic agent approved for use in asthma in the United States is *ipratropium bromide*, a derivative of atropine that blocks muscarinic receptors in the airways.
2. Anticholinergic aerosols offer only marginal benefits in acute asthma and are used as combination therapy with SABA (e.g., albuterol).
3. The dosing regimen for aerosolized ipratropium is shown in Table 24.1. Ipratropium can be mixed with albuterol for nebulizer treatments, and a premixed preparation of albuterol and ipratropium is commercially available for nebulizers and MDIs.
4. Systemic absorption of ipratropium is minimal, and there is little risk of anticholinergic side effects (e.g., tachycardia, dry mouth, blurred vision, urinary retention).
5. Ipratropium has no proven benefit beyond the first few hours of treatment, and it *should not be used for daily maintenance therapy in asthma* (1).

TABLE 24.1 Drug Regimens for Acute Exacerbations of Asthma

Drug	Dosing Regimens
Albuterol	Dosing: 2.5-5 mg (or 4-8 puffs) every 20 min for 3 doses, then if needed, continue hourly doses, or start continuous inhalation at 5-15 mg/h, for up to 3 h. Maintenance dose is 2.5 mg (or 2 puffs) every 4-6 h. Comment: Aggressive dosing can elevate lactate levels.
Levalbuterol	Dosing: 1.25-2.5 mg (or 4-8 puffs) every 20 min for 3 doses, then if needed, continue hourly doses for up to 3 h. Maintenance dose is 1.25 mg (or 2 puffs) every 4-6 h. Comment: No proven benefit over albuterol.
Ipratropium	Dosing: 0.5 mg every 20 min for 3 doses, then as needed. Can be added (0.5 mg/h) to continuous inhalation of albuterol. Comment: Use only if initial response to albuterol is not satisfactory, but do not continue use after admission to hospital.

From Asthma and COPD in the ICU. In: Marino PL. *Marino's The ICU Book.* 5th ed. Wolters Kluwer; 2025:374-89. Table 23.2.

Aerosol Intolerance

For the occasional patient that does not tolerate bronchodilator aerosols (usually because of excessive coughing), consider one of the following regimens (8):

1. *Epinephrine:* 0.3-0.5 mg subcutaneously every 20 min for 3 doses. Having both β_1 and β_2 effects, it can be associated with hypertension, tachycardia, and other cardiac dysrhythmias.
2. *Terbutaline:* 0.25 mg subcutaneously every 20 min for 3 doses. Primarily a β_2-agonist it is rapidly effective without the cardiac stimulating effects of epinephrine (16).

3. Following the initial bronchodilator response, patients are more likely to tolerate aerosol treatments.

Corticosteroids

Systemic corticosteroid therapy treats the airway inflammation and may improve mortality (17).

1. *Relevant Observations:* The following observations about steroid therapy in acute asthma deserve mention:
   a. There is no difference in efficacy between oral and intravenous steroids (5).
   b. The beneficial effects of steroids are often not apparent for 6 to 12 h after therapy is started (4,18), and thus steroid therapy will not influence the clinical course of asthma in the emergency department.
   c. There is no dose-response relationship for steroids in acute asthma (i.e., no evidence that larger steroid doses produce greater responses) (19).
   d. A 10-day course of steroids can be stopped abruptly, without a tapering dose (20).
2. *Recommendations:* The recommendations for systemic steroid therapy in acute asthma are summarized in Table 24.2. (5,20). Inhaled corticosteroids can be added when the acute episode begins to resolve and should continue for at least a few weeks after resolution to prevent relapses (21).

Other Considerations

- *Magnesium:* Intravenous magnesium has mild bronchodilator effects (as "nature's calcium channel blocker"), and magnesium sulfate in a dose of 2 grams IV over 15-30 min has been shown to improve lung function and reduce hospital admissions in patients who respond poorly to initial bronchodilator therapy (4-5).

TABLE 24.2　Recommendations for Steroid Therapy

Acute Exacerbation of Asthma[1]
Indication: Unsatisfactory bronchodilator response after 1 h.
Route: Oral route preferred.
Dose: 40-80 mg daily in 1 or 2 divided doses, using prednisone (for PO) or methylprednisolone (for IV).
Duration: Continue until resolution of signs and symptoms. No taper necessary if duration < 10 days.

Acute Exacerbation of COPD[2]
Indication: Admission to hospital.
Route: Oral route preferred.
Dose: 40 mg prednisone equivalent per day
Duration: Continue for 5 days.

[1]Gayen S, Dachert S, Lashari BH, et al. Critical care management of severe asthma exacerbations. J Clin Med 2024;13.

[2]Agusti A, Celli BR, Criner GJ, et al. Global Initiative for Chronic Obstructive Lung Disease 2023 Report: GOLD Executive Summary. Am J Respir Crit Care Med 2023;207:819-37.

- *Ketamine:* Ketamine is a dissociative anesthetic that lacks the cardiovascular and respiratory depression of most anesthetics (22), and has two effects that impact asthmatic exacerbations: 1) the sedative effects lessen anxiety and reduce the respiratory rate, air trapping, and hyperinflation (17,22); and 2) ketamine also has sympathomimetic effects, including β_2 activity, causing direct bronchodilation. Evidence supporting the use of ketamine in acute asthma is minimal (17,23).
- *Leukotriene Receptor Antagonists (LRAs):* LRAs, such as montelukast, benralizumab, and mepolizumab, have both bronchodilator and anti-inflammatory effects and may have a role in improving pulmonary function in acute asthma exacerbations (data is limited) (5).
- *Helium-Oxygen Mixture (Heliox):* The helium component of this gas mixture decreases airflow resistance. Heliox

use is due to limited data and expense. The admixture of oxygen is limited to 30% making its use in hypoxic patients challenging (17).
- *ABGs:* Arterial blood gas analysis is advised for patients who show little or no clinical improvement after one hour of aggressive bronchodilator therapy. A normal $PaCO_2$ in acute asthma is evidence of respiratory failure (because the minute ventilation is high, which should lower the arterial $PaCO_2$), and hypercapnia is a sign that ventilatory assistance may be necessary.
- *Antibiotics:* Asthma exacerbations are often triggered by viral upper respiratory tract infections, and antibiotic therapy is *not advised unless there is evidence of a bacterial infection* (8,21).

Noninvasive Ventilation

Although not an alternative to intubation and mechanical ventilation, noninvasive ventilation (NIV) can be effective in correcting the hypercapnia and avoiding intubation and mechanical ventilation (4). The indications and contraindications for NIV are shown in Table 24.3 (5,17).

ACUTE EXACERBATION OF COPD

An acute exacerbation of COPD simply stated is, "worsening respiratory symptoms needing additional therapy" (3). The majority of COPD exacerbations are triggered by a pulmonary infection, followed by air pollution, and medical noncompliance (3,17).

Pathophysiology

Like asthma, COPD is also an inflammatory disease. However, in contrast to asthma, COPD is typically diagnosed at a later age as inflammatory processes have led to pulmonary fibrosis, worsening compliance, and a typically fixed airway obstruction (17,24).

TABLE 24.3 Indications and Contraindications for Noninvasive Ventilation

Indications	Contraindications
• Tachypnea >25/min	• Altered mental status
• Hypercapnia but <60 mmHg	• High aspiration risk
• Accessory muscle use	• Hemodynamic instability
• FEV_1 <50% predicted following two (2) consecutive nebulized bronchodilator treatments	• Inability to clear secretions
	• Lack of proper seal of mask
• Invasive Mechanical Ventilation not appropriate	• Lack of properly trained staff

Adapted from Johnston C, Nixon P. Asthma and chronic obstructive pulmonary disease in the intensive care unit. Anaesth Intensive Care 2022;23:628-34 and Gayen S, Dachert S, Lashari BH, et al. Critical care management of severe asthma exacerbations. J Clin Med 2024;13.

Bronchodilator Therapy

1. Bronchodilator therapy for acute exacerbations of COPD involves the same aerosolized drugs used for acute asthma, but with different dosing regimens (Table 24.4), and different expectations (i.e., unlike asthma, COPD is characterized by poor bronchodilator responsiveness, so bronchodilator therapy has much less influence on outcomes in COPD).
2. Ipratropium is used as combination therapy when the response to short-acting β-agonists is less than satisfactory (which is usually the case in COPD), although at least three clinical studies do not support this practice (25).

Corticosteroids

A brief course of corticosteroid therapy is recommended for all hospital admissions with acute exacerbation of COPD, and the recommended dosing is 40 mg prednisone equivalent daily for 5 days (20).

TABLE 24.4	Drug Regimens for Acute Exacerbations of COPD
Drug	**Dosing Regimens**
Albuterol	Dosing: 2.5-5 mg by nebulizer, or 2-8 puffs by MDI with spacer, every 4-6 h. Comment: MDI is favored over nebulizer because of equivalent bronchodilator response at a much lower dose.
Levalbuterol	Dosing: 1.25-2.5 mg by nebulizer, or 2-8 puffs by MDI with spacer, every 4-6 h. Comment: More potent form of albuterol, but has no proven advantage.
Ipratropium	Dosing: 0.5 mg by nebulizer, or 2-8 puffs by MDI with spacer, every 4-6 h. Comment: Use as combination therapy only when response to short-acting β_2-agonists is less than satisfactory.

From Asthma and COPD in the ICU. In: Marino PL. *Marino's The ICU Book*. 5th ed. Wolters Kluwer; 2025:374-89. Table 23.4.

Antibiotic Therapy

Bacterial pathogens are responsible for about half of the airway infections in acute exacerbations of COPD (26).

Indications

Clinical practice guidelines recommend antibiotics when either of the following conditions is satisfied (27):

- Increased volume and purulence of sputum
- Noninvasive or mechanical ventilation

Antibiotics

Streptococcus pneumoniae and *Hemophilus influenzae* are the most frequent isolates in the sputum of hospitalized patients with COPD with *Pseudomonas aeruginosa* prominent in ventilator-dependent patients (28-29).

- Antibiotic choices should be based on these isolates and local bacterial resistance patterns (20).
- Antibiotics for mechanically ventilated patients should provide coverage for *Pseudomonas aeruginosa* pending culture and sensitivity results, e.g., cefepime (28-29).
- The duration of antibiotic therapy is typically 5-7 days (20).

Oxygen Therapy

1. In cases of severe COPD with chronic hypercapnia, high concentrations of inhaled O_2 can promote further increases in arterial PCO_2. This is not due to a decrease in ventilatory drive (23), as believed, but may be from CO_2 unloading by hemoglobin.
2. The best practice in this situation is to use the lowest FiO_2 (fractional concentration of inhaled fractional concentration of inhaled oxygen) that achieves an O_2 saturation by pulse oximetry (SpO_2) of 88-90%.
3. Monitor the mental status closely after initiating O_2 therapy, because a decrease in consciousness most likely signals progressive hypercapnia (CO_2 narcosis), and mandates immediate intubation and mechanical ventilation.

Noninvasive Ventilation

1. Noninvasive ventilation (NIV) has been successful in avoiding intubation in about 75% of patients with hypercapnic respiratory failure from COPD exacerbations (see Chapter 20: Dysrhythmias, Table 20.1) (30).
2. See Chapter 20: Dysrhythmias for more information on NIV.

MECHANICAL VENTILATION

Mechanical ventilation is required in <5% of hospitalized patients with acute asthma (31), but in >50% of patients with exacerbation of COPD (32). The following are some of the major considerations regarding positive pressure ventilation in these patients.

Dynamic Hyperinflation

1. In normal subjects, exhalation is completed before the end of expiration, and the end-expiratory pressure in the alveoli is equivalent to atmospheric (zero reference) pressure. This is illustrated in the lower pressure-volume loop in Figure 24.5.

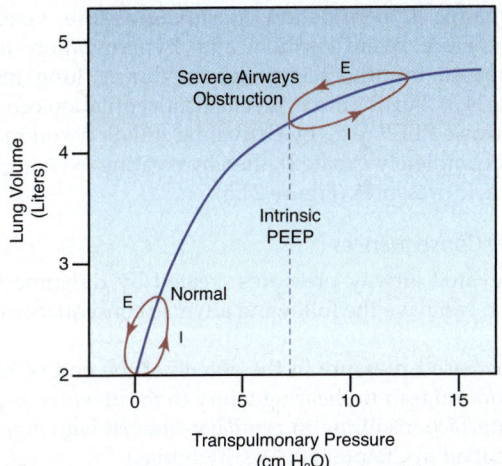

FIGURE 24.5. Pressure-volume curves showing the effects of dynamic hyperinflation. The hysteresis loops show the pressure and volume changes for a single breath. I = inspiration, E = expiration. See text for further explanation. (From Asthma and COPD in the ICU. In: Marino PL. *Marino's The ICU Book*. 5th ed. Wolters Kluwer; 2025:374-89. Figure 23.4.)

2. In patients with severe airway obstruction from asthma or COPD, exhalation is prolonged and is not completed before the next inhalation. This results in hyperinflation (called *dynamic hyperinflation*), and the trapped gas in the alveoli creates a positive end-expiratory pressure (PEEP), which is called *intrinsic PEEP* (33). This is illustrated by the upper pressure-volume loop in Figure 24.5.
3. Note that, in the presence of intrinsic PEEP, the respiratory muscles must generate higher transpulmonary pressures

to inflate the lungs (partly to overcome intrinsic PEEP, and partly because breathing occurs on a flat portion of the pressure-volume curve). This increases the work of breathing.

Positive Pressure Ventilation

Because of the shift in the pressure-volume curves caused by dynamic hyperinflation, positive-pressure ventilation will generate overdistention and hyperinflation leading to increased intrathoracic pressures during lung inflation (Figure 24.3). Furthermore, mechanical ventilation can add to the intrinsic PEEP (e.g., by delivering inflation volumes that are not completely exhaled), thereby creating even higher intrathoracic pressures (Figure 24.5).

Adverse Consequences

The elevated airway pressures created by dynamic hyperinflation can have the following adverse consequences:

- Increased pressure in the alveoli at the end of inspiration can lead to shearing injury to the alveolar–capillary interface, resulting in *ventilator-induced lung injury* (described in Chapter 20: Dysrhythmias).
- Increased alveolar pressure can also cause rupture of alveoli, with escape of air into the lung parenchyma or pleural space (i.e., *barotrauma*).
- Increased mean intrathoracic pressure can reduce cardiac output by increasing right ventricular afterload and decreasing right ventricular filling.

Monitoring

Dynamic Hyperinflation

Dynamic hyperinflation can be implicated by monitoring the expiratory airflow visualizing the *Flow-Time* graphics display during mechanical ventilation (Figure 24.2). The normal flow waveforms in the upper panel show that the expiratory flow ceases before the next lung inflation, while the flow waveforms in the lower panel show that expiratory flow is continuing when the next lung inflation is delivered. *The presence of expiratory flow at the end of expiration is evidence of dynamic hyperinflation* (Figure 24.3).

Ventilator Strategies

The following strategies are designed to limit dynamic hyperinflation and intrinsic PEEP during mechanical ventilation.

1. Ventilate with low tidal volumes (6 mL/kg predicted body weight) using the *lung protective ventilation* protocol described in Chapter 18: Inflammatory Shock.
2. Maximize the time for exhalation with the following measures:
   a. Avoid rapid respiratory rates (with sedation, if possible, or temporary neuromuscular paralysis, if necessary).
   b. Increase the inspiratory flow rate, if necessary, so that lung inflation accounts for only one-third of the respiratory cycle (i.e., I:E ratio of 1:2).

References

1. Krishnan V, Diette GB, Rand CS, et al. Mortality in patients hospitalized for asthma exacerbations in the United States. Am J Respir Crit Care Med 2006;174:633-8.
2. MacIntyre N, Huang YC. Acute exacerbations and respiratory failure in chronic obstructive pulmonary disease. Proc Am Thorac Soc 2008;5:530-5.
3. Prediletto I, Giancotti G, Nava S. COPD exacerbation: why it is important to avoid ICU admission. J Clin Med 2023;12.
4. Talbot T, Roe T, Dushianthan A. Management of acute life-threatening asthma exacerbations in the intensive care unit. Appl Sci 2024;14:693.
5. Gayen S, Dachert S, Lashari BH, et al. Critical care management of severe asthma exacerbations. J Clin Med 2024;13.
6. Chakraborty RK, Chen RJ, Basnet S. Status Asthmaticus. In: StatPearls. Treasure Island (FL): StatPearls Publishing; 2024.

7. Gorrieri G, Scudieri P, Caci E, et al. Goblet cell hyperplasia requires high bicarbonate transport to support mucin release. Sci Rep 2016;6:36016.
8. National Asthma Education and Prevention Program. Expert Panel Report 3: Guidelines for the Diagnosis and Management of Asthma: U.S. Department of Health and Human Services. Updated 2020. Accessed September 15, 2024. https://www.nhlbi.nih.gov/health-topics/guidelines-fordiagnosis-management-of-asthma
9. Salmeron S, Brochard L, Mal H, et al. Nebulized versus intravenous albuterol in hypercapnic acute asthma. A multicenter, double-blind, randomized study. Am J Respir Crit Care Med 1994; 149:1466-70.
10. Dutta EJ, Li JT. Beta-agonists. Med Clin North Am 2002;86:991-1008.
11. Jat KR, Khairwa A. Levalbuterol versus albuterol for acute asthma: a systematic review and meta-analysis. Pulm Pharmacol Ther 2013; 26:239-48.
12. Peters SG. Continuous bronchodilator therapy. Chest 2007;131:286-9.
13. Bodenhamer J, Bergstrom R, Brown D, et al. Frequently nebulized beta-agonists for asthma: effects on serum electrolytes. Ann Emerg Med 1992;21:1337-42.
14. Truwit JD. Toxic effects of drugs used in the ICU. Toxic effects of bronchodilators. Crit Care Clin 1991;7(3):639-57.
15. Lewis LM, Ferguson I, House SL, et al. Albuterol administration is commonly associated with increases in serum lactate in patients with asthma treated for acute exacerbation of asthma. Chest 2014;145:53-9.
16. Ebert TJ. Autonomic nervous system pharmacology. In: Hemmings HC, Egan TD, editors. *Pharmacology and Physiology for Anesthesia*. Elsevier; 2019. p. 282-99.
17. Johnston C, Nixon P. Asthma and chronic obstructive pulmonary disease in the intensive care unit. Anaesth Intensive Care 2022;23:628-34.
18. Shefrin AE, Goldman RD. Use of dexamethasone and prednisone in acute asthma exacerbations in pediatric patients. Can Fam Physician 2009;55:704-6.
19. Rodrigo G, Rodrigo C. Corticosteroids in the emergency department therapy of acute adult asthma: an evidence-based evaluation. Chest 1999;116:285-95.
20. Agusti A, Celli BR, Criner GJ, et al. Global Initiative for Chronic Obstructive Lung Disease 2023 Report: GOLD Executive Summary. Am J Respir Crit Care Med 2023;207:819-37.
21. Lazarus SC. Clinical practice. Emergency treatment of asthma. N Engl J Med 2010;363:755-64.
22. Orhurhu VJ, Vashisht R, Claus LE, Cohen SP. Ketamine Toxicity. In: StatPearls. Treasure Island (FL): StatPearls Publishing; 2024.

23. La Via L, Sanfilippo F, Cuttone G, et al. Use of ketamine in patients with refractory severe asthma exacerbations: systematic review of prospective studies. Eur J Clin Pharmacol 2022;78:1613-22.
24. Hudler A, Holguin F, Sharma S. Pathophysiology of asthma-chronic obstructive pulmonary disease overlap. Immunol Allergy Clin North Am 2022;42:521-32.
25. Walters JA, Gibson PG, Wood-Baker R, et al. Systemic corticosteroids for acute exacerbations of chronic obstructive pulmonary disease. Cochrane Database Syst Rev 2009:CD001288.
26. Suau SJ, DeBlieux PM. Management of acute exacerbation of asthma and chronic obstructive pulmonary disease in the emergency department. Emerg Med Clin North Am 2016;34:15-37.
27. Rabe KF, Hurd S, Anzueto A, et al. Global strategy for the diagnosis, management, and prevention of chronic obstructive pulmonary disease: GOLD executive summary. Am J Respir Crit Care Med 2007;176:532-55.
28. Beasley V, Joshi PV, Singanayagam A, et al. Lung microbiology and exacerbations in COPD. Int J Chron Obstruct Pulmon Dis 2012;7:555-69.
29. Restrepo MI, Sibila O, Anzueto A. Pneumonia in patients with chronic obstructive pulmonary disease. Tuberc Respir Dis (Seoul) 2018;81:187-97.
30. Boldrini R, Fasano L, Nava S. Noninvasive mechanical ventilation. Curr Opin Crit Care 2012;18:48-53.
31. Leatherman J. Mechanical ventilation for severe asthma. Chest 2015;147:1671-80.
32. Hoo GW, Hakimian N, Santiago SM. Hypercapnic respiratory failure in COPD patients: response to therapy. Chest 2000;117:169-77.
33. Blanch L, Bernabe F, Lucangelo U. Measurement of air trapping, intrinsic positive end-expiratory pressure, and dynamic hyperinflation in mechanically ventilated patients. Respir Care 2005;50:110-23; discussion 23-4.

Acute Respiratory Distress Syndrome

Chapter 25

Acute respiratory distress syndrome (ARDS) is a diffuse inflammatory injury of the lungs leading to hypoxia that is not caused by cardiac disease. It is responsible for 10% of ICU admissions and 25% of cases of prolonged mechanical ventilation worldwide (1). The understanding of the immunopathology of ARDS continues to emerge, including not only the participation of neutrophils, but also macrophages, T-helper cells, and other immunologic mechanisms (2-3). This inflammation causes worsening of lung compliance and alveolar damage leading to alveolar edema (protein-rich fluid) that fills the distal airspaces and impairs pulmonary gas exchange. Importantly, ARDS is not a primary disorder but is a consequence of a variety of direct pulmonary injury and non-pulmonary injury (indirect) causes, as well as infectious and noninfectious conditions (1-7). Many of the etiologies of ARDS are listed in Table 25.1.

TABLE 25.1 Examples of Etiologies for ARDS

Direct Pulmonary Injury	Indirect Pulmonary Injury
• Pneumonia	• Extrapulmonary sepsis
• Aspiration	• Severe trauma
• Traumatic contusion	• COVID-19
• Inhalation injury	• Blood transfusion
• Near-drowning	• Shock
• Fat embolism	• Pancreatitis

ARDS = acute respiratory distress syndrome.

DIAGNOSTIC CRITERIA

The hallmark of ARDS is refractory hypoxemia resulting from alveolar edema, ventilation-perfusion mismatch, and intrapulmonary shunting.

Clinical Criteria That Apply to All ARDS Categories

- *Risk Factors and Origin of Edema*. ARDS is not primarily or exclusively attributable to cardiac pulmonary edema. It is precipitated by some predisposing factors, as shown in Table 25.1 (8).
- *Timing*. Onset of hypoxic respiratory failure <1 week of predisposing risk factor.
- *Chest Imaging*. Bilateral opacities on chest radiography.

Diagnostic Criteria for Specific ARDS Categories

The diagnostic criteria for specific ARDS categories are shown in Table 25.2 (8). These criteria are based on the partial pressure of oxygen in the arterial blood (PaO_2) to fraction of inspired oxygen (FiO_2) ratio (P/F ratio) and separated into intubated and nonintubated patients. Intubated patients are further categorized into mild, moderate, and severe. In "resource-limited" settings, i.e., limited arterial blood or no available arterial blood gas analysis, oxygen saturation (SpO_2) to FiO_2 ratios may be used as an acceptable alternative to the P/F ratio (9-10).

Radiographic Appearance

Chest X-ray

The characteristic appearance of ARDS on a portable chest x-ray is shown in Figure 25.1. The infiltrate has a fine granular or ground-glass appearance and is diffusely distributed throughout both lungs. Also note the lack of a prominent pleural effusion, which helps to distinguish ARDS from cardiogenic pulmonary edema.

TABLE 25.2	Diagnostic Criteria for Specific ARDS Categories	
Nonintubated ARDS	**Intubated ARDS (P/F Ratio)**	**Resource-Limited Settings**
P/F <300 or SpO$_2$:FiO$_2$ <315 (if SpO$_2$ <97%) on HFNO with >30 L/min flow or NIV/CPAP with at least 5 cm H$_2$O end-expiratory pressure	Mild: P/F ratio 201-300 mm Hg	SpO$_2$:FiO$_2$ <315 (if SpO$_2$ <97%) Neither PEEP nor a minimum flow rate of O$_2$ is required in resource-limited setting.
	Moderate: 101-200 mm Hg	
	Severe: <100 mm Hg	

ARDS = acute respiratory distress syndrome; CPAP = continuous positive airway pressure; FiO$_2$ = fraction of inspired oxygen; HFNO = high flow nasal oxygen; NIV = noninvasive ventilation; PEEP = positive end expiratory pressure; P/F ratio = PaO$_2$/FiO$_2$; SpO$_2$ = pulse oximetry.

From Matthay MA, Arabi Y, Arroliga AC, et al. A new global definition of acute respiratory distress syndrome. Am J Respir Crit Care Med 2024;209:37-47.

Computed Tomography Chest

Although portable chest x-rays frequently show an apparent homogeneous pattern of lung infiltration in ARDS, computed tomography (CT) images reveal that the lung infiltration in ARDS is more heterogeneous with dependent regions worse (11-12). This is shown in the CT image in Figure 25.2.

The Wedge Pressure

The pulmonary artery occlusion pressure (wedge pressure) has been used to distinguish between ARDS and cardiogenic pulmonary edema, i.e., a wedge pressure ≤18 mm Hg is considered evidence of ARDS (13). This is problematic because the wedge pressure is not a measure of capillary hydrostatic pressure. Although the wedge pressure is no longer a required

CHAPTER 25 ■ Acute Respiratory Distress Syndrome 421

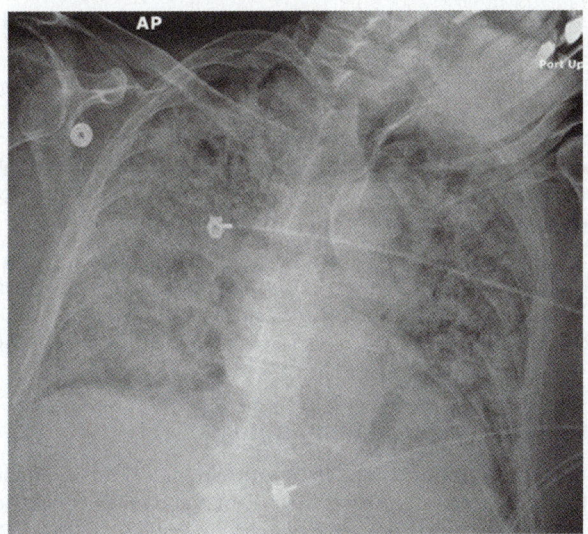

FIGURE 25.1. Portable chest radiograph showing characteristic appearance of acute respiratory distress syndrome (ARDS).

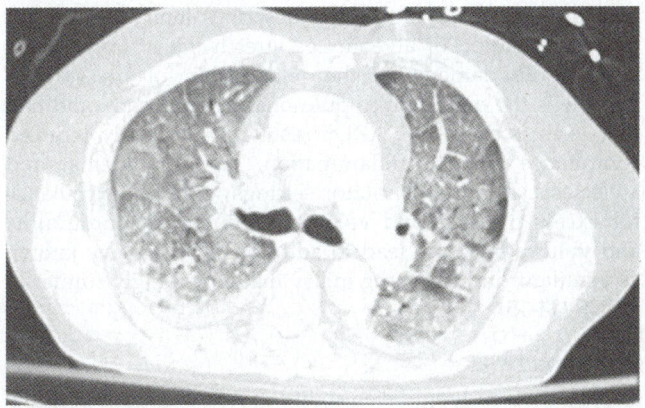

FIGURE 25.2. Computed tomography findings of acute respiratory distress syndrome (ARDS).

measurement in the diagnosis of ARDS, the limitations of this measurement deserve mention.

MECHANICAL VENTILATION

As mentioned earlier in this chapter, about 80% of patients with ARDS require mechanical ventilation (1). There are two general goals of mechanical ventilation in ARDS:

1. Limit the stretch imposed on the distal airspaces during lung inflation (barotrauma and volutrauma).
2. Prevent the distal airspaces from collapsing during lung deflation (atelectrauma).

Ventilator-Induced Lung Injury

One of the most important discoveries in critical care medicine in the last quarter-century is the role of mechanical ventilation as a source of lung injury, particularly in patients with ARDS.

Barotrauma and Volutrauma

Barotrauma refers to injury as a result of excess alveolar pressure, whereas volutrauma describes injury as a result of overdistention of alveoli, i.e., stretch injury from excess volume. Fundamentally, the relationship of pressure to volume is the definition of pulmonary compliance, and neither term is exclusive. ARDS results in markedly reduced compliance due to inflammation, alveolar edema, and atelectasis. Routine ventilator settings without surveillance for excess pressure and volume relationships (barotrauma and volutrauma) can lead to additional lung injury known as ventilator-induced lung injury that is strikingly similar to ARDS (14-15).

Atelectrauma

The decrease in lung distensibility in ARDS can result in the collapse of small airways at the end of expiration. When this occurs, the cyclic opening and closing of small airways during mechanical ventilation may be the result of high-velocity shear forces, traumatic to the alveolar membrane, called atelectrauma, another cause of ventilator-induced lung injury (16).

Lung Protective Ventilation

As shown in Table 25.3, the ARDS Clinical Network (ARDSNet), a network created by the National Heart, Lung, and Blood Institute (NHLBI) and the National Institutes of Health (NIH), has developed a "Lung Protective Ventilation" protocol considering pressure and volume relationships to limit the risk of barotrauma and volutrauma, and positive end-expiratory pressure (PEEP) to limit the risk of atelectrauma (17).

TABLE 25.3 Protocol for Lung Protective Ventilation in ARDS

First Stage	1. Calculate patient's predicted body weight (PBW)†. Males: PBW = 50 + [2.3 × (height in inches − 60)] Females: PBW = 45.5 + [2.3 × (height in inches − 60)] 2. Set initial tidal volume (V_T) at 8 mL/kg PBW. 3. Add positive end-expiratory pressure(PEEP) of 5 cm H_2O. 4. Select the lowest FiO_2 that achieves an SpO_2 of 88-95%. 5. Reduce V_T by 1 mL/kg every 2 h until V_T = 6 mL/kg.
Second Stage	1. When V_T = 6 mL/kg, measure plateau pressure (P_{plat}). 2. If P_{plat} >30 cm H_2O decrease V_T in 1 mL/kg increments until P_{plat} <30 cm H_2O or V_T = 4 mL/kg.
Third Stage	1. Monitor blood gases for respiratory acidosis. 2. If pH = 7.15-7.30, increase respiratory rate (RR) until pH >7.30 or RR = 35. 3. If pH <7.15, increase RR to 35. If pH is still <7.15, increase V_T in 1 mL/kg increments until pH >7.15.
Optimal Goals	V_T = 6 mL/kg, P_{plat} ≤30 cm H_2O, SpO_2 = 88-95%, pH = 7.30-7.45.

ARDS = acute respiratory distress syndrome.
†Predicted body weight is the weight associated with normal lung volumes.

Adapted from Acute Respiratory Distress Syndrome Network; Brower RG, Matthay MA, et al. Ventilation with lower tidal volumes as compared with traditional tidal volumes for acute lung injury and the acute respiratory distress syndrome. N Engl J Med 2000;342:1301-8.

Lung protective ventilation has been shown to improve survival rates in ARDS (18), although this is not a consistent observation (19). The principal factor that seems to determine the success or failure of this ventilatory method is the ability to keep the end-inspiratory plateau (alveolar) pressure <30 cm H_2O.

The Plateau Pressure

One goal of lung protective ventilation is an end-inspiratory plateau pressure (P_{plat}) ≤30 cm H_2O. A P_{plat} >30 cm H_2O can result in alveolar overdistention and ventilator-induced lung injury. The P_{plat} is described in greater detail in Chapter 27: Conventional Mechanical Ventilation and depicted graphically in Figure 27.5. The P_{plat}, measured with an inspiratory hold at the end of inspiration, is essentially the alveolar pressure.

Positive End-Expiratory Pressure

For a more detailed description of this pressure, see Chapter 27: Conventional Mechanical Ventilation. Lung protective ventilation employs PEEP of at least 5 cm H_2O to prevent the collapse of small airways at the end of expiration. The goal is to prevent atelectrauma. Increased PEEP (>8 cm H_2O) is generally reserved for cases where the concentration of inhaled O_2 (FiO_2) is at potentially toxic levels (>60%). It is important to be aware that P_{plat} may increase as PEEP increases.

Permissive Hypercapnia

Lung protective ventilator strategies, e.g., low tidal volume (V_T), can make maintaining normal PCO_2 levels challenging. Allowing a "controlled" level of hypercapnia, "permissive hypercapnia," can be lung protective. A consequence of increasing the respiratory rate is a decrease in I-time, which can increase P_{plat}, decrease mean airway pressure, and oxygenation. The limits of tolerance to hypercapnia are unclear (20), but clinical trials of permissive hypercapnia show that an arterial PCO_2 of 60-70 mm Hg and an arterial pH of 7.2-7.25 are safe for most patients (21).

Pressure Control Inverse Ratio Ventilation

The normal inspiratory time (I-time) to expiration time (E-time), the I:E ratio, is 1:3. PC-IRV "reverses" this ratio to increase the I-time (at the same time decreasing the expiratory time). Using pressure control, the increased I-time may result in an increase in V_T with no change in the P_{plat}. Another method to increase I-time using pressure control is to decrease the rate. Again, this can increase the V_T with no change in the P_{plat} but may increase $PaCO_2$ (see permissive hypercapnia above). The increase in I-time increases mean airway pressure improving oxygenation and recruitment (22). Reversing the I:E comes with the risk of dynamic hyperinflation and air-trapping. This can be avoided by guiding the I:E following the flow-time graphics on the mechanical ventilator (see a more detailed discussion of *Dynamic Hyperinflation* in Chapter 24: Severe Asthma and COPD in the ICU.)

Airway Pressure Release Ventilation

Airway pressure release ventilation (APRV) involves prolonged periods of spontaneous breathing at relatively high airway pressures (to open collapsed alveoli), interspersed with brief periods of rapid lung deflation (to facilitate CO_2 removal) (23). Because APRV involves spontaneous breathing, high-level continuous positive airway pressure (CPAP) is used instead of PEEP. APRV improves arterial oxygenation gradually, over 24 h (23), but there is no survival benefit (24).

Adjunctive Measures

Fluid Management

Clinical studies have shown that conservative fluid management strategies in patients with ARDS can reduce the duration of mechanical ventilation and improve survival rates (25). The goal is oxygen delivery (hemodynamics) and minimizing pulmonary edema risk.

Neuromuscular Blockade

Early continuous neuromuscular blockade (NMB) may be useful by negating patient-ventilator dyssynchrony, however, the data regarding a mortality benefit is unclear (26-28). Sedation should be optimized prior to initiating NMB and train-of-four twitch maintained to maximal 1-of-4 to avoid excessive paralysis. Extended use (>48 h), especially in combination with corticosteroids, may increase risk for myopathy of critical illness and mortality (29).

Corticosteroid Therapy

The use of corticosteroids in ARDS may decrease mortality (28,30), however, the optimal dosing, timing, and duration remain uncertain (31). The Society of Critical Care Medicine

TABLE 25.4 Common Corticosteroid Dosing Regimens for ARDS

Early ARDS (within 24 h)	• Dexamethasone 20 mg IV daily for 5 d, then 10 mg IV daily for 5 d until extubation
Early ARDS (within 72 h)	• Methylprednisolone 1 mg/kg IV bolus, then » Days 1-14: 1 mg/kg/d continuous infusion » Days 15-21: 0.5 mg/kg/d » Days 22-25: 0.25 mg/kg/d » Days 26-28: 0.125 mg/kg/d • If extubated between days 1 and 15 then advance to day 15 of regimen
Unresolving ARDS (7-21 d)	• Methylprednisolone 2 mg/kg IV bolus, then » Days 1-14: 2 mg/kg/d divided every 6 h » Days 15-21: 1 mg/kg/d » Days 22-28: 0.5 mg/kg/d » Days 29-30: 0.25 mg/kg/d » Days 31-32: 0.125 mg/kg/d • If extubated before day 14, then advance to day 15 of regimen drug therapy

ARDS = acute respiratory distress syndrome.

From Chaudhuri D, Nei AM, Rochwerg B, et al. 2024 focused update: Guidelines on use of corticosteroids in sepsis, acute respiratory distress syndrome, and community-acquired pneumonia. Crit Care Med 2024;52:e219-e33.

makes a "suggested" recommendation of corticosteroids in critically ill patients with ARDS (30). Table 25.4 lists common corticosteroid regimens.

Prone Positioning

The American Thoracic Society, European Society of Intensive Care Medicine, and Society of Critical Care Medicine strongly recommend prone positioning (12-18 h daily) (32). This maneuver improves arterial oxygenation by improving ventilation-perfusion matching, and reducing the risk of ventilator-induced lung injury (because lung inflation is more homogeneous) (32). Unstable spine fractures are an absolute contraindication to prone positioning. Relative contraindications include unstable pelvic fractures, intracranial hypertension, hemodynamic instability, and massive hemoptysis (33-34). Complications are uncommon but include pressure ulcers and mainstem bronchus intubation (34-35).

Recruitment Maneuvers

ARDS patients have dependent atelectasis compounded by the increased lung weight from pulmonary edema. Recruitment maneuvers (RMs) are deliberate (temporary) increases in airway pressures to recruit collapsed alveoli to improve oxygenation (36-38). A variety of RMs have been described such as a continuous high driving pressure (i.e., CPAP of 40 cm H_2O × 40 s) and progressive incremental PEEP.

Extracorporeal Membrane Oxygenation

Veno-venous extracorporeal membrane oxygenation (ECMO) is a "suggested" recommendation for severe ARDS by the American Thoracic Society (28). Venous blood is pumped through a membrane oxygenator and returned to the venous system facilitating both oxygenation and CO_2 removal. ECMO serves as an adjunct (rather than replacement) for mechanical ventilation, and ventilation of the lungs is achieved at lower airway pressures to reduce the risk of ventilator-induced lung injury (39). See Chapter 30: Extracorporeal Membrane Oxygenation.

References

1. Bellani G, Laffey JG, Pham T, et al. Epidemiology, patterns of care, and mortality for patients with acute respiratory distress syndrome in intensive care units in 50 countries. JAMA 2016;315:788-800.
2. Diamond M, Peniston HL, Sanghavi DK, Mahapatra S. Acute Respiratory Distress Syndrome. In: StatPearls. Treasure Island (FL): StatPearls Publishing; 2025.
3. Wong JJM, Leong JY, Lee JH, et al. Insights into the immunopathogenesis of acute respiratory distress syndrome. Ann Transl Med 2019;7:504.
4. Gibson PG, Qin L, Puah SH. COVID-19 acute respiratory distress syndrome (ARDS): clinical features and differences from typical pre-COVID-19 ARDS. Med J Aust 2020;213:54-6 e1.
5. Kao SJ, Yeh DY, Chen HI. Clinical and pathological features of fat embolism with acute respiratory distress syndrome. Clin Sci (Lond) 2007;113:279-85.
6. Ruan SY, Huang CT, Chien YC, et al. Etiology-associated heterogeneity in acute respiratory distress syndrome: a retrospective cohort study. BMC Pulm Med 2021;21:183.
7. Shah J, Rana SS. Acute respiratory distress syndrome in acute pancreatitis. Indian J Gastroenterol 2020;39:123-32.
8. Matthay MA, Arabi Y, Arroliga AC, et al. A new global definition of acute respiratory distress syndrome. Am J Respir Crit Care Med 2024;209:37-47.
9. Janipalli VP, Moturi PK. Comparison of SpO2/FiO2 ratio and PaO2/FiO2 ratio as diagnostic criteria in patients with ALI and ARDS. J Evid Based Med Healthc 2020;7:2520-25.
10. Kumar A, Aggarwal R, Khanna P, et al. Correlation of the SpO_2/FiO_2 (s/f) ratio and the PaO_2/FiO_2 (p/f) ratio in patients with COVID-19 pneumonia. Medicina intensiva 2022;46:408.
11. Grieser C, Goldmann A, Steffen IG, et al. Computed tomography findings from patients with ARDS due to influenza A (H1N1) virus-associated pneumonia. Eur J Radiol 2012;81:389-94.
12. Hashimoto H, Yamamoto S, Nakagawa H, et al. Predictive value of computed tomography for short-term mortality in patients with acute respiratory distress syndrome: a systematic review. Sci Rep 2022;12:9579.
13. Bernard GR, Artigas A, Brigham KL, et al. The American-European consensus conference on ARDS. Definitions, mechanisms, relevant outcomes, and clinical trial coordination. Am J Respir Crit Care Med 1994;149:818-24.
14. Rayner-Hartley E, Miller PE, Burstein B, et al. The basics of ARDS mechanical ventilatory care for cardiovascular specialists. Can J Cardiol 2020;36:1675-9.

15. Silva PL, Scharffenberg M, Rocco PRM. Understanding the mechanisms of ventilator-induced lung injury using animal models. Intensive Care Med Exp 2023;11:82.
16. Gattinoni L, Quintel M, Marini JJ. Volutrauma and atelectrauma: Which is worse? Crit Care 2018;22:264.
17. Thompson BT, Bernard GR. ARDS Network (NHLBI) studies: successes and challenges in ARDS clinical research. Crit Care Clin 2011;27:459-68.
18. Acute Respiratory Distress Syndrome Network; Brower RG, Matthay MA, et al. Ventilation with lower tidal volumes as compared with traditional tidal volumes for acute lung injury and the acute respiratory distress syndrome. N Engl J Med 2000;342:1301-8.
19. Fan E, Needham DM, Stewart TE. Ventilatory management of acute lung injury and acute respiratory distress syndrome. JAMA 2005;294:2889-96.
20. Nassar B. Should we be permissive with hypercapnia? Ann Am Thorac Soc 2022;19:165-6.
21. Hickling KG, Walsh J, Henderson S, Jackson R. Low mortality rate in adult respiratory distress syndrome using low-volume, pressure-limited ventilation with permissive hypercapnia: a prospective study. Crit Care Med 1994;22:1568-78.
22. Sembroski E, Sanghavi DK, Bhardwaj A. Inverse Ratio Ventilation. In: StatPearls. Treasure Island (FL): StatPearls Publishing; 2025.
23. Kallet RH. Patient-ventilator interaction during acute lung injury, and the role of spontaneous breathing: part 2: airway pressure release ventilation. Respir Care 2011;56:190-203; discussion 203-6.
24. Tonelli AR, Zein J, Adams J, Ioannidis JP. Effects of interventions on survival in acute respiratory distress syndrome: an umbrella review of 159 published randomized trials and 29 meta-analyses. Intensive Care Med 2014;40:769-87.
25. Lee J, Corl K, Levy MM. Fluid therapy and acute respiratory distress syndrome. Crit Care Clin 2021;37:867-75.
26. National Heart, Lung, and Blood Institute PETAL Clinical Trials Network; Moss M, Huang DT, et al. Early neuromuscular blockade in the acute respiratory distress syndrome. N Engl J Med 2019;380:1997-2008.
27. Ho ATN, Patolia S, Guervilly C. Neuromuscular blockade in acute respiratory distress syndrome: a systematic review and meta-analysis of randomized controlled trials. J Intensive Care 2020;8:12.
28. Qadir N, Sahetya S, Munshi L, et al. An update on management of adult patients with acute respiratory distress syndrome: an official American Thoracic Society clinical practice guideline. Am J Respir Crit Care Med 2024;209:24-36.
29. Lin C, Chao WC, Pai KC, et al. Prolonged use of neuromuscular blocking agents is associated with increased long-term mortality

in mechanically ventilated medical ICU patients: a retrospective cohort study. J Intensive Care 2023;11:55.
30. Chaudhuri D, Nei AM, Rochwerg B, et al. 2024 focused update: guidelines on use of corticosteroids in sepsis, acute respiratory distress syndrome, and community-acquired pneumonia. Crit Care Med 2024;52:e219-e33.
31. Kuperminc E, Heming N, Carlos M, Annane D. Corticosteroids in ARDS. J Clin Med 2023;12.
32. Fan E, Del Sorbo L, Goligher EC, et al. An official American Thoracic Society/European Society of Intensive Care Medicine/Society of Critical Care Medicine clinical practice guideline: mechanical ventilation in adult patients with acute respiratory distress syndrome. Am J Respir Crit Care Med 2017;195:1253-63.
33. Bein T, Grasso S, Moerer O, et al. The standard of care of patients with ARDS: ventilatory settings and rescue therapies for refractory hypoxemia. Intensive Care Med 2016;42:699-711.
34. Rampon GL, Simpson SQ, Agrawal R. Prone positioning for acute hypoxemic respiratory failure and ARDS: a review. Chest 2023;163:332-40.
35. Bloomfield R, Noble DW, Sudlow A. Prone position for acute respiratory failure in adults. Cochrane Database Syst Rev 2015; 2015:CD008095.
36. Borges JB, Okamoto VN, Matos GF, et al. Reversibility of lung collapse and hypoxemia in early acute respiratory distress syndrome. Am J Respir Crit Care Med 2006;174:268-78.
37. Fan E, Brodie D, Slutsky AS. Acute respiratory distress syndrome: advances in diagnosis and treatment. JAMA 2018;319:698-710.
38. Hodgson CL, Tuxen DV, Davies AR, et al. A randomised controlled trial of an open lung strategy with staircase recruitment, titrated peep and targeted low airway pressures in patients with acute respiratory distress syndrome. Crit Care 2011;15:R133.
39. Ventetuolo CE, Muratore CS. Extracorporeal life support in critically ill adults. Am J Respir Crit Care Med 2014;190:497-508.

SECTION VII
RESPIRATORY MANAGEMENT

Chapter 26
Noninvasive Ventilation

This chapter describes the fundamentals of using pressure-assisted breathing techniques that do not require endotracheal intubation. The effects of positive pressure breathing on cardiac performance are also briefly reviewed.

METHODS OF NONINVASIVE VENTILATION

Continuous Positive Airway Pressure

When breathing with continuous positive airway pressure (CPAP), the pressure at the end of expiration is *positive* relative to the atmospheric pressure, and the positive pressure (usually 5-10 cm H_2O) is maintained during the respiratory cycle. This pressure helps to prevent collapse of the small airways at the end of expiration and increases the end-expiratory volume. This is demonstrated in Figure 26.1.

Clinical Uses

The principal use of CPAP is in patients with obstructive sleep apnea, where the positive pressure prevents the inspiratory collapse of the pharynx that causes an obstruction to airflow (1-2). CPAP has also been successful in managing patients with acute cardiogenic pulmonary edema (3). CPAP provides only limited pressure support, and it is rarely used to manage patients with acute respiratory failure.

Bilevel Positive Pressure Ventilation

Noninvasive ventilation (NIV) is a patient-triggered, pressure-targeted mode of ventilation that provides two "levels" of pressure to support breathing. This bilevel mode

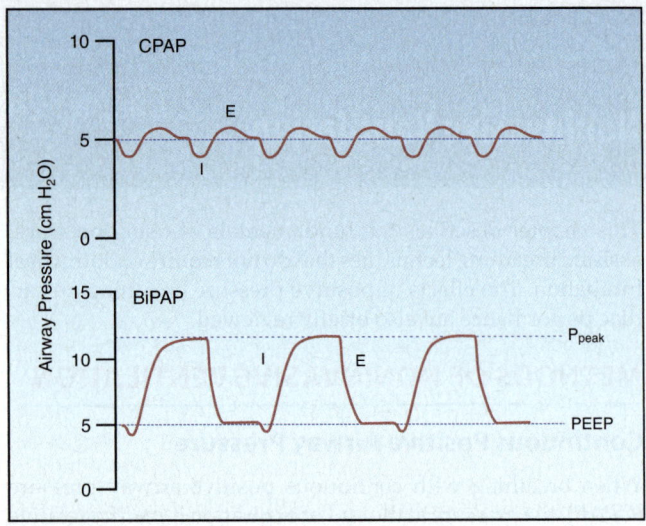

FIGURE 26.1. Airway pressure waveforms for continuous positive airway pressure (CPAP) and bilevel positive airway pressure (BiPAP). These waveforms show a spontaneous breathing pattern with a positive end-expiratory pressure (PEEP) of 5 cm H_2O. (From Noninvasive Ventilation. In: Marino PL. *Marino's The ICU Book*. 5th ed. Wolters Kluwer; 2025:428-40. Figure 26.1.)

of ventilation is also known bilevel ventilation or *BiPAP*; *however*, this is a proprietary name (registered as a trademark name by Philips Respironics) and is used sparingly here. The *first* pressure augments tidal volumes to help with work of breathing and the *second* pressure is positive end-expiratory pressure (PEEP) to prevent airways collapse (4-5). This is illustrated in Figure 26.1. The patient triggers each positive-pressure lung inflation (indicated by the negative pressure swings), and the inspiratory pressure gradually rises until it reaches a preselected pressure. Exhalation then proceeds until the pressure reaches a preselected PEEP. Peak inspiratory pressures are typically 10-20 cm H_2O, and PEEP levels are usually 5-10 cm H_2O. Higher pressures are generally not advised because they are poorly tolerated and promote leaks around the face mask.

Other Methods

Pressure support ventilation (PSV) and proportional assist ventilation (PAV) are alternative patient-triggered methods that are rarely used for NIV.

Face Masks

The emergence of NIV is largely due to advances in the design of the mask interface. Low-level CPAP can be delivered by nasal masks, but full-face masks are required for bilevel NIV (Figure 26.2), and the face masks must be tight-fitting to minimize leaks.

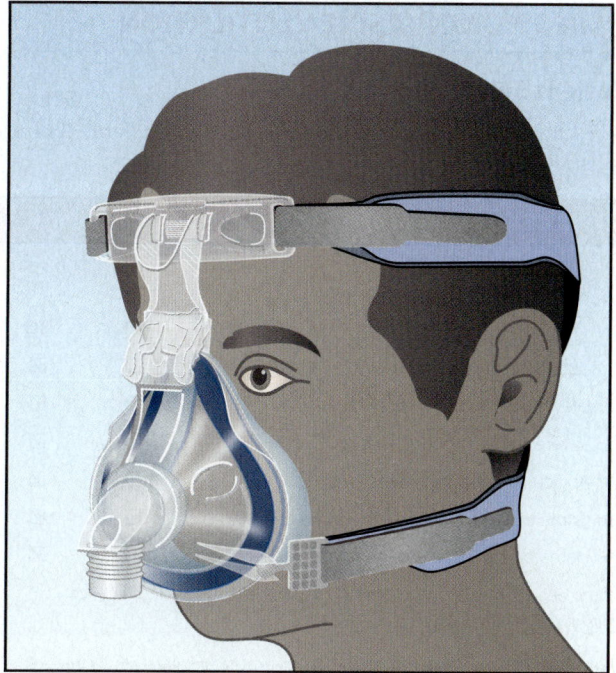

FIGURE 26.2. A tightly secured face mask used for noninvasive ventilation. (From Noninvasive Ventilation. In: Marino PL. *Marino's The ICU Book*. 5th ed. Wolters Kluwer; 2025:428-40. Figure 26.3.)

In addition to general discomfort, masks can cause skin breakdown at points of contact, (i.e., the bridge of the nose). "Mask intolerance" is a significant source (15-20%) of failed attempts to prevent intubation with NIV (6-8).

The Helmet

An alternative to tight-fitting face masks is available with a device called a "helmet," which is a transparent hood that encloses the entire head and has a soft collar that provides a seal at the neck. Some reports have demonstrated fewer intubations and lower mortality, but more studies are necessary to determine the clinical effectiveness of this modality (8).

USING NONINVASIVE VENTILATION

Patient Selection

NIV can be used safely if the criteria listed in Table 26.1 are satisfied.

TABLE 26.1 Checklist for Noninvasive Ventilation

Are any of the following conditions present in a patient who presents with acute respiratory failure?

	YES	NO
1. Agonal breathing	☐	☑
2. Life-threatening circulatory collapse	☐	☑
3. Severe agitation or uncontrolled seizures	☐	☑
4. An acute confusional state	☐	☑
5. Coma with inadequate airway protection	☐	☑
6. Hematemesis or persistent vomiting	☐	☑

If the answer is NO to all of the above, the patient is a candidate for noninvasive ventilation.

From Noninvasive Ventilation. In: Marino PL. *Marino's The ICU Book*. 5th ed. Wolters Kluwer; 2025:428-40. Table 26.1.

NIV is a consideration in any case of acute respiratory failure that does not meet the criteria in Table 26.1. However, *the likelihood of success* (i.e., preventing intubation) *is dependent on the type of respiratory failure* (i.e., hypercapnic or purely hypoxemic respiratory failure), *and the underlying illness*.

Hypercapnic Respiratory Failure

The most successful use of NIV is in patients with acute hypercapnic respiratory failure from an acute exacerbation of chronic obstructive pulmonary disease (COPD) (9). The benefits of NIV in this condition are shown in Figure 26.3.

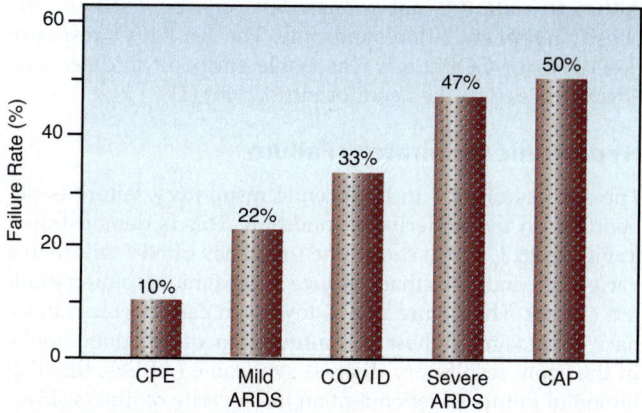

FIGURE 26.3. The failure rate of noninvasive ventilation in common conditions that cause acute hypoxemic respiratory failure. CPE = cardiogenic pulmonary edema; ARDS = acute respiratory distress syndrome; CAP = community acquired pneumonia. (Data from References 10, 12-14.)

As a result, *NIV is recommended as a first-line therapy for acute exacerbations of COPD that are associated with acute hypercapnic respiratory failure* (4,8). NIV does not have this benefit when the hypercapnia is chronic (4).

Evaluating the Response

About 10-20% of COPD patients with acute hypercapnia will not respond favorably to NIV (9). These patients can be identified by checking the $PaCO_2$ after 1 h of NIV and comparing it to the baseline $PaCO_2$. *Failure of the $PaCO_2$ to decrease significantly (e.g., by at least 10%) after 1 h of NIV is evidence of a poor response* (10). Altered mentation (e.g., from hypercapnia) should not be used as an early indication of NIV failure because this sign takes longer to resolve. Intubation is indicated when NIV fails.

Obesity Hypoventilation Syndrome

Although data are not robust, NIV can be used for the obesity hypoventilation syndrome. The 1-h $PaCO_2$ response described for COPD is a reasonable endpoint to determine effectiveness (i.e., the need for intubation) (11).

Hypoxemic Respiratory Failure

The success of NIV in hypoxemic respiratory failure is dependent on the underlying condition. This is demonstrated in Figure 26.3, which shows the frequency of NIV failure in a variety of conditions that produce hypoxemic respiratory failure (12-15). The failure rate is lowest in cardiogenic pulmonary edema and highest in community-acquired pneumonia. In the acute respiratory distress syndrome (ARDS), the likelihood of failure is dependent on the severity of illness (13).

Evaluating the Response

Failure to increase the PaO_2/FiO_2 ratio after 1 h of NIV is evidence of a poor response; i.e., NIV failure and the need for endotracheal intubation (12).

Cardiogenic Pulmonary Edema

Both CPAP and NIV are highly successful (and equally effective) in cardiogenic pulmonary edema (16). This benefit is not limited to improvements in lung function because *positive intrathoracic pressure can increase cardiac stroke output* (9,17). This is illustrated in Figure 26.4.

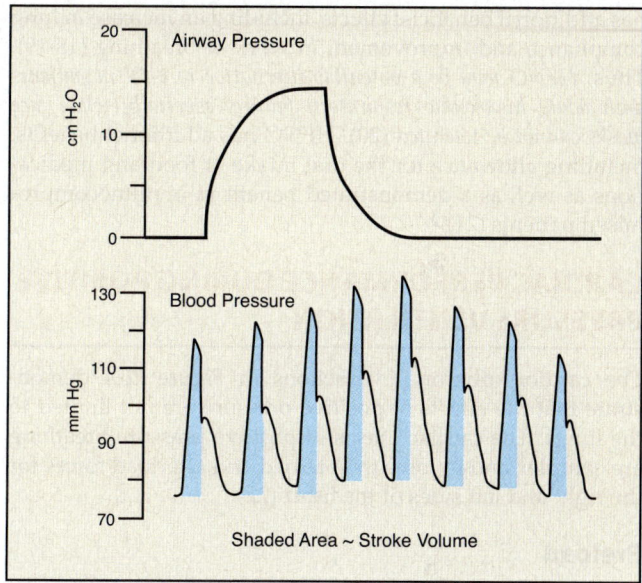

FIGURE 26.4. Changes in arterial pressure associated with a positive pressure breath. The shaded areas in the arterial pressure waveforms (which are proportional to stroke volume) show the increase in arterial pressure which also reflects an increase in cardiac stroke output. (From Noninvasive Ventilation. In: Marino PL. *Marino's The ICU Book*. 5th ed. Wolters Kluwer; 2025:428-40. Figure 26.6.)

The effect shown in Figure 26.4 is largely the result of a decrease in left ventricular afterload. An increase in intrathoracic pressure reduces the pressure gradient between the aorta and the thoracic cavity, thereby lessening the force the left ventricle needs to exert to eject blood during systole.

High Flow Nasal Oxygen

High-flow nasal oxygen (HFNO) is traditionally used for cases of hypoxemic respiratory failure when the hypoxemia is refractory to conventional methods of O_2 inhalation. HFNO has additional beneficial effects, including an increase in lung compliance and improvement in work of breathing (18-19). Thus, *HFNO may be a potential alternative to NIV in patients with acute hypoxemic respiratory failure, especially when face masks cannot be tolerated* (20). HFNO has additional benefits, including allowance for the oral intake of food and medications as well as a demonstrated benefit in immunocompromised patients (21).

CARDIAC PERFORMANCE DURING POSITIVE PRESSURE VENTILATION

The cardiorespiratory interactions in Figure 26.4 demonstrate that the effects of positive pressure are not limited to the lungs. The cardiac effects of positive pressure breathing are complex and involve the preload and afterload forces for the right and left sides of the heart (22).

Preload

The term "preload" refers to a force that stretches a resting muscle to a new length. Positive intrathoracic pressure can reduce ventricular preload (end-diastolic volume) in several ways, as shown in Figure 26.5.

Thus, higher levels of positive pressure ventilation present a threat to cardiac filling—a state potentially analogous to hypovolemia (16). Thus, avoidance of hypovolemia is imperative during positive pressure ventilation, especially when high pressures are required for lung inflation.

Afterload

The term "afterload" refers to the force that must be overcome by muscle contraction. Unlike the preload force, which facilitates muscle contraction, the afterload force opposes muscle

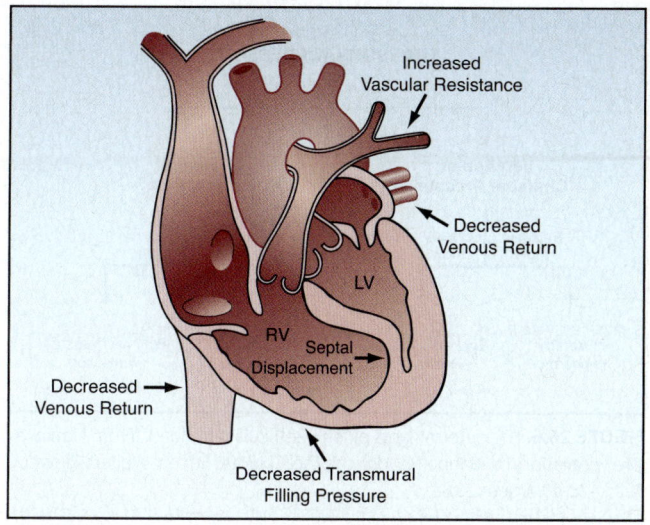

FIGURE 26.5. The different ways that positive intrathoracic pressure can decrease filling of the right (RV) and left ventricles (LV). (From Noninvasive Ventilation. In: Marino PL. *Marino's The ICU Book*. 5th ed. Wolters Kluwer; 2025:428-40. Figure 26.7.)

contraction. The determinants of left ventricular afterload are shown in Figure 26.6.

Afterload is a transmural pressure and is a function of the pleural pressure surrounding the heart: i.e.,

Afterload = Chamber Pressure − Pleural Pressure   (26.1)

The Effect of Positive Pressure Ventilation on Afterload

Negative pleural pressure during spontaneous breathing *increases* left ventricular afterload by *opposing* inward movement of the ventricular wall during systole. This explains why the systolic blood pressure decreases during a spontaneous inspiration. *Pulsus paradoxus* (i.e., a drop in systolic blood pressure by >10 mm Hg) may occur in conditions associated with exaggerated inspiratory efforts (e.g., asthma) (23).

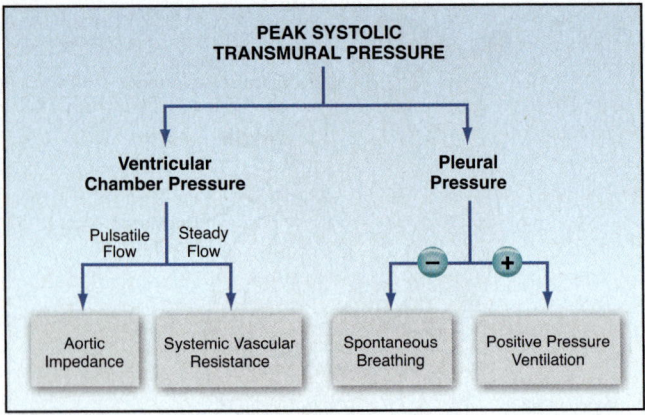

FIGURE 26.6. The determinants of left ventricular afterload. (From Noninvasive Ventilation. In: Marino PL. *Marino's The ICU Book*. 5th ed. Wolters Kluwer; 2025:428-40. Figure 26.8.)

Alternatively, *positive* intrathoracic pressure can *decrease* left ventricular afterload by *promoting* the inward movement of the ventricle during systole. This action is one of the proposed mechanisms for the benefit of positive intrathoracic pressure in patients with heart failure receiving NIV and cardiac arrest (i.e., the ability of chest compressions to promote cardiac output—the thoracic pump model) (24).

Overall Effect on Cardiac Output

The overall effect of positive pressure ventilation on cardiac output is determined by the balance between preload and afterload. This balance is determined by three factors: *the intravascular volume, the level of intrathoracic pressure, and the presence of absence of cardiac dysfunction.*

Role of Cardiac Function

Normal Heart. The normal heart operates on the steep portion of the preload curve and the flat portion of the afterload curve (see Figure 17.2 in Chapter 17: Cardiogenic Shock). Hence, a *decrease in preload has a greater influence on cardiac output than a decrease in afterload*, so positive pressure ventilation is more likely to impair cardiac output (due to impedance of cardiac filling). *In patients with normal cardiac function, it is essential to maintain intravascular volume to support venous return during positive pressure ventilation.*

Heart Failure. The failing heart operates on the flat portion of the preload curve and the steep portion of the afterload curve. In this *situation, a decrease in afterload has a greater influence on cardiac output than a decrease in preload*, so positive pressure ventilation is more likely to enhance cardiac output, assuming the patient is euvolemic. *This explains the benefit of CPAP and NIV in cardiogenic pulmonary edema.*

References

1. Rochwerg B, Brochard L, Elliott MW, et al. Official ERS/ATS clinical practice guideline: noninvasive ventilation for acute respiratory failure. Eur Respir J 2017;50:1602426.
2. Patil SP, Ayappa IA, Caples SM, et al. Treatment of adult obstructive sleep apnea with positive air-way pressure: an American Academy of Sleep Medicine clinical practice guideline. J Clin Sleep Med 2019;15(2):335-43.
3. Gray A, Goodacre S, Newby DE, et al. for the 3CPO Trialists. Noninvasive ventilation in acute cardio-genic pulmonary edema. N Engl J Med 2008;359:142-51.
4. Munshi L, Mancebo J, Brochard LJ. Noninvasive respiratory support for adults with acute respiratory failure. N Engl J Med 2022;387:1688-98.
5. Hess DR. Ventilator waveforms and the physiology of pressure support ventilation. Respir Care 2005;50:166-86.
6. Kramer N, Meyer TJ, Meharg J, et al. Randomized, prospective trial of noninvasive positive pressure ventilation in acute respiratory failure. Am J Respir Crit Care Med 1995;151:1799-806.
7. Thille AW, Balen F, Carteaux G, et al. Oxygen therapy and noninvasive respiratory supports in acute hypoxemic respiratory failure: a narrative review. Ann Intensive Care 2024;14(1):158.
8. Osadnik CR, Tee VS, Carson-Chahhoud KV, et al. Non-invasive ventilation for the management of acute hypercapnic respiratory failure due to exacerbation of chronic obstructive pulmonary disease. Cochrane Database Syst Rev 2017:CD004104.
9. Baratz DM, Westbrook PR, Shah PK, et al. Effect of nasal continuous positive airway pressure on cardiac output and oxygen delivery in patients with congestive heart failure. Chest 1992;102:1397-401.

10. Antón A, Güell R, Gómez J, et al. Predicting the result of noninvasive ventilation in severe acute exacerbations of patients with chronic airflow obstruction. Chest 2000;117:828-33.
11. Carillo A, Ferrer M, Gonzalez-Diaz G, et al. Noninvasive ventilation in acute hypercapnic respiratory failure cause by obesity hypoventilation syndrome and chronic obstructive pulmonary disease. Am J Respir Crit Care Med 2012;186:1279-85.
12. Antonelli M, Conti G, Moro ML, et al. Predictors of failure of noninvasive positive pressure ventilation in patients with acute hypoxemic respiratory failure: a multi-center study. Intensive Care Med 2001;27:1718-28.
13. Bellani G, Laffey JG, Pham T, et al. Noninvasive ventilation of patients with acute respiratory distress syndrome: insights from the LUNG SAFE study. Am J Respir Crit Care Med 2017;195:67-77.
14. Nair PR, Haritha D, Behera S, et al. Comparison of high-flow nasal cannula and noninvasive ventilation in acute hypoxemic respiratory failure due to severe COVID-19 pneumonia. Respir Care 2021;66:1824-30.
15. Berbenetz N, Wang Y, Brown J, et al. Non-invasive positive pressure ventilation (CPAP or bilevel NPPV) for cardiogenic pulmonary edema. Cochrane Database Syst Rev 2019:CD005351.
16. Pinsky MR. Why knowing the effects of positive-pressure ventilation on venous, pleural, and pericardial pressures is important to the bedside clinician? Crit Care Med 2014;42(9):2129-31.
17. Michard F. Changes in arterial pressure during mechanical ventilation. Anesthesiology 2005;103:419-28.
18. Nishimura M. High-flow nasal cannula oxygen therapy in adults: physiological benefits, indications, clinical benefits, and adverse effects. Respir Care 2016;61:529-41.
19. Mauri T, Turrini C, Eronia N, et al. Physiologic effects of high-flow nasal cannula in acute hypoxemic respiratory failure. Am J Resp Crit Care Med 2017;195:1207-15.
20. Frat J-P, Thille AW, Mercat A, et al. for the FLORALI Study Group and the REVA Network. High-flow oxygen through nasal cannula in acute hypoxemic respiratory failure. N Engl J Med 2015;372:2185-95.
21. Frat J-P, Ragot S, Girault C, et al. for the REVA Network. Effect of non-invasive oxygenation strategies in immunocompromised patients with severe acute respiratory failure: a post-hoc analysis of a randomised trial. Lancet Respir Med 2016;4:646-52.
22. Pinsky MR. Cardiopulmonary interactions: physiological basis and clinical applications. Annals ATS 2018;15:S45-S48.
23. Hamzaoui O, Monnet X, Teboul J-L. Pulsus paradoxus. Eur Respir J 2013;42:1696-705.
24. Redberg RF, Tucker KJ, Cohen TJ, et al. Physiology of blood flow during cardiopulmonary resuscitation. A transesophageal echocardiographic study. Circulation 1993;88(2):534-42.

Chapter 27

Conventional Mechanical Ventilation

This chapter describes the general framework for *initiating* and managing conventional "invasive" mechanical ventilation for patients with acute hypoxic and/or hypercarbic respiratory failure. The term "invasive" denotes the use of an artificial airway: an endotracheal tube, cricothyrotomy, or tracheostomy. Descriptions of airway management are detailed in Chapter 2: Airway Management.

CORE MECHANICAL VENTILATOR SETTINGS

There are four core ventilator settings that are a part of all modes of mechanical ventilation:

1. **Tidal volume (V_t)** is the amount of air that moves in and out of the lungs with each breath. Too much V_t results in overdistention and barotrauma, which is important for gas exchange (O_2 and CO_2). To avoid barotrauma, V_t should be set at 6 mL/kg predicted body weight or maintaining the plateau pressure (P_{plat}) <30 cm H_2O, i.e., "lung protective strategy" (1-2). Details of how different mechanical ventilatory modes accomplish V_t are described in the section that follows, "Methods of Lung Inflation."
2. **Respiratory rate (RR)** is simply breaths per minute. Along with V_t, RR is a principal determinant of minute ventilation (V_e):

$$V_e = RR \times V_t$$

Alveolar ventilation (VA) includes physiologic dead space which is the amount of ventilation that *does not* participate in gas exchange (3):

$$VA = RR \times (V_t - \text{dead space})$$

a. Physiologic dead space is the sum of anatomic dead space and alveolar dead space.
b. *Anatomic dead space* is the volume of air in the respiratory tract that conduct air flow but do not participate in gas exchange, i.e., trachea, bronchioles, ventilator tubing (4).
c. *Alveolar dead space* refers to alveoli that are ventilated but not perfused, e.g., decreased cardiac output, emphysema, shunts, pulmonary emboli, etc. VA directly affects $PaCO_2$ levels with increases in VA leading to decreases in $PaCO_2$. At a constant VA and stable CO_2 production, a rise in $PaCO_2$ denotes an increase in dead space. Increasing V_t is more effective in improving VA than RR (5).
3. **Fraction of inspired oxygen (FiO_2)** is the percentage of oxygen in inspired gas. The optimal FiO_2 should aim to achieve a minimum oxygen saturation (or pulse oximetry) of 93% in patients without pulmonary disease and possibly 88% in those with chronic obstructive pulmonary disease (COPD) (6). A target oxygen saturation of 100% is not associated with improved outcomes and risks oxygen toxicity and worsening lung injury (7-9). Excess oxygen creates oxygen free radicals that damage alveolar membranes, worsening lung injury. A pulse oximetry (SpO_2) of 100% could have a PO_2 of 100 mm Hg or as high as the 400s!
4. **Positive end-expiratory pressure (PEEP)**

PEEP

Alveolar Collapse

During mechanical ventilation, there is a tendency for the distal airspaces to collapse at the end of expiration in dependent lung regions (10), and this is magnified in patients with obstructive airway disease (e.g., COPD) and lung injury that reduce the distensibility of the lungs and decrease surfactant (e.g., acute respiratory distress syndrome [ARDS]). This has two adverse consequences:

1. Alveoli that remain collapsed cannot participate in gas exchange
2. Distal airspaces that repetitively close and open with each respiratory cycle can generate shear forces that damage the airway epithelium. This form of lung injury is called *atelectrauma* (1).

To prevent alveolar collapse at the end of expiration, PEEP (usually 5 cm H_2O) is routinely applied to the airways during mechanical ventilation to prevent alveolar collapse and maintain the functional residual capacity (FRC). This pressure is created by a pressure-relief valve in the expiratory limb of the ventilator circuit, which allows exhalation to proceed until a preselected pressure is reached, and PEEP is then maintained until the next inspiration.

Alveolar Recruitment

In diffuse infiltrative lung diseases, like ARDS, increases in PEEP to levels above those used to prevent alveolar collapse can be effective in opening collapsed alveoli (*alveolar recruitment*) to improve arterial oxygenation.

- The use of increased PEEP levels is generally reserved for cases where the concentration of inhaled O_2 (FiO_2) is at potentially toxic levels (>60%).
- If increased PEEP is used to improve arterial oxygenation, the P_{plat} should not exceed 30 cm H_2O, to limit the risk of ventilator-induced lung injury (11).

Influence on Airway Pressures

The influence of PEEP on airway pressures using pressure control ventilation (PCV) is shown in Figure 27.1. Note that the addition of PEEP increases both the end-inspiratory alveolar pressure, and the mean airway pressure, (hence, arterial oxygenation). Thus, the pressure control setting *is additive* to the PEEP setting and needs a target of 6 mL/kg V_t or P_{plat} ≤30 cm H_2O to avoid barotrauma.

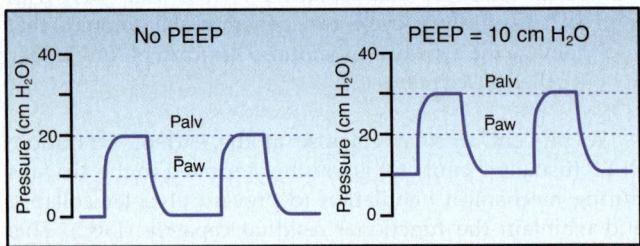

FIGURE 27.1. Airway pressure waveforms during pressure control ventilation showing the effects of positive end-expiratory pressure (PEEP) on end-inspiratory alveolar pressure (Palv) and mean airway pressure (Paw).

The increase in mean airway pressure determines the tendency for PEEP to decrease cardiac output (see section that follows).

Hemodynamic Effects

It is prudent for the provider to be aware that PEEP can have a variable impact on cardiac output via changes in intrathoracic pressures, transpulmonary pressures, and alterations in pulmonary circulation pressure impacting venous returns resulting in decrease cardiac output (12). These effects can be exaggerated by hypovolemia, chest wall compliance, and poor pulmonary compliance (e.g., ARDS). Figure 27.2 illustrates opposing effects of PEEP, arterial oxygenation, and cardiac output (13).

Because of the tendency of PEEP to decrease cardiac output, some measure of cardiac output is appropriate when using higher than usual levels of PEEP (e.g., >10 cm H_2O).

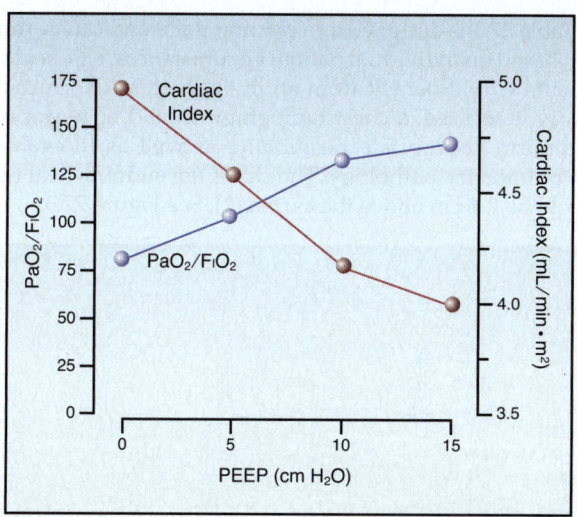

FIGURE 27.2. The opposing effects of positive end-expiratory pressure (PEEP) on arterial oxygenation (PaO_2/FiO_2) and cardiac output. (Data from Reference 13.)

INITIAL MECHANICAL VENTILATOR SETTINGS

Unless a depolarizing neuromuscular blocking agent, like succinylcholine, is used, most patients who are intubated with neuromuscular blockade, sedation, and analgesia will need full ventilatory support for up to 30 min. Suggested initial ventilator settings after intubation are shown in Table 27.1.

TABLE 27.1	Suggested Initial Ventilator Settings
Mode of Ventilation: Assist Control	
Tidal Volume	6-8 mL/kg PBW
Respiratory Rate	12-20 breaths per minute
Fraction of Inspired oxygen (FiO_2)	100%
Positive End-Expiratory Pressure (PEEP)	5 cm H_2O

PBW = predicted body weight.

Table 27.1 is designed as a starting point and can be modified based on individual patient circumstances, e.g., acidotic patients would benefit from an initial higher RR. Once the airway is secured, a chest radiograph should be performed to confirm appropriate positioning as well as to evaluate any pulmonary pathology. The tip of the endotracheal tube should be 2-6 cm above the carina (2). See Figure 27.3.

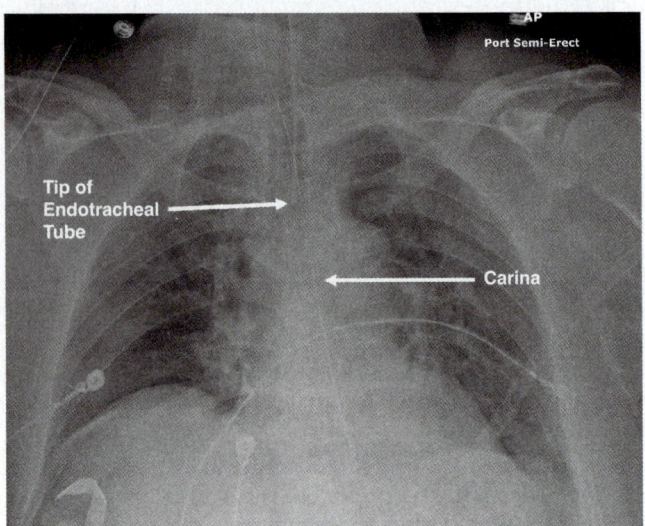

FIGURE 27.3. Postintubation chest radiograph.

Arterial blood gas should be obtained within 15-30 min to assess acid-base status, oxygenation, and ventilation. Choice of ventilator mode and the titration of mechanical ventilator settings can then be targeted to optimize oxygenation, optimize ventilation, and avoid barotrauma.

METHODS OF LUNG INFLATION

Volume versus Pressure Control

There are two basic modes of mechanical ventilation based on the method used to inflate the lungs.

With *volume control ventilation* (VCV), the inflation (tidal) volume is preselected, and the lungs are inflated at a constant flow rate until the desired volume is delivered. Examples include assist control, intermittent mandatory ventilation, pressure-regulated volume control, and volume support ventilation.

With *PCV*, the inflation pressure is preselected, and high flow rates are used at the onset of lung inflation to achieve the desired inflation pressure quickly. The flow rate decelerates during lung inflation, and the inspiratory time is adjusted to allow the flow rate to fall to zero at the end of inspiration.

Airway Pressures

Alveolar Pressure

Note in Figure 27.4 that the peak airway pressure (Paw), measured at the end of inspiration, is higher with volume control than pressure control, but the alveolar pressure (Palv) at end inspiration is the same with both methods of lung inflation.

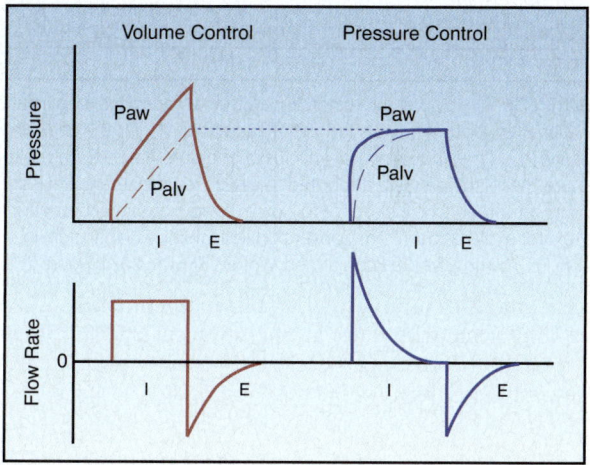

FIGURE 27.4. Pressure changes during a single ventilator breath with volume control and pressure control methods of lung inflation, at equivalent inflation (tidal) volumes. Changes in airway pressure (Paw) indicated by the *solid lines*, and changes in alveolar pressure (Palv) indicated by the *dashed lines*. I = inspiration, E = expiration.

The peak pressure (P_{peak}) at the end of inspiration is the pressure needed to overcome both airway resistance, and the elastic recoil force (lung compliance) of the lungs and chest wall. An inspiratory hold (about 1 s) allows the "recoil" of the lung indicating the compliance of the lung (as opposed to stiffness and minimal recoil). This is the P_{plat}. See Figure 27.5.

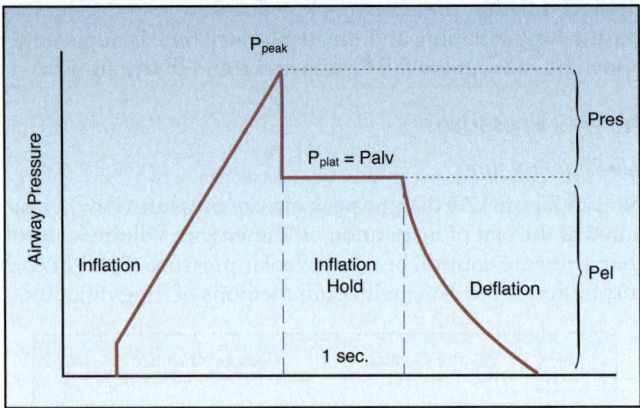

FIGURE 27.5. Airway pressure profile for a volume-controlled lung inflation with a brief end-inspiratory occlusion (inflation hold). P_{peak} is the peak airway pressure, P_{plat} is the end-inspiratory occlusion pressure, Palv is the alveolar pressure, Pres is the pressure attributed to airway resistance, and Pel is the pressure attributed to the elastic recoil force of the lungs and chest wall. See text for explanation. (From Conventional Mechanical Ventilation. In: Marino PL. *Marino's The ICU Book*. 5th ed. Wolters Kluwer; 2025. Figure 27.2.)

The difference between the peak and plateau pressure is the pressure needed to overcome airway resistance (Pres). Because there is no airflow during the inflation hold maneuver, the P_{plat} is essentially equivalent to the alveolar pressure at the end of inspiration (P_{plat} = Palv). As reflection of the pressures (stress) imposed on the walls of the alveoli by the inflation (tidal) volume, the P_{plat} should be maintained <30 cm H_2O to avoid ventilator-induced lung injury (2). Alveolar injury from overdistension is called *volutrauma* (1).

Static Compliance

Static compliance (Cstat) is a measure of the expansion of the lungs and chest when pressure is applied during a period of no flow (end inspiration). This is calculated using the formula:

$$Cstat = V_t / (P_{plat} - PEEP)$$

Normal Cstat is 50-70 mL/cm H_2O and can be used to assess current pulmonary mechanics, direct therapies (e.g., optimize PEEP), and assess therapeutic interventions.

The Preferred Mode of Ventilation

Either method of lung inflation can be used effectively. Table 27.2 provides a summary of commonly used modes of mechanical ventilation.

TABLE 27.2 Commonly Used Modes of Mechanical Ventilation

	Distinctions	Comments
Assist Control (A/C)	Fixed V_t and rate Patient can trigger breaths over breath fixed rate and will receive full V_t each breath.	May be more comfortable early in "air hunger" Uncontrolled tachypnea can result in severe respiratory alkalosis (pH >7.55) or dynamic hyperinflation.
Intermittent Mandatory Ventilation (IMV)	Fixed V_t and rate Patient can trigger breaths between set rate, but V_t limited to patient's intrinsic negative inspiratory force.	Higher work of breathing than A/C, PSV can be added to further augment triggered breaths.
Pressure Regulated Volume Control (PRVC)	Fixed V_t and rate Hybrid mode that delivers set V_t with variable inspiratory pressures.	Similar to IMV
Pressure Control Ventilation (PCV)	Fixed inspiratory pressure limit and rate. V_t will vary with compliance; can also run in IMV	Improvement in compliance can be observed with increasing V_t on stable PCV settings.
Pressure Support Ventilation (PSV)	The patient triggered breath is pressure augmented allowing the patient to determine duration of lung inflation and ultimate V_t.	Low support (5-8 cm H_2O) commonly used with small levels of PEEP (≤5 cm H_2O) for spontaneous breathing trials Can be added to the spontaneous breaths in IMV No backup rate for apnea, needs apnea alarm
Volume Support Ventilation (VSV)	Fixed V_t breaths triggered by patient's spontaneous effort	No backup rate for apnea, needs apnea alarm

References

1. Gattinoni L, Quintel M, Marini JJ. Volutrauma and atelectrauma: Which is worse? Crit Care 2018;22:264.
2. Mora Carpio AL, Mora JI. Ventilator Management. In: StatPearls. Treasure Island (FL): StatPearls Publishing; 2025.
3. Intagliata S, Rizzo A, Gossman W. Physiology, Lung Dead Space. In: StatPearls. Treasure Island (FL): StatPearls Publishing; 2025.
4. Quinn M, St Lucia K, Rizzo A. Anatomy, Anatomic Dead Space. In: StatPearls. Treasure Island (FL): StatPearls Publishing; 2025.
5. Hallett S, Toro F, Ashurst JV. Physiology, Tidal Volume. In: StatPearls. Treasure Island (FL): StatPearls Publishing; 2025.
6. Fuentes S, Chowdhury YS. Fraction of Inspired Oxygen. In: StatPearls. Treasure Island (FL): StatPearls Publishing; 2025.
7. Cumpstey AF, Oldman AH, Martin DS, et al. Oxygen targets during mechanical ventilation in the ICU: a systematic review and meta-analysis. Crit Care Explor 2022;4:e0652.
8. Semler MW, Casey JD, Lloyd BD, et al. Oxygen-saturation targets for critically ill adults receiving mechanical ventilation. N Engl J Med 2022;387:1759-69.
9. Singer M, Young PJ, Laffey JG, et al. Dangers of hyperoxia. Crit Care 2021;25:440.
10. Harris RS. Pressure-volume curves of the respiratory system. Respir Care 2005;50:78-99.
11. Mercat A, Richard JC, Vielle B, et al. Positive end-expiratory pressure setting in adults with acute lung injury and acute respiratory distress syndrome: a randomized controlled trial. JAMA 2008;299:646-55.
12. Joseph A, Petit M, Vieillard-Baron A. Hemodynamic effects of positive end-expiratory pressure. Curr Opin Crit Care 2024;30:10-9.
13. Gainnier M, Michelet P, Thirion X, et al. Prone position and positive end-expiratory pressure in acute respiratory distress syndrome. Crit Care Med 2003;31:2719-26.

Ventilator-Associated Pneumonia

Chapter 28

The clinical approach to pneumonia in the mechanically ventilated patient can be described by one word: *problematic*. Both diagnosis and treatment are fraught with challenges. Clinical presentations are nonspecific, e.g., radiologic infiltrates are common in mechanically ventilated patients, the ability to identify offending organisms is limited, and the emergence of multidrug resistant organisms remains a challenge.

This chapter presents the clinical decisions regarding pneumonias that appear after 48 h of mechanical ventilation (i.e., *ventilator-associated pneumonias [VAPs]*).

VAP is defined as onset >48 h after intubation. Hospital-acquired pneumonia is defined as onset >48 h after hospitalization not associated with mechanical ventilation (1).

GENERAL INFORMATION

1. Pneumonia is the most common nosocomial infection in ICU patients (2), with an incidence of 5-40% of patients mechanically ventilated for >48 h (3).
2. Unlike community-acquired pneumonias, where the predominant pathogens are pneumococci, atypical organisms, and viruses (4), three-quarters of the responsible pathogens in VAP are gram-negative aerobic bacilli and *Staphylococcus aureus* (Table 28.1) (5-8).
3. The mortality rate associated with VAP varies widely, from 0-65% (9-10), and there are claims that VAP is not a life-threatening illness (9). However, VAP-associated mortality rates must be viewed with caution because of the tendency for overdiagnosis of VAP (11).

TABLE 28.1 Common Isolates in Ventilator-Associated Pneumonia

Gram-Negative Microorganisms	Gram-Positive Microorganisms
• *Klebsiella* species • *Enterobacter* species • *Pseudomonas aeruginosa* • *Acinetobacter* species • *Escherichia coli*	• *Staphylococcus aureus* • Methicillin-sensitive *Staph aureus* (MSSA) • Methicillin-resistant *Staph aureus* (MRSA)

PREVENTIVE MEASURES

Aspiration of pathogenic organisms from the oropharynx is believed to be the inciting event in most cases of VAP. The pathogens that most often colonize the oropharynx in ICU patients are gram-negative aerobic bacilli, which explains the predominance of these pathogens in VAP. Specific interventions to address this mechanism are discussed.

Routine Oral Hygiene

Acting on the concept that VAP begins with the aspiration of pathogens, the Centers for Disease Control and Prevention (CDC) has developed clinical practices for routine oral hygiene. Endotracheal tubes prevent mouth closure, promoting desiccation of the mucosal surfaces of the mouth. Evidence-based practices (12) regarding oral hygiene include the following:

Brushing
- Teeth
- Gums
- Tongue

Moistening (every 2-4 h)
- Oral mucosa
- Lips

Both 0.05% cetylpyridinium chloride and 0.12% chlorhexidine gluconate can be used as antiseptic rinses for brushing and moisturizing application. Application swabs and toothbrushes are available with suction attachments to prevent pooling and aspiration of oral rinse during treatment (Figure 28.1).

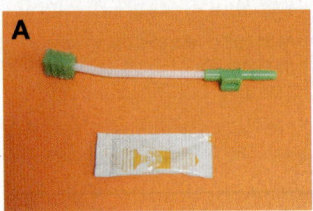 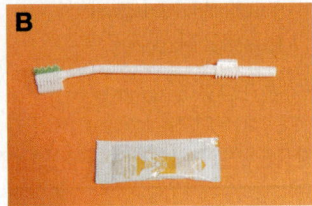

FIGURE 28.1. Suction swab and suction toothbrush. (A) Suction swab with 7 mL packet of 0.05% cetylpyridinium antiseptic cleansing and moisturizing oral rinse. (B) Suction toothbrush with 7 mL packet of 0.05% cetylpyridinium antiseptic cleansing and moisturizing oral rinse.

Selective Decontamination

A common practice in Europe, selective decontamination is the administration of an oral paste and administering a gastric suspension of nonabsorbable antibiotics up to four times daily in an attempt to decrease colonization of pathogens in the oropharynx and upper gastrointestinal tract. This practice has not resulted in an improvement in mortality (13-14).

Routine Airway Care

The inner surface of artificial airways (endotracheal and tracheostomy tubes) rapidly develops a biofilm colonized with pathogenic organisms (6). Passing a suction catheter through the tubes can dislodge these organisms and introduce pathogens into the lower airways (15). Because of this risk, *endotracheal suctioning is not recommended as a routine procedure* and should be used only when necessary to clear secretions from the airways (16).

Clearing Subglottic Secretions

1. *Inflation of the cuff of endotracheal tubes does not create a watertight seal and does not prevent aspiration of mouth secretions into the lower airways.* Aspiration of saliva and liquid tube feedings has been documented in over 50% of patients with tracheostomies, and the aspiration is clinically silent in most cases (17).
2. Concern about aspiration around inflated cuffs prompted the introduction of specialized endotracheal tubes equipped with a suction port just above the cuff. The suction port is connected to a source of continuous suction (usually not exceeding -20 cm H_2O) to clear the secretions that accumulate in the subglottic region, as illustrated in Figure 28.2.
3. Clinical studies have shown a significant reduction in the incidence of VAP when subglottic secretions are cleared using these specialized endotracheal tubes (18-19).

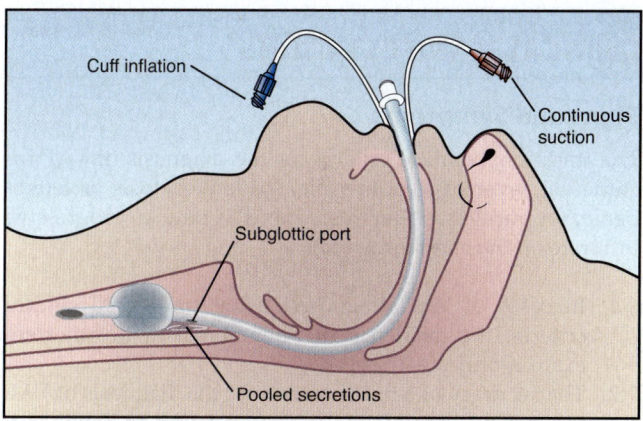

FIGURE 28.2. Endotracheal tube with a suction port placed just above the cuff to clear secretions that accumulate in the subglottic region

Ventilator Bundles

Advocated by the Institute for Healthcare Improvement, "bundles" are a compilation of interventions that when used together will improve outcomes. An example of a ventilator bundle is shown in Table 28.2 (12,20-22).

TABLE 28.2 Ventilator Bundle

- Maintain HOB 30-45°
- Avoid gastric distention
- Encourage early mobilization
- "Sedation vacations"
- Assess readiness to wean
- Use cuffed ETT with inline suctioning
- Avoid acid suppression if possible
- Routine oral care
- Q 2-4 h moistening of oral mucosa
- Brush teeth, gums, and tongue BID
- Hand hygiene
- Subglottic suctioning with expected mechanical ventilation >72 h

HOB = head of bed; ETT = endotracheal tube; Q = every; BID = twice daily.

CLINICAL MANIFESTATIONS

Signs and Symptoms

The traditional clinical criteria for the diagnosis of VAP include: (a) fever or hypothermia, (b) leukocytosis or leukopenia, (c) purulent secretions, and (d) a new or progressive infiltrate on the chest x-ray (23).

1. In cases of VAP diagnosed using traditional clinical criteria, the incidence of pneumonia on postmortem exam is only 30-40% (11).
2. The accuracy of clinical criteria for the diagnosis of VAP verified by lung biopsy is demonstrated in Table 28.3. Table 28.3, as well as the results of two studies that used autopsy evidence of pneumonia to evaluate the premortem diagnosis of VAP based on clinical findings (24-25), demonstrate that *the diagnosis of VAP is not possible using clinical criteria alone.*

TABLE 28.3	Diagnostic Value of Clinical Findings in VAP Verified by Lung Biopsy		
	Sensitivity	Specificity	Diagnostic Odds Ratio[†]
Fever	66%	54%	2.3
Leukocytosis	64%	59%	2.6
Purulent Secretions	77%	39%	2.1
Infiltrate on Chest X-Ray	89%	26%	2.8

[†]The odds of a positive test in a patient with the disease relative to the odds of a positive test in a patient without the disease. A reliable test has an odds ratio of ≥10.

Data from Fernando SM, Tran A, Cheng W, et al. Diagnosis of ventilator-associated pneumonia in critically ill adult patients–a systematic review and meta-analysis. Intensive Care Med 2020;46:1170-9.

Chest Radiography

The diagnostic value of portable chest x-rays in detecting pneumonia is shown in Table 28.3 (26). Pulmonary infiltrates are common in mechanically ventilated patients from a wide variety of causes besides pneumonia, e.g., atelectasis, pulmonary edema, pulmonary aspiration, acute respiratory distress syndrome, lung hemorrhage, and contusion (in trauma). Note that the poor specificity (26%) means that pneumonia accounts for one-quarter to one-third of pulmonary infiltrates seen on chest x-ray.

TABLE 28.4	Diagnostic Performance of Portable Chest X-rays and Ultrasound		
	Sensitivity	Specificity	Accuracy
Alveolar Consolidation			
Portable CXR	38%	89%	49%
Ultrasound	100%	78%	95%
Pleural Effusion			
Portable CXR	65%	81%	69%
Ultrasound	100%	100%	100%

Data from Xirouchaki N, Magkanas E, Vaporidi K, et al. Lung ultrasound in critically ill patients: comparison with bedside chest radiography. Intensive Care Med 2011;37:1488-93.

A Simple Take-Home for the Diagnosis of VAP

The concomitant presence of the three following criteria are (3):

1. Clinical suspicion
2. New or progressive and persistent radiologic infiltrate
3. Positive lower respiratory tract microbiological cultures

MICROBIOLOGICAL EVALUATION

The diagnosis of VAP rests heavily on identifying a responsible pathogen, and the variety of methods used for this purpose are described next.

Blood Cultures

Blood cultures have a limited value in the diagnosis of VAP because they are positive in only 15% of cases (27), however, bacteremia VAP is associated with a higher mortality (28). They can also be helpful in identifying the causative pathogen when respiratory cultures are unrevealing.

Gram Stain

Quality Gram stains are considered a "best practice" by the Agency for Healthcare Research and Quality (AHRQ) (27). They are helpful in guiding empiric antibiotic therapy pending species identification and antibiotic sensitivities. For example, the absence of gram-positive organisms makes it less likely MRSA will be cultured (29).

A quality sputum Gram stain can be defined as:

- The presence of >10 squamous epithelial cells per low-power field (×100) indicates that the specimen is contaminated with mouth secretions and is not an appropriate specimen for culture (30).
- The presence of neutrophils in tracheal aspirates is not evidence of infection because neutrophils can make up

20% of the cells recovered from a routine mouthwash (31). The neutrophils should be present in abundance to indicate infection, i.e., >25 neutrophils per low-power field (×100) can be used as evidence of infection (32).

MRSA Polymerase Chain Reaction

Nasal screening of Methicillin-resistant *Staph aureus* (MRSA) using polymerase chain reaction (PCR) is a molecular test that has a high sensitivity in identifying MRSA colonization in ICU patients (33). Its utility in de-escalating empiric anti-MRSA antibiotics for VAP has demonstrated a poor positive predictive value but an excellent negative predictive value. Its use to de-escalate anti-MRSA should be limited to culture-negative patients with VAP (34-35).

Endotracheal Aspirates

The recommended approach to suspected VAP involves aspiration of respiratory secretions through an endotracheal or tracheostomy tube (1,27). These specimens can be contaminated with mouth secretions that are aspirated into the upper airway. Gram stains can be used to screen the quality of the specimen (see previous section).

Qualitative Cultures

The standard culture method for tracheal aspirates provides a qualitative assessment of the presence or absence of organisms. These cultures have a high sensitivity (usually >90%) but a very low specificity (15-40%) for the diagnosis of VAP (36). Thus, *a negative qualitative culture can help to exclude the diagnosis of VAP, but a positive culture is not reliable for identifying the culprit pathogen.*

Quantitative Cultures

For quantitative cultures of tracheal aspirates (where growth density is reported), the threshold growth for the diagnosis of VAP is 10^5 colony-forming units per mL (CFU/mL). This threshold has a sensitivity and specificity of about 75% for the diagnosis of VAP (36-37). The conclusion of a Cochrane Review of over 5,000 articles comparing qualitative versus quantitative respiratory cultures did not show any significant differences in mortality, antibiotic usage, length of ICU stay (38), or clinical advantage to either approach.

Invasive Specimen Sampling

Lung biopsies or the use of bronchoscopy is considered an "invasive" technique for pulmonary specimen acquisition along with a protected brush specimen (discussion to follow) as opposed to tracheal aspirates which are considered "noninvasive" (1).

Bronchoalveolar Lavage

Despite "standardizations" from organizations such as the American Thoracic Society and the British Thoracic Society there is much variability in how Bronchoalveolar Lavage (BAL) is performed (39). BAL is performed by wedging the bronchoscope in a distal airway and performing a lavage with sterile physiologic saline. Aliquots of 20-60 mL are instilled. A minimum lavage volume of 100 mL with retrieval of at least 30% instilled volume is recommended as an adequate sample for culture (40).

Quantitative Cultures

The threshold for a positive BAL culture is 10^4 CFU/mL (1,27).

The reported sensitivity and specificity of BAL cultures are shown in Table 28.5 (36-37,41). Because BAL cultures have the highest specificity, they are most likely to identify the presence of VAP.

Intracellular Organisms

Inspection of BAL specimens for intracellular organisms can help in guiding initial antibiotic therapy until culture results are available.

When intracellular organisms are present in >3% of the cells in the lavage fluid, the likelihood of pneumonia is over 90% (42).

This inspection requires special processing and staining and will require a specific request for the microbiology lab to perform the inspection.

TABLE 28.5 Culture Methods for the Diagnosis of VAP

	Tracheal Aspirate		Bronchoalveolar Lavage
	Qualitative	Quantitative	
Diagnostic Threshold	Any Growth	$\geq 10^5$ cfu/mL	$\geq 10^4$ cfu/mL
Sensitivity	>90%	~75%	~75%
Specificity	<40%	~75%	~80%

From American Thoracic Society; Infectious Diseases Society of America. Guidelines for the management of adults with hospital-acquired, ventilator-associated, and healthcare-associated pneumonia. Am J Respir Crit Care Med 2005;171:388-416; Cook D, Mandell L. Endotracheal aspiration in the diagnosis of ventilator-associated pneumonia. Chest 2000;117:195S-7S; and Torres A, El-Ebiary M. Bronchoscopic BAL in the diagnosis of ventilator-associated pneumonia. Chest 2000;117:198S-202S.

Invasive

Although generally considered a safe procedure, BAL does have relative contraindications that may vary based on individual patient factors (39). See Table 28.6.

TABLE 28.6 Relative Contraindications to Bronchoalveolar Lavage*

- Severe respiratory distress
- Severe hypoxemia
- Hemodynamic instability
- Coagulopathy
- Recent cardiac event
- Severe uncontrolled hypertension
- Unprotected airway
- Severe pulmonary hypertension
- Active respiratory tract bleeding
- Elevated intracranial pressure

*Contraindications may vary based on individual patient factors, institutional protocols, and clinical context.

From Patel PH, Antoine MH, Sankari A, Ullah S. Bronchoalveolar Lavage. In: StatPearls. Treasure Island (FL): StatPearls Publishing; 2024.

In addition, the bronchoscopy feature of a BAL offers the therapeutic aspect of directed suctioning for clearance of secretions.

BAL Without Bronchoscopy

BAL can also be performed without the aid of bronchoscopy using a sheathed catheter. This catheter (COMBICATH, KOL Bio-Medical) is inserted through a tracheal tube and advanced "blindly" until it wedges in a distal airway. An absorbable polyethylene plug at the tip of the catheter prevents contamination while the catheter is advanced. Once wedged, an inner cannula is advanced for the BAL, which is performed with 20 mL of sterile saline. Only 1 mL of BAL aspirate is required for culture and microscopic analysis.

- Nonbronchoscopic BAL (also called mini-BAL) is a safe procedure that can be performed by respiratory therapists (43).
- Despite the inability to direct the catheter to the region of suspected infection, *the yield from quantitative cultures with mini-BAL is equivalent to the yield with bronchoscopic BAL* (37,44).

Protected Specimen Brush (PSB)

A PSB is an attempt to minimize contamination of the pulmonary specimen. A bronchoscope is inserted into the bronchi of the suspected pneumonia. The PSB is then inserted through the bronchoscope. The brush, internal to a sheath, is then inserted into the distal airways to collect the specimen and subsequently pulled back into the sheath so as to not contaminate the specimen. See Figure 28.3.

Quantitative Cultures

The threshold for a positive PBS culture is 10^3 CFU/mL (1,27).

A summary of the thresholds for quantitative cultures are shown in Table 28.7.

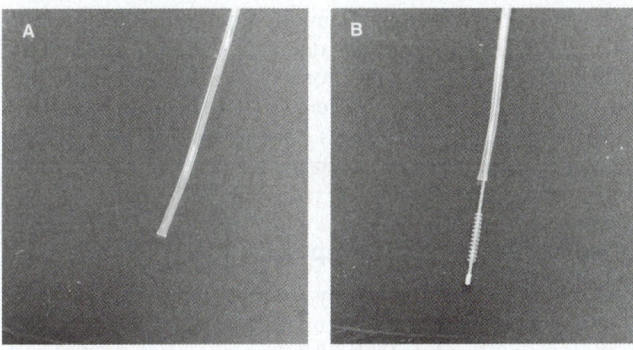

FIGURE 28.3. Protected brush. (A) Brush "protected" within sheath. (B) Brush exposed.

TABLE 28.7	Diagnostic Value of Quantitative Cultures in VAP Verified by Lung Biopsy		
	Tracheal Aspirate	Protected Brush Specimen	Bronchoalveolar Lavage
Threshold (CFU/mL)	10^5	10^3	$\geq 10^4$
Sensitivity	76%	61%	71%
Specificity	68%	77%	80%
Diagnostic Odds Ratio[†]	6.6	5.1	9.6

[†]The odds of a positive test in a patient with the disease relative to the odds of a positive test in a patient without the disease. A reliable test has an odds ratio of 10 or higher.

From Fernando SM, Tran A, Cheng W, et al. Diagnosis of ventilator-associated pneumonia in critically ill adult patients—a systematic review and meta-analysis. Intensive Care Med 2020;46:1170-9.

ANTIMICROBIAL THERAPY

Antimicrobial therapy for pneumonia accounts for half of all antibiotic use in the ICU, and 60% of this antibiotic use is for suspected pneumonias that are not confirmed by bacteriologic studies (45). There is evidence that the mortality rate in VAP is increased by delays in initiating appropriate antibiotic therapy (46), so prompt initiation of empiric antimicrobial therapy is considered essential. A critical point, however, is to obtain cultures prior to the initiation of antibiotics as to not interfere with the accuracy of culture data, which stated above is already not perfect (27,47).

Empiric Antibiotic Therapy

Empiric antimicrobial therapy for VAP can be divided into low-risk and high-risk for antimicrobial resistance. Risk factors are outlined in Table 28.8.

TABLE 28.8 Risk Factors for an Unfavorable Outcome

- Late-onset VAP (>5 days after admission)
- Septic shock
- Prior infection with MRSA or a multidrug-resistant organism
- Hospital antibiogram in which 25% of isolates are resistant organisms
- Antibiotic exposure within 90 days

From Kalil AC, Metersky ML, Klompas M, et al. Management of adults with hospital-acquired and ventilator-associated pneumonia: 2016 clinical practice guidelines by the Infectious Diseases Society of America and the American Thoracic Society. Clin Infect Dis 2016;63:e61-e111.

Empiric antibiotic regimens for suspected VAP are shown in Table 28.9.

De-escalation

When a responsible pathogen is identified the empiric antibiotic regimen can be "de-escalated," meaning either stopping one or more empiric regimen or changing to an antibiotic with a narrower antimicrobial spectrum.

Duration of Antibiotic Therapy

One week of antimicrobial therapy is adequate for most cases of VAP. Individual clinical responses may increase or decrease duration (1).

TABLE 28.9 Empiric Antibiotic Regimens for Suspected VAP

Low-Risk Patients	High-Risk Patients
A. MSSA and gram-negative (including antipseudomonal) coverage with any of the following: 1. Cefepime 2. Levofloxacin 3. Piperacillin/Tazobactam	A. MRSA coverage with: 1. Vancomycin or 2. Linezolid B. Gram-negative and antipseudomonal coverage with a β-lactam agent: 1. Piperacillin/Tazobactam or 2. Cefepime or 3. Meropenem C. Gram-negative and antipseudomonal coverage with a non-β-lactam agent[§]: 1. Levofloxacin or 2. An aminoglycoside

[§]Include regimen C only if there is a high risk of infection with multidrug-resistant organisms.

MSSA = methicillin-sensitive *Staphylococcus aureus*.

From Torres A, El-Ebiary M. Bronchoscopic BAL in the diagnosis of ventilator-associated pneumonia. Chest 2000;117:198S-202S and Kalil AC, Metersky ML, Klompas M, et al. Management of adults with hospital-acquired and ventilator-associated pneumonia: 2016 clinical practice guidelines by the Infectious Diseases Society of America and the American Thoracic Society. Clin Infect Dis 2016;63:e61-e111.

TABLE 28.10 Thresholds for Culture Specimens for the Diagnosis of Pneumonia

- Endotracheal aspirate >10^5 CFU/mL
- Bronchoalveolar Lavage >10^4 CFU/mL
- Protected Brush Specimen >10^3 CFU/mL
- Lung biopsy (tissue) >10^4 CFU/g of tissue

PARAPNEUMONIC EFFUSIONS

Pleural effusions are present in up to 50% of bacterial pneumonias (48). These *parapneumonic effusions* (Table 28.11) are more likely to be detected by ultrasound than by portable chest x-rays (Table 28.4).

TABLE 28.11	Classification of Parapneumonic Effusions		
	Character of Effusion	Pleural Fluid Analysis	Chest Tube
Category 1	<10 mm in thickness	Thoracentesis not necessary	No
Category 2	>10 mm thick but <50% of hemithorax, free-flowing	pH >7.20, Glucose >60 mg/dL, negative Gram stain & culture	No
Category 3	Loculated, or fills >50% of hemithorax	pH <7.20, Glucose <60 mg/dL, positive Gram stain or culture	Yes
Category 4	Purulent	Same as Category 3	Yes

From Light RW. Parapneumonic effusions and empyema. Proc Am Thorac Soc 2006;3:75-80 and Shen KR, Bribiesco A, Crabtree T, et al. The American Association of Thoracic Surgery consensus guidelines for the management of empyema. J Thorac Cardiovasc Surg 2017;153:e129-46.

When culture results are negative or a quantitative culture does not meet the diagnostic threshold (Table 28.10), antibiotics should be discontinued (1,11,27).

Thoracentesis

Thoracentesis is generally advised for all parapneumonic effusions except small, free-flowing effusions in patients who are not severely ill or are responding to antimicrobial therapy. Ultrasound guidance is advised for aspiration of pleural fluid, especially in ventilator-dependent patients.

The following pleural fluid studies are needed to guide decisions regarding drainage of the effusion (49).

1. Gram stain and culture
2. pH (measured with a blood gas analyzer)
3. Glucose concentration (if pH measurement is unavailable)

Other pleural fluid studies (e.g., cell count, protein, lactate dehydrogenase) are not necessary.

Indications for Drainage

The presence of any of the following is an indication for drainage of a parapneumonic effusion (49-50):

1. Effusions that are large (≥ half the hemithorax) or loculated.
2. Purulent pleural aspirate
3. Presence of organisms on Gram stain, or positive culture
4. Pleural fluid pH <7.2
5. Pleural fluid glucose <60 mg/dL (if the pH measurement is not available)

Drainage

Tube thoracostomy is used for pleural fluid drainage (at least initially). Small-bore chest tubes (10-14 French) are advised, because they are less painful, and they are as effective as large-bore tubes in most cases (50).

Intrapleural Fibrinolysis

For loculated pleural effusions or empyema, intrapleural administration of a fibrinolytic agent can facilitate chest tube drainage and reduce the need for surgical drainage (51). The success of intrapleural fibrinolysis has not been consistent, but the following regimen has demonstrated a 78% success rate for complete resolution, with only 6% requiring decortication (51).

Administer *tissue plasminogen activator* (4 mg) in 50 mL normal saline via the chest tube and clamp for 12 h. If not resolved, may repeat one time.

Surgical Drainage

Surgical drainage is indicated when other therapies (i.e., antibiotics, chest tube drainage, intrapleural fibrinolysis) fail after 5-7 days (49-50). Video-assisted thoracoscopic surgery (VATS) is preferred because it is minimally invasive, but thoracotomy with pleural decortication is occasionally required.

References

1. Kalil AC, Metersky ML, Klompas M, et al. Management of adults with hospital-acquired and ventilator-associated pneumonia: 2016 clinical practice guidelines by the Infectious Diseases Society of America and the American Thoracic Society. Clin Infect Dis 2016;63:e61-e111.
2. Edwardson S, Cairns C. Nosocomial infections in the ICU. Anaesthesia & Intensive Care Medicine 2019;20:14-8.
3. Papazian L, Klompas M, Luyt CE. Ventilator-associated pneumonia in adults: a narrative review. Intensive Care Med 2020;46:888-906.
4. Regunath H, Oba Y. Community-acquired Pneumonia. In: StatPearls. Treasure Island (FL): StatPearls Publishing; 2024.
5. Chastre J, Wolff M, Fagon JY, et al. Comparison of 8 vs 15 days of antibiotic therapy for ventilator-associated pneumonia in adults: a randomized trial. JAMA 2003;290:2588-98.
6. Howroyd F, Chacko C, MacDuff A, et al. Ventilator-associated pneumonia: pathobiological heterogeneity and diagnostic challenges. Nat Commun 2024;15:6447.
7. Kohbodi GA, Rajasurya V, Noor A. Ventilator-associated Pneumonia. In: StatPearls. Treasure Island (FL): StatPearls Publishing; 2024.
8. Koulenti D, Tsigou E, Rello J. Nosocomial pneumonia in 27 ICUs in Europe: perspectives from the EU-VAP/CAP study. Eur J Clin Microbiol Infect Dis 2017;36:1999-2006.
9. Bregeon F, Ciais V, Carret V, et al. Is ventilator-associated pneumonia an independent risk factor for death? Anesthesiology 2001;94:554-60.
10. Muscedere J, Dodek P, Keenan S, et al. Comprehensive evidence-based clinical practice guidelines for ventilator-associated pneumonia: prevention. J Crit Care 2008;23:126-37.
11. Wunderink RG. Clinical criteria in the diagnosis of ventilator-associated pneumonia. Chest 2000;117:191S-4S.
12. Gupta A, Gupta A, Singh TK, Saxsena A. Role of oral care to prevent VAP in mechanically ventilated Intensive Care Unit patients. Saudi J Anaesth 2016;10:95-7.
13. Myburgh JA, Seppelt IM, et al; SuDDICU Investigators ANZICSCTG. selective decontamination of the digestive tract on hospital mortality in critically ill patients receiving mechanical ventilation: a randomized clinical trial. JAMA 2022;328:1911-21.
14. Wittekamp BHJ, Oostdijk EAN, Cuthbertson BH, et al. Selective decontamination of the digestive tract (SDD) in critically ill patients: a narrative review. Intensive Care Med 2020;46:343-9.
15. Adair CG, Gorman SP, Feron BM, et al. Implications of endotracheal tube biofilm for ventilator-associated pneumonia. Intensive Care Med 1999;25:1072-6.

16. American Association for Respiratory Care. AARC clinical practice guidelines. Endotracheal suctioning of mechanically ventilated patients with artificial airways 2010. Respir Care 2010;55:758-64.
17. Elpern EH, Scott MG, Petro L, Ries MH. Pulmonary aspiration in mechanically ventilated patients with tracheostomies. Chest 1994;105:563-6.
18. Agency for Healthcare Research and Quality. Subglottic Secretion Drainage Endotracheal Tube Facts. 2017. https://www.ahrq.gov/hai/tools/mvp/modules/technical/subglottic-fact-sheet.html
19. Muscedere J, Rewa O, McKechnie K, et al. Subglottic secretion drainage for the prevention of ventilator-associated pneumonia: a systematic review and meta-analysis. Crit Care Med 2011;39:1985-91.
20. Centers for Disease Control and Prevention. Ventilator-associated Pneumonia Basics. 2024. https://www.cdc.gov/ventilator-associated-pneumonia/about/
21. Klompas M, Li L, Kleinman K, et al. Associations between ventilator bundle components and outcomes. JAMA Intern Med 2016; 176:1277-83.
22. Wip C, Napolitano L. Bundles to prevent ventilator-associated pneumonia: How valuable are they? Curr Opin Infect Dis 2009;22:159-66.
23. Kollef MH. Ventilator-associated complications, including infection-related complications: the way forward. Crit Care Clin 2013;29:33-50.
24. Fagon JY, Chastre J, Hance AJ, et al. Detection of nosocomial lung infection in ventilated patients. Use of a protected specimen brush and quantitative culture techniques in 147 patients. Am Rev Respir Dis 1988;138:110-6.
25. Timsit JF, Misset B, Goldstein FW, et al. Reappraisal of distal diagnostic testing in the diagnosis of ICU-acquired pneumonia. Chest 1995;108:1632-9.
26. Fernando SM, Tran A, Cheng W, et al. Diagnosis of ventilator-associated pneumonia in critically ill adult patients—a systematic review and meta-analysis. Intensive Care Med 2020;46:1170-9.
27. Agency for Healthcare Research and Quality. Best Practices in the Diagnosis and Treatment of Ventilator-Associated Pneumonia. 2019. https://www.ahrq.gov/antibiotic-use/acute-care/diagnosis/vap.html
28. Ferreira-Coimbra J, Ardanuy C, Diaz E, et al. Ventilator-associated pneumonia diagnosis: a prioritization exercise based on multi-criteria decision analysis. Eur J Clin Microbiol Infect Dis 2020;39:281-6.
29. Ranzani OT, Motos A, Chiurazzi C, et al. Diagnostic accuracy of Gram staining when predicting staphylococcal hospital-acquired pneumonia and ventilator-associated pneumonia: a systematic review and meta-analysis. Clin Microbiol Infect 2020;26:1456-63.

30. Centers for Disease Control and Prevention; National Healthcare Safety Network. Ventilator-Associated Event (VAE). 2024. https://www.cdc.gov/nhsn/pdfs/pscmanual/10-vae_final.pdf
31. Rankin JA, Marcy T, Rochester CL, et al. Human airway macrophages. A technique for their retrieval and a descriptive comparison with alveolar macrophages. Am Rev Respir Dis 1992;145:928-33.
32. Wong LK, Barry AL, Horgan SM. Comparison of six different criteria for judging the acceptability of sputum specimens. J Clin Microbiol 1982;16:627-31.
33. Lewis AD, Bridwell MR, Hambuchen MD, et al. Correlation of MRSA polymerase chain reaction (PCR) nasal swab in ventilator-associated pneumonia, lung abscess, and empyema. Diagn Microbiol Infect Dis 2023;105:115836.
34. Buckley MS, Kobic E, Yerondopoulos M, et al. Comparison of methicillin-resistant staphylococcus aureus nasal screening predictive value in the intensive care unit and general ward. Ann Pharmacother 2023;57:1036-43.
35. Dangerfield B, Chung A, Webb B, Seville MT. Predictive value of methicillin-resistant Staphylococcus aureus (MRSA) nasal swab PCR assay for MRSA pneumonia. Antimicrob Agents Chemother 2014;58:859-64.
36. Cook D, Mandell L. Endotracheal aspiration in the diagnosis of ventilator-associated pneumonia. Chest 2000;117:195S-7S.
37. American Thoracic Society; Infectious Diseases Society of America. Guidelines for the management of adults with hospital-acquired, ventilator-associated, and healthcare-associated pneumonia. Am J Respir Crit Care Med 2005;171:388-416.
38. Berton DC, Kalil AC, Teixeira PJ. Quantitative versus qualitative cultures of respiratory secretions for clinical outcomes in patients with ventilator-associated pneumonia. Cochrane Database Syst Rev 2014;2014:CD006482.
39. Patel PH, Antoine MH, Sankari A, Ullah S. Bronchoalveolar Lavage. In: StatPearls. Treasure Island (FL): StatPearls Publishing; 2024.
40. Meyer KC, Raghu G, Baughman RP, et al. An official American Thoracic Society clinical practice guideline: the clinical utility of bronchoalveolar lavage cellular analysis in interstitial lung disease. Am J Respir Crit Care Med 2012;185:1004-14.
41. Torres A, El-Ebiary M. Bronchoscopic BAL in the diagnosis of ventilator-associated pneumonia. Chest 2000;117:198S-202S.
42. Veber B, Souweine B, Gachot B, Chevret S, Bedos JP, Decre D, et al. Comparison of direct examination of three types of bronchoscopy specimens used to diagnose nosocomial pneumonia. Crit Care Med 2000;28:962-8.
43. Kollef MH, Bock KR, Richards RD, Hearns ML. The safety and diagnostic accuracy of minibronchoalveolar lavage in patients with suspected ventilator-associated pneumonia. Ann Intern Med 1995;122:743-8.

44. Campbell GD Jr. Blinded invasive diagnostic procedures in ventilator-associated pneumonia. Chest 2000;117:207S-11S.
45. Bergmans DC, Bonten MJ, Gaillard CA, et al. Indications for antibiotic use in ICU patients: a one-year prospective surveillance. J Antimicrob Chemother 1997;39:527-35.
46. Iregui M, Ward S, Sherman G, et al. Clinical importance of delays in the initiation of appropriate antibiotic treatment for ventilator-associated pneumonia. Chest 2002;122:262-8.
47. Levy MM, Evans LE, Rhodes A. The surviving sepsis campaign bundle: 2018 update. Intensive Care Med 2018;44:925-8.
48. Light RW. Parapneumonic effusions and empyema. Clin Chest Med 1985;6:55-62.
49. Colice GL, Curtis A, Deslauriers J, et al. Medical and surgical treatment of parapneumonic effusions: an evidence-based guideline. Chest 2000;118:1158-71.
50. Ferreiro L, San Jose ME, Valdes L. Management of parapneumonic pleural effusion in adults. Arch Bronconeumol 2015;51:637-46.
51. Townsend A, Raju H, Serpa KA, et al. Tissue plasminogen activator with prolonged dwell time effectively evacuates pleural effusions. BMC Pulm Med 2022;22:464.

Liberation from Mechanical Ventilation

Chapter 29

This chapter describes the process of evaluating the readiness, weaning, and extubation from mechanical ventilation and the difficulties that can occur during the transition to unassisted breathing (1-5).

READINESS EVALUATION

Simply stated, "readiness" is the improvement of the clinical cause of the respiratory failure within clinical parameters to breath spontaneously without mechanical support. The indication for the initiation of mechanical ventilation may or may not be of a primary pulmonary etiology and commonly there are multisystem issues beyond pulmonary function that can affect the ability to liberate from mechanical ventilation such as sepsis, cardiac dysfunction, severe deconditioning from prolonged critical illness, neurologic impairment, anxiety, and so forth. Table 29.1 lists readiness parameters for spontaneous breathing trial.

TABLE 29.1 Readiness Criteria
Resolution/significant improvement of the acute phase of disease
SpO_2 ≥90% with FiO_2 ≤50%
PEEP ≤8 cm H_2O
$PaCO_2$ normal or at baseline
Hemodynamically stable
Awake to easily arousable

FiO_2 = fraction of inspired oxygen; $PaCO_2$ = partial pressure of carbon dioxide; PEEP = positive end-expiratory pressure; SpO_2 = oxygen saturation.

From El-Khatib MF, Bou-Khalil P. Clinical review: liberation from mechanical ventilation. Crit Care 2008;12(4):221.

WEANING

The management of ventilator-dependent patients should include a daily evaluation for signs that ventilatory support may be decreased or even no longer necessary.

When the conditions for readiness are met the patient is removed from the ventilator for a spontaneous breathing trial to assess "predictors of success" (also known as "weaning parameters"). See Table 29.2 (3).

TABLE 29.2	Measurements Used to Predict a Successful Trial of Spontaneous Breathing	
Measurement	Threshold for Success	Likelihood Ratios[ɛ]
Tidal Volume (V_T)	4-6 mL/kg	0.7-3.8
Respiratory Rate (RR)	30-38 bpm	1.0-3.8
RR/V_T Ratio	60-105 bpm/L	0.8-4.7
Maximum Inspiratory Pressure (PI_{max})	−15 to −30 cm H_2O	0-3.2

[ɛ]The likelihood ratio is the likelihood that the measurement will predict success, divided by the likelihood that the measurement will predict failure.

From MacIntyre NR. Evidence-based assessments in the ventilator discontinuation process. Respir Care 2012; 57:1611-8.

Note the wide range of likelihood ratios in Table 29.2, which indicates that each of the weaning parameters can have a poor predictor value in individual patients. As a result, the emerging consensus is that weaning parameters are not necessary, and trials of spontaneous, unassisted breathing can begin when the readiness criteria in Table 29.1 are satisfied.

Spontaneous Breathing Trial

The traditional approach to discontinuing mechanical ventilation emphasizes a gradual reduction in ventilatory support (over hours to days), and this creates unnecessary delays in removing ventilatory support for patients who are capable of unassisted breathing. (This delayed approach is evident in the practice of placing patients back on a ventilator at night to "rest them".) In contrast, spontaneous breathing trials (SBTs) are conducted with minimal to no ventilatory support, so that patients capable of unassisted breathing can be rapidly identified. There are two methods for conducting an SBT.

T-Piece Trial

1. The endotracheal tube is disconnected from the mechanical ventilator and connected to a T-shaped adapter with high-flow O_2 (Figure 29.1).

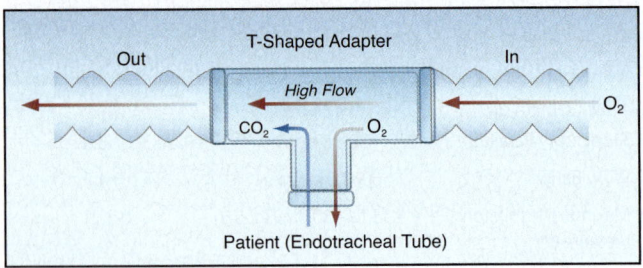

FIGURE 29.1. The design of the breathing circuit for spontaneous breathing trials while totally disconnected from the ventilator (also called T-piece weaning because of the T-shaped adapter in the circuit). See text for further explanation. (From Discontinuing Mechanical Ventilation. In: Marino PL. *Marino's The ICU Book*. 5th ed. Wolters Kluwer; 2025:485-96. Figure 30.3.)

2. The high-flow rate in this circuit achieves three goals: (1) it promotes comfortable breathing in patients with increased ventilatory demands, (2) it prevents the patient from inhaling low O_2 gas from the expiratory limb of the circuit, and (3) it carries exhaled CO_2 away from the patient, and thereby prevents CO_2 rebreathing.
3. The major disadvantage of the T-piece weaning trials is the inability to monitor the patient's tidal volume (V_T) and respiratory rate (RR).

Pressure Support Ventilation Trial

SBTs are often conducted while the patient breathes through the ventilator circuit.

1. Low-level Pressure Support Ventilation (PSV) (5 cm H_2O) is used to counteract the resistance to breathing through the endotracheal tube and ventilator circuit but does not augment the patient's V_T.
2. The advantage of this method is the ability to detect apnea as well as to monitor the patient's V_T and RR, which allows for the early detection of rapid, shallow breathing (indicated by an increase in the RR/V_T ratio), which is a sign of ventilatory failure (6).

Which Method is Preferred?

There is no evidence of superiority for either method of spontaneous breathing in predicting successful extubation, however, PSV trials may shorten the weaning process (7-8).

Success versus Failure

A majority of patients (~80%) who tolerate SBTs for 2 h can be removed from the ventilator (3-4). Failure to tolerate spontaneous breathing is usually signaled by one or more of the following:

1. Signs of respiratory distress, e.g., agitation, rapid breathing, and use of accessory muscles of respiration.
2. Signs of respiratory muscle weakness, e.g., paradoxical inward movement of the abdominal wall during inspiration.
3. Progressive hypoxemia or hypercapnia.
4. Stridor, a sign of airway compromise.

Rapid Breathing

Rapid breathing during SBTs can be the result of anxiety rather than ventilatory failure (9). This is an important distinction because it is possible to manage anxiety without terminating the SBT trial (see section that follows).

Tidal Volumes. Monitoring the V_T can be useful in distinguishing anxiety from ventilatory failure, i.e., anxiety produces *hyperventilation*, which is characterized by an increase in the RR and an unchanged or increased V_T, whereas ventilatory failure is typically associated with rapid, shallow breathing (i.e., the RR is increased but the V_T is decreased) (6). Therefore, *rapid breathing without an associated decrease in V_T can represent anxiety and not ventilatory failure.*

Using Opiates. If anxiety is suspected as the cause of rapid breathing, administration of an anxiolytic agent should be considered, rather than terminating the SBT. Opiates can be useful in this setting because they are particularly effective in curbing the sensation of dyspnea (10). Contrary to the pervasive fear of opiate use in COPD, opiates have been used safely for the relief of dyspnea in patients with advanced COPD (10).

FAILURE OF SPONTANEOUS BREATHING TRIAL

Factors other than intrinsic pulmonary disease can contribute to a failed trial of spontaneous breathing, and the principal ones are described in the section that follows.

Acute Cardiac Dysfunction

Cardiac dysfunction can develop during a trial of spontaneous breathing (11-12) and can contribute to failed weaning trials by promoting pulmonary congestion, known as weaning-induced pulmonary edema (WIPO), and decreasing the strength of diaphragmatic contractions (13).

Potential sources of cardiac dysfunction in this situation include the following:

- Negative intrathoracic pressure, which increases left ventricular afterload (14)
- Hyperinflation and intrinsic PEEP from rapid breathing, which increases right ventricular afterload
- Silent myocardial ischemia (15)

Cardiac Assessment

In addition to cardiac ultrasound and pulmonary artery catheterization, the following methods can be used to assess cardiac dysfunction in patients who fail spontaneous breathing trials.

1. *Venous O_2 Saturation Saturation (SvO_2)*: Monitoring the mixed SvO_2 has been used to detect changes in cardiac output during trials of spontaneous breathing (11). The central venous O_2 saturation ($ScvO_2$) is a suitable alternative to SvO_2 and is more easily monitored.
2. *β-type natriuretic peptide (BNP)*: Plasma levels of BNP are significantly increased when cardiac dysfunction develops during SBTs (16), and further, that increased BNP levels are associated with weaning failure (11). Therefore, monitoring BNP levels can be useful in patients who are failing SBTs.

Management

Once the determination of the cardiac cause of weaning failure is determined, appropriate therapy can be initiated. Suggested treatment options are shown in Figure 29.2.

Respiratory Muscle Weakness

Respiratory muscle weakness is a common concern in patients who fail repeated attempts to wean from mechanical ventilation, but the prevalence of muscle weakness as a cause of failed wean attempts is unclear.

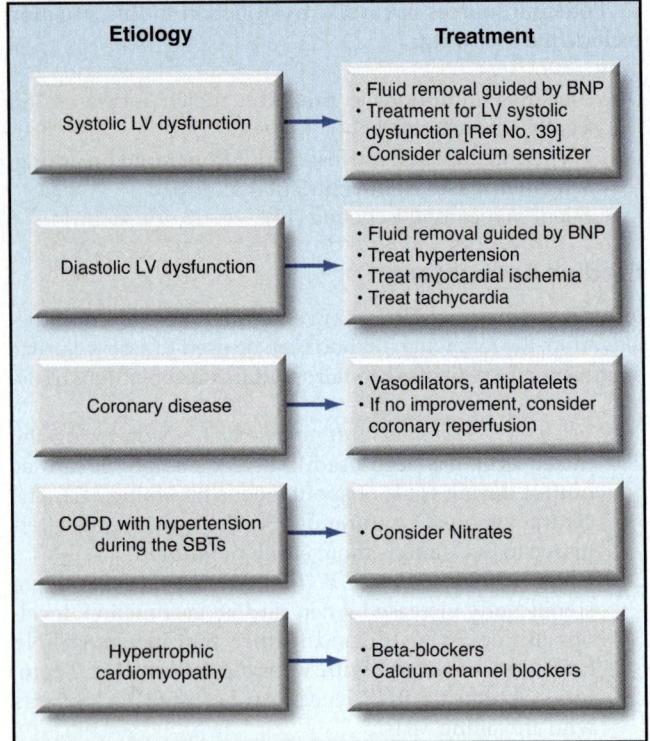

FIGURE 29.2. Suggested treatment options for weaning failure of cardiovascular origin. (From Routsi C, Stanopoulos I, Kokkoris S, et al. Weaning failure of cardiovascular origin: how to suspect, detect and treat—a review of the literature. Ann Intensive Care 2019;9:6.)

Predisposing Conditions

Potential sources of respiratory muscle weakness include controlled mechanical ventilation (especially during neuromuscular paralysis), electrolyte depletion (magnesium and phosphorous), prolonged steroid therapy, and *critical illness neuromyopathy*. This latter condition is an inflammatory-mediated polyneuropathy and/or myopathy that typically appears in patients with septic shock and multiorgan failure and is recognized when patients fail to wean from mechanical ventilation (17).

Monitoring

The standard measure of respiratory muscle strength in the ICU is the *maximum inspiratory pressure* (PI_{max}), which is the negative pressure generated by a maximum inspiratory effort against a closed airway (18-19).

The normal values of PI_{max} can vary widely, but mean values of –120 cm H_2O and –84 cm H_2O have been reported for adult men and women, respectively (18).

Spontaneous breathing is threatened, and acute CO_2 retention is a risk, when the PI_{max} drops below –30 cm H_2O (Table 29.2).

EXTUBATION

Once the patient has demonstrated "readiness" for liberation from mechanical ventilation, the next step is to remove the endotracheal tube. The patient should be "ready" for removal from mechanical ventilation *and* an endotracheal tube.

Airway Protection

Prior to extubation, the strength of the gag and cough reflexes should be checked to determine the patient's ability to protect the airways from aspirated secretions and food particles.

Postextubation Laryngeal Edema

As many as 10% of extubations are followed by signs of respiratory insufficiency that mandates reintubation (20). Most reintubations are the result of traumatic laryngeal edema from the endotracheal tube, which has a reported incidence of 1.5-26.3% (20). Contributing factors include difficult or prolonged intubation, endotracheal tube size, and self-extubations.

Cuff-Leak Test

The endotracheal tube cuff is deflated, and a leak of exhaled V_T is detected. A small leak or lack of a leak may demonstrate increased airway risk. However, there are multiple confounding factors such as endotracheal tube size to trachea size and no standards for "amount of leak" to decide with proceeding with extubation. Although the presence of a leak is reassuring, absence does not preclude successful extubation (21). The American Thoracic Society (ATS) and the American College of Chest Physicians (ACCP) Clinical Practice Guideline recommends performing a cuff-leak test in patients deemed high risk of postintubation stridor and if failed cuff-leak suggest administering systemic steroids at least 4 h prior to extubation (22).

Pre-Extubation Administration of Systemic Steroids

Multiple studies have shown that pretreatment with systemic steroids, starting 12-24 h prior to extubation, can reduce the incidence of clinically significant laryngeal edema after extubation (22-23). The effective steroid regimens are as follows:

- *Methylprednisolone*: 20 mg IV every 4 h, starting 12 h before extubation (total of 4 doses) (24)
- *Dexamethasone*: 5 mg IV every 6 h, starting 24 h prior to extubation (total of 4 doses) (25)

Postextubation Stridor

Postextubation stridor occurs in <10% of extubations (26) when the airway narrowing exceeds 50% (20). The sound is much more pronounced during inspiration (because the negative intrathoracic pressure during inspiration is transmitted to the larynx and causes slight narrowing of the airway). When stridor develops, it's apparent within 30 min of extubation in a majority (80%) of cases (27).

Management

If postextubation stridor is accompanied by signs of respiratory insufficiency, immediate reintubation is required. Otherwise, the following measures can be considered:

1. *Aerosolized epinephrine*: Inhalation of an epinephrine aerosol (2.5 mL of 1% epinephrine) is used to promote vasoconstriction and thereby reduce laryngeal edema (20). However, this is an unproven practice in adults.
2. *Steroids*: Postextubation corticosteroids are recommended for laryngeal edema (20), even though this has not been studied. The preventive steroid regimens mentioned earlier (e.g., dexamethasone, 5 mg IV every 6 h for 24 h) have been suggested for this purpose (20).

Noninvasive Ventilation and High-Flow Nasal Oxygen

Attitudes towards the use of noninvasive ventilation (both continuous positive airway pressure [CPAP] and bilevel positive airway pressure [BiPAP]) and high-flow nasal oxygen applied postextubation are varied (28). Multiple studies have suggested that they may reduce postextubation respiratory failure (29-31).

References

1. El-Khatib MF, Bou-Khalil P. Clinical review: liberation from mechanical ventilation. Crit Care 2008;12(4):221.
2. Ferrera MC, Hayes MM. How I teach: liberation from mechanical ventilation. ATS Sch 2023;4:372-84.
3. Macintyre NR. Evidence-based assessments in the ventilator discontinuation process. Respir Care 2012;57:1611-8.
4. MacIntyre NR, Cook DJ, Ely EW Jr, et al. Evidence-based guidelines for weaning and discontinuing ventilatory support: a collective task force facilitated by the American College of Chest Physicians; the American Association for Respiratory Care; and the American College of Critical Care Medicine. Chest 2001;120:375S-95S.
5. Nitta K, Okamoto K, Imamura H, et al. A comprehensive protocol for ventilator weaning and extubation: a prospective observational study. J Intensive Care 2019;7:50.

6. Krieger BP, Isber J, Breitenbucher A, et al. Serial measurements of the rapid-shallow-breathing index as a predictor of weaning outcome in elderly medical patients. Chest 1997;112:1029-34.
7. Na SJ, Ko RE, Nam J, et al. Comparison between pressure support ventilation and T-piece in spontaneous breathing trials. Respir Res 2022;23:22.
8. Thille AW, Gacouin A, Coudroy R, et al. Spontaneous-breathing trials with pressure-support ventilation or a T-Piece. N Engl J Med 2022;387:1843-54.
9. Bouley GH, Froman R, Shah H. The experience of dyspnea during weaning. Heart Lung 1992;21:471-6.
10. Raghavan N, Webb K, Amornputtisathaporn N, O'Donnell DE. Recent advances in pharmacotherapy for dyspnea in COPD. Curr Opin Pharmacol 2011;11:204-10.
11. Routsi C, Stanopoulos I, Kokkoris S, et al. Weaning failure of cardiovascular origin: how to suspect, detect and treat—a review of the literature. Ann Intensive Care 2019;9:6.
12. Vignon P. Cardiopulmonary interactions during ventilator weaning. Front Physiol 2023;14:1275100.
13. Nishimura Y, Maeda H, Tanaka K, et al. Respiratory muscle strength and hemodynamics in chronic heart failure. Chest 1994;105:355-9.
14. Teboul JL. Weaning-induced cardiac dysfunction: Where are we today? Intensive Care Med 2014;40:1069-79.
15. Srivastava S, Chatila W, Amoateng-Adjepong Y, et al. Myocardial ischemia and weaning failure in patients with coronary artery disease: an update. Crit Care Med 1999;27:2109-12.
16. Grasso S, Leone A, De Michele M, et al. Use of N-terminal pro-brain natriuretic peptide to detect acute cardiac dysfunction during weaning failure in difficult-to-wean patients with chronic obstructive pulmonary disease. Crit Care Med 2007;35:96-105.
17. Shepherd S, Batra A, Lerner DP. Review of critical illness myopathy and neuropathy. Neurohospitalist 2017;7:41-8.
18. Bruschi C, Cerveri I, Zoia MC, et al. Reference values of maximal respiratory mouth pressures: a population-based study. Am Rev Respir Dis 1992;146:790-3.
19. Mier-Jedrzejowicz A, Brophy C, Moxham J, Green M. Assessment of diaphragm weakness. Am Rev Respir Dis 1988;137:877-83.
20. Pluijms WA, van Mook WN, Wittekamp BH, Bergmans DC. Postextubation laryngeal edema and stridor resulting in respiratory failure in critically ill adult patients: updated review. Crit Care 2015;19:295.
21. Fisher MM, Raper RF. The 'cuff-leak' test for extubation. Anaesthesia 1992;47:10-2.
22. Girard TD, Alhazzani W, Kress JP, et al. An Official American Thoracic Society/American College of Chest Physicians Clinical Practice Guideline: liberation from mechanical ventilation in critically ill adults. Rehabilitation protocols, ventilator liberation protocols, and cuff leak tests. Am J Respir Crit Care Med 2017;195:120-33.

23. Feng IJ, Lin JW, Lai CC, et al. Comparative efficacies of various corticosteroids for preventing postextubation stridor and reintubation: a systematic review and network meta-analysis. Front Med (Lausanne) 2023;10:1135570.
24. Francois B, Bellissant E, Gissot V, et al. 12-h pretreatment with methylprednisolone versus placebo for prevention of postextubation laryngeal oedema: a randomised double-blind trial. Lancet 2007;369:1083-9.
25. Lee CH, Peng MJ, Wu CL. Dexamethasone to prevent postextubation airway obstruction in adults: a prospective, randomized, double-blind, placebo-controlled study. Crit Care 2007;11:R72.
26. Saeed F, Lasrado S. Extubation. [Updated 2023 Feb 9]. In: StatPearls [Internet]. Treasure Island (FL): StatPearls Publishing; 2025 Jan-. Available from: https://www.ncbi.nlm.nih.gov/books/NBK539804/
27. Khamiees M, Raju P, DeGirolamo A, et al. Predictors of extubation outcome in patients who have successfully completed a spontaneous breathing trial. Chest 2001;120:1262-70.
28. Nuzzo EA, Kahn JM, Girard TD. Provider perspectives on preventive postextubation noninvasive ventilation for high-risk intensive care unit patients. Ann Am Thorac Soc 2020;17:246-9.
29. Basoalto R, Damiani LF, Jalil Y, et al. Physiological effects of highflow nasal cannula oxygen therapy after extubation: a randomized crossover study. Ann Intensive Care 2023;13:104.
30. Boscolo A, Pettenuzzo T, Sella N, et al. Noninvasive respiratory support after extubation: a systematic review and network meta-analysis. Eur Respir Rev 2023;32.
31. Thille AW, Muller G, Gacouin A, et al. Effect of Postextubation highflow nasal oxygen with noninvasive ventilation vs high-flow nasal oxygen alone on reintubation among patients at high risk of extubation failure: a randomized clinical trial. JAMA 2019;322:1465-75.

# Extracorporeal Membrane Oxygenation

Chapter 30

There are currently >600 centers worldwide providing extracorporeal life support (ECLS) in the form of venovenous (VV) and venoarterial (VA) extracorporeal membrane oxygenation (ECMO) (1). The use of VV ECMO for respiratory failure has increased substantially over the past decade, following increased use during the 2009 influenza A (H1N1) pandemic (2). A comprehensive review of ECMO management is far beyond the scope of this text, as there are many excellent references available, including resources provided by the Extracorporeal Life Support Organization (https://www.elso.org) (3). The focus of this chapter is to introduce concepts regarding indications, physiology, and general management for patients requiring VV or VA ECMO.

VENOVENOUS ECMO

Indications

Current survival rates to discharge for patients requiring VV ECMO approach 60%, depending on the indication (3-4). VV ECMO is indicated for patients with a high predicated mortality due to severe, acute, reversible respiratory failure that is refractory to conventional medical management (5-8). A list of indications and contraindications for VV ECMO is provided in Table 30.1.

Several clinical calculators are available to predict survival following VV ECMO (e.g., the RESP, PRESET, ECMOnet scores) (9-11).

Physiology

VV ECMO is designed to provide respiratory support and "lung rest" by circumventing the lungs in cases of severe acute respiratory failure (see Chapter 25: Acute Respiratory

TABLE 30.1 Indications for VV ECMO

Indications	Relative Contraindications

• Hypoxemic respiratory failure with:
  • PaO_2 <100 mm Hg with FiO_2 ≥80%, and P_{plat} ≥30 cm H_2O or P_1 ≥30 cm H_2O (APRV)
• Hypercarbic respiratory failure
• $PaCO_2$ >60 with pH <7.25, or inability to adequately ventilate with P_{plat} ≤30 or P_1 ≥30 (APRV)
• On ventilator ≤7 days
• <65 years of age
• Reversable form of ARDS
• Specific conditions:
  • Acute eosinophilic pneumonia
  • Diffuse alveolar hemorrhage
  • Severe asthma
  • Thoracic trauma (e.g., severe pulmonary contusion)
  • Severe inhalational injury
  • Large bronchopleural fistula
  • Peri-lung transplant
	• Preadmission home O_2 use for severe lung disease
	• Terminal disease with low 1 year survival rates
	• Patient unwilling to accept blood products
	• Underlying cirrhosis (child class C or MELD ≥30)
	• Abdominal compartment syndrome (if treated adequately, may be considered)
	• Uncontrolled hemorrhage
	• Severe traumatic brain injury (case by case discussion)
	• Contraindication to anticoagulation
	• Mechanical ventilation for >7 days with P_{plat} >30 cm H_2O and FiO_2 >90%

APRV = Airway Pressure Release Ventilation; ARDS = Acute Respiratory Distress Syndrome; ECMO = extracorporeal membrane oxygenation; MELD = Model for End-Stage Liver Disease; VV = venovenous.

From References 3, 8.

Distress Syndrome) and providing enhanced oxygenation and removal of CO_2 (5-8). VV ECMO drains blood from the venous system (usually the inferior vena cava) and shunts blood to an oxygenator (Figure 30.1).

A membrane oxygenator facilitates the delivery of O_2 and the removal of CO_2, returning oxygenated blood back to the venous system. Various configurations can be used for venous drainage (outflow) and blood return (inflow), with three common configurations shown in Figure 30.2.

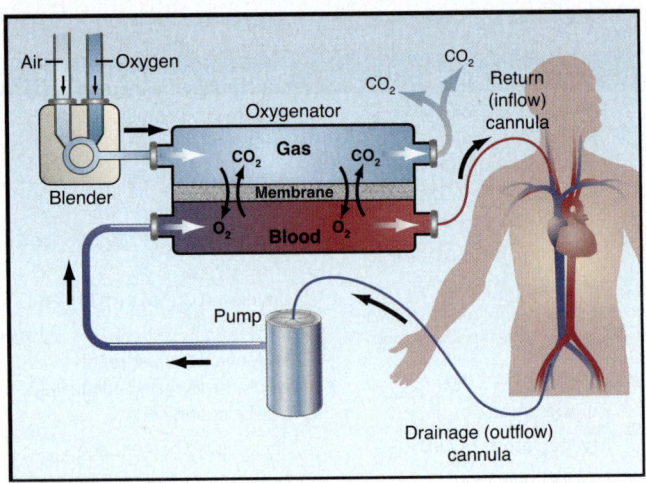

FIGURE 30.1. VV ECMO. See text for explanation.

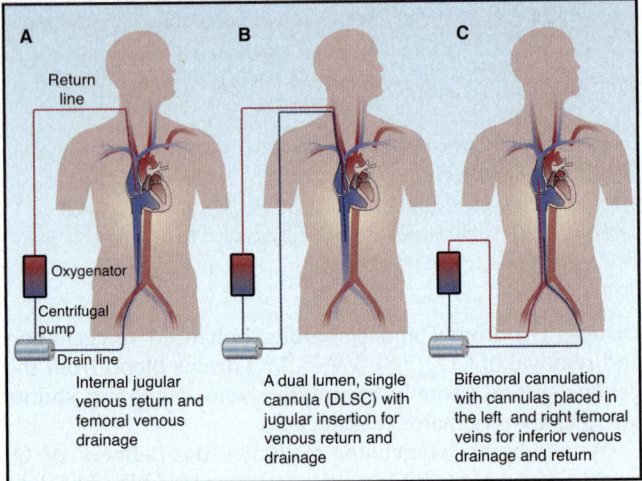

FIGURE 30.2. Three of the most common venous configurations for drainage of deoxygenated blood and return of oxygenated blood from the VV ECMO circuit.

Oxygenation

VV ECMO blood flow rates and hemoglobin can be adjusted to achieve systemic O_2 delivery (8). Oxygenation in VV ECMO depends on the arterial oxygen content (CaO_2) (see Chapter 15: Approaches to Clinical Shock), the percentage of hemoglobin saturated in arterial blood with oxygen (SaO_2), blood flow through the ECMO circuit, the size of the cannulas (i.e., "rated flow"), and FiO_2 provided by mechanical ventilation (5-8). An initial blood flow rate when a patient is initiated on VV ECMO is usually 2 L/min, with a gradual titration upwards to a goal of 4-5 L/min, targeting a flow of 50-60 mL/kg/min. Blood flow rates and hemoglobin can be adjusted to achieve systemic oxygen delivery rates of at least 300 mL/m^2/min (8). When a patient is on VV ECMO, *SaO_2 ranges of 60-90% are acceptable* because only a portion of the venous return from the patient is captured by the ECMO circuit. The return of oxygenated blood from the oxygenator, when mixed with the patient's native blood flow, results in an SaO_2 that is always <100% in patients with severe respiratory failure (8).

CO_2 Removal

The "sweep gas" flow rate through the oxygenator controls the amount of CO_2 removal. Sweep gas rates of 2-9 L/min are typical, although higher rates are occasionally required for the most severe cases of acute lung injury (7). An initial sweep gas flow rate of 2 L/min is used upon initiation of VV ECMO, with adjustments as needed to lower the partial pressure of CO_2 in arterial blood ($PaCO_2$) and normalize the pH, with an eventual $PaCO_2$ goal of 35-45 mm Hg (7). In cases of right heart dysfunction, a lower $PaCO_2$ goal (35-40 mm Hg) is used to avoid increases in right ventricular afterload caused by increased pulmonary vascular resistance (exacerbated by hypercarbia). Rapid lowering of $PaCO_2$ can cause neurological injury from cerebral vasoconstriction; hence, the rate of $PaCO_2$ decrease should not exceed 20 mm Hg/h (7).

Hemodynamics

The hypoxemia and hypercarbia that precede cannulation for VV ECMO often cause hemodynamic derangements (7). VV ECMO does not provide *direct* support to the right or left ventricle, but when acidemia, hypercarbia, and hypoxemia are corrected, VV ECMO may *indirectly* lead to hemodynamic improvements (7). Prior to and following cannulation, inotropic and vasopressor support is often required. During cannulation, arrhythmias are frequent (due to guidewire placement and catheter manipulation), occasionally requiring intervention (see Chapter 20: Dysrhythmias). When VV ECMO is initiated, significant vasopressor support may be required to mitigate vasoplegia resulting from a systemic inflammatory response caused by exposure to the ECMO circuit (7). Unrecognized hemorrhage due to cannulation complications should be rapidly ruled out if hypotension persists.

General Management Considerations

General management considerations are listed in Table 30.2.

Troubleshooting

Although there are many potential complications related to the use of VV ECMO (3,8), two of the more common complications are discussed here.

Chatter and Suck-down

"Chatter," also known as "chugging," is caused by venous drainage insufficiency that occurs when there is partial or complete cannula occlusion (12). VV ECMO drainage insufficiency may occur in cases of hypovolemia or catheter malposition. Judicious titration of IV fluids may help correct chatter, but excessive fluid administration should be avoided. Suck-down can occur when ECMO flows drop precipitously (i.e., <1-2 L/min from baseline). Suck-down can result in abrupt cessation of ECMO flow, air embolization, and hemolysis (8). The treatment

TABLE 30.2 General Management Considerations for Patients Supported with VV ECMO

Initial ventilator settings
- Pressure control mode with an inspiratory pressure of 20 cm H_2O
- PEEP 10 cm H_2O
- FiO_2 40%
- Inspiratory time ~1.5 seconds
- Consider an inspiratory pressure of 25 cm H_2O with PEEP of 15 cm H_2O if proning

Hemoglobin (Hgb) goal
- Once stabilized on ECMO, Hgb = 7 mg/dL
- If PaO_2 <60 mm Hg, consider increasing Hgb goal to 9 or 10 mg/dL

Platelet goal
- 40,000/μL (assuming no bleeding)

aPTT goal
- 45-55 s when on heparin

Hemolysis monitoring
- Daily LDH and plasma hemoglobin

Daily labs
- Lactate and liver function enzymes only if indicated (i.e., liver dysfunction or injury; septic or hemorrhagic shock)
- Complete blood count, basic metabolic panel with calcium, magnesium, phosphorous
- Arterial blood gas (every 12 h)
- Coagulation studies if on heparin (every 12 h)

Prone positioning
- 1st prone session: 8 h to ensure no significant hemodynamic issues or skin breakdown
- Assuming no issues, all subsequent proning sessions should be for 16 h.
- A chest radiograph is indicated only when supine (unless there is an acute issue)
- Patients should be supinated during the morning hours to allow for patient care / exams
- Proning continues until lack of evidence for improvement

TABLE 30.2 (continued)

Right heart dysfunction
- Epinephrine at 0.04 µg/kg/min and inhaled epoprostenol pending a formal echocardiograph
- Once right heart dysfunction is resolved or ruled out, both agents are weaned off

Fluid management
- Diuresis is generally indicated whenever possible using furosemide, an ECMO hemoconcentrator or continuous renal replacement therapy
- A net negative balance of 1-2 L/day is targeted, as tolerated

ECMO = extracorporeal membrane oxygenation; LDH = lactate dehydrogenase; VV = venovenous.

for suck-down is to decrease the ECMO pump speed while adjusting the ventilator as necessary to provide oxygenation and ventilation. Fluids and repositioning are often required before increasing the pump speed back to baseline. Bedside ultrasound can be very useful for assessing catheter position as well as dynamic indices that can be used to guide the titration of fluids (see Chapter 7: Bedside Echocardiography) (13).

Refractory Hypoxemia

Hypoxemia may occur during VV ECMO (14). Table 30.3 lists steps to consider for the management of refractory hypoxemia during VV ECMO.

Weaning

There are many approaches to weaning from VV ECMO. One approach is described in Table 30.4.

VENOARTERIAL ECMO

Indications

VA ECMO is a form of ECLS that provides complete biventricular circulatory support as well as simultaneous

TABLE 30.3 Management of Refractory Hypoxemia During VV ECMO

Steps	Interventions
1	Increase blood O_2 content (CaO_2). • Increase ECMO flow (L/min, up to the maximum rated flow per cannula size). • Increase blood oxygen-carrying capacity (i.e., transfuse RBCs for a higher Hgb goal).
2	Reduce recirculation. • Adjust cannulas, if necessary. • Note: This step can be considered simultaneously during Step 1.
3	Reduce O_2 consumption (VO_2). • Increase sedation. • Consider neuromuscular blockade. • Therapeutic hypothermia (~36°C)
4	Manipulate cardiac output/improve ventilation-perfusion matching. • Initiate a trial of prone positioning, if not already attempted. • Titrate β-blockers (metoprolol or propranolol).
5	Consider VA ECMO or an extra drainage cannula. • Place an additional drainage cannula to capture more cardiac output to send to the oxygenator. • Consider VA ECMO only if the cause of refractory hypoxemia is related to severe myocardial dysfunction.

ECMO = extracorporeal membrane oxygenation; Hgb = hemoglobin; RBC = red blood cell; VA = venoarterial; VV = venovenous.

From References 8, 14.

gas exchange (15). The principal indication for VA ECMO is cardiogenic shock that has failed to respond to standard medical therapy (see Chapter 17: Cardiogenic Shock) (3,15-18). VA ECMO is also indicated for other causes of acute cardiac failure (i.e., poisonings) that require temporary mechanical support for acute cardiac failure (3,15-19). Indications for VA ECMO are listed in Table 30.5.

TABLE 30.4	**Approach to Weaning from VV ECMO**
Step	**Objective / Intervention(s)**
1	**Resolution of the underlying cause** **Return of adequate lung function** • Gradually adjust the ventilator to lung-protective settings (i.e., tidal volume <6-8 mL/predicted body weight, FiO_2 <40%, PPlt <30 cm H_2O, PEEP <10 cm H_2O).
2	**Ensure ventilation will be adequate off VV ECMO** • Decrease the sweep gas flow gradually to 0.5 or 1.0 L/min. • Confirm that an SpO_2 ≥92% or PaO_2 ≥70 mm Hg can be achieved without additional ventilator support. • Monitor ABGs and the chest radiograph.
3	**Recirculation trial** • Turn the sweep gas flow to 0 L/min. • Periodically monitor $ETCO_2$, SpO_2, and ABGs. • Confirm a stable PaO_2 >70 mm Hg and acceptable pH without excessive work of breathing or increased ventilator settings. • Recirculation trials vary per institution; a conservative approach is to maintain a recirculation trial for at least 24 h before decannulation.
4	**Decannulation** • Have blood available for transfusion (at least 2 U of RBCs, typed and crossed). • Hold heparin for at least 1-2 h (institution-specific). • If a jugular venous cannula is present, place in the Trendelenburg position during decannulation (to prevent air emboli). • Prepare to hold pressure after placement of sutures (institution-specific; many centers recommend at least 20 min of continuous pressure to the cannulation site). • Check for deep venous thromboses 24 h after decannulation.

ABG = arterial blood gas; ECMO = extracorporeal membrane oxygenation; Hgb = hemoglobin; PPlt = plateau pressure; VV = venovenous.

TABLE 30.5   Indications and Contraindications for VA ECMO

Indications	Contraindications (Absolute)
• Cardiogenic shock • Primary graft failure post heart transplant • COVID-19 infection • Massive pulmonary embolism • Cardiotoxic drug intoxication • Refractory ventricular arrhythmias • Myocarditis • Peripartum cardiomyopathy • Sepsis-induced cardiomyopathy • Postcardiotomy shock • Sudden cardiac arrest • Acute decompensated pulmonary vascular disease • ECPR	• Severe aortic insufficiency • Aortic dissection • Irreversible noncardiac origin organ failure (i.e., end-stage malignancy, anoxic brain injury) • Advanced age • Lack of a transition to well-defined end point • Severe coagulopathy* • Contraindication to anticoagulation* • Severe peripheral vascular disease* • Immunocompromised status* • Mechanical ventilation ≥7 days* • Comorbid conditions that decrease the probability of recovery*

*Relative contraindication.

ECMO = extracorporeal membrane oxygenation; ECPR = extracorporeal cardiopulmonary resuscitation; VA = venoarterial.

From References 3, 15-19.

The SAVE Score (https://www.elso.org/savescore/index.html) calculator can be used to predict survival for patients receiving VA ECMO for refractory cardiogenic shock (20).

Physiology

VA ECMO is a form of ECLS that uses the same equipment as VV ECMO (i.e., centrifugal flow pump, heat exchanger, membrane oxygenator) but with a venous drainage cannula and *arterial inflow* cannula. Various configurations are possible for cannulation (i.e., central, axillary), with the most common peripheral configuration (femorofemoral) shown in Figure 30.3.

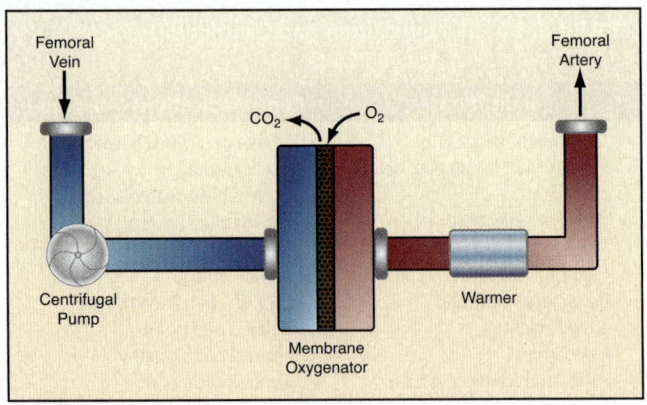

FIGURE 30.3. Schematic for a VA ECMO circuit. (From Cardiogenic Shock. In: Marino PL. *Marino's The ICU Book*. 5th ed. Wolters Kluwer; 2025:257-70. Figure 16.5.)

Initial Setting

Pump speeds are incrementally titrated upward to achieve flows of 3-4 L/min, while monitoring for signs of end-organ perfusion. Sweep gas flow is adjusted to maintain oxygenation (1-10 L/min) and a normal pH, as described for VV ECMO; however, unlike VV ECMO, *the sweep gas flow is never decreased <0.5 L/min as this can cause regional alkalemia because VA ECMO bypasses the lungs.*

Consequences of Retrograde Flow

The femorofemoral configuration involves removal of blood from the venous system and return of oxygenated blood in a *retrograde* manner into the aorta (15,21). While removal of blood from the venous system can often decompress the right heart (improving right-sided hemodynamics), retrograde arterial return can cause significant increases in left ventricular afterload and left ventricular distention (16). Strategies to decompress or "vent" the left ventricle include mechanical unloading of the left ventricle using percutaneous transaortic assistant devices (i.e., a microaxial flow pump [Impella;

Abiomed, Danvers, MA]), intra-aortic balloon pumps, or atrial septostomy with or without an atrial drainage cannula (16-22).

General Management Considerations

Critical care management considerations for VA ECMO are summarized in Table 30.6.

Troubleshooting

VA ECMO is highly nuanced and requires management by a specialized team using institution-specific guidelines to ensure safety and a consistent approach. This section describes a few common complications that require prompt recognition by the intensive care unit (ICU) team.

Differential Hypoxemia

Differential hypoxemia occurs in patients with femoral arterial return (i.e., retrograde perfusion) when left ventricular performance improves (as may occur with the addition of a ventricular assist device for unloading), with the outflow overcoming the retrograde flow from the ECMO circuit. Blood saturated with O_2 from the ECMO circuit perfuses the lower body while poorly oxygenated blood ejected from the left ventricle can cause cerebral and cardiac ischemia. This hemodynamic phenomenon is known as "dual circulation," "north-south syndrome," or "harlequin syndrome," and may occur in >8% of patients supported with VA ECMO (15,24). This condition is most common when pulmonary function is impaired, causing a caudad shift of the "mixing cloud" of oxygenated and deoxygenated blood (Figure 30.4).

Detection. Differential hypoxemia is detected by monitoring oxygenation (PaO_2 and SpO_2) in the right upper extremity because this reflects blood flow to the innominate artery and carotid arch; a gradient >15% between the right and left radial arteries is suggestive of the syndrome (15).

TABLE 30.6	General Critical Care Monitoring and Management Considerations for Patients on VA ECMO
Cardiovascular Monitoring	• The right radial artery should be used for blood gas and arterial blood pressure monitoring (allows earlier detection of upper-body hypoxemia). • PA catheters (Chapter 9) and echocardiography (Chapter 7) are used extensively. • Doppler vascular monitoring and NIRS are used to detect lower extremity ischemia. • Lactate and SvO_2 are monitored to assure adequate O_2 delivery.
Cardiovascular Management	• Lack of pulsatility on the arterial waveform may be caused by inadequate preload, poor myocardial function, or excessive VA ECMO support. • See Chapters 11 and 17 for management strategies.
Respiratory Management	• A tidal volume of 6-8 mL/kg/predicted body weight is used. • For patients with concomitant pulmonary disease, management is as described for VV ECMO (Tables 30.2 and 30.3). • For patients without pulmonary disease, mechanical ventilation may not be required.
Neurological Monitoring	• Sedation and analgesia targeting a RASS of 0 is recommended to accurately assess neurologic status (Chapter 5). • Cerebral NIRS, optic nerve sheath diameter (US), EEG, and head CT should be used in patients with a poor neurological exam or declining neurological function (to detect intracerebral hemorrhage or cerebral hypoxemia).

TABLE 30.6	**(continued)**
Hematological Management	• A protocolized (institution-specific) anticoagulation strategy should be used, typically targeting an aPTT at least twice the control (a higher goal than in VV ECMO). • Common coagulation goals if using heparin are aPTT 60-90 s, anti-Xa 0.3-0.7 IU/mL. • General goals in the nonbleeding patient: Hgb ≥7.0 mg/dL, platelets ≥50,000 × 10^9/L, fibrinogen ≥1 g/L, INR <3 • Alternative anticoagulants may be used (i.e. bivalirudin)
Renal and Fluid Management	• A daily net negative or net even fluid balance is desirable. • AKI is common in VA ECMO and CRRT may be required (see Chapter 33)

AKI = acute kidney injury; aPTT = activated partial thromboplastin time; CRRT = continuous renal replacement therapy; CT = computed tomography; ECMO = extracorporeal membrane oxygenation; EEG = electroencephalography; NIRS = near infrared spectroscopy; RASS = Richmond Agitation-Sedation Scale; US = ultrasound; VA = venoarterial; VV = venovenous.

From References 16-23.

Management. Differential hypoxemia is managed by increasing the circuit flow, optimizing mechanical ventilation (i.e., adding PEEP, increasing FiO$_2$), adding a second inflow cannula (to inject oxygenated blood directly into the right atrium), or switching to central or upper extremity cannulation (15-17,24).

Lower Extremity Ischemia

Ipsilateral lower extremity ischemia is a known complication of VA ECMO and may occur in 13-35% of patients (15-17,25). Signs include pallor, coolness, and gangrene in the affected extremity. Most centers place a distal extremity perfusion catheter after cannulation to prevent this complication. Monitoring with Doppler ultrasound and NIRS can

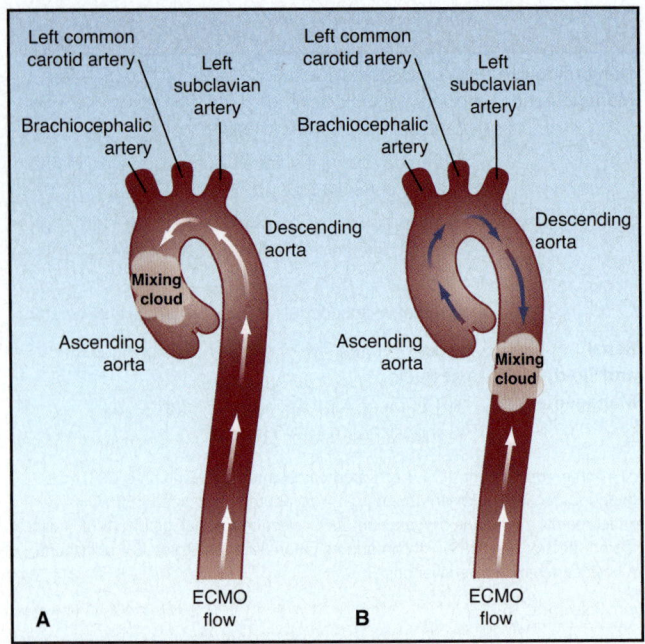

FIGURE 30.4. Explanation of differential oxygenation in VA ECMO. **A.** VA ECMO provides retrograde flow of oxygenated blood (black arrows) up to the aortic root, perfusing the carotid and coronary arteries. **B.** A mixing cloud exists when the left ventricular function improves (but lung function does not), pumping poorly oxygenated blood to the carotid and coronary arteries. Oxygenated blood from VA ECMO retrograde flow perfuses the lower extremities and lower branches of the aorta but does not reach the branches of the aortic arch.

facilitate early detection. The differential diagnosis of limb ischemia in the patient supported by VA ECMO should also include acute thrombosis, cardiogenic shock, hypothermia, and vasoconstriction (15-17).

Other Complications

The rates of other complications associated with VA ECMO are listed in Table 30.7.

TABLE 30.7 Complication Rates in VA ECMO

Complication	Rate
Acute brain injury (all types)	13-19%
Acute kidney injury	45-85%
Bleeding	30-79%
Hyperbilirubinemia	Up to 12%
Infections (all)	Up to 65%
Infection at access site	7-20%
Intracerebral hemorrhage	5-9%
Ischemic stroke	4-9%
Thrombosis	Up to 22%

ECMO = extracorporeal membrane oxygenation; VA = venoarterial; VV = venovenous.

From References 15-17, 26.

Weaning

The precise criteria for weaning from VA ECMO are frequently driven by institutional experience (15-17). The decision to decannulate requires multidisciplinary, with input from both the ICU team and cardiothoracic surgeons. VA ECMO support is generally decreased incrementally by 0.5-1.0 L/min until a flow rate of 1.0-1.5 L/min is achieved, with stable hemodynamics (i.e., MAP >60-65 mm Hg with only low-dose inotropes or vasopressors; left ventricular ejection fraction >30%) (15). In difficult-to-wean patients, a systematic approach evaluating arrhythmias, blood pressure, contractility, coronary perfusion, mechanical heart dysfunction, and extracardiac organ function (i.e., pulmonary, inflammation, endocrine) has been described (27).

EXTRACORPOREAL CARDIOPULMONARY RESUSCITATION

Extracorporeal cardiopulmonary resuscitation (ECPR) involves the application of VA ECMO for patients in refractory cardiac arrest (21,28-29). Indications are discussed in Chapter 22: Cardiac Arrest. The goal is to establish VA ECMO flow within 60 min of arrest (28-29). Once the VA ECMO flow is >3 L/min, mechanical compressions can be discontinued. Because coronary atherosclerotic disease is the most common cause of cardiac arrest, most experts recommend emergent coronary angiography after cannulation (28-29).

COMPARISON OF ECMO TECHNIQUES

Table 30.8 compares salient features of VV ECMO, VA ECMO, and ECPR.

TABLE 30.8	Comparison of VV and VA ECMO and ECPR		
Parameter	VV	VA	ECPR
Circulatory support	No	Yes	Yes
Removal of CO_2	Yes	Yes	Yes
Oxygenation	Yes	Yes	Yes
Risk of air emboli	Moderate	High	High
Risk of bleeding	Moderate	High	High
Primary indication	Respiratory support (ARDS)	Cardiac support (cardiogenic shock)	Cardiac arrest

ARDS = acute respiratory distress syndrome; ECMO = extracorporeal membrane oxygenation; ECPR = extracorporeal cardiopulmonary resuscitation; VA = venoarterial; VV = venovenous.

References

1. 2024 ELSO Reports. Extracorporeal Life Support Organization (ELSO). Updated October 2024. Accessed February 14, 2025. https://www.elso.org/registry/internationalsummaryandreports/reports.aspx
2. Australia and New Zealand Extracorporeal Membrane Oxygenation (ANZ ECMO) influenza investigators, Davies A, Jones D, et al. Extracorporeal membrane oxygenation for 2009 influenza A(H1N1) acute respiratory distress syndrome. JAMA 2009;302(17):1888-95.

3. MacLaren G, Brodie D, Lorusso R, et al. *Extracorporeal Life Support: the ELSO Red Book*. 6th ed. Extracorporeal Life Support Organization; 2022.
4. Chandel A, Fabyan KD, Mendelsohn S, et al. Prevalence and survival of prolonged venovenous extracorporeal membrane oxygenation for acute respiratory distress syndrome: an analysis of the Extracorporeal Life Support Organization registry. Crit Care Med 2024;52(6):869-77.
5. Brodie D, Bacchetta M. Extracorporeal membrane oxygenation for ARDS in adults. N Engl J Med 2011;365(20):1905-14.
6. Makdisi G, Wang IW. Extracorporeal membrane oxygenation (ECMO): review of a lifesaving technology. J Thorac Dis 2015;7(7):E166-76.
7. Geetha S III, Verma N, Chakole V. A comprehensive review of Extracorporeal Membrane Oxygenation: the lifeline in critical moments. Cureus 2024;16(1):e53275.
8. Tonna JE, Abrams D, Brodie D, et al. Management of adult patients supported with venovenous extracorporeal membrane oxygenation (VV ECMO): guideline from the Extracorporeal Life Support Organization (ELSO). ASAIO J 2021;67(6):601-10.
9. Schmidt M, Bailey M, Sheldrake J, et al. Predicting survival after extracorporeal membrane oxygenation for severe acute respiratory failure. The Respiratory Extracorporeal Membrane Oxygenation Survival Prediction (RESP) score. Am J Respir Crit Care Med 2014;189(11):1374-82.
10. Hilder M, Herbstreit F, Adamzik M, et al. Comparison of mortality prediction models in acute respiratory distress syndrome undergoing extracorporeal membrane oxygenation and development of a novel prediction score: the PREdiction of Survival on ECMO Therapy-Score (PRESET-Score). Crit Care 2017;21(1):301.
11. Pappalardo F, Pieri M, Greco T, et al. Predicting mortality risk in patients undergoing venovenous ECMO for ARDS due to influenza A (H1N1) pneumonia: the ECMOnet score. Intensive Care Med 2013;39(2):275-81.
12. Zakhary B, Vercaemst L, Mason P, et al. How I manage drainage insufficiency on extracorporeal membrane oxygenation. Crit Care 2020;24(1):151.
13. Douflé G, Dragoi L, Morales Castro D, et al. Head-to-toe bedside ultrasound for adult patients on extracorporeal membrane oxygenation. Intensive Care Med 2024;50(5):632-45.
14. Montisci A, Maj G, Zangrillo A, et al. Management of refractory hypoxemia during venovenous extracorporeal membrane oxygenation for ARDS. ASAIO J 2015;61(3):227-36.
15. Koziol KJ, Isath A, Rao S, et al. Extracorporeal membrane oxygenation (VA-ECMO) in management of cardiogenic shock. J Clin Med 2023;12(17):5576.

16. Lorusso R, Shekar K, MacLaren G, et al. ELSO interim guidelines for venoarterial extracorporeal membrane oxygenation in adult cardiac patients. ASAIO J 2021;67(8):827-44.
17. Tsangaris A, Alexy T, Kalra R, et al. Overview of veno-arterial extracorporeal membrane oxygenation (VA-ECMO) support for the management of cardiogenic shock. Front Cardiovasc Med 2021;8:686558.
18. Rihal CS, Naidu SS, Givertz MM, et al. 2015 SCAI/ACC/HFSA/STS clinical expert consensus statement on the use of percutaneous mechanical circulatory support devices in cardiovascular care. J Am Coll Cardiol 2015;65(19):e7-e26.
19. Upchurch C, Blumenberg A, Brodie D, et al. Extracorporeal membrane oxygenation use in poisoning: a narrative review with clinical recommendations. Clin Toxicol (Phila) 2021;59(10):877-87.
20. Schmidt M, Burrell A, Roberts L, et al. Predicting survival after ECMO for refractory cardiogenic shock: the survival after veno-arterial-ECMO (SAVE)-score. Eur Heart J 2015;36(33):2246-56.
21. Powell E, Keller AP, Galvagno SM Jr. Advanced critical care techniques in the field. Crit Care Clin 2024;40(3):463-80.
22. Cevasco M, Takayama H, Ando M, et al. Left ventricular distension and venting strategies for patients on venoarterial extracorporeal membrane oxygenation. J Thorac Dis 2019;11(4):1676-83.
23. McMichael ABV, Ryerson LM, Ratano D, et al. 2021 ELSO adult and pediatric anticoagulation guidelines. ASAIO J 2022;68(3):303-10.
24. Rupprecht L, Lunz D, Philipp A, et al. Pitfalls in percutaneous ECMO cannulation. Heart Lung Vessel 2015;7(4):320-6.
25. Cheng R, Hachamovitch R, Kittleson M, et al. Complications of extracorporeal membrane oxygenation for treatment of cardiogenic shock and cardiac arrest: a meta-analysis of 1,866 adult patients. Ann Thorac Surg 2014;97(2):610-6.
26. Cho SM, Hwang J, Chiarini G, et al. Neurological monitoring and management for adult extracorporeal membrane oxygenation patients: Extracorporeal Life Support Organization Consensus guidelines. ASAIO J 2024;70(12):e169-e181.
27. Meuwese CL, Brodie D, Donker DW. The ABCDE approach to difficult weaning from venoarterial extracorporeal membrane oxygenation. Crit Care 2022;26(1):216.
28. Tonna JE, Cho SM. Extracorporeal cardiopulmonary resuscitation. Crit Care Med 2024;52(6):963-73.
29. Richardson ASC, Tonna JE, Nanjayya V, et al. Extracorporeal cardiopulmonary resuscitation in adults. Interim guideline consensus statement from the Extracorporeal Life Support Organization. ASAIO J 2021;67(3):221-8.

SECTION VIII
ACID-BASE DISORDERS

Chapter 31
Acid-Base Analysis

This chapter presents a structured approach to the identification of acid-base disorders based on the relationships between the pH, partial pressure of carbon dioxide (PCO_2), and bicarbonate (HCO_3) concentration in extracellular fluid (plasma). Several outstanding reviews on this topic are listed in the bibliography (1-5).

CLASSIFICATION OF ACID-BASE DISORDERS

The pH is a logarithmic function of the hydrogen ion concentration in extracellular fluid [H^+]. Changes in pH are not linear; for example, changes in pH in an acidotic range can be approximately 2.5 times greater than in an alkalotic range. The [H^+] is determined by the PCO_2/HCO_3 ratio, and this ratio identifies all the primary acid-base disorders and compensatory responses, as shown in Table 31.1.

TABLE 31.1 Primary Acid-Base Disorders and Compensatory Responses

$\Delta [H^+] \sim \Delta PCO_2 / \Delta HCO_3$

Primary Disorder	Primary Change	Compensatory Response†
Respiratory Acidosis	↑ PCO_2	↑ HCO_3
Respiratory Alkalosis	↓ PCO_2	↓ HCO_3
Metabolic Acidosis	↓ HCO_3	↓ PCO_2
Metabolic Alkalosis	↑ HCO_3	↑ PCO_2

From Acid-Base Analysis. In: Marino PL. *Marino's The ICU Book*. 5th ed. Wolters Kluwer; 2025:499-510. Table 31.1.

Primary Acid-Base Disorders

A change in either the PCO_2 or HCO_3 will cause a change in the [H⁺] (reflecting a change in pH). The pH is *decreased* (higher [H⁺]) in acidemia and *increased* (lower [H⁺]) in alkalemia. When a change in PCO_2 initiates the change in [H⁺], the condition is called a *respiratory* acid-base disorder: an increase in PCO_2 is a *respiratory acidosis*, and a decrease in PCO_2 is a *respiratory alkalosis*. When a change in HCO_3 initiates the change in [H⁺], the condition is called a *metabolic* acid-base disorder: a decrease in HCO_3 is a *metabolic acidosis*, and an increase in HCO_3 is a *metabolic alkalosis*.

Compensatory Responses

Compensatory responses are designed to limit the change in [H⁺] produced by the primary acid-base disorder, and this is accomplished by altercations of the partial pressure of CO2 in the arterial blood $(PaCO_2)/HCO_3$. For example, if the primary change is an increase in $PaCO_2$ (respiratory acidosis), the compensatory response will be an increase in HCO_3, which limits the final change in [H⁺]. It is important to emphasize that *compensatory responses limit, but do not correct, the change in [H⁺] produced by the primary acid-base disorder*. The expected compensatory changes in each of the primary acid-base disorders are shown in Figure 31.1.

Responses to Metabolic Acid-Base Disorders

Metabolic Acidosis

The response to metabolic acidosis is an increase in tidal volume and respiratory rate (minute ventilation), which is mediated by peripheral chemoreceptors in the carotid body, causing a subsequent decrease in $PaCO_2$. This response appears in 30-120 minutes. Using a normal $PaCO_2$ of 40 mm Hg and a normal HCO_3 of 24 mEq/L, the following equation defines the magnitude of the response (1):

$$\text{Expected PaCO}_2 = 40 - [1.2 \times (24 - \text{current HCO}_3)] \quad (31.1)$$

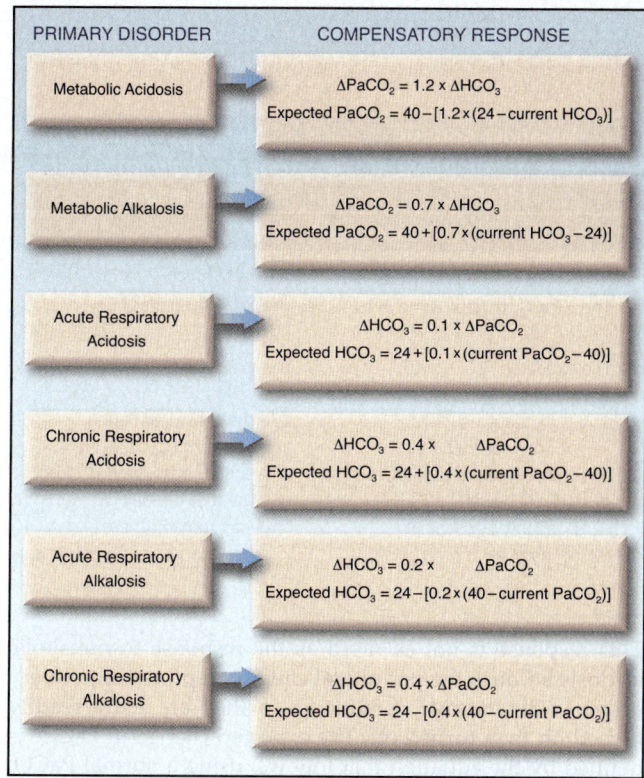

FIGURE 31.1. Predictive equations for evaluating secondary responses to primary acid-base disorders. All equations are from reference 1. (From Acid-Base Analysis. In: Marino PL. *Marino's The ICU Book*. 5th ed. Wolters Kluwer; 2025:499-510. Figure 31.1.)

Examples of expected changes in metabolic disorders are listed in Table 31.2.

Metabolic Alkalosis

The compensatory response to metabolic alkalosis is a *decrease* in minute ventilation, which increases the $PaCO_2$.

TABLE 31.2	Examples of Compensatory Changes in Metabolic Acidosis and Metabolic Alkalosis
Metabolic Acidosis *Assume a plasma HCO_3 of 14 mEq/L*	**Metabolic Alkalosis** *Assume a plasma HCO_3 of 40 mEq/L*
$\Delta PaCO_2 = 1.2 \times \Delta HCO_3$	
1. The ΔHCO_3 is 24 − 14 = 10 mEq/L.	1. The ΔHCO_3 is 40 − 24 = 16 mEq/L.
2. The $\Delta PaCO_2$ is 1.2 × 10 = 12 mm Hg.	2. The $\Delta PaCO_2$ is 0.7 × 16 = 11 mm Hg.

3. The expected $PaCO_2$ is 40 − 12 = 28 mm Hg.
  a. If the measured $PaCO_2$ >28 mm Hg, there is a *secondary respiratory acidosis*.
  b. If the measured $PaCO_2$ is <28 mm Hg, there is a *secondary respiratory alkalosis*.
	3. The expected $PaCO_2$ is 40 + 11 = 51 mm Hg.
	  a. If the measured $PaCO_2$ is >51 mm Hg, there is a *secondary respiratory acidosis*.
	  b. If the measured $PaCO_2$ is <51 mm Hg, there is a *secondary respiratory alkalosis*.

This response is not as rapid as the response to metabolic acidosis because the peripheral chemoreceptors are not very active under normal conditions, so they are more readily turned on than turned off. The expected change in $PaCO_2$ is defined by the equation that follows, using a normal $PaCO_2$ of 40 mm Hg and a normal HCO_3 of 24 mEq/L (1):

$$\text{Expected } PaCO_2 = 40 + [0.7 \times (\text{current } HCO_3 - 24)] \qquad (31.2)$$

Examples of compensatory changes for metabolic alkalosis are shown in Table 31.2.

Responses to Respiratory Acid-Base Disorders

The compensatory response to primary changes in $PaCO_2$ occurs in the kidneys, where HCO_3 reabsorption in the proximal tubules changes in the same direction as the change in $PaCO_2$. This renal response is slow and can take up to two or three days. Because of this delay, respiratory disorders are classified as acute or chronic (compensated).

Acute Respiratory Disorders

Acute changes in $PaCO_2$ have a minor effect on the plasma HCO_3, as described by the equations that follow (1):

For acute respiratory *acidosis*:

$$\Delta HCO_3 = 0.1 \times \Delta PaCO_2 \qquad (31.3)$$

For acute respiratory *alkalosis*:

$$\Delta HCO_3 = 0.2 \times \Delta PaCO_2 \qquad (31.4)$$

Examples of expected changes in $PaCO_2$ and HCO_3 in respiratory acid-base disorders are provided in Table 31.3.

TABLE 31.3 Examples of Compensatory Responses in Respiratory Acidosis and Respiratory Alkalosis

Acute Respiratory Disorders	Chronic Respiratory Disorders
Acute respiratory acidosis: $\Delta HCO_3 = 0.1 \times \Delta PaCO_2$ *Acute respiratory alkalosis:* $\Delta HCO_3 = 0.2 \times \Delta PaCO_2$	*Chronic respiratory acidosis:* Expected $HCO_3 = 24 + [0.4 \times (\text{current } PaCO_2 - 40)]$ *Chronic respiratory alkalosis:* Expected $HCO_3 = 24 - [0.4 \times (40 - \text{current } PaCO_2)]$

1. For an acute increase in $PaCO_2$ of 20 mm Hg:
  a. The ΔHCO_3 is $0.1 \times 20 = 2$ mEq/L for an *acute respiratory acidosis*.
  b. The ΔHCO_3 is $0.2 \times 20 = 4$ mEq/L for an *acute respiratory alkalosis*.
 	
Note: Neither of these changes would be clinically significant.
	1. Assuming an increase in $PaCO_2$ to 60 mm Hg that persists for at least a few days:
	  a. The $\Delta PaCO_2$ is $60 - 40 = 20$ mm Hg.
	  b. The ΔHCO_3 is $0.4 \times 20 = 8$ mEq/L.
	  c. The expected HCO_3 is $24 + 8 = 32$ mEq/L.

STEPWISE APPROACH TO ACID-BASE ANALYSIS

The following is a structured, rule-based approach to the diagnosis of primary, secondary, and mixed acid-base disorders using reference ranges for arterial pH, PCO_2, and HCO_3:

$$pH = 7.36\text{-}7.44$$

$$PCO_2 = 36\text{-}44 \text{ mm Hg}$$

$$HCO_3 = 22\text{-}26 \text{ mEq/L}$$

Step 1. Identify the Primary Acid-Base Disorder

- **Rule 1.** If the $PaCO_2$ and pH are both abnormal, compare the directional change.
  - **Rule 1a.** If the $PaCO_2$ and pH change in the same direction, there is a primary metabolic acid-base disorder.
  - **Rule 1b.** If the $PaCO_2$ and pH change in opposite directions, there is a primary respiratory acid-base disorder.
- **Rule 2.** When the $PaCO_2$ is abnormal, but the pH is normal, the condition can be called a *mixed* metabolic and respiratory disorder. The directional change in $PaCO_2$ identifies the type of respiratory disorder, and the metabolic disorder is then in the opposite direction. Compensatory responses do not fully correct the primary acid-base change.

Step 2. Identify Secondary Acid-Base Disorders

- **Rule 3.** For a primary metabolic disorder, determine the expected $PaCO_2$.
  - **Rule 3a.** If the measured $PaCO_2$ is higher than expected, there is a secondary respiratory acidosis.

- **Rule 3b**. If the measured $PaCO_2$ is lower than expected, there is a secondary respiratory alkalosis.
- **Rule 4**. For a primary respiratory disorder, determine the expected HCO_3 for both acute and chronic (compensated) conditions. If the measured HCO_3 is between the expected HCO_3 for the acute and chronic conditions, it is a *partially compensated respiratory disorder*.
  - **Rule 4a**. For a primary respiratory acidosis:
    - If the HCO_3 is less than the expected HCO_3 for the acute condition, there is a secondary metabolic acidosis.
    - If the HCO_3 is higher than expected for the chronic condition, there is a secondary metabolic alkalosis.
  - **Rule 4b**. For a primary respiratory alkalosis:
    - If the HCO_3 is higher than expected for the acute condition, there is a secondary metabolic alkalosis.
    - If the HCO_3 is lower than expected for the chronic condition, there is a secondary metabolic acidosis.

Step 3: Use the "Gaps" to Evaluate a Metabolic Acidosis

The use of measurements called "gaps" can help to uncover the underlying cause of the acidosis. These are described in the next section.

The three-step process described above enables precise classification of acid-base disorders and should be used to definitively identify primary and secondary disorders. An alternative simplified approach using "rules of thumb" is presented in Table 31.4 (2).

THE GAPS

The anion gap, delta gap, and osmolal gap can help identify secondary disorders and narrow the differential diagnosis.

SECTION VIII ■ Acid-Base Disorders

TABLE 31.4 Simplified Approach for Recognizing Primary Acid-Base Disorders Without Using a Nomogram or Calculator

Step	Assessment	Rationale
1	Assess the direction of pH change (assume an average pH of 7.40). Example: If the pH is <7.40, then an elevated PCO_2 (respiratory acidosis) or a lowered HCO_3 (metabolic acidosis) would be the primary abnormality.	Over time, the pH approaches but does not completely normalize in primary acid-base disorders.
2	Calculate the anion gap. If >20 mmol/L, there is a primary metabolic acidosis (regardless of pH or HCO_3 concentration).	The body does not generate an anion gap larger enough to compensate for a primary disorder.
3	Calculate the excess anion gap. Assume a normal anion gap value of 12 mmol/L and add this to the measured HCO_3 concentration. If the sum is >30 mmol/L, there is an underlying metabolic alkalosis. If the sum is <24 mmol/L, there is an underlying non-anion gap metabolic acidosis.	One mmol of unmeasured acid should normally titrate 1 mmol of HCO_3 (+ Δ anion gap = – Δ [HCO_3]).

From Haber RJ. A practical approach to acid-base disorders. West J Med 1991;155(2):146-51.

The Anion Gap

The anion gap (AG) is a rough approximation of the amount of unmeasured anions in extracellular fluid (2, 6-7). Equation 31.5 provides a simple method for calculating the AG.

$$AG = (Na) - (CL + HCO_3) \tag{31.5}$$

The reference range for the AG is 8-12 mEq/L, but because electrolyte measurements can differ in clinical laboratories, the reference AG published by the laboratory should be used (6-7). Determinants of the AG are listed in Table 31.5.

TABLE 31.5 Determinants of the Anion Gap	
Unmeasured Anions	**Unmeasured Cations**
Albumin (15 mEq/L)	Calcium (5 mEq/L)
Organic Acids (5 mEq/L)	Potassium (4.5 mEq/L)
Phosphate (2 mEq/L)	
Sulfate (1 mEq/L)	Magnesium (1.5 mEq/L)
Total UA: (23 mEq/L)	Total UC: (11 mEq/L)
Anion Gap = UA − UC = 12 mEq/L	

From Acid-Base Analysis. In: Marino PL. *Marino's The ICU Book*. 5th ed. Wolters Kluwer; 2025:499-510. Table 31.2.

Influence of Albumin

Albumin is a weak acid, and when present in low concentrations can mask the presence of other unmeasured anions, such as lactate. Equation 31.6 is used to calculate the corrected AG in ICU patients with hypoalbuminemia (which is common in ICU patients):

$$\text{Corrected AG} = \text{AG} + [2.5 \times (4.5 - \text{albumin})] \quad (31.6)$$

Using the Anion Gap

The AG can be used to identify the underlying mechanism of a metabolic acidosis. Table 31.6 lists causes of metabolic acidosis based on the AG.

The Delta Gap

The delta gap is the ratio of the increase in the anion gap to the decrease in plasma HCO_3, and is described by the following equation:

$$\text{AG Excess}/HCO_3 \text{ Deficit} = (\text{AG} - 12) / (24 - HCO_3) \quad (31.7)$$

where 12 is normal AG (mEq/L) and 24 is the normal plasma HCO_3 (in mEq/L). This ratio is sometimes called the

TABLE 31.6 Cause of Metabolic Acidosis Based on the Anion Gap

High Anion Gap	Normal Anion Gap
L-lactic acid	Diarrhea
D-*lactic acid*	Isotonic saline infusion
Ketoacids	Early renal insufficiency
Ethylene glycol (oxalic acid)	Renal tubular acidosis
Methanol (formic acid)	Acetazolamide
Pyroglutamic acid[†]	Ureteroenterostomy
Salicylate toxicity	
Advanced renal failure	

[†]Also known as 5-oxoproline and associated with chronic acetaminophen ingestion.
From Acid-Base Analysis. In: Marino PL. *Marino's The ICU Book*. 5th ed. Wolters Kluwer; 2025:499-510. Table 31.3

"*gap-gap*" because it involves *two* gaps (the AG excess and the HCO_3 deficit). The delta gap is useful for identifying mixed acid-base disorders (8).

Mixed Metabolic Acidoses

In metabolic acidoses caused by non-volatile acids (e.g., high AG metabolic acidosis), the increase in the anion gap should be equivalent to the decrease in plasma HCO_3 (i.e., the delta gap should be 1). However, if there is a second source of acidosis that is associated with a normal AG (e.g., hyperchloremic) acidosis, the decrease in HCO_3 is greater than the increase in AG, and the delta gap ratio falls below 1.0. Therefore, *in the presence of a high AG metabolic acidosis, a delta gap <1 indicates the co-existence of a normal AG (hyperchloremic) metabolic acidosis* (9).

Diabetic Ketoacidosis

Diabetic ketoacidosis (DKA) is initially associated with a high AG metabolic acidosis with a delta gap = 1. As saline is given for the management of DKA, a normal AG metabolic acidosis can develop, and the plasma HCO$_3$ decreases relative to the AG, resulting in a delta gap <1 (9). Thus, *monitoring the plasma HCO$_3$ alone will suggest the DKA is not resolving, while the delta gap provides an accurate assessment of the changing acid-base status.*

Metabolic Acidosis and Alkalosis

When alkali is added in the presence of a high AG acidosis, the decrease in plasma HCO$_3$ is less than the increase in AG, and the delta gap is >1. Therefore, *in the presence of a high AG metabolic acidosis, a delta gap >1 indicates the co-existence of a metabolic alkalosis* (2,10).

Osmolar Gap

The osmolality of plasma (Posm) can be both calculated and measured. Equation 31.8 is a calculation for Posm:

$$\text{Posm} = 2 \times [\text{Na}^+] + \frac{\text{Glucose}}{18} + \frac{\text{BUN}}{2.8} \qquad (31.8)$$

The Posm can also be measured, and the difference between the measured and calculated plasma osmolality (i.e., the *osmolal gap*) is normally <10 mOsm/kg (11).

Detecting Hidden Solutes

When extra solutes are added to extracellular fluid, the measured Posm will increase, while the calculated Posm will be unaffected (i.e., the osmolal gap will *increase*). An elevated osmolal gap may indicate the presence of unmeasured acids (e.g., D-lactic acid, oxalic acid, formic acid, salicylates, pyroglutamic acid [associated with chronic acetaminophen ingestion]) (12).

STEWART APPROACH

An alternative approach to acid-base interpretation assesses three independent factors: the PaCO$_2$, the strong ion difference (SID), and the total amount of weak acids (13-15). The SID can be calculated using Equation 31.9:

$$SID = [Na^+] + [K^+] + [Ca^{2+}] + [Mg^{2+}] - [Cl^-] - [UA^-] \quad (31.9)$$

where [UA$^-$] represents the concentration of unmeasured anions (like lactate and ketoacids), and a normal value is between 38 and 42 mEq/L (13,15-16). The Stewart approach enables a quantitative overall assessment of acid-base status, accounting for anion and cation concentrations. Using the Stewart approach, acidosis is associated with a *decreased SID* and is observed in disorders where *cations are decreased* (i.e., hypokalemia, hyponatremia) or where *anions are increased* (i.e., hyperchloremia, lactate). Alkalosis is associated with an *increased SID* and is seen in disorders where *cations are increased* (i.e., hyperkalemia, hypercalcemia, hypernatremia) or where *anions are decreased* (see Chapters 34-37). Further details regarding the theory and application of the Stewart approach are beyond the scope of this text, but several excellent references are available (13-16) as well as an online calculator (https://www.acidbase.org/).

References

1. Adrogué HJ, Madias NE. Secondary responses to altered acid-base status: the rules of engagement. J Am Soc Nephrol 2010;21:920-3.
2. Haber RJ. A practical approach to acid-base disorders. West J Med 1991;155(2):146-51.
3. Adrogué HJ, Madias NE. Management of life-threatening acid-base disorders. N Engl J Med 1999;340(3):247.
4. Adrogué HJ, Madias NE. Management of life-threatening acid-base disorders. Second of two parts. N Engl J Med 1998;338(2):107-11.
5. Kaplan LJ, Frangos S. Clinical review: acid-base abnormalities in the intensive care unit—part II. Crit Care 2005;9(2):198-203.
6. Fenves AZ, Emmett M. Approach to patients with high anion gap metabolic acidoses: core curriculum 2021. Am J Kidney Dis 2021;78:590-600.
7. Emmet M, Narins RG. Clinical use of the anion gap. Medicine 1977;56:38-54.
8. Rastegar A. Use of the delta AG/delta HCO$_3$ ratio in the diagnosis of mixed acid-base disorders. J Am Soc Nephrol 2007;18:2429-31.

9. Paulson WD. Anion gap bicarbonate relationship in diabetic ketoacidosis. Am J Med 1986;81:995-1000.
10. Narins RG, Emmett M. Simple and mixed acid base disorders: a practical approach. Medicine 1980;59:161-87.
11. Turchin A, Seifter JL, Seely EW. Clinical problem-solving. Mind the gap. N Engl J Med 2003;349:1465-9.
12. Purssell RA, Lynd LD, Koga Y. The use of the osmole gap as a screening test for the presence of exogenous substances. Toxicol Rev 2004;23:189-202.
13. Story DA. Acid-base analysis in the operating room: a bedside stewart approach. Anesthesiology 2023;139(6):860-7.
14. Stewart PA. Modern quantitative acid-base chemistry. Can J Physiol Pharmacol 1983;61:1444-61.
15. Stewart PA. Whole-body acid-base balance. In: Kellum JA, Elbers PWG, eds. *Stewart's Textbook of Acid Base*. 2nd ed. AcidBase.org, 2009:181-197.
16. Morgan TJ. The Stewart approach—one clinician's perspective. Clin Biochem Rev 2009;30(2):41-54.

Lactic Acidosis and Ketoacidosis

Chapter 32

This chapter focuses on the two most prominent acid-base disorders encountered in the ICU: lactic acidosis and ketoacidosis.

LACTIC ACIDOSIS

Misconceptions

There are a few misconceptions concerning lactate in the critically ill.

Lactate ≠ Anaerobic Metabolism

Contrary to various traditional teachings, the production of lactate is not driven solely by anaerobic metabolism (1). During conditions of metabolic stress, lactate serves as an oxidative fuel when glucose is limited, providing up to 60% of the energy needs of the myocardium (2) and 30% of the energy needs of the brain (3). Lactate is more than just the end-product of glycolysis and an inert energy donor; lactate is a powerful marker for energy regulation, immune modulation, mitochondrial activity and ischemic tissue injury (4).

Lactate Is Not an Acid

The relationship between lactate production and acidosis remains poorly understood. The end-product of glycolysis is the lactate anion, which is not an acid. The chemical reaction that produces lactate consumes hydrogen ions, and the hydrogen ions associated with lactate production are attributed to hydrolysis of adenosine triphosphate (ATP) during glycolysis (5-6). Furthermore, hyperlactatemia can exist without an associated acidosis (7).

Prognostic Value

The normal lactate concentration in blood is ≤2 mmol/L. Regardless of its origins or function, plasma lactate levels have prognostic significance in critically ill patients. In hemorrhagic shock, failure of lactate to normalize over 24 h has been strongly correlated with organ failure and death as shown in Figure 32.1 (8).

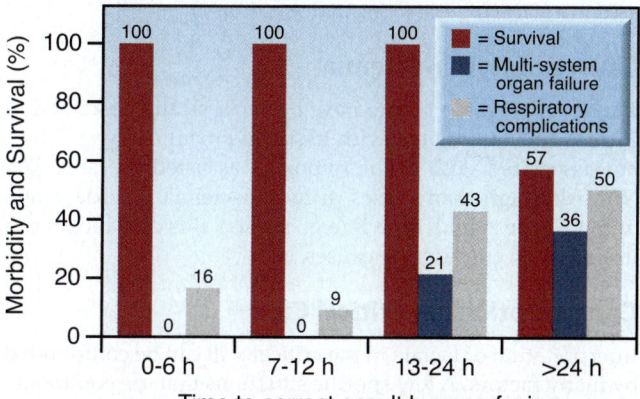

FIGURE 32.1. The "silver day." When lactate fails to decrease in patients with hemorrhagic shock, multiple organ function, respiratory complications and mortality increase substantially. (From Blow O, Magliore L, Claridge JA, et al. The golden hour and the silver day: detection and correction of occult hypoperfusion within 24 hours improves outcome from major trauma. J Trauma 1999;47[5]:964-9.)

In critically ill patients in shock, the initial lactate level is directly related to mortality rates (9–10), but the time required for lactate levels to return to normal (i.e., lactate "clearance") has greater predictive value than the initial lactate level (10). *A lactate level >4 mmol/L, with or without hypotension, is highly associated with in-hospital mortality in patients with septic shock* (11). Similar observations (i.e., the need for blood transfusion, mortality) have been observed in hemorrhagic shock patients with lactate levels >4 mmol/L (12–13).

Measurements

Measurements can be obtained using arterial or venous blood samples. If immediate measurements are unavailable, the blood should be placed on ice to retard lactate production by red blood cells. The anion gap (described in Chapter 31: Acid-Base Analysis) should be elevated in lactic acidosis, but there are numerous reports of a normal anion gap in patients with lactic acidosis (14). As a result, *the anion gap should not be used as a screening test for lactic acidosis*.

Causes of Hyperlactemia

Causes of elevated lactate have been classically described as Type A (i.e., associated with tissue hypoxia) or Type B (i.e., not associated with tissue hypoxia), as listed in Table 32.1 (15). Although many cases of hyperlactemia include a mix of both Type A and Type B (e.g., sepsis), this classification is useful when considering causes.

Considerations in Critical Care

Interpretation of lactate in the critically ill can be confounded by many factors. A few specific situations that are commonly encountered are briefly described in the sections that follow.

Septic Shock

Sepsis and septic shock are the most common causes of hyperlactatemia in the critically ill. The source of elevated lactate is a combination of increased pyruvate and a defect in O_2 utilization in the mitochondria. *However, tissue oxygenation is often not impaired and may actually be increased* (1,16-17).

Thiamine Deficiency

The total body stores of thiamine are limited; thiamine deficiency can develop rapidly in the critically ill due to inadequate nutrition, acute metabolic stress, alcohol abuse, or sepsis (18). Lactic acidosis can be severe in cases of thiamine deficiency because thiamine pyrophosphate is a co-factor for pyruvate dehydrogenase. This enzyme is responsible in

TABLE 32.1 Causes of Hyperlactemia

Type A (Clinical Evidence of Tissue Hypoxia)	Type B (No Evidence of Tissue Hypoxia)
- Shock (septic*, cardiogenic, hypovolemic, etc.) - Regional hypoperfusion (mesenteric ischemia) - Severe hypoxemia - Poisonings (cyanide, carbon monoxide, iron) - Severe muscle activity (seizures, asthma, exercise)	*Association with underlying diseases* - Liver disease - Sepsis - Diabetes mellitus - Malignancy - Thiamine deficiency - Pheochromocytoma *Drugs/toxins* - Biguanides (e.g., metformin) - Epinephrine (or other adrenergic agonists) - Ethanol - Methanol - Ethylene glycol - Propylene glycol - Sorbitol - Fructose - Salicylates - Acetaminophen - Isoniazid - Linezolid *Inborn errors of metabolism* - Glucose-6-diphosphatase deficiency - Pyruvate carboxylase deficiency - Fructose-1-6-diphosphatase deficiency - Pyruvate dehydrogenase deficiency - Oxidative phosphorylation defects *Miscellaneous causes:* - Hypoglycemia - D-lactic acidosis (e.g., short bowel syndrome)

*See Chapters 15 and 18; lactate is an unreliable indicator of tissue hypoxia in sepsis.

From Blow O, Magliore L, Claridge JA, et al. The golden hour and the silver day: detection and correction of occult hypoperfusion within 24 hours improves outcome from major trauma. J Trauma 1999;47(5):964-9.

converting pyruvate into acetyl coenzyme A (a key step in the citric acid [Krebs] cycle within the mitochondria), and when inhibited, favors lactate production (Figure 32.2) (19).

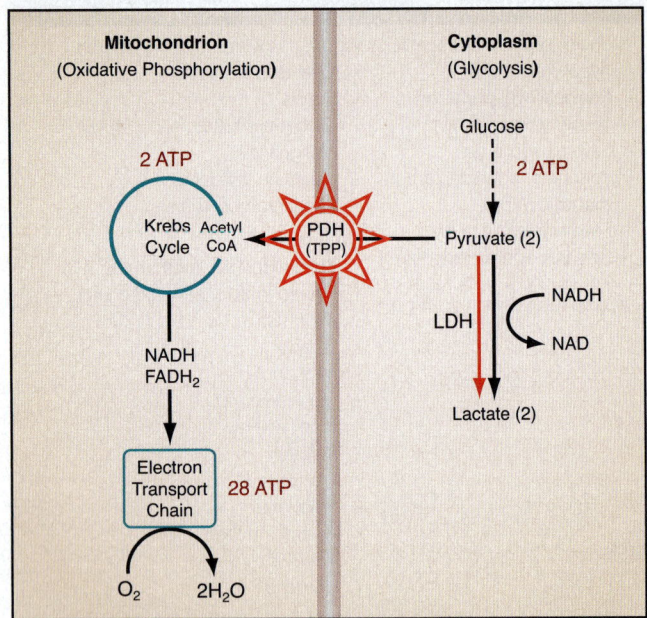

FIGURE 32.2. Inhibition of pyruvate dehydrogenase (PDH) in sepsis. When pyruvate cannot enter the mitochondria, the pathway shifts to the production of more lactate. TPP-thiamine pyrophosphate, a necessary cofactor for PDH. (Adapted from Marino PL. Is tissue hypoxia a common cause of death? In: *Oxygen: Creating a New Paradigm*. Wolters Kluwer; 2021:39-54. Figure 4.1.)

Commonly Used ICU Drugs

Epinephrine. Epinephrine increases Na+/K+/ATPase enzyme activity through β2-receptor stimulation, thereby increasing the metabolic rate of glycolysis, and generating more pyruvate and lactate (20).

Linezolid. Hyperlactemia is rarely associated with the use of linezolid, but when this complication occurs, the mortality approaches 25% (21).

Toxidromes. Lactic acidosis is often found with various intoxications, including carbon monoxide, cyanide, and propylene glycol (see Chapter 51: Nonpharmaceutical Poisons). Propylene glycol is found in intravenous (IV) preparations of lorazepam, diazepam, esmolol, nitroglycerin, and phenytoin.

Other Sources

Other common sources of hyperlactemia in the ICU include hepatic insufficiency (from reduced lactate clearance) (22), acute asthma (from enhanced lactate production by respiratory muscles or albuterol [β2-receptor activation]) (23), generalized seizures (from hypermetabolism) (24), and hematologic malignancies (25).

ALKALI THERAPY IN LACTIC ACIDOSIS

The goal of therapy in lactic acidosis is to correct the underlying cause of the abnormality. The use of alkalizing agents like sodium bicarbonate is of questionable value because these agents do not address the underlying cause and may be counterproductive (26).

Bicarbonate

Bicarbonate Is an Ineffective Buffer

Sodium bicarbonate is frequently ineffective for raising the plasma pH in lactic acidosis because *bicarbonate is not an effective buffer in the usual pH range of extracellular fluid* (26-28). This is demonstrated in Figure 32.3 which shows the range of optimal extracellular buffer effectiveness, which lies in the pH range of 5.1-7.1 (28).

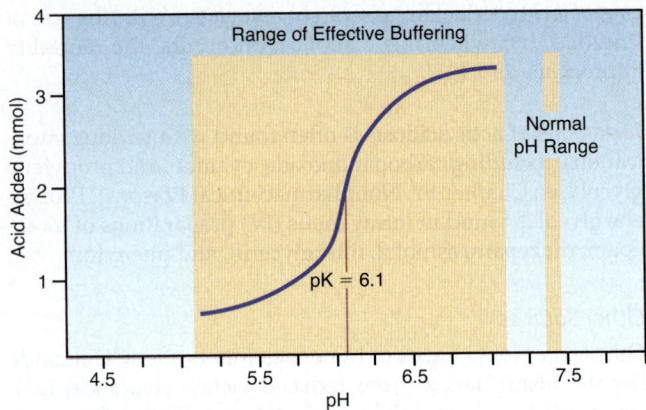

FIGURE 32.3. The titration curve for the carbonic acid-bicarbonate buffer system. The yellow shaded area indicates the effective pH range for the bicarbonate buffer system, which does not coincide with the physiological pH range of extracellular fluid. (From Lactic Acidosis and Ketoacidosis. In: Marino PL. *Marino's The ICU Book*. 5th ed. Wolters Kluwer; 2025:511-25. Figure 32.2.)

Bicarbonate Is Counterproductive

Bicarbonate infusions generate CO_2 (hypercarbia), which enters cells and the cerebrospinal fluid, lowering the intracellular pH and cerebrospinal fluid pH (29-30). Bicarbonate infusions can also increase blood lactate levels through an alkalosis-induced increase in lactate production (30).

Effect on Vasopressor Pharmacology

An often cited claim is that vasopressors are inhibited in academic conditions; hence, sodium bicarbonate is thought to help enhance vasopressor effectiveness by raising the pH. However, the observation of impaired myocardial contractility in acidosis is based on *in vitro* preclinical experiments (31). Acidemia, *in vivo*, is accompanied by an *increase* in cardiac output owing to stimulation for catecholamine release (32). Following administration of sodium bicarbonate, blood pressure is often increased, but this may be from the osmotic load of the preparation (i.e., 2,000 mOsm/L) rather than correction of the pH. No clinical trial has established the level at which pH becomes deleterious for hemodynamics, although many (not all) experts recommend bicarbonate therapy for severe lactic acidosis when the pH is ≤7.1 and/or the plasma HCO_3 is ≤5 mEq/L (30,33-34).

Dosing

Bicarbonate therapy is probably most helpful in patients with lactic acidosis and renal insufficiency, where part of the problem is renal loss of HCO_3. The bicarbonate deficit can be estimated with the following equation (30):

$$HCO_3 \text{ deficit (mEq)} = 0.6 \times \text{wt (kg)} \times (15 - \text{measured } HCO_3) \quad (32.1)$$

Half of the deficit can be replaced, and if this results in hemodynamic improvement, the infusion can be continued to maintain the HCO_3 at 15 mEq/L.

Tris-Hydroxymethyl Aminomethane

An alternative to sodium bicarbonate is the alkalizing agent tris-hydroxymethyl aminomethane (THAM). THAM has been shown to correct acidosis with an efficacy equivalent to sodium bicarbonate but with less hypernatremia and hypercarbia (35). Adverse effects of THAM include hypoglycemia, hyperkalemia, ventilatory depression, and tissue damage with extravasation (35). THAM can be dosed using the following general guide:

$$\text{Tromethamine solution (mL of 0.3 M) required} = \text{Body Weight (kg)} \times \text{Base Deficit (mEq/L)} \times 1.1 \quad (32.2)$$

KETOACIDS

When carbohydrates are not available for metabolic energy production, there is a breakdown of triglycerides in adipose tissue to generate fatty acids, which are transported to the liver and metabolized to form three ketones (i.e., acetoacetate, β-hydroxybutyrate, and acetone) (Figure 32.4). These ketones are released from the liver and can be used as oxidative fuels by vital organs such as the heart and central nervous system.

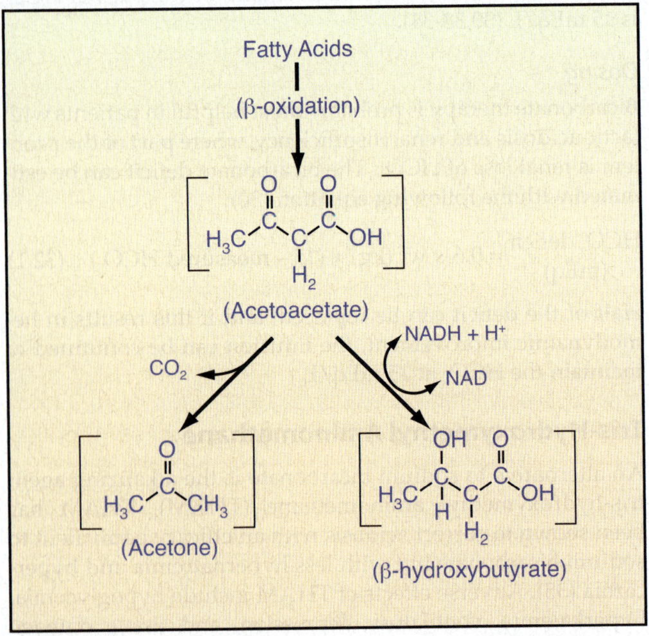

FIGURE 32.4. Ketogenesis in the liver, which occurs in response to diminished availability of glucose. Acetone is a ketone but is not a ketoacid. (From Lactic Acidosis and Ketoacidosis. In: Marino PL. *Marino's The ICU Book*. 5th ed. Wolters Kluwer; 2025:511-25. Figure 32.3.)

Acetoacetate and β-hydroybutyrate are strong acids that produce a decrease in plasma pH when their plasma concentrations reach 3 mmol/L (36). The colorimetric laboratory test for detecting ketoacids (the nitroprusside reaction) does not reliably detect β-hydroybutyrate. Other "ketone meters" must be used to detect β-hydroybutyrate, which is often the most predominant pathological ketoacid in diabetic ketoacidosis (DKA) (37).

DIABETIC KETOACIDOSIS

DKA can occur in patients with either type 1 or type 2 diabetes mellitus (38). The most common precipitating factors in DKA are inappropriate insulin dosing and concurrent illness (e.g., infection).

Clinical Features

The features of DKA proposed by the American Diabetes Association are listed in Table 32.2 (39-45).

Management

The management of DKA is summarized in Table 32.3.

Volume Resuscitation

Volume deficits in DKA are significant, averaging 50-100 mL/kg (i.e., 4-8 L for a 175 lb adult) (39). The traditional resuscitation fluid of choice in DKA has been 0.9% saline, but balanced salt solutions such as Plasma-Lyte or Ringer's lactate are preferred as these preparations have been shown to hasten resolution of the acidosis in DKA (46-47). The plasma bicarbonate HCO_3 can remain in the acidotic range if 0.9% saline is used because of the high chloride concentration (154 mEq/L) that causes a hyperchloremic (normal anion gap) metabolic acidosis.

Insulin

Because insulin adsorbs to IV tubing, the bolus insulin dose should be injected directly into the vein, and the initial 10 mL of infusate should be run through the IV line before the insulin drip is started. Correction to euglycemia is not recommended because of the risk of hypoglycemia (i.e., "overshoot").

Following correction of the acidosis (i.e., the anion gap normalizes and the plasma HCO_3 is >18 mEq/L), subcutaneous insulin can be started, although the insulin infusion should be continued for at least one hour after the first subcutaneous dose to prevent rebound hyperglycemia. Insulin-dependent

TABLE 32.2 Diagnostic Features and Caveats Associated with the Diagnosis of DKA

Diagnostic Criteria	Caveats
• Blood glucose >250 mg/dL • Plasma HCO_3 <18 mEq/L • Plasma pH ≤7.30 • Elevated anion gap • Evidence of ketones in blood or urine	• The blood glucose is <250 mg/dL in about 3% of cases of DKA (euglycemic diabetic ketoacidosis). This is most common in pregnancy, starvation, and in patients using sodium-glucose cotransporter-2 (SGLT2) inhibitors. • The anion gap may be normal in some cases of DKA due to renal excretion of ketones and increased chloride reabsorption in the renal tubules. • Leukocytosis can be caused by ketonemia and thus is not a reliable marker for infection in DKA. • Troponin I levels may be falsely elevated in up to 27% of patients with DKA. • The plasma sodium concentration decreases by 2.4 mEq/L for every 100 mg/dL increase in the plasma glucose concentration (this may mask dehydration, which is almost universal in DKA). • The plasma sodium, not the corrected value, should be used to calculate the anion gap because hyperglycemia has a dilutional effect on the plasma sodium concentration.

DKA = diabetic ketoacidosis.

From References 39-45.

TABLE 32.3 Management of DKA

I. Intravenous Fluids
1. Start with a balanced crystalloid fluid (e.g., Ringer's lactate) and infuse at a rate of 15-20 mL/kg/h (or 1 L/h) for a few hours.
2. When patient stabilizes, decrease rate to 250 mL/h.
3. When blood glucose falls to ≤250 mg/dL, change IV fluid to 5% dextrose in 0.45% saline and reduce rate to 150-200 mL/h.
4. Continue IV fluids until patient can tolerate oral fluids.
5. *Note:* In cases of euglycemic ketoacidosis, 5% dextrose should be added to all IV fluids.

II. Insulin
1. Start insulin only if plasma K^+ >3.3 mEq/L.
2. Use regular insulin, start with a bolus of 0.1 U/kg, and inject directly into vein (insulin adsorbs to IV tubing). Then infuse at 0.1 U/kg/h (run first 10 mL through IV tubing and discard).
3. Adjust rate, if needed, for a decrease in blood glucose of 100 mg/dL/h.
4. When blood glucose falls to ≤250 mg/dL, decrease rate to 0.05 U/kg/h.
5. Continue infusion until anion gap normalizes and plasma HCO_3 >18 mEq/L. Then transition to subQ insulin, but continue infusion for at least 1 h after first subQ dose.

DKA = diabetic ketoacidosis.

From Lactic Acidosis and Ketoacidosis. In: Marino PL. *Marino's The ICU Book*. 5th ed. Wolters Kluwer; 2025:511-25. Table 32.3.

patients can be restarted on their usual outpatient regimen. Patients new to insulin should receive 0.5-0.8 U/kg/day with half given as a long-acting preparation (e.g., glargine) and the remaining half as a short-acting preparation (e.g., lispro), in divided doses, to cover meals (48).

Potassium

Potassium depletion is universal in DKA, and the average deficit is 3-5 mEq/kg (49). Initial plasma K^+ levels are normal in most patients with DKA due to concomitant acidosis, so the presence of hypokalemia at the time of presentation indicates severe K⁺ depletion (49). *Insulin should not be started if the initial plasma K⁺ is <3.3 mEq/L because insulin drives K⁺ into cells, precipitating life-threatening hypokalemia.* Recommendations for K⁺ repletion in DKA are shown in Table 32.4.

TABLE 32.4 Potassium Replacement in DKA	
Plasma K⁺	Recommendation
<3.3 mEq/L	Hold insulin infusion and give 40 mEq K⁺ per hour IV until the plasma K⁺ >3.3 mEq/L.
3.3-4.0 mEq/L	Give 20 mEq K⁺ per hour IV.
4.0-5.5 mEq/L	Give 10 mEq K⁺ per hour IV.
>5.5 mEq/L	Check plasma K⁺ every 2 h.

DKA = diabetic ketoacidosis.

From Lowie BJ, Bond MC. Diabetic ketoacidosis. Emerg Med Clin N Am 2023;41:677-86.

Phosphate and Bicarbonate

Phosphate depletion is common in DKA, but replacement has no documented benefit and is not recommended unless the phosphate falls to <1 mg/dL (39,49). Bicarbonate therapy is not recommended in DKA (48-49).

ALCOHOLIC KETOACIDOSIS

Clinical Presentation

Alcoholic ketoacidosis (AKA) occurs in chronic, malnourished alcoholics, and may manifest 1-3 days after a period of heavy binge drinking (50-51). Patients with AKA often present with nausea, vomiting, and abdominal pain (50). Electrolyte deficits are common (e.g., hyponatremia, hypokalemia, hypophosphatemia, hypomagnesemia, hypoglycemia) and the acid base picture is usually mixed with a high anion gap metabolic acidosis, ketonemia, hyperlactatemia, and alkalemia (from protracted vomiting) (51).

Diagnosis

The diagnosis of AKA is suggested by the history, evidence of dehydration, an elevated anion gap, and the presence of ketones in the serum or urine *without hyperglycemia*. β-hydroxybutyrate may not be detected unless specific tests are ordered as described previously (37). Lactate elevations are often mild and blood alcohol levels may be negative (50). Pancreatitis should be ruled out in patients complaining of abdominal pain (see Chapter 39: Acute Pancreatitis).

Management

The management of AKA is straightforward. An infusion of dextrose-containing IV fluids is all that is required to correct hypovolemia and acidosis while promoting renal clearance of ketones (50-51). The ketoacidosis typically resolves in <24 h. Other electrolyte disorders are corrected as needed (see Chapters 35-37).

References

1. Marino PL. Is tissue hypoxia a common cause of death? In: *Oxygen: Creating a New Paradigm*. Wolters Kluwer; 2021:39-54
2. Ferguson BS, Rogatzki MJ, Goodwin ML, et al. Lactate metabolism: historical context, prior misinterpretations, and current understanding. Europ J Appl Physiol 2018;118:691-728.
3. van Hall G, Strømstead M, Rasmussen P, et al. Blood lactate is an important energy source for the human brain. J Cereb Blood Flow Metab 2009;29:1121-9.
4. Sun S, Li H, Chen J, Qian Q. Lactic acid: no longer an inert and end-product of glycolysis. Physiology (Bethesda) 2017;32(6):453-63.
5. Robergs R, O'Malley B, Torrens S, Siegler J. The missing hydrogen ion, part 2: where the evidence leads to. Sports Med Health Sci 2024;6:94-100.
6. Robergs RA, Farzenah G, Parker D. Biochemistry of exercise-induced metabolic acidosis. Am J Physiol Regul Integr Comp Physiol 2004;287:R502-R516.
7. Dargent A, Wallet F, Friggeri A, et al. Lactic alkalosis in intensive care: a red flag? Crit Care 2023;27:184.
8. Blow O, Magliore L, Claridge JA, et al. The golden hour and the silver day: detection and correction of occult hypoperfusion

within 24 hours improves outcome from major trauma. J Trauma 1999;47(5):964-9.
9. Trzeciak S, Dellinger RP, Chansky ME, et al. Serum lactate as a predictor of mortality in patients with infection. Intensive Care Med 2007;33:970-7.
10. McNelis J, Marini CP, Jurkiewicz A, et al. Prolonged lactate clearance is associated with increased mortality in the surgical intensive care unit. Am J Surg 2001;182:481-5.
11. Casserly B, Phillips GS, Schorr C, et al. Lactate measurements in sepsis-induced tissue hypoperfusion: results from the Surviving Sepsis Campaign database. Crit Care Med 2015;43(3):567-73.
12. Zadorozny EV, Weigel T, Stone A, et al. Prehospital lactate is associated with the need for blood in trauma. Prehosp Emerg Care 2022;26(4):590-9.
13. Galvagno SM Jr, Sikorski RA, Floccare DJ, et al. Prehospital point of care testing for the early detection of shock and prediction of lifesaving interventions. Shock 2020;54(6):710-6.
14. Iberti TS, Liebowitz AB, Papadakos PJ, et al. Low sensitivity of the anion gap as a screen to detect hyperlactatemia in critically ill patients. Crit Care Med 1990;18:275-7.
15. Cohen RD, Woods HF. *Clinical and Biochemical Aspects of Lactic Acidosis*. Blackwell Scientific Publications; 1976.
16. Gore DC, Jahoor F, Hibbert JM, DeMaria EJ. Lactic acidosis during sepsis is related to increased pyruvate production, not deficits in tissue oxygen availability. Ann Surg 1996;224:97-102.
17. Fink MP. Cytopathic hypoxia. Crit Care Clin 2001;17:219-38.
18. Attaluri P, Castillo A, Edriss H, Nugent K. Thiamine deficiency: an important consideration in critically ill patients. Am J Med Sci 2018;356(4):382-90.
19. Campbell CH. The severe lacticacidosis of thiamine deficiency: acute, pernicious or fulminating beriberi. Lancet 1984;1:446-9.
20. Levy B. Use of pressors in the management of septic shock. Lancet 2007;370(9602):1827-8.
21. Mao Y, Dai D, Jin H, Wang Y. The risk factors of linezolid-induced lactic acidosis. Medicine 2018;97:36.
22. Kruse JA, Zaidi SAJ, Carlson RW. Significance of blood lactate levels in critically ill patients with liver disease. Am J Med 1987;83:77-82.
23. Mountain RD, Heffner JE, Brackett NC, Sahn SA. Acid-base disturbances in acute asthma. Chest 1990;98:651-5.
24. Lipka K, Bülow HH. Lactic acidosis following convulsions. Acta Anaesthesiol Scand 2003;47(5):616-8.
25. Friedenberg AS, Brandoff DE, Schiffman FJ. Type B lactic acidosis as a severe metabolic complication of lymphoma and leukemia: a case series from a single institution and literature review. Medicine (Baltimore) 2007;86:225-32.

26. Forsythe SM, Schmidt GA. Sodium bicarbonate for the treatment of lactic acidosis. Chest 2000;117:260-7.
27. Graf H, Arieff AI. The use of sodium bicarbonate in the therapy of organic acidoses. Intensive Care Med 1986;12:286-8.
28. Comroe JH. *Physiology of Respiration*. Yearbook Medical Publishers; 1974.
29. Rhee KY, Toro LO, McDonald GG, et al. Carbicarb, sodium bicarbonate, and sodium chloride in hypoxic lactic acidosis. Chest 1993;104:913-8.
30. Rose BD. *Clinical Physiology of Acid Base and Electrolyte Disorders*. 4th ed. McGraw Hill; 1994.
31. Sonnett J, Pagani FD, Baker LS, et al. Correction of intramyocardial hypercarbic acidosis with sodium bicarbonate. Circ Shock 1994;42:163-73.
32. Mehta PM, Kloner RA. Effects of acid base disturbance, septic shock, and calcium and phosphorous abnormalities on cardiovascular function. Crit Care Clin 1987;3:747-58.
33. Kimmoun A, Novy E, Auchet T, et al. Hemodynamic consequences of severe lactic acidosis in shock states: from bench to bedside. Crit Care 2015;19(1):175.
34. Boyd JH, Walley KR. Is there a role for sodium bicarbonate in treating lactic acidosis from shock? Curr Opin Crit Care 2008;14:379-83.
35. Radosevich MA, Wieruszewski PM, Wittwer ED. Tris-hydroxymethyl aminomethane in critically ill adults: a systematic review. Anesth Analg 2023;137(5):1007-18.
36. Cartwright MM, Hajja W, Al-Khatib S, et al. Toxigenic and metabolic causes of ketosis and ketoacidotic syndromes. Crit Care Clin 2012;601-31.
37. Plüdderman A, Hemeghan C, Price C, et al. Point-of-care blood test for ketones in patients with diabetes: primary care diagnostic technology update. Br J Clin Pract 2011;61:530-1.
38. Elendu C, David JA, Udoyen AO, et al. Comprehensive review of diabetic ketoacidosis: an update. Ann Med Surg (Lond) 2023; 85(6):2802-7.
39. American Diabetes Association. Hyperglycemic crisis in diabetes. Diabetes Care 2004;27(Suppl):S94-S102.
40. Long B, Lentz S, Koyfman A, Gottlieb M. Euglycemic diabetic ketoacidosis: etiologies, evaluation, and management. Am J Emerg Med 2021;44:157-160.
41. Gamblin GT, Ashburn RW, Kemp DG, Beuttel SC. Diabetic ketoacidosis presenting with a normal anion gap. Am J Med 1986;80: 758-60.
42. Slovis CM, Mork VG, Slovis RJ, Brain RP. Diabetic ketoacidosis and infection: leukocyte count and differential as early predictors of serious infection. Am J Emerg Med 1987;5:1-5.

43. AlMallah M, Zuberi O, Arida M, Kim HE. Positive troponin in diabetic ketoacidosis without evident acute coronary syndrome predicts adverse cardiac events. Clin Cardiol 2008;31:67-71.
44. Hillier TA, Abbott RD, Barrett EJ. Hyponatremia: evaluating the correction factor for hyperglycemia. Am J Med 1999;106:399-403.
45. Matz R. Calculating the anion gap in patients with DKA: use the measured or a corrected value? J Crit Illness 1999;14:535.
46. Ramanan M, Attokaran A, Murray L, et al. Sodium chloride or Plasmalyte-148 evaluation in severe diabetic ketoacidosis (SCOPE-DKA): a cluster, crossover, randomized, controlled trial. Intensive Care Med 2021;47:1248-57.
47. Self WH, Evans CS, Jenkins CA, et al. Clinical effects of balanced crystalloids vs saline in adults with diabetic ketoacidosis: a subgroup analysis of cluster randomized clinical trials. JAMA Netw Open 2020;3:e2024596.
48. Lowie BJ, Bond MC. Diabetic ketoacidosis. Emerg Med Clin N Am 2023;41:677-86.
49. Charfen MA, Fernandez-Frackelton M. Diabetic ketoacidosis. Emerg Med Clin N Am 2005;23:609-28.
50. Long B, Lentz S, Gottlieb M. Alcoholic ketoacidosis: etiologies, evaluation, and management. J Emerg Med 2021;61:658-65.
51. McGuire LC, Cruickshank AM, Munro PT. Alcoholic ketoacidosis. Emerg Med J 2006;23:417-20.

SECTION IX

RENAL & ELECTROLYTE DISORDERS

Chapter 33

Acute Kidney Injury

Acute kidney injury (AKI), affects as many as 60% of all ICU patients (1). Approximately 15% of ICU patients with AKI require renal replacement therapy (RRT) and as many as 60% of ICU patients who develop AKI do not survive (2-3). This chapter presents diagnostic criteria for AKI, followed by descriptions of inciting conditions, and concludes with a description of renal replacement therapies.

DIAGNOSTIC CRITERIA

The Kidney Disease Improving Global Outcomes (KDIGO) group has established diagnostic criteria for AKI, as shown in Table 33.1 (4).

TABLE 33.1 Diagnostic Criteria for Acute Kidney Injury

The diagnosis of acute kidney injury (AKI) requires <u>one of the following</u> conditions:

1. An increase in serum creatinine of ≥0.3 mg/dL (≥26.5 µmol/L) within 48 h.
2. An increase in serum creatinine to ≥1.5 times baseline within the previous 7 days.
3. Urine volume <0.5 mL/kg/hr (ideal body weight) for 6 h.

From Khwaja A. KDIGO clinical practice guidelines for acute kidney injury. Nephron Clin Pract 2012;120(4):c179-c184.

This definition combines prior definitions, including the Risk, Injury, Failure, Loss of kidney function, and End-stage kidney disease (RIFLE) score (5), providing greater parity and simplicity for clinical use (6).

Limitations

Limitations in the diagnostic criteria for AKI are the following (6):

1. Oliguria (i.e., urine output <0.5 mL/kg/hr) can be an appropriate physiological adjustment to decreased renal perfusion.
2. There is a lack of agreement about the minimum increase in serum creatinine required for the diagnosis of AKI.
3. The serum creatinine can be misleading (described in the section that follows).

Serum Creatinine

Creatinine is the traditional marker for glomerular filtration rate (GFR), but with the following limitations:

1. Creatinine in blood is derived from creatinine in muscle and is thus influenced by muscle mass and the rate of creatinine production in muscle. Critically ill patients lose about 2% of their muscle mass each day (7) and creatinine production is decreased in sepsis (8).
2. The serum creatinine level is influenced by changes in plasma volume.
3. Creatinine may not increase for 24-48 h following an insult (50% of renal function must be lost before serum creatinine increases).
4. Creatinine can increase without a true loss in function (i.e., hemoconcentration from diuresis, drug-induced inhibition of tubular secretion).

Popular formulas for estimating the GFR based on creatinine are shown in Figure 33.1.

Estimates of GFR based on serum creatinine consistently overestimate the true GFR in critically ill patients (9-10). This has important implications not only for assessing the presence and degree of AKI but also for the appropriate dosing of drugs based on GFR estimates.

Cockroft-Gault Formula

$$\text{GFR} = \frac{(140 - \text{Age}) \times \text{wt (kg)} \times (0.85 \text{ if Female})}{72 \times \text{Serum Creatinine (mg/dL)}} \text{ (mL/min)}$$

MDRD Formula

$$\text{GFR} = 186 \times \text{Serum Creatinine (mg/dL)}^{-1.154} \times \text{Age}^{-0.203} \times (0.74 \text{ if Female})$$

Units expressed as mL/min/1.73 m², where 1.73 m² is the body surface area of an adult who weighs 63 kg (139 lbs) and has a height of 1.7 m (5 ft, 6 in).

FIGURE 33.1. Popular formulas for estimating the glomerular filtration rate (GFR) based on the serum creatinine level. MDRD = Modification of Diet in Renal Disease. (From Acute Kidney Injury. In: Marino PL. *Marino's The ICU Book*. 5th ed. Wolters Kluwer; 2025:537-67. Figure 34.1.)

Biomarkers

Serum and urine biomarkers have advantages over serum creatinine and urine output in delineating the etiology, pathophysiology, anatomical site of injury, mechanisms, and severity of injury in AKI (11). Biomarkers indicating renal *function* (e.g., cystatin C, proenkephalin A), *stress* (e.g., Dickkopf-3, insulin-like growth binding protein 7), and *damage* (e.g., alanine aminopeptidase, CC-motif chemokine ligand 14) are becoming more widely available, though adoption has been slow, with no current consensus recommendations advocating routine use (11).

Chronic Kidney Disease

Chronic kidney disease (CKD) is defined by the presence of kidney damage (i.e., evidenced by biopsy, imaging findings, biomarkers, or urine studies) *or* decreased kidney function (i.e., decreased GFR) *for at least three months or greater* (12). In patients admitted to the ICU with a history of established

CKD, it is important to understand the stage of disease so patients with the most severe disease and greatest risk for progression and complications can be identified. CKD is staged according to GFR and levels of albuminuria (Table 33.2).

TABLE 33.2 Stages of Chronic Kidney Disease

GFR Stages	GFR (mL/min/1.73 m^2)	Terminology
G1	≥90	Normal or high
G2	60-89	Mildly decreased
G3a	45-59	Mildly to moderately decreased
G3b	30-44	Moderately to severely decreased
G4	15-29	Severely decreased
G5	<15	Kidney failure (add "D" if treated by dialysis)

Albuminuria Stages	Albumin Excretion Rate (mg/day)	Terminology
A1	>30	Normal to mildly increased
A2	30-300	Moderately increased
A3	>300	Severely increased*

CKD = chronic kidney disease. The etiology for CKD is not accounted for in this system.

*May be subdivided into nephrotic and non-nephrotic for risk prediction, differential diagnosis, and management.

From International Society of Nephrology. Chapter 1: definition and classification of CKD. Kidney Int Suppl (2011) 2013;3(1):19-62.

CAUSES OF ACUTE KIDNEY INJURY

The common causes of AKI are listed in Table 33.3.

Sepsis

Sepsis is the leading cause for AKI in ICU patients (13). The principal mechanism is inflammation, including oxidative injury that involves both the capillary endothelium in the glomerulus and the epithelial lining of the renal tubules (i.e., acute tubular necrosis [ATN]) (14).

TABLE 33.3 Common Causes of Acute Kidney Injury

Mechanism	Conditions
Inflammation	Major Surgery Multisystem Trauma Sepsis†
Hemodynamic Compromise	Cardiac Arrest Heart Failure Hemorrhage Increased Abdominal Pressure Liver Failure
Nephrotoxic	Radiocontrast Dye Rhabdomyolysis Nephrotoxic Drugs & Toxins

†The leading cause of acute kidney injury in the ICU.

From Acute Kidney Injury. In: Marino PL. *Marino's The ICU Book*. 5th ed. Wolters Kluwer; 2025:537-67. Table 34.2.

Other Inflammatory Causes

Multisystem trauma and major surgery are other conditions where AKI may be induced because of inflammation, although hemodynamic factors may also be involved, as discussed below. AKI has been reported in over 50% of patients after liver transplantation, in 18% of patients following cardiac surgery, and in 13% of patients undergoing major abdominal surgery (13).

Cardiorenal Syndrome

The association between heart failure and renal impairment is known as *cardiorenal syndrome* (15). See Chapter 19: Acute Heart Failure(s). AKI associated with heart failure has been attributed to both a *decrease in renal perfusion pressure* and an *increase in central venous pressure* (16). Venous congestion is more likely in cases of chronic, decompensated heart failure (17).

Hypotension

Flow through the glomerulus is determined by the difference between the mean arterial pressure and the renal venous pressure (Pā – Pv). This is known as the *glomerular filtration pressure*. The net filtration pressure across the glomerulus (i.e., the *filtration gradient*), is the difference between the glomerular filtration pressure and the pressure in the proximal renal tubules (P_{PT}), as shown in the following equation:

$$\text{Filtration Gradient} = (P\bar{a} - Pv) - P_{PT} \quad (33.1)$$

These relationships predict that *GFR will decrease with conditions that cause a decrease in mean arterial pressure* (i.e., hypovolemia, hemorrhage, sepsis, or heart failure, as discussed in Chapters 16-19). GFR will also decrease when there is an *increase in venous pressure* (discussed below) or an *increase in pressure in the proximal tubules* (Figure 33.2).

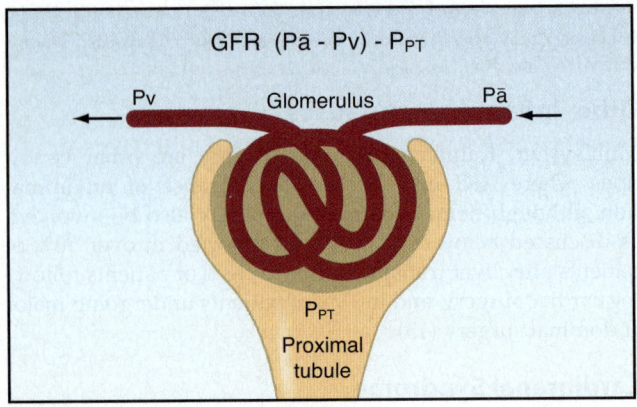

FIGURE 33.2. Schematic depiction of the pressures that influence the glomerular filtration rate (GFR). Pā = mean arterial pressure, Pv = venous pressure, P_{PT} = pressure in the proximal tubules. (From Acute Kidney Injury. In: Marino PL. *Marino's The ICU Book*. 5th ed. Wolters Kluwer; 2025:537-67. Figure 34.2.)

Abdominal Compartment Syndrome

Abdominal compartment syndrome (ACS) is defined as an increase in intra-abdominal pressure (IAP) (>20 mm Hg) that is associated with new organ dysfunction (18). *ACS is often overlooked as a cause of AKI in ICU patients* (19). When the IAP is increased, the pressure in the proximal tubules becomes equivalent, thus preventing blood flow to the kidney. The pressure equalization between the IAP and proximal tubules may explain why *oliguria is one of the first signs of ACS*. Another common and under-recognized cause of increased IAP is excessive crystalloid resuscitation, which can raise the IAP by promoting edema in the abdominal organs, especially the bowel.

Hepatorenal Syndrome

AKI has been reported in 50% of patients with end-stage liver disease (20). AKI in this setting can be the result of hypovolemia or sepsis, or as the result of the hepatorenal syndrome (HRS), a condition caused by diversion of blood flow away from the kidneys due to a combination of renal vasoconstriction and splanchnic vasodilation (21). *In any patient with end-stage liver disease and AKI, HRS should be suspected if no other cause of AKI is apparent.* Diagnostic criteria for HRS are listed in Table 33.4. The prognosis for HRS is poor, with liver transplantation being the definitive treatment.

Nephrotoxins

A variety of drugs can precipitate AKI, as shown in Table 33.5.

Radiocontrast Dye

Iodinated contrast agents have long been perceived as a cause of AKI in critically ill patients, but more recent studies have revealed that these agents *do not increase the incidence of AKI in critically ill patients* (24). Furthermore, iodinated contrast agents do not worsen renal function in patients with pre-existing AKI (25), though use is considered risky in patients with CKD and a GFR <30 mL/min/1.73 m² (26).

TABLE 33.4 Diagnostic Criteria for Hepatorenal Syndrome

Clinical Parameter	Comment
Known cirrhosis with ascites	Ascites is diagnosed with a combination of the physical exam and imaging (usually abdominal ultrasound).
Acute Kidney Injury (AKI)	Any increase in serum creatinine by ≥0.3 mg/dL within 48 h or any increase in creatinine >1.5 times baseline. Urine output criteria is not used because urine volume is often low in patients with cirrhosis and ascites.
No alternative causes for AKI	• No shock. • No nephrotoxic drugs. • No proteinuria or hematuria. • Normal renal ultrasound findings. • Lack of improvement in renal function following a trial of two days of volume expansion with IV 25% albumin (1 g/kg of body weight per day up to 100 g/day, given once or twice daily in divided doses), *without* the addition of diuretics.

From Angeli P, Gines P, Wong F, et al. Diagnosis and management of acute kidney injury in patients with cirrhosis: revised consensus recommendations of the International Club of Ascites. Gut 2015;64(4):531-7.

Prevention. Despite favorable data regarding radiocontrast agents, current consensus statements recommend the following for *prevention* of worsening renal function (26):

1. Prophylactic 0.9% saline infusions are recommended for radiocontrast dye injections in patients with AKI, or in patients with an estimated GFR <30 mL/min/1.73 m^2. This recommendation does not necessarily apply to patients with heart failure.
2. The infusion should begin 1 h prior to the radiographic study and should continue for 3-12 h after the study. There is no firm recommendation regarding the amount of volume to be infused.

TABLE 33.5 Drugs Most Often Implicated in Acute Kidney Injury

Mechanism	Offending Drugs
Altered Renal Hemodynamics	*Most Cited:* Nonsteroidal antiinflammatory agents (NSAIDs) *Others:* ACE inhibitors, angiotensin receptor blockers, cyclosporine, tacrolimus
Osmotic Nephropathy	*Most Cited:* Hydroxyethyl starches *Others:* Mannitol, IV immunoglobulins
Renal Tubular Injury	*Most Cited:* Aminoglycosides *Others:* Amphotericin B, antiretrovirals, cisplatin
Interstitial Nephritis	*Most Cited:* Antimicrobials (penicillins, cephalosporins, sulfonamides, vancomycin, macrolides) *Others:* Anticonvulsants (phenytoin, valproic acid), H$_2$ blockers, NSAIDs, proton pump inhibitors

From Bentley ML, Corwin HL, Dasta J. Drug-induced acute kidney injury in the critically ill adult: recognition and prevention strategies. Crit Care Med 2010;38(Suppl 6):S169-74.

Rhabdomyolysis

Release of myoglobin from injured muscle (i.e., rhabdomyolysis) can damage renal tubular epithelial cells and cause AKI (27). Rhabdomyolysis is diagnosed using the criteria in Table 33.6.

TABLE 33.6 Diagnostic Criteria for Rhabdomyolysis

Triggering factors (trauma, crush injury, compartment syndrome, heat injury [i.e., heat stroke], prolonged immobilization, extreme exertion, intoxication)
OR
Symptoms and signs to include muscle weakness and dark-colored urine
OR
Urinalysis demonstrating myoglobinuria (presence of <3 red blood cells per high powered field on microscopic examination or a urine myoglobin level >20 µg/L)
AND
Marked elevation of the serum creatinine kinase (i.e., typically >5,000 U/L)

Derived from Zimmerman JL, Shen MC. Rhabdomyolysis. Chest 2013;144:1058-65 and Huerta-Alardín AL, Varon J, Marik PE. Bench-to-bedside review: Rhabdomyolysis—an overview for clinicians. Crit Care 2005;9(2):158-69.

Management

The following measures are recommended to prevent or limit myoglobinuric renal injury (27-29):

1. Volume resuscitation to promote renal tubular flow is the most effective measure for preventing or limiting myoglobin nephrotoxicity. A 0.9% saline can be given in a volume of 10-20 mL/kg initially, and then infused to maintain a urine output of at least 1 mg/kg/hr. This strategy should be abandoned if oliguria persists as fluid overload will ensue (30-32).
2. Increasing the urine pH >6.5 may potentially prevent heme-protein (i.e. Tamm-Horsfall protein) and uric acid precipitation, intratubular cast formation, and the release of free iron from myoglobin. This can be accomplished by infusing 1 L of 0.9% saline alternating with 1 L of 0.45% saline + 50 mEq sodium bicarbonate at a high infusion rate (500 mL/hr). The benefits of this approach remain unproven (30-31).
3. Diuresis with mannitol or furosemide has been used to promote renal tubular flow, but diuresis is risky and counterproductive to the planned fluid resuscitation (32).

Data supporting alkaline diuresis and/or prophylactic mannitol for the prevention of renal failure, mortality, or the need for dialysis for the treatment of rhabdomyolysis are lacking. As many as 30% of patients with rhabdomyolysis will require RRT (33).

DIAGNOSTIC CONSIDERATIONS

Ultrasound

Point-of-care ultrasound (POCUS) can be helpful for detecting evidence for CKD (i.e., unusually small kidneys) and for identifying post-renal obstruction (i.e., hydronephrosis).

Renal Indices

Table 33.7 lists urinary tests that can help determine if the source of AKI is renal hypoperfusion or renal tubular injury (34).

TABLE 33.7 Urinary Indices for the Evaluation of AKI

Measure	Renal Hypoperfusion	Renal Tubular Injury
Spot Urine Sodium	<20 mEq/L	>40 mEq/L
Fractional Excretion of Sodium	<1%	>12%
Fractional Excretion of Urea	<35%	>50%
Urine Osmolality	>500 mOsm/kg	300-400 mOsm/kg
U/P Osmolality	>1.5	1-1.3

U/P = urine-to-plasma ratio.

From Acute Kidney Injury. In: Marino PL. *Marino's The ICU Book*. 5th ed. Wolters Kluwer; 2025:537-67. Table 34.2.

Each of these indices has limitations and urinary biomarkers are likely to supersede these measures soon (10-11).

Urine Sodium

The "spot" urine sodium is *low* (<20 mEq/L) in conditions where sodium reabsorption occurs (i.e., hypovolemia) and *high* (>40 mEq/L) when renal tubular injury is present, which results in impaired sodium reabsorption and increased urinary sodium losses. The urine sodium can be *paradoxically high* in states of hypovolemia if there is ongoing diuretic therapy or if the patient has chronic renal disease.

Fractional Excretion of Sodium

The fractional excretion of sodium (FENa) is considered a more accurate measure of renal tubular function than the spot urine sodium. The FENa is expressed by the following equation:

$$\text{FENa (\%)} = \frac{U/P\,[Na]}{U/P\,[Cr]} \qquad (33.2)$$

where U/P is the urine-to-plasma ratio for sodium and creatinine concentrations. In conditions associated with renal hypoperfusion, the FENa is <1% reflecting *sodium conservation*; when tubular injury is present the FENa is typically >2% reflecting an *increase in urinary sodium excretion*. The FENa, like the spot urine sodium, can be elevated (>1%) in diuretic therapy and chronic renal insufficiency. The FENa can also be falsely *low* (<1%) in patients with acute tubular injury from sepsis or in rhabdomyolysis (36).

Fractional Excretion of Urea

The fractional excretion of urea (FEUrea) is conceptionally similar to the FENa, and is expressed by the following equation:

$$\text{FEU (\%)} = \frac{U/P\,[Urea]}{U/P\,[Cr]} \qquad (33.3)$$

Where U/P is the urine-to-plasma ratio for urea and creatinine concentrations, the FEUrea is *low* (<35%) with renal hypoperfusion, and *high* (>50%) with renal tubular injury. The FEUrea is not affected by diuretics (37), which is the major advantage over the FENa, although the FEUrea is not superior to the FENa for differentiating intrinsic from prerenal AKI (34).

MANAGEMENT

General Considerations

Fluid Challenge

An initial intervention for patients with AKI is a volume challenge, usually with 500 mL of a crystalloid fluid infused over 10-15 minutes (the *rate* of infusion is more important than the *volume*). This intervention may help rule out renal hypoperfusion as a contributing factor (see Chapter 11: Fluid Management).

Diuretics

A trial of intravenous furosemide is a reasonable intervention to mitigate fluid accumulation in AKI, *but diuretics should never be given to increase urine output if renal hypoperfusion is a contributing factor*. A positive response to furosemide does *not* improve renal function (38).

Low-Dose Dopamine

Dopamine can promote renal vasodilation at low doses (2 µg/kg/min), but the use of low-dose dopamine is *not recommended* because it does not improve renal function and may decrease splanchnic perfusion (39).

Renal Replacement Therapy

About 15% of ICU patients receive renal replacement therapy (RRT) for management of AKI (2). The usual indications include: (a) severe acidosis, (b) symptomatic uremia (e.g., encephalopathy or uremic pericarditis), (c) volume overload, (d) life-threatening, refractory hyperkalemia, and (e) removal of toxins (40-43). There are several RRT techniques available as depicted in Figure 33.3. An in-depth discussion about RRT is beyond the scope of this text, and the descriptions that follow are limited to an overview of hemodialysis and hemofiltration. References are provided for more detailed

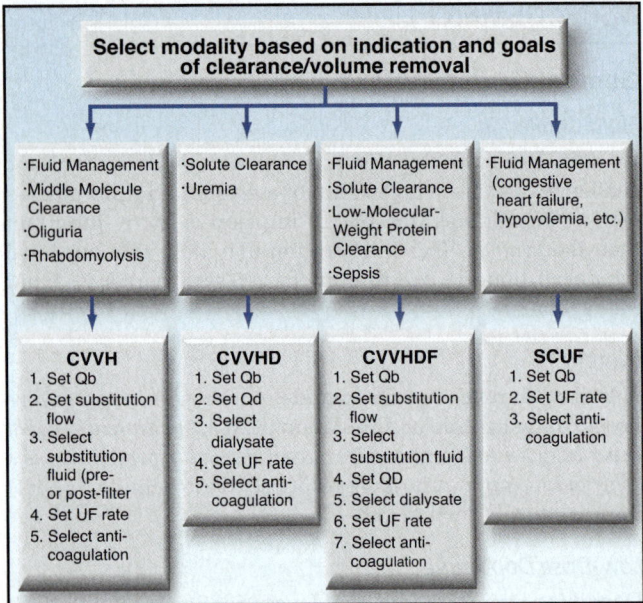

FIGURE 33.3. Techniques, indications, and suggested initial settings for RRT modalities used in the ICU. CVVH = continuous venovenous hemofiltration, CVVHD = continuous venovenous hemodialysis, CVVHDF = continuous venovenous hemodiafiltration, SCUF = slow continuous ultrafiltration, Qb = blood flow rate, QD = dialysate flow rate, UF = ultrafiltration. (From Galvagno SM Jr, Hong CM, Lissauer ME, et al. Practical considerations for the dosing and adjustment of continuous renal replacement therapy in the intensive care unit. J Crit Care 2013;28[6]:1019-26.)

descriptions of how to select and adjust RRT in the ICU (40-43).

The mechanism of fluid and solute removal by each of the RRT techniques is shown in Figure 33.4.

Intravenous Access

Large-bore, central venous catheters like the one in Figure 33.5 are required for hemodialysis in the ICU.

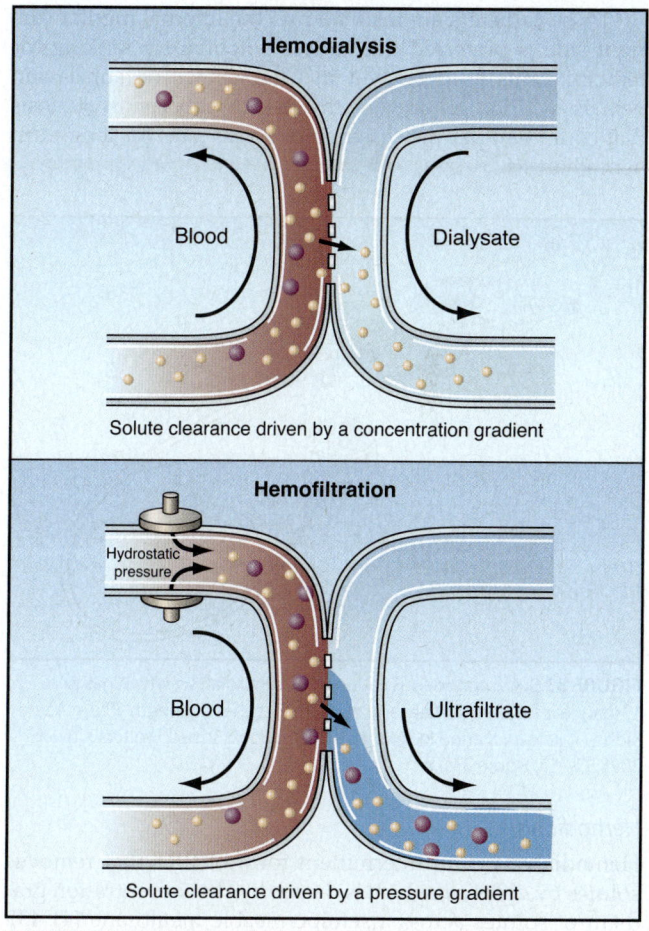

FIGURE 33.4. Mechanisms of solute clearance by hemodialysis and hemofiltration. The smaller particles represent small solutes (e.g., urea), which can be cleared by both techniques, while the larger particles represent larger solutes (e.g., toxins) that can be cleared by hemofiltration, but not by hemodialysis. (From Acute Kidney Injury. In: Marino PL. *Marino's The ICU Book*. 5th ed. Wolters Kluwer; 2025:537-67. Figure 34.4.)

These catheters are inserted into the internal jugular (the right side is preferred due to less potential for kinking) or femoral veins as described in Chapter 1. The subclavian vein is avoided to prevent the risk of subclavian stenosis that could hamper the selection of access sites for long-term hemodialysis.

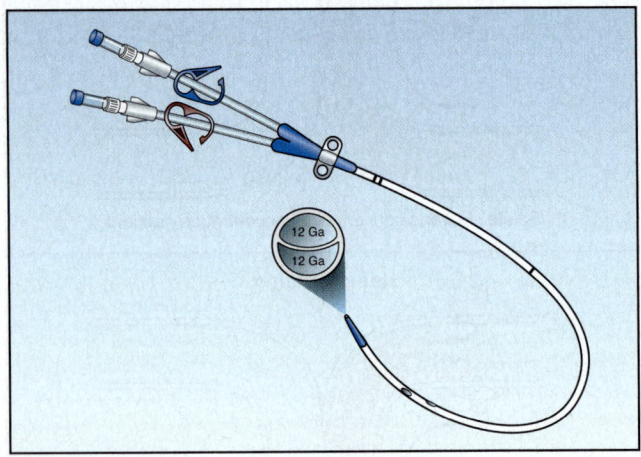

FIGURE 33.5. Central venous catheter for hemodialysis, which has two 12-gauge infusion channels, and is 20 cm (8 inches) in length. (From Acute Kidney Injury. In: Marino PL. *Marino's The ICU Book*. 5th ed. Wolters Kluwer; 2025:537-67. Figure 34.5.)

Hemodialysis

Hemodialysis is an intermittent form of RRT that removes solutes by *diffusion*, which is driven by the concentration gradient of solutes across a semipermeable membrane (41-43). To maintain the concentration gradient, *countercurrent exchange* is used, where blood and dialysis fluid are driven in opposite directions across the dialysis machine. A blood pump is used to move blood in one direction at a rate (Qb) of 200-300 mL/min, while the dialysis fluid on the other side of the membrane moves at a higher rate (QD=500-800 mL/min).

Advantages. The principal benefit of hemodialysis is rapid clearance of small solutes. Only a few hours are required to remove life-threatening concentrations of potassium or nitrogenous waste. Each session lasts about 4 h, and 2-3 liters of fluid can be removed per session.

Disadvantages. Fluid removal is limited (up to 3 L/h) and hypotension is possible in patients who are hemodynamically unstable. Intracranial pressure increase during intermittent RRT can cause *dialysis disequilibrium syndrome*, a rare but potentially life-threatening disorder, with mortality rates as high as 65% (44). This complication can be avoided by using continuous RRT modalities, as listed in Figure 33.3.

Hemofiltration

Hemofiltration removes solutes by convection, where a hydrostatic pressure gradient is established to move a solute-containing fluid across a semipermeable membrane. The bulk movement of fluid "drags" the solute across the membrane (i.e., *solvent drag*) (41-43). Hemofiltration can remove large volumes of fluid (up to 3 L/h), but the rate of small solute clearance is much slower than during hemodialysis. Thus, hemofiltration must be performed continuously (Continuous Renal Replacement Therapy [RRT]) to provide effective solute clearance.

Advantages. Continuous venovenous hemofiltration (CVVH) is the most popular hemofiltration method. The advantages of CVVH include the following: (a) improved tolerance in hemodynamically unstable patients, (b) the ability to remove large volumes of fluid, and (c) the ability to remove drugs and toxins (40-43). CVVH, when used with specialized filters, also has the potential to remove inflammatory cytokines and other mediators from the blood, although such *blood purification* methods have yet to demonstrate a definitive clinical advantage (45-46).

Disadvantages. The major disadvantage of hemofiltration is the slow removal of small solutes, which is not well-suited for clearing nitrogenous waste or for life-threatening hyperkalemia. CRRT modalities are also more labor-intensive for nursing staff and potentially more expensive, although some studies have shown that there is an economic rationale for using CRRT preferentially for ICU patients with AKI and fluid overload (47).

References

1. Hoste EA, Bagshaw SM, Bellomo R, et al. Epidemiology of acute kidney injury in critically ill patients: the multinational AKI-EPI study. Intensive Care Med 2015;41:1411-23.
2. Bellomo R, Baldwin I, Ronco C, Kellum JA. ICU-based renal replacement therapy. Crit Care Med 2021;49:406-18.
3. Verma S, Kellum JA. Defining acute kidney injury. Crit Care Clin 2021;37:251-66.
4. Khwaja A. KDIGO clinical practice guidelines for acute kidney injury. Nephron Clin Pract 2012;120(4):c179-c184.
5. Bellomo R, Ronco C, Kellum JA, et al. for the Acute Dialysis Quality Initiative workgroup. Acute renal failure-definition, outcome measures, animal models, fluid therapy and information technology needs: the Second International Consensus Conference of the Acute Dialysis Quality Initiative (ADQI) Group. Crit Care 2004; 8(4):R204-R212.
6. Lopes JA, Jorge S. The RIFLE and AKIN classifications for acute kidney injury: a critical and comprehensive review. Clin Kidney J 2013; 6(1):8-14.
7. Puthucheary ZA, Rawal J, McPhail M, et al. Acute skeletal muscle wasting in critical illness. JAMA 2013;310:1591-600.
8. Doi K, Yuen PS, Eisner C, et al. Reduced production of creatinine limits its use as a marker of kidney injury in sepsis. J Am Soc Nephrol 2009;20:1217-21.
9. Sangla F, Marti PE, Verissimo T, et al. Measured and estimated glomerular filtration rate in the ICU: a prospective study. Crit Care Med 2020;48:e1232-41.
10. Ravn B, Rimes-Stigare C, Bell M, et al. Creatinine versus cystatin C based glomerular filtration rate in critically ill patients. J Crit Care 2019;52:136-40.
11. Ostermann M, Legrand M, Meersch M, et al. Biomarkers in acute kidney injury. Ann Intensive Care 2024;14(1):145.
12. International Society of Nephrology. Chapter 1: Definition and classification of CKD. Kidney Int, Suppl (2011) 2013;3(1):19-62.
13. Kellum JA, Prowle R. Paradigms of acute kidney injury in the intensive care setting. Nat Rev Nephrol 2018;4:217-30.

14. Wang Z, Holthoff JH, Seely KA, et al. Development of oxidative stress in the peritubular capillary microenvironment mediates sepsis-induced renal microcirculatory failure and acute kidney injury. Am J Pathol 2012;180:505-16.
15. Ajibowo AO, Okobi OE, Emore E, et al. Cardiorenal syndrome:a literature review. Cureus 2023;15(7):e41252.
16. Damman K, van Deursen VM, Navis G, et al. Increased central venous pressure is associated with renal dysfunction and mortality in a broad spectrum of patients with cardiovascular disease. J Am Coll Cardiol 2009;53:582-8.
17. Mullens W, Abrahams Z, Francis GS, et al. Importance of venous congestion for worsening of renal function in advanced decompensated heart failure. J Am Coll Cardiol 2009;53:589-96.
18. Malbrain ML, Cheatham ML, Kirkpatrick A, et al. Results from the international conference of experts on intra-abdominal hypertension and abdominal compartment syndrome. I. definitions. Intensive Care Med 2006;32(11):1722-32.
19. Copur S, Berkkan M, Hasbal NB, et al. Abdominal compartment syndrome: an often overlooked cause of acute kidney injury. J Nephrol 2022;35:1595-1603.
20. Tandon P, James MT, Abraides JG, et al. Relevance of new definitions to incidence and prognosis of acute kidney injury in hospitalized patients with cirrhosis: a retrospective, population-based cohort study. PLoS One 2016;11:e0160394.
21. Kemichian S, Francoz C, Durans S, et al. Hepatorenal syndrome. Crit Care Clin 2021;37:321-34.
22. Angeli P, Gines P, Wong F, et al. Diagnosis and management of acute kidney injury in patients with cirrhosis: revised consensus recommendations of the International Club of Ascites. Gut 2015;64(4):531-7.
23. Bentley ML, Corwin HL, Dasta J. Drug-induced acute kidney injury in the critically ill adult: recognition and prevention strategies. Crit Care Med 2010;38(Suppl 6):S169-74.
24. Ehrmann S, Quartin A, Hobbs BP, et al. Contrast-associated acute kidney injury in the critically ill: systematic review with bayesian meta-analysis. Intensive Care Med 2017;43:785-94.
25. Ehmann MR. Mitchell J, Levin S, et al. Renal outcomes following intravenous contrast administration in patients with acute kidney injury: a multi-site retrospective propensity-adjusted analysis. Intensive Care Med 2023;49:205-15.
26. Davenport MS, Perazella MA, Yee J, et al. Use of intravenous iodinated contrast media in patients with kidney disease: consensus statements from the American College of Radiology and the National Kidney Foundation. Radiology 2020;294:660-8.
27. Zimmerman JL, Shen MC. Rhabdomyolysis. Chest 2013; 144:1058-65.

28. Huerta-Alardín AL, Varon J, Marik PE. Bench-to-bedside review: Rhabdomyolysis—an overview for clinicians. Crit Care 2005;9(2):158-69.
29. Petejova N, Martinek A. Acute kidney injury due to rhabdomyolysis and renal replacement therapy: a critical review. Crit Care 2014;18:224.
30. Scharman EJ, Troutman WG. Prevention of kidney injury following rhabdomyolysis: a systematic review. Ann Pharmacother 2013; 47(1):90-105.
31. Zager RA. Rhabdomyolysis and myohemoglobinuric acute renal failure. Kidney Int 1996;49(2):314-26.
32. Sever MS, Vanholder R; RDRTF of ISN Work Group on Recommendations for the Management of Crush Victims in Mass Disasters. Recommendation for the management of crush victims in mass disasters. Nephrol Dial Transplant 2012;27 Suppl 1:i1-i67.
33. Sharp LS, Rozycki GS, Feliciano DV. Rhabdomyolysis and secondary renal failure in critically ill surgical patients. Am J Surg 2004; 188:801-6.
34. Abdelhafez MO, Alhroob AA, Abu Hawilla MO, et al. Utility of fractional excretion of urea in acute kidney injury with comparison to fractional excretion of sodium: a systematic review and meta-analysis. Am J Med Sci 2024;368(3):224-34.
35. Steiner RW. Interpreting the fractional excretion of sodium. Am J Med 1984;77:699-702.
36. Seethapathy H, Fenves AZ. Fractional excretion of sodium (FENa): an imperfect tool for a flawed question. Clin J Am Soc Nephrol 2022;17(8):1218.
37. Gottfried J, Wiesen J, Raina R, Nally JV Jr. Finding the cause of acute kidney injury: which index of fractional excretion is better? Clev Clin J Med 2012;79:121-6.
38. van der Voort PH, Boerma EC, Koopmans M, et al. Furosemide does not improve renal recovery after hemofiltration for acute renal failure in critically ill patients: a double blind randomized controlled trial. Crit Care Med 2009;37:533-8.
39. Holmes CL, Walley KR. Bad medicine: low-dose dopamine in the ICU. Chest 2003;123:1266-75.
40. Bagshaw SM, Wald R. Starting kidney replacement therapy in critically ill patients with acute kidney injury. Crit Care Clin 2021;37:409-32.
41. Galvagno SM Jr, Hong CM, Lissauer ME, et al. Practical considerations for the dosing and adjustment of continuous renal replacement therapy in the intensive care unit. J Crit Care 2013;28(6):1019-26.
42. Teixeira JP, Neyra JA, Tolwani A. Continuous KRT: a contemporary review. Clin J Am Soc Nephrol 2023;18(2):256-69.
43. Tolwani A. Continuous renal-replacement therapy for acute kidney injury. N Engl J Med 2012;367(26):2505-14.

44. Parsons AD, Sanscrainte C, Leone A, et al. Dialysis disequilibrium syndrome and intracranial pressure fluctuations in neurosurgical patients undergoing renal replacement therapy: systematic review and pooled analysis. World Neurosurg 2023;170:2-6.
45. O'Reilly P, Tolwani A. Renal replacement therapy III. IHD, CRRT, SLED. Crit Care Clin 2005;21:367-78.
46. Honore PM, Blackman S, Perriens E, et al. Adsorptive therapies in sepsis and inflammation: description of the various adsorptive techniques and their failure to improve outcomes. Rev Invest Clin 2023;75(6):359-76.
47. Ethgen O, Murugan R, Echeverri J, et al. Economic analysis of renal replacement therapy modality in acute kidney injury patients with fluid overload. Crit Care Explor 2023;5(6):e0921.

Sodium and Chloride
Chapter 34

This chapter describes the forces that determine the distribution of total body water, and the importance of sodium in determining these forces, followed by an organized approach for managing disorders of sodium and chloride.

OSMOTIC ACTIVITY

Tonicity

The *effective osmotic activity*, or the *osmotic pressure*, is the force that drives the movement of water between fluid compartments (1). The osmotic activity between two fluid compartments is expressed as tonicity. If the osmotic activity in the two compartments is equal, the fluids are described as *isotonic* (see the left panel of Figure 34.1), and if the osmotic activity differs, the fluid with the higher osmotic activity is described as *hypertonic* and the fluid with the lower osmotic activity is described as *hypotonic* (see the right panel of Figure 34.1).

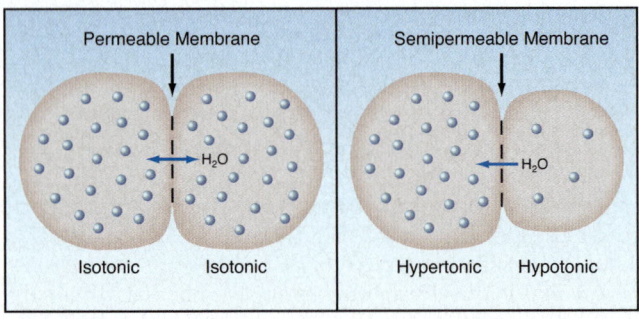

FIGURE 34.1. Illustration of the relationship between osmotic activity and water movement between fluid compartments. (From Sodium. In: Marino PL. *Marino's The ICU Book*. 5th ed. Wolters Kluwer; 2025:552-67. Figure 35.1.)

When the extracellular fluid is *hypertonic*, water moves *out* of cells. When the extracellular fluid is *hypotonic*, water moves *into* cells.

Units of Osmotic Activity

Osmotic activity per volume of *water* is called osmolality and is expressed as mOsm/kg H_2O or mOsm/kg. Plasma is mostly water (95%), so the osmotic activity in plasma is typically expressed as *osmolality*, not *osmolarity* (osmolarity is expressed as osmotic activity per volume of *solution*).

Plasma Osmolality

Normal plasma osmolality is 285-295 (290 ± 5) mOsm/kg H_2O (1-2). Plasma osmolality can be measured or calculated. When measured, the *freezing point depression method* is the "gold standard" test used in laboratories. Plasma osmolality can also be calculated when the concentrations of electrolytes are known using the following equation:

$$Posm = 2 \times Na + \frac{glucose}{18} + \frac{BUN}{2.8} \tag{34.1}$$

where Posm is the plasma osmolality in mOsm/kg/H_2O, Na is the plasma sodium concentration in mEq/L, glucose and BUN are the plasma glucose and urea concentrations in mg/dL, and the factors 18 and 2.8 are the molecular weights of glucose and urea divided by 10, respectively, which converts their concentrations to mOsm/kg/H_2O. The sodium concentration is doubled to account for the negative ions (chloride) that electrically balance sodium. More advanced equations exist that account for all components contributing to osmolality (thereby approximating the calculated osmolality more accurately), but in practice, Equation 34.1 is simple, accurate, and uses serum values that are readily available (2-3).

Importance of Sodium

Sodium is responsible for 98% of the effective plasma osmolality. *The principal factor that determines the distribution of total body water in the intracellular and extracellular fluid compartments is the sodium concentration in extracellular fluid* (plasma).

HYPERNATREMIA

Hypernatremia is defined as a plasma sodium concentration >145 mEq/L. Hypernatremia is a common electrolyte disorder, affecting as many as 25% of ICU patients (4). An approach to diagnosis and management of hypernatremia based on extracellular volume (ECV) is outlined in Figure 34.2.

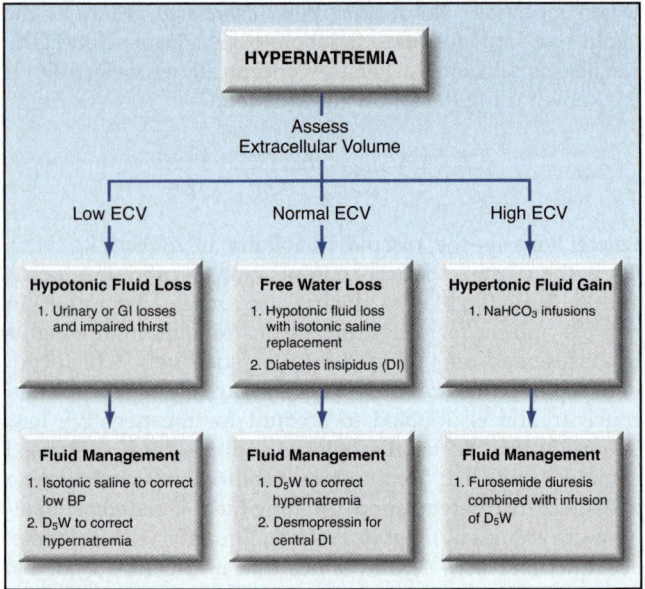

FIGURE 34.2. Flow diagram for hypernatremia based on the extracellular volume (ECV). (From Sodium. In: Marino PL. *Marino's The ICU Book*. 5th ed. Wolters Kluwer; 2025:552-67. Figure 35.2.)

Hypovolemic Hypernatremia

Hypernatremia associated with a low ECV is due to fluid loss that is hypotonic to plasma. The average sodium concentration in fluids that can be lost during an ICU stay is shown in Table 34.1.

Common sources of hypotonic fluid loss in the ICU include diarrhea, vomiting, excessive gastric suctioning, and urinary losses from diuretics or glycosuria.

TABLE 34.1 Average Sodium Concentration in Select Fluids

Normal	Na (mEq/L)	Other	Na (mEq/L)
Gastric Secretions	60	Diuretic Urine	80
Stool	25	Ileostomy Drainage	125
Urine	<10	Inflammatory Diarrhea	75
Sweat	65	Secretory Diarrhea	90

Derived from Gennari FJ, Weise WJ. Acid-base disturbances in gastrointestinal disease. Clin J Am Soc Nephrol 2008;3:1861-8 and Bates GP, Miller VS. Sweat rate and sodium loss during work in the heat. J Occup Med Toxicol 2008;3:4.

Complications

Hypernatremia increases the osmolality of the extracellular fluid, which draws water out of cells and decreases cell volumes; this effect is most prominent in the brain. Acute hypernatremia can cause encephalopathy that can present with lethargy, cognitive impairment, delirium, seizures, and even coma (4). Hypotonic fluid loss only causes hypotension when the fluid losses are severe, because the loss of hypotonic fluids increases the osmotic pressure in plasma, which draws fluid from the interstitial space into the plasma to help maintain intravascular volume (5-6).

Management

Isotonic saline is used to correct hypotension (if fluid losses are severe) but not to correct the hypernatremia (7). Infusion of 5% dextrose in water (D_5W), or the addition of water to enteral tube feeds (e.g., 200 mL every 8 h) can be used. Because hypotonic fluid loss also results in the loss of sodium, 0.45% saline may be more appropriate than D_5W. The optimal rate of correction is not known, but the traditional recommendation has been to *limit the rate of correction to <0.5 mEq/L/h* (faster correction rates have been used safely, without causing cerebral edema) (8).

Normovolemic Hypernatremia

Hypernatremia in the setting of a normal ECV is usually the result of water loss without significant sodium loss. This condition occurs frequently in the ICU when the replacement fluid is hypertonic to the fluid that is lost.

Diabetes Insipidus

Diabetes insipidus (DI) is a disorder of renal water conservation and is characterized by loss of urine that is largely devoid of solute (9). *The underlying problem in DI is loss of the effect of the antidiuretic hormone (ADH)*, which is released by the posterior pituitary gland, and promotes water reabsorption in the distal renal tubules. There are three types of DI:

1. *Central DI* is caused by failure of the posterior pituitary to release ADH. Central DI occurs after surgical resection of pituitary tumors, traumatic brain injury, subarachnoid hemorrhage, and autoimmune diseases (9).
2. *Nephrogenic DI* is characterized by impaired renal responsiveness to ADH. Causes in ICU patients include drugs (e.g., amphotericin, aminoglycosides, lithium) and hypokalemia (10). Nephrogenic DI may also occur during recovery phase for acute tubular necrosis (ATN).
3. *Gestational DI* is the result of an enzyme that is produced by the placenta, inactivating ADH. DI usually manifests in this condition near the end of the second or in the beginning of the third trimester (11).

Diagnosis. The hallmark of DI is dilute (*hypotonic*) urine with *hypertonic* plasma (i.e., hypernatremia and plasma osmolality >300 mOsm/L). Urine output is typically >50 mL/kg/24 h (>3 L in 24 h). In central DI, the urine osmolality is often below 200 mOsm/L, whereas in nephrogenic DI, the urine osmolality is higher (200-500 mOsm/L) (12). The diagnosis of DI is based on the response of the urine osmolality to fluid restriction. Failure of the urine osmolality to rise by >30 mOsm/L in the first few hours of complete fluid restriction will identify a case of DI. The response to vasopressin can then differentiate central from nephrogenic DI (i.e., in central DI, the urine osmolality *increases* ≥50% after vasopressin; the urine osmolality is *unchanged* after vasopressin administration in nephrogenic DI).

Management. Desmopressin, a synthetic analog of vasopressin, is the drug of choice for *central* DI. The parenteral route is recommended in ICU patients as only 5% of the drug is absorbed from the GI tract (13). The initial parenteral dose of desmopressin is 1 µg by subcutaneous injection every 12 h, or 2 µg by IV injection every 12 h (12-13). For *nephrogenic* DI, removal of the offending drug is the initial recommended action. Nonsteroidal anti-inflammatory drugs (NSAIDs) can increase renal responsiveness to ADH in nephrogenic DI because NSAIDs inhibit prostaglandins, which block the actions of ADH. Indomethacin (2 mg/kg/day) has been described as effective in pediatric populations (14).

Hypervolemic Hypernatremia

Hypernatremia with a high ECV can be the result of bicarbonate infusions but is more frequently associated with excessive infusions of isotonic saline.

Management

In patients with normal renal function, excess sodium and water are excreted rapidly. When renal sodium excretion is impaired, a diuretic (i.e., furosemide) may be necessary, but diuresis should be accompanied by an infusion of D_5W because the urinary sodium concentration during furosemide diuresis (~80 mEq/L) is less than the plasma sodium concentration, thereby potentially aggravating the hypernatremia.

HYPONATREMIA

Hyponatremia (plasma sodium <135 mEq/L) is considered the most common electrolyte abnormality in clinical practice (15). Figure 34.3 depicts a diagnostic approach to hyponatremia, using urine osmolality and urine sodium.

Pseudohyponatremia

A spurious decrease in measured plasma sodium is called *pseudohyponatremia* and is caused by marked increases in protein or lipid levels in blood (i.e., which cause an increase in the nonaqueous or solid phase of plasma, decreasing the measured plasma sodium concentration when measured in the clinical laboratory) (16). Pseudohyponatremia becomes significant when plasma protein levels are ≥12 g/dL (normal range is 5.5-8 g/dL) and triglyceride levels are ≥1,500 mg/dL (normal range is 25-175 mg/dL). Clinical conditions that can produce pseudohyponatremia are listed in Table 34.2.

Diagnosis

Pseudohyponatremia can be diagnosed by measuring the plasma osmolality, which will be normal (285-295 mOsm/kg H_2O) with pseudohyponatremia, and will be reduced (<275 mOsm/kg H_2O) with true hyponatremia.

Hyperglycemia

Hyperglycemia is another potential cause of pseudohyponatremia. When glucose does not readily enter cells, the subsequent hyperglycemia draws fluid out of cells. This increases the aqueous phase of plasma and has a dilutional effect on sodium. The corrected sodium in hyperglycemia is expressed with the following equation:

$$\text{Corrected [Na]} = \text{Measured [Na]} + \left[2.4 \times \frac{\text{glucose} - 100 \text{ (mg/dL)}}{100 \text{ (mg/dL)}} \right] \quad (34.2)$$

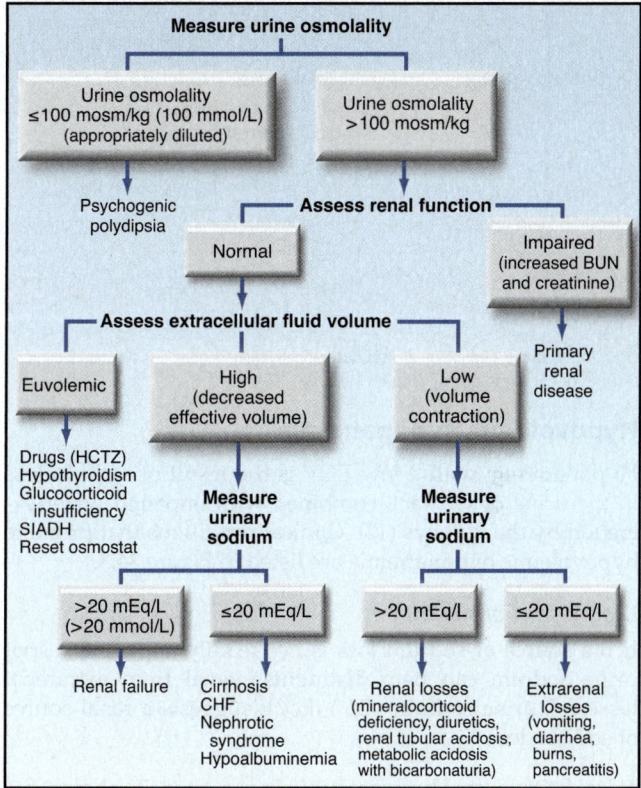

FIGURE 34.3. A diagnostic approach for differentiating causes of hyponatremia.

TABLE 34.2	Clinical Conditions Associated with Pseudohyponatremia
Mechanism	Conditions
Hyperproteinemia	HIV Disease
	Immunoglobulin Infusions
	Monoclonal Gammopathies
	Multiple Myeloma
	Waldenström's Macroglobulinemia
Hypertriglyceridemia	Alcohol Abuse
	Diabetic Ketoacidosis
	Hyperlipidemias (types I and V)
	Pancreatitis
	Type 2 Diabetes (poorly controlled)
Hypercholesterolemia	Biliary Obstruction
	Hepatitis
	Intrahepatic Cholestasis
	Primary Biliary Cirrhosis

From Aziz F, Sam R, Lew SQ, et al. Pseudohyponatremia: mechanism, diagnosis, clinical associations and management. J Clin Med 2023;12:4076.

Hypovolemic Hyponatremia

Hyponatremia with a low ECV is the result of sodium loss in the urine or GI tract, combined with impaired water excretion by the kidneys (17). Clinical conditions that promote hypovolemic hyponatremia are listed in Figure 34.3.

Diagnostic Considerations

If the source of sodium loss is not readily apparent, a spot urine sodium can help distinguish renal from extrarenal losses. A urine sodium >20 mEq/L suggests a renal source of sodium loss.

Thiazide Diuretics. Hypernatremia is reported in about one-third of patients being treated with a thiazide diuretic (18). The mechanism for this hyponatremia is complex and beyond the intent of this chapter.

Adrenal Insufficiency. *Primary* adrenal insufficiency involves *mineralocorticoid* deficiency, which promotes renal sodium wasting. The hyponatremia usually appears in the chronic, not acute, form of the disease. *Secondary* adrenal insufficiency originates in the hypothalamus or pituitary and is a deficiency of *glucocorticoids* and is not associated with hyponatremia.

Cerebral Salt Wasting. Cerebral salt wasting is a condition of urinary sodium loss and hyponatremia associated with neurological disorders such as subarachnoid hemorrhage, traumatic brain injury (see Chapter 45: Traumatic Brain Injury), acute inflammatory demyelinating polyradiculoneuropathy (AIDP, also known as Guillain-Barre syndrome), and neurosurgery (19).

Normovolemic Hyponatremia

Hyponatremia with a normal ECV is the result of water retention with minimal sodium loss. Etiologies are listed in Figure 34.3.

Diagnostic Considerations

The urine osmolality can help differentiate causes of normovolemic hyponatremia. In the syndrome of inappropriate ADH (SIADH) secretion, urine osmolality will be concentrated as evidenced by a higher urine osmolality (300-500 mOsm/kg H_2O). The urine osmolality is low in psychogenic polydipsia (<200 mOsm/kg H_2O).

SIADH. The SIADH release is diagnosed by a combination of hypotonic plasma, inappropriately concentrated urine (urine osmolality >100 mOsm/kg H_2O), and an elevated urine sodium (>20 mEq/L) (20). SIADH is difficult to distinguish from cerebral salt wasting; the distinguishing feature between the two conditions is the ECV, which is *decreased* with cerebral salt wasting and *normal* with SIADH.

Physiological Stress. Physiological stress can promote the release of adrenocorticotropic hormone (ACTH) from the anterior pituitary and ADH from the posterior pituitary. Stress-induced ADH release may explain the increased finding of hyponatremia in postoperative patients and critically ill patients (15).

Primary Polydipsia. Primary polydipsia (water intoxication) is a cause of hyponatremia that occurs primarily in patients with developmental or psychiatric disorders who consume excessive amounts of dilute fluids (21). Another example of hyponatremia caused by heavy consumption of a dilute fluid is *beer potomania*, which is found in chronic, malnourished alcoholics (22).

Hypothyroidism. Though frequently listed as a consideration in the differential diagnosis for normovolemic hyponatremia, the evidence for hypothyroidism as a cause is not convincing (23). A serum thyroid-stimulating hormone (TSH) assay can be used to rapidly exclude hypothyroidism as a potential etiology.

Hypervolemic Hyponatremia

Hypervolemic hyponatremia is caused when water retention exceeds sodium retention. This condition occurs in advanced heart failure (Chapter 19: Acute Heart Failure[s]), cirrhosis (Chapter 38: Liver Failure), and renal failure (Chapter 33: Acute Kidney Injury). Renal failure is associated with a high urine sodium (>20 mEq/L), and heart failure and cirrhosis are associated with a low urine sodium (<20 mEq/L), except in the presence of active diuretic use.

MANAGEMENT OF HYPONATREMIA

The management of hyponatremia is determined by two factors: the presence or absence of hyponatremic encephalopathy and the ECV.

Hyponatremic Encephalopathy

Hyponatremia results in a hypotonic extracellular fluid, which causes fluid to move across the blood-brain barrier and into the brain parenchyma, culminating in cerebral edema. When this condition causes symptoms, it is called hyponatremic encephalopathy (24). This condition is more likely to appear when the hyponatremia is acute (i.e., develops in <48 h). Symptoms may be nonspecific, but early symptoms usually include nausea, vomiting, headache, and ataxia. *The presence of any symptom that suggests possible cerebral edema (rather than the plasma sodium concentration) is an indication for prompt correction with hypertonic saline* (24).

Hypertonic Saline

The treatment with hypertonic saline (3%) is summarized in Table 34.3.

TABLE 34.3 Hypertonic Saline for Symptomatic Hyponatremia

1. Use 3% NaCL (Na^+ = 153 mEq/L, osmolarity = 1,026 mOsm/L).
2. Give IV bolus doses of 2 mL/kg (or 150 mL), which are repeated every few hours until the symptoms resolve. This regimen can be given via peripheral veins.
3. Assess after the serum Na^+ has increased by 5 mEq/L—if there is no improvement, consider another cause for the symptoms.
4. The following limits are recommended as a preventive measure for osmotic demyelination.
   a. The initial increment in serum Na^+ should not exceed 5 mEq/L in 2 h, or 10 mEq/L in 5 h.
   b. The daily increment in serum Na^+ should not exceed 10 mEq/L on the first day, and 8 mEq/L on subsequent days.
   c. The final plasma Na^+ should not exceed 130 mEq/L.

Derived from Hoorn EJ, Zietse R. Diagnosis and treatment of hyponatremia: compilation of the guidelines. J Am Soc Nephrol 2017;28(5):1340-9 and Achinger SG, Ayus JC. Treatment of hyponatremic encephalopathy in the critically ill. Crit Care Med 2017;45:1762-71.

Each bolus can increase the sodium concentration by as much as 2 mEq/L. The 3% saline solution can be delivered safely through a patent peripheral vein (24-25).

Osmotic Demyelination Syndrome

Correction of the sodium that is too rapid can produce a rare, but devastating neurological disorder caused by osmotic damage to the myelin sheath of brainstem neurons (26). This *osmotic demyelinating syndrome*, also known as *central pontine myelinolysis*, has a biphasic course. The initial presentation includes varying degrees of altered mentation with seizures. Following clinical improvement, a more profound deterioration occurs, with dysarthria, oculomotor dysfunction, quadriparesis, and locked-in syndrome (26-27).

Management

Desmopressin can be used when overcorrection of the serum sodium occurs as shown in Table 34.4.

TABLE 34.4 Desmopressin to Prevent or Reverse Overcorrection of Hyponatremia

Indications:
- If the increment in serum Na$^+$ exceeds the limits listed in Table 34.3.
- If there is an abrupt increase in urine output (e.g., >100 mL/h) during corrective therapy with hypertonic saline.
- As a routine measure in conditions where overcorrection is a risk (see text).

Dose:
- 2 μg by subcutaneous injection every 12 h.

Caveats:
- Desmopressin is not advised when the hyponatremia is due to unregulated release of ADH.
- If there is an abrupt increase in urine output (e.g., >100 mL/h) during corrective therapy with hypertonic saline.
- Fluid restriction is mandatory during R$_x$ with desmopressin.

From Sodium. In: Marino PL. *Marino's The ICU Book*. 5th ed. Wolters Kluwer; 2025:552-67. Table 35.4.

Hypovolemia

Isotonic saline may be used to help with blood pressure and tissue perfusion until the responsible conditions are treated or eliminated.

Normovolemia

Fluid restriction (<500 mL/day) is the usual goal for management of normovolemic hyponatremia. The following drug options are available for SIADH when fluid restriction is not tolerated or possible:

1. Demeclocycline blocks the effects of ADH in the renal tubules. It is given in a dose of 600-1,200 mg daily in divided doses. The maximum effect takes several days and the response is variable. The drug can be nephrotoxic, so renal function must be monitored during use.
2. Conivaptan (intravenous) and tolvaptan (oral) are vasopressin antagonists. Both agents can increase the serum sodium by 6 or 7 mEq/L. In many ICUs, use of these drugs is discouraged because both drugs are expensive.

Hypervolemia

Patients with hypervolemia are both salt and water overloaded, with the water overload exceeding the salt overload. Diuresis with furosemide can help correct this problem, but continued activation of the renin-angiotensin-aldosterone system in heart failure and cirrhosis causes a persistent hyponatremia.

HYPERCHLOREMIA

Chloride is often de-emphasized in electrolyte management, but chloride is a crucial electrolyte that contributes to osmotic pressure, cellular homeostasis, and acid-base balance (see Chapter 31: Acid-Base Analysis) (28-29). The typical range for serum chloride concentrations is 96-106 mmol/L (29). Table 34.5 lists common causes of hyperchloremia.

TABLE 34.5	Causes of Hyperchloremia
Cause	Mechanism
Excessive Saline Administration	The concentration of chloride in 0.9% saline is 154 mEq/L. • This supraphysiological dose can lead to hyperchloremia when 0.9% saline is administered in excess. • This phenomenon is usually associated with a non-anion gap acidosis caused by excessive chloride ions (see Chapter 31).
Acid Base Disorders	• Excessive chloride ions decrease the strong ion difference, contributing to metabolic acidosis. • Acidosis and hyperchloremia are exacerbated in renal failure or diabetic ketoacidosis.
Impaired Renal Function	• Dysfunction in tubular reabsorption can impair chloride excretion.
Excessive Sodium Intake (without water)	• Hyperchloremia results from excessive chloride intake.

Derived from Sagar N, Lohiya S. A comprehensive review of chloride management in critically ill patients. Cureus 2024;16(3):e55625 and Nagami GT. Hyperchloremia—why and how. Nefrologia 2016;36(4):347-53.

Physiological Consequences

Hyperchloremia is a strong marker for worsening organ function and adverse outcomes in ICU patients. A serum chloride level >110 mEq/L has been shown to have an independent association with increased odds of ICU mortality in sepsis patients (30-32). Hyperchloremia has also been shown to be associated with AKI and multiple organ dysfunction. Hyperchloremia has been shown to have direct adverse effects on renal function and cardiac output (depressed myocardial contractility) (29).

Management

Hyperchloremia can be prevented by limiting the use of isotonic saline and using dynamic indicators to carefully guide fluid resuscitation (see Chapter 11: Fluid Management). If associated acidosis is severe, renal replacement therapy may be indicated (see Chapter 33: Acute Kidney Injury).

HYPOCHLOREMIA

Hypochloremia is defined as a serum concentration of chloride <96 mmol/L (29). Causes of hypochloremia are listed in Table 34.6.

TABLE 34.6	Causes of Hypochloremia
Cause	Mechanism
Fluid Losses	• GI tract losses (i.e., vomiting and diarrhea) represent a significant cause. • Primary adrenal insufficiency and the use of diuretics can also be contributory.
Metabolic Alkalosis	• Hypochloremia is often associated with metabolic alkalosis, primarily due to the loss of hydrochloric acid. • Excessive administration of bicarbonate or other alkaline substances can contribute to an alkalotic state.
Syndromes and Disorders	• Certain syndromes are associated with abnormalities in chloride transport mechanisms. • Bartter syndrome and other salt-wasting tubulopathies can cause hypochloremia and hypokalemia.

Derived from Sagar N, Lohiya S. A comprehensive review of chloride management in critically ill patients. Cureus 2024;16(3):e55625 and Nagami GT. Hyperchloremia—why and how. Nefrologia 2016;36(4):347-53.

Management

Hypochloremia rarely presents as an isolated electrolyte abnormality. Hence, the etiology of fluid loss or metabolic alkalosis (i.e., vomiting, diarrhea, diuresis) should be addressed. Judicious volume replacement with crystalloids is indicated to correct hypovolemia. Edematous patients who are hypokalemic and alkalotic will not respond to fluid administration; potassium repletion alone often helps correct both alkalosis and associated electrolyte derangements.

References

1. Rasouli M. Basic concepts and practical equations on osmolality: biochemical approach. Clin Biochem 2016;49(12):936-41.
2. Fazekas AS, Funk GC, Klobassa DS, et al. Evaluation of 36 formulas for calculating plasma osmolality. Intensive Care Med 2013; 39(2):302-8.
3. Martín-Calderón JL, Bustos F, Tuesta-Reina LR, et al. Choice of the best equation for plasma osmolality calculation: comparison of fourteen formulae. Clin Biochem 2015;48(7-8):529-33.
4. Chand R, Chand R, Goldfarb D. Hypernatremia in the intensive care unit. Curr Opin Nephrol Hypertens 2022;31:199-204.
5. Gennari FJ, Weise WJ. Acid-base disturbances in gastrointestinal disease. Clin J Am Soc Nephrol 2008;3:1861-8.
6. Bates GP, Miller VS. Sweat rate and sodium loss during work in the heat. J Occup Med Toxicol 2008;3:4.
7. Al-Absi A, Gosmanova EO, Wall BM. A clinical approach to the treatment of chronic hypernatremia. Am J Kidney Dis 2012;60: 1032-8.
8. Chauhan K, Pattharanitima P, Patel N, et al. Rate of correction of hypernatremia and health outcomes in critically ill patients. Clin J Am Soc Nephrol 2019;14(5):656-63.
9. Tomkins M, Lawless S, Martin-Grace J, et al. Diagnosis and management of central diabetes insipidus in adults. J Clin Endocrinol Met 2022;107:2701-15.
10. Garofeanu CG, Weir M, Rosas-Arellano MP, et al. Causes of reversible nephrogenic diabetes insipidus: a systematic review. Am J Kidney Dis 2005;45:626-37.
11. Ananthakrishnan S. Gestational diabetes insipidus: diagnosis and management. Best Pract Res Clin Endocrinol Metab 2020;34:101384.
12. Sterns RH. Disorders of plasma sodium—causes, consequences, and correction. N Engl J Med 2015;372(1):55-65.

13. Oiso Y, Robertson GL, Nørgaard JP, Juul KV. Clinical review: treatment of neurohypophyseal diabetes insipidus. J Clin Endocrinol Metab 2013;98(10):3958-67.
14. Libber S, Harrison H, Spector D. Treatment of nephrogenic diabetes insipidus with prostaglandin synthesis inhibitors. J Pediatr 1986;108:305-11.
15. Spasovski G, Vanholder R, Allolio B, et al. Clinical practice guideline on diagnosis and management of hyponatremia. Intensive Care Med 2014;40:320-31.
16. Aziz F, Sam R, Lew SQ, et al. Pseudohyponatremia: mechanism, diagnosis, clinical associations and management. J Clin Med 2023; 12:4076.
17. Hoorn EJ, Zietse R. Diagnosis and treatment of hyponatremia: compilation of the guidelines. J Am Soc Nephrol 2017;28(5):1340-9.
18. Klhůfek J, Šálek T. Thiazide-associated hyponatremia in internal medicine patients: analysis of epidemiological and biochemical profiles. Postgrad Med 2022;134:487-93.
19. Cui H, He G, Yang S, et al. Inappropriate antidiuretic hormone secretion and cerebral salt-wasting syndromes in neurological patients. Front Neurosci 2019;13:1170.
20. Martin-Grace J, Tomkins M, O'Reilly MW, et al. Approach to the patient: hyponatremia and the syndrome of inappropriate antidiuresis (SIAD). J Clin Endocrinol Metab 2022;107:2362-76.
21. Goldman MB, Luchins DL, Robertson GL. Mechanisms of altered water metabolism in psychotic patients with polydipsia and hyponatremia. N Engl J Med 1988;318:397-403.
22. Sanghvi SR, Kellerman PS, Nanovic L. Beer potomania: an unusual cause of hyponatremia at high risk of complications from rapid correction. Am J Kidney Dis 2007;50:673-80.
23. Wolf P, Beiglböck H, Smaijs S, et al. Hypothyroidism and hyponatremia: rather coincidence than causality. Thyroid 2017; 27:611-5.
24. Achinger SG, Ayus JC. Treatment of hyponatremic encephalopathy in the critically ill. Crit Care Med 2017;45:1762-71.
25. Metheny NA, Moritz ML. Administration of 3% sodium chloride via a peripheral vein. J Infus Nurs 2021;44:94-102.
26. MacMillan TE, Shin S, Topf J, et al. Osmotic demyelination syndrome in patients hospitalized with hyponatremia. NEJM Evid 2023;2(4):EVIDoa2200215.
27. Singh TD, Fugate JE, Rabinstein AA. Central pontine and extrapontine myelinolysis: a systematic review. Eur J Neurol 2014;21:1443-50.
28. Lehrich RW, Greenberg A. Hyponatremia and the use of vasopressin receptor antagonists in critically ill patients. J Intensive Care Med 2012;27:207-18.
29. Sagar N, Lohiya S. A comprehensive review of chloride management in critically ill patients. Cureus 2024;16(3):e55625.

30. Nagami GT. Hyperchloremia—why and how. Nefrologia 2016; 36(4):347-53.
31. Neyra JA, Canepa-Escaro F, Li X, et al. Association of hyperchloremia with hospital mortality in critically ill septic patients. Crit Care Med 2015;43(9):1938-44.
32. Yeh P, Pan Y, Sanchez-Pinto LN, Luo Y. Hyperchloremia in critically ill patients: association with outcomes and prediction using electronic health record data. BMC Med Inform Decis Mak 2020; 20(Suppl 14):302.

Potassium

Chapter 35

This chapter describes the causes and consequences of abnormalities in the plasma potassium concentration.

PHYSIOLOGY

Potassium Distribution

There is a marked difference between intracellular and extracellular potassium (K^+), with 98% of the total body K^+ located inside cells, and only 2% remaining in the extracellular fluid (1-3). The relationship between total body K^+ and serum (plasma) K^+ is shown in Figure 35.1 (4-5).

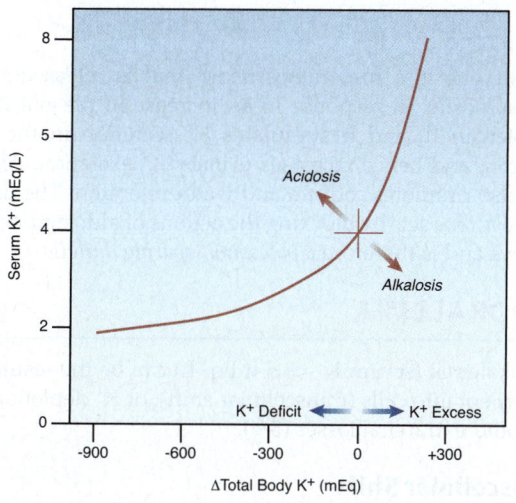

FIGURE 35.1. Relationship between the serum potassium concentration and total body potassium. (Redrawn from Brown RS. Extrarenal potassium homeostasis. Kidney Int 1986;30:116-27.)

The portion of the curve in Figure 35.1 is relatively flat in the region of K⁺ deficiency. For a given change in serum K⁺, the change in total body K⁺ is twofold greater with K⁺ depletion (hypokalemia) than with K⁺ excess (hyperkalemia) (5). The larger K⁺ deficit associated with hypokalemia is due to the large pool of intracellular K⁺ that can replenish extracellular K⁺ (and help to maintain serum K⁺) when K⁺ is lost.

Potassium Excretion

Small amounts of K⁺ are lost in stool (5-10 mEq/day) and sweat (0-10 mEq/day), but the majority of K⁺ loss is in urine (40-120 mEq/day, depending on K⁺ intake) (1). K⁺ excretion in urine is primarily a function of K⁺ secretion in the distal nephron, which is controlled by plasma K⁺ and, primarily, aldosterone. When renal function is normal, the capacity for renal K⁺ excretion is great enough to prevent a sustained rise in serum K⁺ in response to an increased K⁺ load (1).

Aldosterone

Aldosterone is a mineralocorticoid that is released by the adrenal cortex in response to an increase in plasma K⁺ and angiotensin II, and it stimulates K⁺ secretion in the distal nephron, and hence increases urinary K⁺ excretion. Aldosterone also promotes sodium and water retention. The diuretic *spironolactone* acts by blocking the actions of aldosterone in the kidneys and is therefore a *potassium-sparing diuretic*.

HYPOKALEMIA

Hypokalemia (serum K⁺ <3.5 mEq/L) can be the result of K⁺ movement into cells (transcellular shift), or K⁺ depletion from renal and extrarenal losses (3-6).

Transcellular Shift

The movement of K⁺ into cells is facilitated by β_2-adrenergic receptors on cell membranes in muscle, and this explains the decrease in serum K⁺ associated with *inhaled β_2-agonist bronchodilators* (e.g., albuterol) (7). This effect is mild (≤0.5 mEq/L) in the usual therapeutic doses (7) but is more significant when inhaled β_2-agonists are used in combination with diuretics (8). Other factors that promote K⁺ movement into cells include *alkalosis* (respiratory or metabolic), *hypothermia* (accidental or induced), and *insulin*. Alkalosis has a variable and unpredictable effect on serum K⁺ (9). Hypothermia causes a transient drop in serum K⁺ that resolves with rewarming (10).

Potassium Depletion

K⁺ depletion can be the result of K⁺ loss via the kidneys or gastrointestinal tract. The site of K⁺ loss (renal or extrarenal) is usually clinically evident but can be evaluated more precisely by measuring spot urine K⁺ and chloride concentrations, as shown in Figure 35.2.

The leading cause of renal K⁺ loss is *diuretic therapy*. *Magnesium depletion* impairs K⁺ reabsorption in the renal tubules and *may play a very important role in promoting K⁺ depletion* in critically ill patients, particularly those receiving diuretics (see Chapter 36: Magnesium) (11). The major cause of extrarenal K⁺ loss is *diarrhea*, with K⁺ losses that can reach 400 mEq daily in severe cases (12).

Clinical Manifestations

Severe hypokalemia (serum K⁺ <2.5 mEq/L) can be associated with diffuse muscle weakness (3), but in most cases, hypokalemia is asymptomatic.

ECG Changes

Abnormalities in the ECG are the major manifestation of hypokalemia and can be present in 50% of cases (13). The ECG abnormalities include prominent U waves (>1 mm in height), flattening and inversion of T waves, and prolongation of the QT interval, but these changes can also be seen in many other conditions, including left ventricular hypertrophy and QT

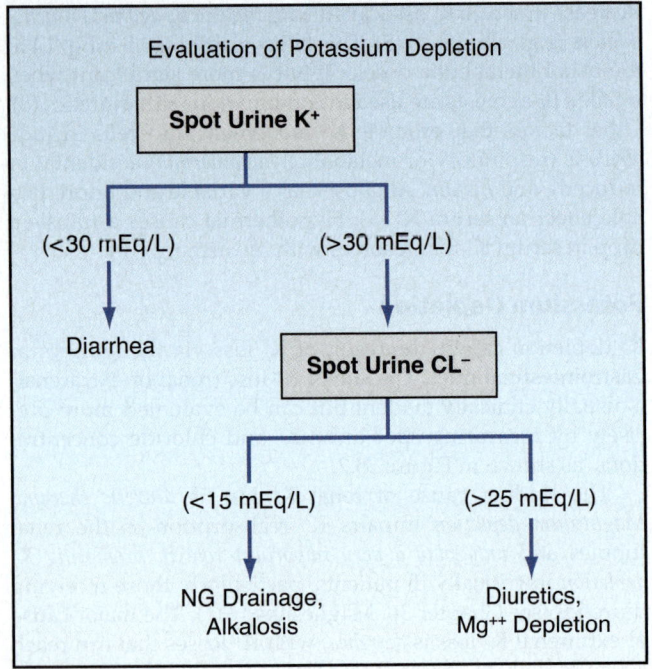

FIGURE 35.2. Evaluation to identify the site of potassium loss. (From Potassium. In: Marino PL. *Marino's The ICU Book*. 5th ed. Wolters Kluwer; 2025:568-79. Figure 36.3.)

prolongation. *Hypokalemia alone is not a risk for serious arrhythmias;* however, hypokalemia can increase the risk of serious arrhythmias from other conditions (e.g., myocardial ischemia) (3).

Management

Elimination of Intracellular Shifts or Deficits

The first step in management is to remove or treat any condition that promotes K^+ shifts (e.g., alkalosis). The estimated K^+ deficits associated with progressive hypokalemia are shown in Table 35.1.

TABLE 35.1	Estimated Potassium Deficits in Hypokalemia[†]		
Serum K+ (mEq/L)	K+ Deficit (mEq)	Serum K+ (mEq/L)	K+ Deficit (mEq)
3.4	35	2.9	210
3.3	70	2.8	245
3.2	105	2.7	280
3.1	140	2.6	315
3.0	175	2.5	350

[†]Estimates based on a lean body weight of 70 kg and a total body K+ of 50 mEq/kg.

From Potassium. In: Marino PL. *Marino's The ICU Book.* 5th ed. Wolters Kluwer; 2025:568-79. Table 36.1.

Potassium Replacement

K+ chloride is the most common replacement solution which is available as a concentrated solution (1-2 mEq/mL) in ampules containing 10, 20, 30, and 40 mEq of K+. These solutions are *extremely hyperosmotic* (the 2 mEq/mL solution has an osmolarity of 4,000 mOsm/L) and *must be diluted* (14). A K+ phosphate solution is also available that contains 4.5 mEq K+ and 3 mmol phosphate per mL and may be considered in conditions associated with concomitant phosphate depletion (e.g., diabetic ketoacidosis).

Rate of Replacement

The standard method of intravenous K+ replacement is to add 20 mEq of K+ to 100 mL of isotonic saline and infuse over 1 h (15). The *maximum rate* of intravenous K+ replacement is usually set at *20-40 mEq/h* (15), but *dose rates as high as 100 mEq/h have been used safely* (16). Infusion through a large, central vein is preferred because of the irritating properties of the hyperosmotic KCL solutions; however, delivery into the superior vena cava is not recommended if the desired rate of replacement exceeds 20 mEq/h because there is a risk (poorly described in the literature) of producing asystole.

Response

The serum K⁺ may be slow to correct initially, as predicted by the flat portion of the curve in Figure 35.1. Magnesium depletion promotes urinary K⁺ loss, and *in patients who are magnesium deficient, hypokalemia is often resistant to K⁺ replacement until the magnesium is repleted* (see Chapter 36: Magnesium) (17).

HYPERKALEMIA

While hypokalemia is often well-tolerated, hyperkalemia (serum K^+ >5.5 mEq/L) can be a life-threatening condition.

Mechanisms

Hyperkalemia can be the result of K⁺ release from cells (transcellular shift), or impaired renal excretion of K⁺. If the source of the hyperkalemia is unclear, a spot urine K⁺ can be useful, as *a low urine K^+ (<30 mEq/L) is evidence of impaired renal excretion* (18).

Factitious Hyperkalemia

Factitious hyperkalemia (also called "pseudohyperkalemia") usually originates from hemolysis of red blood cells, but platelets can contribute in the setting of thrombocytosis (platelet count $>500 \times 10^9$/L), and severe leukocytosis can be a factor in patients with lymphoproliferative disorders (19). Factitious hyperkalemia should also be suspected when there is no apparent reason for hyperkalemia. The following factors have been identified as contributing to factitious hyperkalemia (19):

1. Fist-clenching to help identify veins (which can release K⁺ from skeletal muscle) (20).
2. Excessive suction (e.g., with "vacutainers") when withdrawing the blood specimen.
3. Trauma to the specimen during transport in pneumatic tube systems (21).
4. Delays in processing the blood specimen.

If potentially contributing factors are suspected, blood should be redrawn.

Acidosis

The presumed mechanism for the relationship between acidosis and hyperkalemia is competition between H^+ and K^+ for the same site on the membrane pump that moves K^+ into cells. However, the causal link between acidosis and hyperkalemia is being questioned because lactic acidosis is not associated with hyperkalemia (9), and respiratory acidosis has an inconsistent association with hyperkalemia (9).

Tumor Lysis Syndrome

Tumor lysis syndrome is an acute, life-threatening condition that appears within 7 days after the initiation of cytotoxic therapy for selected malignancies (e.g., non-Hodgkin lymphoma). Features include the combination of hyperkalemia, hyperphosphatemia, hypocalcemia, and hyperuricemia, often accompanied by acute kidney injury (22-23). *Hyperkalemia is the most immediate threat to life.*

Drugs

Drugs that either promote K^+ movement out of cells or inhibit renal excretion are listed in Table 35.2.

TABLE 35.2 Drugs that Promote Hyperkalemia	
Promote Transcellular Shift	**Reduce Renal Excretion**
β-Blockers	ACE inhibitors
Digitalis	ARBs
Succinylcholine	Amiloride
	NSAIDs
	Spironolactone
	TMP-SMX

From References 23-27.

Succinylcholine is a short-acting neuromuscular depolarizing agent that deserves special mention because life-threatening increases in serum K^+ have been reported when this drug is used in patients with spinal cord injury or prolonged immobility; an effect attributed to "denervation hypersensitivity" (24-26). The drugs in Table 35.2 that impair renal excretion promote hyperkalemia by inhibiting some aspect of the renin–angiotensin–aldosterone system. An exception is trimethoprim-sulfamethoxazole, which directly inhibits K^+ secretion in the distal tubules.

Blood Transfusion

Hyperkalemia is a recognized (but inconsistent) complication of massive blood transfusion (see Chapter 12: Anemia and Erythrocyte Transfusions). The K^+ concentration in cooled (4° C) stored blood increases steadily over time due to inhibition of the Na^+-K^+ exchange pump in the erythrocyte cell membrane (27-28). The K^+ load in transfused blood is normally cleared by the kidneys, but when systemic blood flow is compromised (which applies to most patients who need massive blood transfusions), renal K^+ excretion is impaired, and the K^+ in blood transfusions will accumulate. The transfusion volume needed to produce hyperkalemia varies, but one study has shown that hyperkalemia begins to appear after transfusion of 7 units of red blood cells (29).

Clinical Consequences

The principal threat with hyperkalemia is heart block and cardiac arrest caused by slowed impulse transmission in the heart from depolarization of cardiac muscle. The expected ECG changes in progressive hyperkalemia are shown in Figure 35.3.

There is no predictable relationship between the severity of hyperkalemia and the presence of ECG changes (30-31). For example, the traditional teaching has been that ECG changes begin to appear when the serum K^+ approaches 6 mEq/L (31), but one clinical study found that only 40% of patients with a serum K^+ above 7 mEq/L had ECG changes (32).

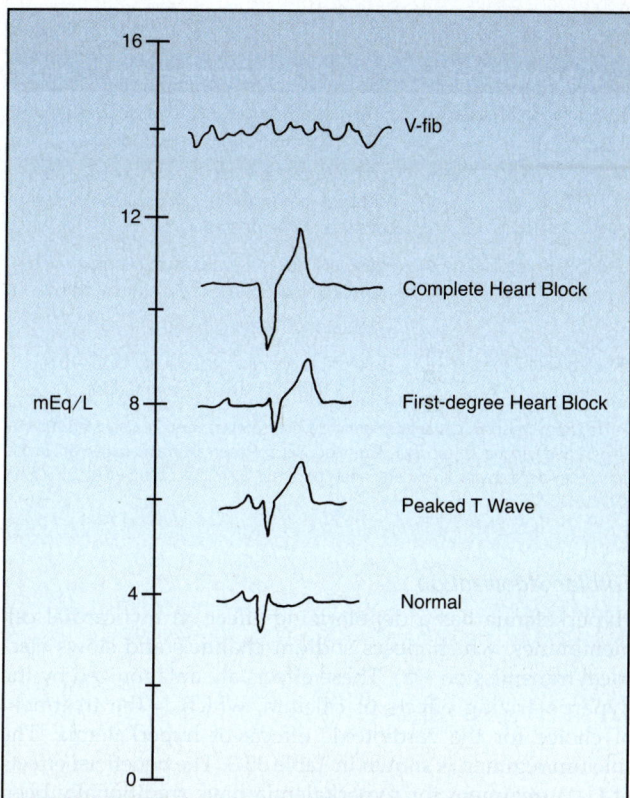

FIGURE 35.3. ECG abnormalities in progressive hyperkalemia. (From Potassium. In: Marino PL. *Marino's The ICU Book*. 5th ed. Wolters Kluwer; 2025:568-79. Figure 36.4.)

Management of Severe Hyperkalemia

Severe hyperkalemia is defined as a serum K^+ >6.5 mEq/L, or any serum K^+ that produces ECG changes (32). The management of this condition has 3 goals as summarized in Table 35.3.

TABLE 35.3	Management of Severe Hyperkalemia
Sequential Goals	Treatment Regimen
1. Cardiac stabilization	• 10% calcium gluconate: 10 mL IV over 3 min, and repeat after 5 min, if necessary. • Use 10% calcium chloride only for circulatory collapse (has triple the calcium [Ca^{++}] content of calcium gluconate).
2. Move K^+ into cells	• Regular insulin: 10 units as an IV bolus, plus 50 mL of 50% dextrose as an IV bolus. • Albuterol: 20 mg as inhaled aerosol.
3. Eliminate Excess K^+	• Sodium zirconium cyclosilicate (SZC): 10 g every 8 h for 48 h, then decrease dose.

Derived from Weisberg L. Management of severe hyperkalemia. Crit Care Med 2008;36: 3246-51 and Rafique R, Peacock F, Armstead T, et al. Hyperkalemia management in the emergency department: an expert panel consensus. J Am Coll Emerg Physicians Open 2021;2:e12572.

Cardiac Stabilization

Hyperkalemia has a depolarizing effect on myocardial cell membranes, which closes sodium channels and slows electrical transmission (33). These effects are antagonized by the hyperpolarizing effects of calcium, which is the treatment of choice for the cardiotoxic effects of hyperkalemia. The calcium regimen is shown in Table 35.3. The beneficial effects of Ca^{++} treatment for hyperkalemia have traditionally been attributed to "membrane stabilization" by restoration of the resting membrane potential (RMP), but more recent data have shown that Ca^{++} treatment for hyperkalemia improves cardiac conduction through calcium channel mediated conduction, rather than improvement in the RMP (34).

Indications. The published indications for calcium include a serum K^+ >6.5 mEq/L (with or without ECG changes), and ECG changes (regardless of the serum K^+) (32). Nevertheless, some prefer to use calcium only when there are concerning ECG changes.

Digitalis Toxicity. Calcium has traditionally been contraindicated for managing the hyperkalemia associated with digitalis toxicity, but retrospective studies have revealed numerous instances where intravenous calcium was given without harm (35).

Movement of K+ into Cells

Insulin-Dextrose. Insulin drives K^+ into skeletal muscle cells by activating the membrane Na^+-K^+ exchange pump, and the insulin-dextrose regimen in Table 35.3 will decrease the serum K^+ by at least 0.6 mEq/L (32). However, this effect is temporary (peak effect at 30-60 min), so measures that promote K^+ elimination should also be initiated.

β_2-Agonists. Inhaled β_2-agonists (e.g., albuterol) produce a small decrease in plasma K^+ (<0.5 mEq/L) in therapeutic doses (7). The dose needed to produce a significant (0.5-1 mEq/L) drop in serum K^+ is at least 4 times the therapeutic dose (32), and this can produce unwanted side effects (e.g., tachycardia). Therefore, these agents should never be used alone for the management of severe hyperkalemia.

Sodium Bicarbonate. Sodium bicarbonate (150 mEq IV in 1 L of D_5W over 3-4 h) has been used to move K^+ into cells by promoting alkalosis, but there are two reasons why bicarbonate use has been discouraged: (*a*) short-term infusions of sodium bicarbonate (<4 h) have no effect on serum K^+ levels in the absence of a metabolic acidosis and (*b*) bicarbonate can form complexes with calcium, which is counterproductive (35). Nevertheless, when patients with severe hyperkalemia have *significant metabolic acidosis* (e.g., pH <7.3 with a serum bicarbonate <17 mmol/L), sodium bicarbonate *should* be part of the treatment because this agent raises extracellular bicarbonate levels, enhancing sodium entry into acidotic skeletal muscle, followed by greater intracellular K^+ uptake (35). Higher doses may be required (body weight [in kg] × 0.5 × bicarbonate deficit per L) (35).

Elimination of Excess Potassium

Cation Exchange Resins. Sodium polystyrene sulfonate or SPS (Kayexalate) is the original cation exchange resin approved for use in severe hyperkalemia. Although once the standard of care for severe hyperkalemia, the use of this has fallen out of favor due to uncertain efficacy, slow onset of action, and reports of necrotic lesions in the bowel linked to its use (35-36).

A newer generation cation exchange resin, SZC (Lokelma) has been shown to be equivalent to SPS for acute management of hyperkalemia (37). The SZC resin does not have the adverse risks associated with SPS. Dosing is described in Table 35.3. A clinically significant effect is reported after one hour (38).

Hemodialysis. The most effective method of K^+ removal is hemodialysis, which can produce a 1 mEq/L drop in serum K^+ after one hour, and a 2 mEq/L drop after 3 h (32). A "rule of 7" has been described to determine the amount of K^+ in the dialysate to be used for a 3-h hemodialysis session (or a longer treatment in a very large or morbidly obese individual) (32,39). It specifies that the sum of the dialysate K^+ concentration and the serum K^+ levels of the patient should be <7 mmol/L (e.g., if a serum K^+ is >7 mmol/L, no additional K^+ is added to the dialysate (32,39).

References

1. Rose BD, Post TW. Potassium homeostasis. In: *Clinical Physiology of Acid-Base and Electrolyte Disorders.* 5th ed. McGraw-Hill; 2001; 372-402.
2. Alfonzo AVM, Isles C, Geddes C, Deighan C. Potassium disorders—clinical spectrum and emergency management. Resusc 2006;70:10-25.
3. Schaefer TJ, Wolford RW. Disorders of potassium. Emerg Med Clin North Am 2005;23:723-47.
4. Brown RS. Extrarenal potassium homeostasis. Kidney Int 1986; 30:116-27.

5. Sterns RH, Cox M, Feig PU, et al. Internal potassium balance and the control of the plasma potassium concentration. Medicine 1981;60:339-54.
6. Glover P. Hypokalemia. Crit Care Resusc 1999;1:239-51.
7. Allon M, Copkney C. Albuterol and insulin for treatment of hyperkalemia in hemodialysis patients. Kidney Int 1990;38:869-72.
8. Lipworth BJ, McDevitt DG, Struthers AD. Prior treatment with diuretic augments the hypokalemic and electrocardiographic effects of inhaled albuterol. Am J Med 1989;86:653-7.
9. Adrogue HJ, Madias NE. Changes in plasma potassium concentration during acute acid-base disturbances. Am J Med 1981;71:456-67.
10. Bernard SA, Buist M. Induced hypothermia in critical care medicine: a review. Crit Care Med 2003;31:2041-51.
11. Salem M, Munoz R, Chernow B. Hypomagnesemia in critical illness. A common and clinically important problem. Crit Care Clin 1991;7:225-52.
12. Gennari FJ, Weise WJ. Acid-base disturbances in gastrointestinal disease. Clin J Am Soc Nephrol 2008;3:1861-8.
13. Stanaszek WF, Romankiewicz JA. Current approaches to management of potassium deficiency. Drug Intell Clin Pharm 1985;19:176-84.
14. Trissel LA. *Handbook on Injectable Drugs.* 13th ed. Bethesda, MD: Amer Soc Health System Pharmacists 2005;1230.
15. Kruse JA, Carlson RW. Rapid correction of hypokalemia using concentrated intravenous potassium chloride infusions. Arch Intern Med 1990;150:613-7.
16. Kim GH, Han JS. Therapeutic approach to hypokalemia. Nephron 2002;92(Suppl 1):28-32.
17. Whang R, Flink EB, Dyckner T, et al. Magnesium depletion as a cause of refractory potassium repletion. Arch Intern Med 1985;145:1686-9.
18. Evans KJ, Greenberg A. Hyperkalemia: a review. J Intensive Care Med 2005;20:272-90.
19. Lábadi Á, Nagy Á, Miseta A, Kovács G. Factitious hyperkalemia in hematologic disorders. Scand J Clin Lab Invest 2016;77:66-72.
20. Don BR, Sebastian A, Cheitlin M, et al. Pseudohyperkalemia caused by fist clenching during phlebotomy. N Engl J Med 1990;322:1290-2.
21. Guiheneuf R, Vuillaume L, Mangalaboyi J, et al. Pneumatic transport is critical for leukemic patients with major leukocytosis: what precautions to measure lactate dehydrogenase, potassium, and aspartate aminotransferase? Ann Clin Biochem 2010;47:94-6.
22. Howard SC, Jones DP, Pui CH. The tumor lysis syndrome. N Engl J Med 2012;364:1844-54.
23. Ponce SP, Jennings AE, Madias N, Harington JT. Drug-induced hyperkalemia. Medicine 1985;64:357-70.

24. Perazella MA. Drug-induced hyperkalemia: old culprits and new offenders. Am J Med 2000;109:307-14.
25. Palmer BF. Managing hyperkalemia caused by inhibitors of the renin-angiotensin-aldosterone system. N Engl J Med 2004;351:585-92.
26. Thomas CM, Thomas J, Smeeton F, Leatherdale BA. Heparin-induced hyperkalemia. Diabetes Res Clin Pract 2008;80:e7-e8.
27. Perazella MA, Mahnensmith RL. Trimethoprim-sulfamethoxazole: hyperkalemia is an important complication regardless of dose. Clin Nephrol 1996;46:187-92.
28. Vraets A, Lin Y, Callum JL. Transfusion-associated hyperkalemia. Transfus Med Rev 2011;25:184-96.
29. Aboudara MC, Hurst FP, Abbott KC, et al. Hyperkalemia after packed red blood cell transfusion in trauma patients. J Trauma 2008;64:S86-S91.
30. Gupta AA, Self M, Mueller M, et al. Dispelling myths and misconceptions about the treatment of acute hyperkalemia. Am J Emerg Med 2022;52:85-91.
31. Montague BT, Ouellette JR, Buller GK. Retrospective review of the frequency of ECG changes in hyperkalemia. Clin J Am Soc Nephrol 2008;3:324-30.
32. Weisberg L. Management of severe hyperkalemia. Crit Care Med 2008;36:3246-51.
33. Rafique R, Peacock F, Armstead T, et al. Hyperkalemia management in the emergency department: An expert panel consensus. J Am Coll Emerg Physicians Open 2021;2:e12572.
34. Piktel JS, Wan X, Kouk S, et al. Beneficial effect of calcium treatment for hyperkalemia is not due to "membrane stabilization". Crit Care Med 2024;52(10):1499-508.
35. Abuelo JG. Treatment of severe hyperkalemia: confronting 4 fallacies. Kidney Int Rep, 2017;3(1):47-55.
36. Harel Z, Harel S, Shah PS, et al. Gastrointestinal adverse events with sodium polystyrene sulfonate (Kayexalate) use: a systematic review. Am J Med 2013;126:264.e9-24.
37. Gonzalez J, Nayyar D. Comparative efficacy of sodium zirconium cyclosilicate and sodium polystyrene sulfonate for acute hyperkalemia: a retrospective chart review. Hosp Pharm 2024;58:159-64.
38. Pacjham DK, Rasmussen HS, Lavin PT, et al. Sodium zirconium cyclosilicate in hyperkalemia. N Engl J Med 2015;372:222-31.
39. Al-Ghamdi G, Hemmelgarn B, Klarenbach S, et al. Dialysate potassium and risk of death in chronic hemodialysis patients. J Nephrol 2010;23(1):33-40.

Magnesium

Chapter 36

This chapter describes the causes and consequences of abnormalities in the serum magnesium concentration.

MAGNESIUM BASICS

Function and Distribution

Magnesium (Mg) is essential for the proper functioning of the Na^+-K^+ exchange pump and plays an important role in the maintenance of cardiac contractile strength and peripheral vascular tone (1-4). Magnesium is distributed in bone (~50%), muscle (~27%) and soft tissues (~20%) *with less than 1% located in plasma*. Consequently, *plasma Mg levels can be normal in the face of total body Mg depletion* (5-6). The normal range of serum Mg in healthy adults is shown in Table 36.1.

TABLE 36.1	Reference Ranges for Serum Magnesium		
	mg/dL	mEq/L	mmol/L
Total Serum Mg	1.7-2.4	1.4-2.0	0.7-1.0
Ionized Mg	-	0.8-1.1	0.4-0.6

From Magnesium. In: Marino PL. *Marino's The ICU Book*. 5th ed. Wolters Kluwer; 2025:580-9. Table 37.2.

Over 60% of the Mg in plasma is in the ionized (active) form, but standard assays measure three fractions of Mg (i.e., ionized, protein bound, chelated with divalent anions), so it is not possible to determine if a lower level of Mg is due to a decrease in the active fraction.

Urinary Magnesium

The serum magnesium level can be normal in patients who are magnesium depleted. Urinary Mg is more specific for identifying early deficiency because only small quantities of Mg are normally excreted in the urine (7-8). Therefore, if urinary Mg excretion falls to negligible levels, deficiency is likely, reflecting renal conservation of Mg. A decrease in urinary Mg is a much earlier indicator of Mg deficiency than plasma Mg, as illustrated in Figure 36.1.

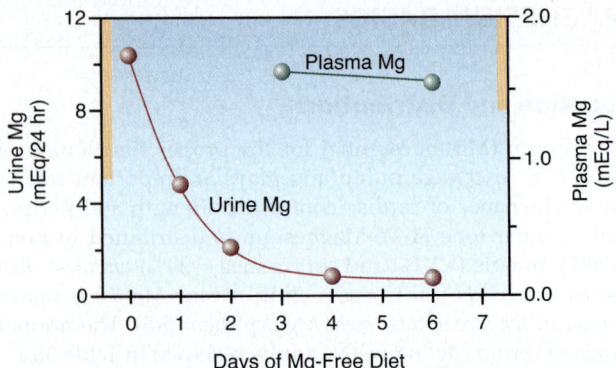

FIGURE 36.1. Urinary magnesium excretion and plasma magnesium levels in a healthy volunteer placed on a magnesium-free diet, illustrating a faster and more precipitous decline in urinary Mg compared to serum Mg levels. Solid bars on the vertical axis represent the normal range for each variable. (Adapted from Shils ME. Experimental human magnesium depletion. Medicine [Baltimore] 1969;48:61-85.)

MAGNESIUM DEFICIENCY

Hypomagnesemia is defined as a total serum Mg <1.7 mg/dL (<0.7 mmol/L) (2-9). Hypomagnesemia is a common electrolyte disorder in the ICU, affecting as many as 65% of patients (2-9). Hypomagnesemia has been associated with a greater risk of mortality, sepsis, mechanical ventilation, and the length of ICU stay in patients admitted to ICU (10).

Predisposing Conditions

The most common predisposing conditions for hypomagnesemia are listed in Table 36.2.

TABLE 36.2 Markers of Possible Magnesium Depletion†

Predisposing Conditions	Clinical Findings
Drug Therapy:	*Electrolyte Disorders:*
Furosemide (50%)	Hypokalemia (40%)
Aminoglycosides (30%)	Hypophosphatemia (30%)
Proton Pump Inhibitors	Hyponatremia (27%)
Insulin	Hypocalcemia (22%)
Alcohol Use Disorder (44%)	*Cardiac Manifestations:*
Diabetes Mellitus	Coronary Ischemia
Diarrhea (secretory)	Arrhythmias
	Digitalis Toxicity
Acute MI (80%)	Hyperactive CNS Syndrome

†Parentheses indicate frequency of associated hypomagnesemia.

From Magnesium. In: Marino PL. *Marino's The ICU Book.* 5th ed. Wolters Kluwer; 2025:580-9. Table 37.3.

Diuretics are a leading cause of Mg deficiency in ICUs and *hypomagnesemia has been reported in up to 50% of patients receiving chronic therapy with furosemide* (11).

Clinical Manifestations

Neurological Signs

There are no specific clinical manifestations of Mg deficiency, although patients with severe deficiency may exhibit neurological signs such as altered mentation, tremors, hyperreflexia, and generalized seizures. *Hyperactive central nervous system syndrome* is magnesium-related and can manifest as ataxia, slurred speech, excessive salivation, diffuse muscle spasms, seizures, and progressive obtundation (12). The symptoms may be triggered by loud noises or bodily contact. This syndrome is associated with reduced Mg levels in cerebrospinal fluid and resolves with Mg infusions. Magnesium is required for transformation of thiamine into thiamine pyrophosphate, so magnesium deficiency can promote *Wernicke's encephalopathy*, even when thiamine intake is adequate (13).

Arrhythmias

The most cited arrhythmia related to magnesium depletion is polymorphic ventricular tachycardia (torsade de pointes), which is discussed in Chapter 20: Dysrhythmias. Magnesium depletion will depolarize cardiac cells and incite arrhythmias. Intravenous Mg can abolish refractory ventricular arrhythmias, even when Mg levels are normal (14). Magnesium deficiency can accompany or exacerbate digitalis cardiotoxicity since both digitalis and Mg deficiency act to inhibit the cardiac Na^+-K^+ exchange pump; hence, intravenous Mg can suppress digitalis-related arrhythmias, even in the absence of a low Mg level (15).

Electrolyte Disorders

Electrolyte disorders frequently accompany hypomagnesemia (see Table 36.2) (16). About half of the patients who develop hypokalemia also have hypomagnesemia, and *the hypokalemia that accompanies Mg depletion can be refractory to K^+ replacement unless the Mg is replaced* (16-17). Hypocalcemia is a well-known manifestation of Mg depletion, presumably due to inhibition of parathyroid hormone (PTH) (18) (see Chapter 37: Calcium and Phosphorus) (16). *As with hypokalemia, the hypocalcemia that accompanies Mg depletion is difficult to correct until Mg is repleted*. Phosphate depletion (see Chapter 37: Calcium and Phosphorus) is a cause, rather than an effect of Mg depletion, due to enhanced renal Mg excretion.

Magnesium Replacement

Table 36.3 lists oral and intravenous Mg preparations and daily requirements.

Absorption of Mg from the GI tract can be erratic in ICU patients, so intravenous Mg is used for replacement. Ringer's solution should not be used as the diluent for magnesium sulfate ($MgSO_4$) because the calcium in Ringer's solutions will counteract the actions of magnesium. Magnesium replacement protocols are described in Table 36.4.

TABLE 36.3 Magnesium Preparations and Daily Requirements

	Elemental Mg
Normal Daily Requirements:	
Adult Males (>30 yrs)	420 mg (35 mEq, 17.5 mmol)
Adult Females (>30 yrs)	320 mg (26 mEq, 13 mmol)
Oral Preparation:	
Magnesium Oxide (400 mg)	241 mg (20 mEq, 10 mmol)
IV Preparation:	
$MgSO_4$	98 mg (8 mEq, 4 mmol)/gram[†]

[†]The magnesium content is for magnesium sulfate heptahydrate ($MgSO_4 \cdot 7 H_2O$), which is the usual $MgSO_4$ preparation.

From Magnesium. In: Marino PL. *Marino's The ICU Book*. 5th ed. Wolters Kluwer; 2025:580-9. Table 37.4.

TABLE 36.4 Intravenous Magnesium Replacement Protocols for Hypomagnesemia

Mild Hypomagnesemia 1-1.4 mEq/L; 1.2-1.7 mg/dL; or 0.5-1.0 mmol/L	Moderate Hypomagnesemia <1 mEq/L; <1.2 mg/dL; or <0.5 mmol/L	Life-Threatening Hypomagnesemia (seizures or serious cardiac arrhythmias (e.g., torsade de pointes))
Assume a total Mg deficit of 1-2 mEq/kg	Add 6 g $MgSO_4$ (48 mEq of Mg) in 250 or 500 mL 0.9 saline and infuse over 3 h	Infuse 2 g $MgSO_4$ (16 mEq, or 8 mmol of Mg) IV over 2-5 min
Because 50% of IV Mg can be lost in urine, assume that the total Mg requirement is twice the Mg deficit	Follow with 5 g $MgSO_4$ (40 mEq of Mg) in 250 or 500 mL 0.9 saline infused over the next 6 h	Follow with 5 g $MgSO_4$ (40 mEq or 20 mmol of Mg) in 250 or 500 mL 0.9 saline infused over the next 6 h
Replace 1 mEq/kg for the first 24 h, and 0.5 mEq/kg daily for the next 3-5 days	Continue with 5 g $MgSO_4$ every 12 h by continuous infusion for the next 5 days	Continue with 5 g $MgSO_4$ every 12 h by continuous infusion for the next 5 days

Note: The $MgSO_4$ used in these protocols is magnesium sulfate heptahydrate ($MgSO_4 \cdot 7 H_2O$). These protocols assume patients have normal renal function.

From Oster JR, Epstein M. Management of magnesium depletion. Am J Nephrol 1988; 8:349-54.

Replacement for Renal Insufficiency

Hypomagnesemia is not common in patients with renal insufficiency, but it can occur with extrarenal losses and a low creatinine clearance (30-50 mL/min). In patients with renal insufficiency, *no more than 50% of the standard replacement protocols should be administered* (Table 36.4) and the serum Mg should be monitored closely (19).

Monitoring Magnesium Replacement

Serum Mg levels will rise after an initial intravenous Mg bolus but will start to fall after 15 min. Therefore, it is important to follow the bolus dose with a continuous infusion. Serum Mg may normalize after 1 to 2 days, but it will take several days to replenish the total body Mg stores. The best indicator of magnesium repletion is the urinary magnesium test (3,20) (see Table 36.5). This test can be used to identify the endpoint of Mg replacement therapy (3,20).

TABLE 36.5 Magnesium Retention Test

Protocol:

1. Add 6 grams $MgSO_4$ (24 mmol or 48 mEq elemental Mg) to 250 mL of isotonic saline and infuse over 1 h.
2. Collect urine for 24 h, beginning with the onset of the magnesium infusion.

Results:

1. Urinary Mg excretion ≤12 mmol (24 mEq) in 24 h (i.e., ≤50% of the infused Mg) is evidence of continued Mg depletion
2. Urinary Mg excretion >19 mmol (38 mEq) in 24 h (i.e., >80% of the infused Mg) indicates sufficient Mg stores.

Magnesium deficiency is likely when less than 50% of the infused Mg is recovered in the urine and is unlikely when more than 80% of the infused Mg is excreted in the urine. This test is not reliable in patients with renal insufficiency.

From Clague JE, Edwards RH, Jackson MJ. Intravenous magnesium loading in chronic fatigue syndrome. Lancet 1992;340:124-5.

HYPERMAGNESEMIA

Prevalence and Causes

Hypermagnesemia is comparatively rare in ICU patients (~5%), and most cases are the result of impaired renal function combined with a source of Mg intake (e.g., use of magnesium-containing antacids or laxatives or Mg infusions for conditions like eclampsia) (3,21-22). *Massive hemolysis* can cause hypermagnesemia because the Mg concentration in erythrocytes is approximately three times greater than in serum (23). Other conditions associated with mild hypermagnesemia are adrenal insufficiency, hyperparathyroidism, and lithium intoxication (3).

Clinical Features

Magnesium has been described as *nature's physiologic calcium blocker* (24), and most of the serious effects of hypermagnesemia are the result of calcium antagonism in the AV conduction system of the heart. The clinical manifestations of progressive hypermagnesemia are listed in Table 36.6.

TABLE 36.6	Serum Magnesium Levels and Expected Clinical Manifestations	
Threshold Serum Mg in mEq/L (mg/dL)	**Clinical Findings**	
>4 (4.9)	Hyporeflexia (mild)	Mild confusion
>5 (6.1)	1st degree AV block Worsening confusion	Lethargy Bradycardia
>10 (12.2)	Complete heart block Severe bradycardia Severe muscle weakness	Delirium Coma Respiratory distress
>13 (15.8)	Cardiac arrest	

Units are mEq/L with mg/dL in parentheses.
From References 2, 21-22.

Management

Emergent hemodialysis (see Chapter 33: Acute Kidney Injury) is the treatment of choice for severe hypermagnesemia (21-22). Intravenous calcium gluconate (1 g IV over 2-3 min.) can be used to antagonize the cardiovascular effects of hypermagnesemia temporarily, until dialysis is started. If fluids are permissible, and some renal function is preserved, aggressive volume infusion combined with furosemide may be effective in reducing the serum magnesium levels in less advanced cases of hypermagnesemia.

References

1. Fiorentini D, Cappadone C, Farruggia G, Prata C. Magnesium: biochemistry, nutrition, detection, and social impact of diseases linked to its deficiency. Nutrients 2021;13:1136.
2. Noronha JL, Matuschak GM. Magnesium in critical illness: metabolism, assessment, and treatment. Intensive Care Med 2002; 28:667-79.
3. Wynne Z, Falat C. Disorders of calcium and magnesium. Emerg Med Clin N Am 2023;41:833-48.
4. Tangvoraphonkchai K, Davenport A. Magnesium and cardiovascular disease. Adv Chronic Kidney Dis 2018;25:251-60.
5. Elin RJ. Assessment of magnesium status. Clin Chem 1987;33: 1965-70.
6. Reinhart RA. Magnesium metabolism. A review with special reference to the relationship between intracellular content and serum levels. Arch Intern Med 1988;148:2415-20.
7. Lowenstein FW, Stanton MF. Serum magnesium levels in the United States, 1971–1974. J Am Coll Nutr 1986;5:399-414.
8. Shils ME. Experimental human magnesium depletion. Medicine (Baltimore) 1969;48:61-82.
9. Tong GM, Rude RK. Magnesium deficiency in critical illness. J Intensive Care Med 2005;20:3-17.
10. Jiang P, Lv Q, Lai T, Xu F. Does hypomagnesemia impact on the outcome of patients admitted to the intensive care unit? A systematic review and meta-analysis. Shock 2017;47(3):288-95.
11. Dyckner T, Wester PO. Potassium/magnesium depletion in patients with cardiovascular disease. Am J Med 1987;82:11-7.
12. Langley WF, Mann D. Central nervous system magnesium deficiency. Arch Intern Med 1991;151:593-6.

13. Longsdale D. Thiamine and magnesium deficiencies: keys to disease. Med Hypotheses 2015;84:120-34.
14. Tzivoni D, Keren A. Suppression of ventricular arrhythmias by magnesium. Am J Cardiol 1990;65:1397-9.
15. Cohen L, Kitzes R. Magnesium sulfate and digitalis-toxic arrhythmias. JAMA 1983;249:2808-10.
16. Hansen BA, Bruserud Ø. Hypomagnesemia in critically ill patients. J Intensive Care 2018;6:21.
17. Whang R, Flink EB, Dyckner T, et al. Magnesium depletion as a cause of refractory potassium repletion. Arch Intern Med 1985; 145:1686-9.
18. Anast CS, Winnacker JL, Forte LR, Burns TW. Impaired release of parathyroid hormone in magnesium deficiency. J Clin Endocrinol Metab 1976;42:707-17.
19. Oster JR, Epstein M. Management of magnesium depletion. Am J Nephrol 1988;8:349-54.
20. Clague JE, Edwards RH, Jackson MJ. Intravenous magnesium loading in chronic fatigue syndrome. Lancet 1992;340:124-5.
21. Adomako EA, Yu ASL. Magnesium disorders: core curriculum 2024. Am J Kidney Dis 2024;83(6):803-15.
22. Van Laecke S. Hypomagnesemia and hypermagnesemia. Acta Clin Belg 2019;74(1):41-7.
23. Elin RJ. Magnesium metabolism in health and disease. Dis Mon 1988;34:161-218.
24. Iseri LT, French JH. Magnesium: nature's physiologic calcium blocker. Am Heart J 1984;108:188-93.

Calcium and Phosphorus — Chapter 37

Calcium and phosphorus have important physiological functions in the human body. Phosphorus participates in aerobic energy production, whereas calcium participates in blood coagulation, neuromuscular transmission, and smooth muscle contraction. Calcium and phosphorus are also responsible for much of the structural integrity of the bony skeleton. This chapter describes the causes and management of abnormalities in plasma calcium and phosphorus concentrations.

CALCIUM BASICS

Calcium is the most abundant electrolyte in the human body, but 99% is in bone (1-2). Parathyroid hormone and vitamin D (calcitriol) promote calcium resorption from bone and thereby maintain plasma calcium levels, while calcitonin from the thyroid gland has the opposite effect and inhibits calcium release from bone.

Plasma Calcium

The calcium in plasma is present in three forms, as shown in Figure 37.1. Approximately half of the calcium is ionized (biologically active, abbreviated as Ca^{++}) and the remainder is either bound to albumin (80%) or complexed with sulfate and phosphate anions (20%) (1-4).

The concentration of total and ionized Ca^{++} in plasma is shown in Table 37.1.

Total vs. Ionized Calcium

The Ca^{++} assay used by most clinical laboratories measures all three fractions of Ca^{++} in plasma, and this can be misleading in patients with hypoalbuminemia. Figure 37.1 shows that a decrease in plasma albumin will decrease the total Ca^{++}

concentration without affecting the ionized Ca++ concentration. Measurement of Ca++ (using ion-specific electrodes) in the clinical laboratory is the only acceptable method for ensuring accuracy.

TABLE 37.1 Normal Ranges for Calcium and Phosphate in Blood

Serum Electrolyte	Traditional Units (mg/dL)	Conversion Factor*	SI Units (mmol/L)
Total Calcium	9.0-10.0	0.25	2.25-2.50
Ionized Calcium	4.6-5.0	0.25	1.15-1.25
Phosphorus	2.5-5.0	0.32	0.8-1.6

*Multiply traditional units by conversion factor to derive SI Units or divide SI Units by conversion factor to derive traditional units.

From Calcium and Phosphorus. In: Marino PL. *Marino's The ICU Book*. 5th ed. Wolters Kluwer; 2025:590-603. Table 38.1.

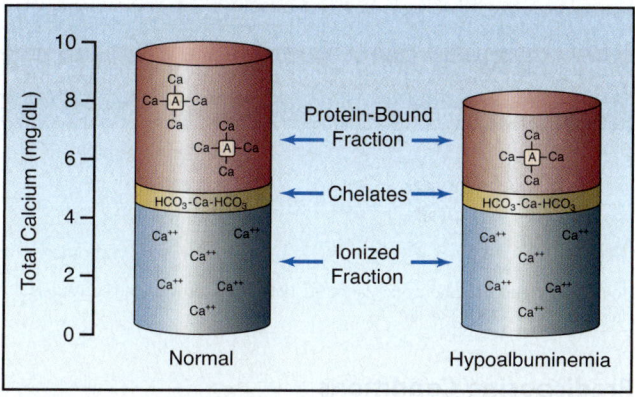

FIGURE 37.1. The three fractions of calcium in plasma and the contribution of each to the total calcium concentration. The column on the right shows how a decrease in plasma albumin can reduce the total plasma calcium without influencing the ionized (active) fraction. (From Calcium and Phosphorus. In: Marino PL. *Marino's The ICU Book*. 5th ed. Wolters Kluwer; 2025:590-603. Figure 38.1.)

Collection Precautions

Precautions are necessary when collecting blood samples for a Ca^{++} measurement. Loss of carbon dioxide from a blood sample could falsely lower the Ca^{++} by increasing Ca^{++} binding to albumin, so it is important to avoid gas bubbles in the blood sample. Anticoagulants (e.g., heparin, citrate, and EDTA) can bind Ca^{++}, so blood samples should not be placed in collection tubes that contain these anticoagulants. Tubes with red stoppers ("red top" tubes) contain silicone and are adequate for measuring ionized Ca^{++} in serum samples.

HYPOCALCEMIA

Ionized hypocalcemia, defined as a plasma Ca^{++} <4.6 mg/dL or <1.7 mmol/L), is extremely common in ICUs (5-7), with one multicenter survey reporting an incidence of 88% in ICU patients (7). The conditions that predispose to ionized hypocalcemia in ICU patients are listed in Table 37.2.

TABLE 37.2 Causes of Ionized Hypocalcemia in the ICU

Most Common	Others
Alkalosis	Massive Transfusion
Magnesium Deficiency	Pancreatitis
Renal Failure	Rhabdomyolysis
Sepsis	Tumor Lysis Syndrome

From Calcium and Phosphorus. In: Marino PL. *Marino's The ICU Book*. 5th ed. Wolters Kluwer; 2025:590-603. Table 38.2.

Predisposing Conditions

Alkalosis

Alkalosis promotes the binding of Ca^{++} to albumin and reduces the fraction of ionized Ca^{++} in blood. Infusions of sodium bicarbonate can also promote ionized hypocalcemia because the infused bicarbonate forms complexes with free Ca^{++}.

Magnesium Depletion

As discussed in Chapter 36: Magnesium, *hypocalcemia from magnesium depletion is refractory to Ca^{++} replacement therapy until magnesium is repleted.*

Systemic Inflammation

Systemic inflammation (i.e., from sepsis) promotes ionized hypocalcemia via actions of cytokines to stimulate calcitonin release and blunt the response to parathormone (5-6).

Renal Failure

Renal failure can lead to ionized hypocalcemia as a result of phosphate retention and impaired conversion of vitamin D to its active form in the kidneys. However, acidosis in renal failure will decrease the binding of Ca^{++} to albumin, which helps to maintain ionized Ca^{++} levels.

Massive Transfusion

Transfusion of red blood cells is an independent predictor of hypocalcemia and is associated with increased mortality (7). The culprit is the citrate anticoagulant used in banked blood, which complexes with Ca^{++}, although other mechanisms may also be responsible (i.e., acidosis, coagulopathy) (8).

Clinical Manifestations

Potential consequences of hypocalcemia include enhanced cardiac and neuromuscular excitability and reduced contractile force in cardiac muscle and vascular smooth muscle; however, *most cases of ionized hypocalcemia in the ICU have no apparent adverse consequences* (5-7).

Neuromuscular

The neuromuscular manifestations of hypocalcemia that are often cited include hyperreflexia, paresthesias, seizures and tetany (9). However, these rarely occur in ICU patients (5-7). *Chvostek's sign* (facial twitching when tapping the facial nerve) is cited as a sign of hypocalcemia, but this sign *has also been* reported in over 50% of healthy subjects with normal Ca^{++} levels (10). *Trousseau's sign* (i.e., carpopedal spasms in the same arm where a blood pressure cuff is inflated to exceed the systolic pressure) is also a potential sign of hypocalcemia (11).

Cardiovascular

Cardiovascular complications such as hypotension, reduced cardiac output, and ventricular ectopic activity are rare and usually only associated with extreme cases of hypocalcemia (i.e., <0.65 mmol/L) (12).

Calcium Replacement Therapy

Intravenous Ca^{++} preparations and recommended dosing regimens are shown in Table 37.3.

TABLE 37.3 Intravenous Calcium Replacement Therapy

Solution	Elemental Ca^{++}	Unit Volume	Osmolarity
10% Calcium chloride	27 mg/mL	10 mL ampules	2,000 mOsm/L
10% Calcium gluconate	9 mg/mL	10 mL ampules	680 mOsm/L

For symptomatic hypocalcemia:

1. Give a bolus dose of 200 mg elemental calcium (e.g., 22 mL of 10% calcium gluconate) in 100 mL isotonic saline over 10 minutes.
2. Follow with a continuous infusion of 1-2 mg/kg per hour for 6-12 h.
3. Monitor ionized calcium levels hourly for the first few hours.

From Calcium and Phosphorus. In: Marino PL. *Marino's The ICU Book*. 5th ed. Wolters Kluwer; 2025:590-603. Table 38.3.

The Ca^{++} solutions for intravenous use are 10% Ca^{++} chloride and 10% Ca^{++} gluconate. *Ca^{++} chloride contains three times more elemental Ca^{++} than Ca^{++} gluconate*, but Ca^{++} gluconate is usually preferred because it has a lower osmolarity and is less irritating when injected.

HYPERCALCEMIA

Hypercalcemia is usually the result of a hyperparathyroidism or malignancy, with malignancy being the usual culprit in ICU patients (13). Malignancies associated with hypercalcemia include multiple myeloma, breast, lung, and ovarian cancer, squamous cell carcinoma of the head and neck, and some lymphomas (14).

Clinical Manifestations

Potential manifestations of hypercalcemia are often nonspecific, but can be organized as follows:

1. *Gastrointestinal:* nausea, vomiting, constipation, and ileus.
2. *Cardiovascular:* hypovolemia, hypotension, and shortened QT interval.
3. *Renal:* polyuria and acute kidney injury.
4. *Neurologic:* confusion, depressed consciousness, and coma.

Manifestations usually begin to appear when the serum Ca^{++} is >12.5 mg/dL (or the ionized Ca^{++} is >3.0 mmol/L), and they are almost always present when the serum Ca^{++} is >14 mg/dL (or the ionized Ca^{++} is >3.5 mmol/L) (14-15). Manifestations are more likely to appear with rapid increases in serum Ca^{++}.

Management

Treatment is indicated when the serum Ca^{++} is >14 mg/dL (or ionized Ca^{++} is >3.5 mmol/L), or when there are neurologic symptoms. The treatment options for hypercalcemia are summarized in Table 37.4.

Loop diuretics like furosemide can increase urinary Ca^{++} excretion, but there is no evidence that intravenous furosemide adds to the benefit of saline infusions (15). Therefore, *furosemide is recommended only to alleviate concomitant volume overload.*

TABLE 37.4	Management of Severe Hypercalcemia
Agent	Dosing Regimens and Comments
Isotonic saline	Dosing: Infuse to maintain a urine output of 100-150 mL/hr. Comment: Can reduce the serum Ca^{++} by 1-2 mg/dL.
Calcitonin	Dosing: 4 Units/kg by subQ injection every 12 h for 24-48 h. Comment: Rapid onset of action (2 h). Tachyphylaxis is common.
Bisphosphonates	Dosing: Zoledronate (4 mg IV over 15 min) or Pamidronate (60-90 mg IV over 4 h). Comment: First-line drugs, but have a delayed onset of action (48 h), and can be nephrotoxic. Zoledronate may be more effective.
Glucocorticoids	Dosing: IV Hydrocortisone (200-400 mg daily) for 3 days, then Prednisone (10-20 mg daily) for 7 days. Comment: Most effective in patients with myeloma and lymphoma.

From Maier JD, Levine SN. Hypercalcemia in the intensive care unit: A review of pathophysiology, diagnosis, and modern therapy. J Intensive Care Med 2015;30:235-52 and Almuradova E, Cicin I. Cancer-related hypercalcemia and potential treatments. Front Endocrinol 2023;14:1039490.

HYPOPHOSPHATEMIA

Inorganic phosphate (PO_4) is predominantly intracellular, where it is used for glycolysis and energy (ATP) production. The normal concentration of PO_4 in plasma is shown in Table 37.1. Hypophosphatemia (serum PO_4 <2.5 mg/dL or <0.8 mmol/L) is present in as many as 80% of ICU patients, and is especially common after major surgery, in multisystem trauma, and fulminant sepsis (16).

Predisposing Conditions

Hypophosphatemia can be the result of reduced phosphate absorption from the gastrointestinal (GI) tract, increased phosphate excretion in the urine, or the transcellular movement of phosphate into cells. In Table 37.5, the mechanisms for common causes of hypophosphatemia in the ICU are described.

TABLE 37.5 Predisposing Conditions and Mechanisms for Hypophosphatemia in the ICU

Condition	Mechanism	Comment
Glucose Loading	As glucose moves into cells, so does PO_4 (presumably because PO_4 is need for glycolysis).	• Most common cause of hypophosphatemia in hospitalized patients. • Can cause refeeding syndrome due to the high carbohydrate concentration in total parenteral nutrition (TPN).
Diabetic Ketoacidosis	Caused by osmotic diuresis from prolonged hyperglycemia, which promotes urinary PO_4 losses. When insulin is given, both glucose and PO_4 are driven intracellularly.	See Chapter 32
Respiratory Alkalosis	A higher intracellular pH accelerates glycolysis. This is accompanied by the movement of glucose and PO_4 into cells.	May be found in over ventilated or hyperventilating patients.
Physiological Stress	Stimulation of β-adrenergic receptors moves PO_4 into cells.	
Systemic Inflammation	High levels of cytokines are associated with lower serum levels of PO_4.	Possible explanations may include increased PO_4 utilization by neutrophils and higher circulating levels of catecholamines.
Phosphate Binders	Aluminum can form insoluble complexes with inorganic phosphates.	May be associated with sucralfate (an aluminum-containing compound).

From References 17-22.

Clinical Manifestations

Oxidative Metabolism

Hypophosphatemia is often clinically silent, even when the PO_4 falls to extremely low levels. Severe PO_4 depletion creates a risk for impaired oxidative metabolism, as demonstrated in Figure 37.2, with the following effects:

1. Impaired myocardial contractility and reduced cardiac output.
2. Association with hemolytic anemia, perhaps due to reduced red blood cell deformability.
3. Depletion of 2,3-diphosphoglycerate, shifting the oxyhemoglobin dissociation curve to the left.
4. Reduced energy availability as the result of decreased production of high-energy phosphate compounds (i.e., ATP).

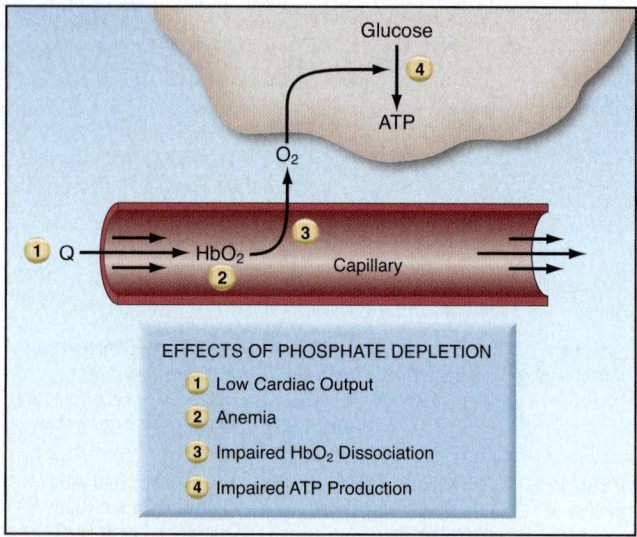

FIGURE 37.2. The effects of hypophosphatemia that threaten oxidative cellular energy production. (From References 21–23.)

Muscle Disorders

Hypophosphatemia is a reported cause of rhabdomyolysis (24) and respiratory muscle weakness (25). In some studies, hypophosphatemia has been found to be an independent risk factor for failure to discontinue mechanical ventilation in ICU patients, with a more pronounced association in patients with chronic obstructive pulmonary disease (26-27).

Phosphate Replacement

Intravenous phosphate replacement is recommended for all patients with severe hypophosphatemia (i.e., serum PO_4 <1.0 mg/dL or 0.3 mmol/L), and for patients with hypophosphatemia of any degree who also have cardiac dysfunction, respiratory failure, or rhabdomyolysis. Phosphate solutions and dosing regimens are listed in Table 37.6.

TABLE 37.6	Phosphate Replacement Therapy	
Solution†	PO_4 Content	Other Content
Sodium Phosphate	93 mg (3 mmol)/mL	Na^+: 4.0 mEq/L
Potassium Phosphate	93 mg (3 mmol)/mL	K^+: 4.3 mEq/L
PO_4 Replacement (IV) by Body Weight			
Serum PO_4 (mg/dL)	40-60 kg	61-80 kg	81-120 kg
<1	30 mmol	40 mmol	50 mmol
1-1.7	20 mmol	30 mmol	40 mmol
1.8-2.5	10 mmol	15 mmol	20 mmol

†If the plasma K^+ is ≥4 mEq/L, use sodium phosphate, and if the plasma K^+ is <4 mEq/L, use potassium phosphate.

From Reference 28.

HYPERPHOSPHATEMIA

The principal cause of hyperphosphatemia in the ICU is end-stage renal disease. Less common causes are tumor lysis syndrome and hypoparathyroidism.

Clinical Manifestations

ICU patients with hyperphosphatemia have a higher risk of all-cause mortality than those without and a higher requirement for continuous renal replacement therapy (29). The consequences of hyperphosphatemia include the formation of insoluble Ca^{++}-phosphate complexes and hypocalcemia, the significance of which is unknown (8).

Management

The management of hyperphosphatemia involves the use of phosphate binders to reduce GI absorption of phosphate. There is no evidence that one type of phosphate binder is superior to the other, though some prefer non-Ca^{++} containing binders because there is a daily limit of Ca^{++} (<800 mg) recommended in patients with chronic kidney disease (30-31). In severe cases associated with acute renal failure, renal replacement may be required (see Chapter 33: Acute Kidney Injury).

Sevelamer

Sevelamer is a non-Ca^{++}-containing phosphate binder that is dosed by PO_4 level as described in Table 37.7. Sevelamer gluconate is preferred to sevelamer hydrochloride because the latter preparation can cause a metabolic acidosis (32).

TABLE 37.7 Dosing of Sevelamer

Serum PO_4 (mg/dL)	Sevelamer Dose
5.6-7.4	800 mg TID
7.5-8.9	1,00-1,600 mg TID
>9	1,600 mg TID

From Scialla JJ, Kendrick J, Uribarri J, et al. State-of-the-art management of hyperphosphatemia in patients with CKD: an NKF-KDOQI controversies perspective. J Kidney Dis 2021;77:132-41.

Calcium Acetate

Ca^{++} acetate (PhosLo) is available in tablets (667 mg per tab) or an oral solution (667 mg/5 mL). The initial dose is 1,334 mg (2 tabs or 10 mL) three times daily, and this can be increased to achieve a serum PO_4 <6 mg/dL, as long as hypercalcemia does not develop (33).

References

1. Baker SB, Worthley LI. The essentials of calcium, magnesium and phosphate metabolism: part I. Physiology. Crit Care Resusc 2002;4:301-6.
2. Wynne Z, Falat C. Disorders of calcium and magnesium. Emerg Med Clin N Am 2023;41:833-48.
3. Smith JD, Wilson S, Schneider HG. Misclassification of calcium status based on albumin-adjusted calcium: studies in a tertiary hospital setting. Clin Chem 2018;64:1713-22.
4. Slomp J, van der Voort PH, Gerritsen RT, et al. Albumin-adjusted calcium is not suitable for diagnosis of hyper- and hypocalcemia in the critically ill. Crit Care Med 2003;31:1389-93.
5. Melchers M, van Zanten ARH. Management of hypocalcemia in the critically ill. Curr Opin Crit Care 2023;29:330-8.
6. Aberegg SK. Ionized calcium in the ICU: should it be measured and corrected? Chest 2016;149:846-55.
7. Byerly S, Inaba K, Biswas S, et al. Transfusion-related hypocalcemia after trauma. World J Surg 2020;44(11):3743-50.
8. Giancarelli A, Birrer KL, Alban RF, et al. Hypocalcemia in trauma patients receiving massive transfusion. J Surg Res 2016;202(1):182-7.
9. Baker SB, Worthley LI. The essentials of calcium, magnesium and phosphate metabolism: part II. Disorders. Crit Care Resusc 2002;4:307-15.
10. Méneret A, Guey S, Degos B. Chvostek sign, frequently found in healthy subjects, is not a useful clinical sign. Neurology 2013;80:1067.
11. van Bussel BCT, Koopmans RP. Trousseau's sign at the emergency department. BMJ Case Rep 2016;2016.
12. Zaloga GP. Hypocalcemia in critically ill patients. Crit Care Med 1992;20:251-62.
13. Maier JD, Levine SN. Hypercalcemia in the intensive care unit: A review of pathophysiology, diagnosis, and modern therapy. J Intensive Care Med 2015;30:235-52.

14. Almuradova E, Cicin I. Cancer-related hypercalcemia and potential treatments. Front Endocrinol 2023;14:1039490.
15. LeGrand S, Leskuski D, Zama I. Narrative review: furosemide for hypercalcemia: an unproven yet common practice. Ann Intern Med 2008;149:259-63.
16. Sin JCK, King L, Ballard E, et al. Hypophosphatemia and outcomes in ICU: A systematic review and meta-analysis. J Intensive Care Med 2021;36:1025-35.
17. Paleologos M, Stone E, Braude S. Persistent, progressive hypophosphataemia after voluntary hyperventilation. Clin Sci (Lond) 2000;98:619-25.
18. Roestel C, Hoeping W, Deckert J. Hypophosphatemia in panic disorder. Am J Psychiatry 2004;161:1499-500.
19. Barak V, Schwartz A, Kalickman I, et al. Prevalence of hypophosphatemia in sepsis and infection: the role of cytokines. Am J Med 1998;104:40-7.
20. Miller SJ, Simpson J. Medication-nutrient interactions: hypophosphatemia associated with sucralfate in the intensive care unit. Nutr Clin Pract 1991;6:199-201.
21. King AL, Sica DA, Miller G, et al. Severe hypophosphatemia in a general hospital population. South Med J 1987;80:831-5.
22. Davis SV, Olichwier KK, Chakko SC. Reversible depression of myocardial performance in hypophosphatemia. Am J Med Sci 1988;295:183-7.
23. Klock JC, Williams HE. Mentzer WC. Hemolytic anemia and somatic cell dysfunction in severe hypophosphatemia. Arch Intern Med 1974;134:360-4.
24. Knochel JP, Barcenas C, Cotton JR, et al. Hypophosphatemia and rhabdomyolysis. J Clin Invest 1978;62:1240-6.
25. Gravelyn TR, Brophy N, Siegert C, et al. Hypophosphatemia-associated respiratory muscle weakness in a general inpatient population. Am J Med 1988;84:870-6.
26. Alsumrain MH, Jawad SA, Imran NB, et al. Association of hypophosphatemia with failure-to-wean from mechanical ventilation. Ann Clin Lab Sci 2010;40(2):144-8.
27. Zhao Y, Li Z, Shi Y, et al. Effect of hypophosphatemia on the withdrawal of mechanical ventilation in patients with acute exacerbations of chronic obstructive pulmonary disease. Biomed Rep 2016;4(4):413-6.
28. Taylor BE, Huey WY, Buchman TG, et al. Treatment of hypophosphatemia using a protocol based on patient weight and serum phosphorus level in a surgical intensive care unit. J Am Coll Surg 2004;198:198-204.
29. Zheng WH, Yao Y, Zhou H, et al. Hyperphosphatemia and outcomes in critically ill patients: a systematic review and meta-analysis. Front Med (Lausanne) 2022;9:870637.

30. Scialla JJ, Kendrick J, Uribarri J, et al. Management of hyperphosphatemia in patients with CKD: an NKF-KDOQI controversies perspective. J Kidney Dis 2021;77:132-41.
31. Sevelamer. In: *Drug Information Handbook*. 24th ed. Lexi-Comp Inc.; 2015;1821-2.
32. Brezina B, Quinibi WY, Nolan CR. Acid loading during treatment with sevelamer hydrochloride: mechanisms and clinical implications. Kidney Int Suppl 2004;66(90):S39-S45.
33. Calcium Acetate. In: *Drug Information Handbook*. 24th ed. Lexi-Comp Inc.; 2015;318-9.

SECTION X
THE ABDOMEN AND PELVIS

Chapter 38
Liver Failure

There are two types of liver failure:

1. Acute (fulminant) liver failure
2. Acute-on-chronic liver failure

ACUTE LIVER FAILURE

Acute liver failure (ALF) occurs without prior liver disease and is an uncommon disorder (annual incidence is <10 per million). Acetaminophen is the leading cause of ALF in the United States, responsible for 50% of cases, and drug-induced hepatitis and viral hepatitis are the two most common etiologies of ALF (1). Other causes include ischemic hepatitis, other drugs (e.g., cocaine), heat stroke, and others (2). About 20% of cases are idiopathic (3).

ACUTE-ON-CHRONIC LIVER FAILURE

Acute-on-chronic liver failure (ACLF) is *not* decompensated liver cirrhosis; it is characterized by a triggering event resulting in severe deterioration of liver function, extrahepatic organ failure, and is associated with high short-term mortality (4-5). Examples of precipitating events are shown in Table 38.1 (2,4).

CLINICAL FEATURES

Both types of liver failure share similar clinical features with some differences.

TABLE 38.1 Examples of Triggering Events for ACLF

Hepatic Causes	Non-Hepatic Causes
• Alcohol binge consumption* • Liver surgery (including TIPS) • Reactivation of viral hepatitis	• Infection* • Major surgery • Drug-induced

ACLF = acute-on-chronic liver failure; TIPS = transjugular intrahepatic portosystemic shunt.

Estimated 40-50% unrecognized triggering event.

*Most common.

Clinical Features of Acute Liver Failure (3)

- A dominant feature is hepatic encephalopathy, which appears within 8 weeks of symptom onset, and can raise intracranial pressure (6).
- Variceal hemorrhage is less common in patients with portal hypertension than in those with ACLF.
- Severity of liver injury is reflected in decreases in coagulation factors (e.g., prothrombin time or elevated international normalized ratio [INR]) and total bilirubin reflecting hepatocellular function (6).
- N-acetylcysteine (NAC), used to treat acute acetaminophen overdose, has been demonstrated to improve clinical outcomes in non-acetaminophen-related liver failure (7). Treatment in non-acetaminophen-related liver failure should be extended beyond the 72-h recommendation for acetaminophen overdose (8). (See Table 38.2.)

Clinical Features of Acute-on-Chronic Liver Failure

- Characterized by organ failure and systemic inflammation (6)
- Portal hypertension is prominent, and variceal hemorrhage is common. Hemorrhage and shock may be the trigger for the acute aspect of this liver failure.
- Ascites is prominent, and there is a risk of spontaneous bacterial peritonitis and hepatorenal syndrome.

TABLE 38.2 Intravenous NAC Acetaminophen Overdose

1. Regimen:

Use 20% NAC (200 mg/mL) for each of the doses below and infuse in sequence.

1. 150 mg/kg in 200 mL D_5W over 1 h
2. 50 mg/kg 500 mL D_5W over 4 h
3. 100 mg/kg in 1,000 mL D_5W over 16 h

Total Dose: 300 mg/kg over 21 h

2. NAC Stopping Criteria:

1. Plasma acetaminophen <10 µg/mL
2. AST/ALT normal for patient, or decreased by 25-50%.
3. INR <2.0
4. Patient feeling well

a. If NAC stopping criteria are not satisfied, continue IV NAC at a rate of at least 6.25 mg/kg/h.

b. Recheck criteria every 12-24 h and continue NAC until criteria are satisfied.

NAC = N-acetylcysteine.

From References 12 and 13.

ACETAMINOPHEN OVERDOSE

A single dose of activated charcoal is best administered within 1 h of ingestion (9-11) but at least within 4 h, hopefully in the emergency department prior to intensive care unit (ICU) admission. Notably gastric lavage is no longer recommended per the US and Canada Consensus Statement (12). NAC administration is based on acetaminophen levels but should be started regardless of ingestion >30 g or acetaminophen level will take >8 h. Although NAC can be administered orally, intravenous is preferred (12). Intravenous regimen is shown in Table 38.2. Treatment with NAC proceeds in two stages (12). The first stage involves a 21-h infusion of NAC, which is given in three separate aliquots, for a total dose of 300 mg/kg (13). This is followed by an evaluation of four criteria of treatment, which are listed in Table 38.2 as the "NAC Stopping Criteria."

The NAC infusion is continued at a dosage rate of at least 6.25 mg/kg/h (12) if these goals are not reached, and goals are reevaluated again after 12-24 h. The NAC infusion is maintained until the goals have been achieved.

NAC treatment of acetaminophen overdose is nearly 100% protective if NAC is administered within 8-10 h of ingestion; however, treatment with NAC should proceed if >12 h (9).

HEPATORENAL SYNDROME

Hepatorenal syndrome (HRS) is a functional renal failure (i.e., occurs without intrinsic renal disease) that occurs in patients with cirrhosis and ascites, especially those with spontaneous bacterial peritonitis or sepsis from another source (14). HRS is rapid onset characterized by doubling of the serum creatinine in <2 weeks and is associated with a 50% mortality within 2 weeks.

Pathogenesis

HRS is caused by hemodynamic alterations in splanchnic and renal circulation. Cirrhosis and portal hypertension are associated with splanchnic vasodilation, and the neurohumoral (renin-angiotensin system) response to this vasodilation results in vasoconstriction in the kidneys (14-15). The renal vasoconstriction makes the glomerular filtration rate vulnerable to small decreases in cardiac output.

Diagnosis

The diagnostic criteria for HRS are shown in Table 38.3 (16). These criteria include evidence of acute kidney injury (an increase in serum creatinine ≥0.3 mg/dL within 48 h) that does not respond to albumin infusions (volume resuscitation) and no other likely source of acute kidney injury (i.e., circulatory shock or nephrotoxic drugs) (14,17).

TABLE 38.3 Diagnostic Criteria for Hepatorenal Syndrome

1. Cirrhosis with ascites
2. Increase in SCr of ≥0.3 mg/dL within 48 h, or SCr ≥1.5 times baseline
3. No response to diuretic withdrawal and 2 days of fluid challenges with albumin (1 g/kg/day).
4. No evidence of shock and no recent use of nephrotoxic drugs
5. No signs of structural kidney injury:
   a. Absence of proteinuria (>500 mg/day).
   b. Absence of hematuria (>50 RBCs per high power field).
   c. Normal findings on renal ultrasound.

SCr = serum creatinine; RBC = red blood cell.

From Simonetto DA, Gines P, Kamath PS. Hepatorenal syndrome: pathophysiology, diagnosis, and management. BMJ 2020;370:m2687.

Management

HRS can be remarkably challenging as the understanding of HRS continues to evolve. The classifications of two types (type-1 HRS and type-2 HRS) are no longer used (18). Acute kidney injury (AKI) is common in critically ill patients. Concomitant pressures on an already fragile HRS kidney, such as sepsis and hypovolemia, clearly confound the impact of therapeutic measures. For example, terlipressin, a vasopressin analog used for HRS, has had mixed results. A 25-year literature review found norepinephrine as effective as terlipressin in reversing HRS (19). Thus, the management of AKI/HRS needs to be pragmatic with considerations of many clinical factors, i.e., hypovolemia, sepsis.

Pharmaceutical options for HRS are shown in Table 38.4 (16).

Continuous renal replacement therapy (CRRT) not only is used for the usual indications for renal failure but also can impact severe hepatic encephalopathy (20).

Liver transplantation is the only cure (15).

> **TABLE 38.4** Pharmaceutical Treatments for Hepatorenal Syndrome
>
> 1. Albumin (25%): 20-40 g daily
> 2. Splanchnic vasoconstriction with one of the following:
>   a. Terlipressin: 1 mg IV every 4-6 h, or infuse at 84 µg/h (2 mg/day)
>   b. Norepinephrine: 5-40 µg/min by continuous infusion
>   c. Octreotide (100-200 µg subQ) plus midodrine (7.5-15 mg PO) three times daily.

From Simonetto DA, Gines P, Kamath PS. Hepatorenal syndrome: pathophysiology, diagnosis, and management. BMJ 2020;370:m2687.

SPONTANEOUS BACTERIAL PERITONITIS

Twenty-five to 30% of patients with ascites will develop spontaneous bacterial peritonitis (SBP) (21-22), a bacterial infection of the ascitic fluid that occurs without an obvious source of bacteria. The current belief is that the bacteria come from the "translocation" of enteric organisms from the gastrointestinal (GI) tract. This presumption is supported by the typical pathogens isolated from SBP: gram-negative aerobic bacilli in 75% of cases, and gram-positive aerobic cocci (especially streptococci) in 25% of cases (23). Importantly, SBP can be a trigger for ACLF.

Clinical Features

Clinical features include fever, abdominal pain, and rebound tenderness in at least 50% of patients, but the condition can be asymptomatic in one-third of patients (23).

SBP should be suspected in cirrhotic patients who present with acute deterioration.

Diagnostic Evaluation and Management

Diagnostic evaluation requires peritoneal fluid culture. A polymorphonuclear leukocyte count of ≥250 cells/mm^3 in the peritoneal fluid is presumptive evidence of infection and an indication to begin empiric antimicrobial therapy. The preferred antibiotic is *cefotaxime* (2 g IV every 8 h), or another third-generation cephalosporin (24).

In patients who do not respond to antibiotic therapy, a secondary source of peritonitis, such as diverticulitis or appendicitis, should be taken into consideration.

The mortality rate in SBP is 30-40% despite adequate antibiotic coverage (25). About one-third of patients with SBP develop the HRS (26), which might explain the high mortality rate.

HEPATIC ENCEPHALOPATHY

The hallmark of the advanced stages of liver failure is an encephalopathy that is characterized by cerebral edema and increased intracranial pressure. Ammonia (NH_3) has been identified as a key factor in the pathogenesis of hepatic encephalopathy (HE) (27-30).

Pathogenesis

The normal clearance of NH_3 by conversion to urea in the liver is impaired in liver failure, and the resulting increase in plasma NH_3 eventually leads to accumulation of NH_3 in the brain, where it is taken up by astrocytes and used to convert glutamate to glutamine, i.e.,

$$\text{glutamate} + NH_3 + ATP \rightarrow \text{glutamine} + ADP \quad (38.1)$$

The intracellular accumulation of glutamine creates an osmotic force that draws water into the astrocytes, thereby promoting cerebral edema (27).

Diagnostic Evaluation

Clinical Features

The clinical features of grading for HE are described in Table 38.5 (20).

The earliest signs of encephalopathy include personality changes, altered cognition, and asterixis (irregular

TABLE 38.5	Grading of Hepatic Encephalopathy: The West Haven System
Grade	Features
Grade 1	• Short attention span • Personality change
Grade 2	• Apathy or lethargy • Disoriented to time
Grade 3	• Stuporous but responsive • Disoriented to place and time
Grade 4	• Coma

From Weissenborn K. Hepatic encephalopathy: definition, clinical grading and diagnostic principles. Drugs 2019;79(Suppl 1):S5-S9.

movements produced by sustained dorsiflexion of the wrist), whereas disorientation and depressed consciousness become prominent as the encephalopathy progresses. Extrapyramidal signs (e.g., rigidity, parkinsonian tremor) are common in HE, and a positive Babinski sign can be observed (30). Focal neurological deficits and seizures are uncommon in HE (30).

Overall, clinical features of HE are nonspecific (including asterixis, which can be observed with metabolic encephalopathies and drug overdoses), and the diagnosis is made by excluding other causes of altered mentation (31).

Serum Ammonia (NH_3)

Despite the importance of NH_3 in the pathogenesis of HE, monitoring serum NH_3 levels has a limited role in HE.

- The major role for serum NH_3 levels is in ALF, where there is a good correlation between NH_3 levels and both the presence and severity of HE, the risk for increased intracranial pressure, and an independent risk factor for mortality (3,20,31).

- *In patients with cirrhosis, serum NH_3 levels may be chronically elevated and less reliable for both detecting HE and determining the severity of illness (31-32). This is demonstrated by the results of one study (29), which showed that serum NH_3 levels were normal in >50% of cirrhotic patients with HE.*

Reducing the Ammonia Burden

The principal site of NH_3 production is the lower GI tract, where NH_3 is a byproduct of protein degradation, and urease-producing gut microbes promote the breakdown of urea to generate additional NH_3. The following measures are used to reduce the NH_3 burden from the bowel.

Lactulose

Lactulose is a nonabsorbable disaccharide that is metabolized by gut microbes to form short-chain fatty acids, and the resulting acidification of the bowel lumen has two advantages: (1) it promotes the conversion of NH_3 to NH_4^+ (ammonium), which is less easily absorbed from the gut, and (2) its low pH eradicates urease-producing microbes (30,33).

Lactulose Dosing. 10-30 g orally or enterally (e.g., nasogastric tube) 2-4 times daily targeting 2 semisoft bowel movements per day; may be given as retention enema, 200 g in 700 mL water for 1 h; can be repeated every 4-6 h (31,33-34)

Polyethylene Glycol

Polyethylene glycol is an alternative to lactulose in critically ill patients with overt HE.

Polyethylene Glycol Dosing. 4 L enterally over 4 h (35)

Rifaximin

Rifaximin is a nonabsorbable antibiotic resulting in high concentrations in the intestinal lumen targeting NH_3-producing bacteria.

Rifaximin Dosing. 550 mg orally twice daily or 400 mg orally 3 times daily (31)

Continuous Renal Replacement Therapy (CRRT)
CRRT can rapidly lower serum NH_3 levels (20,31,36).

Liver Transplantation
Liver transplantation is the ultimate fix for HE; transplantation can usually reverse the cognitive impairment associated with HE (31).

Closure of Porto-Systemic Shunts
Closure of portosystemic shunts, such as a transjugular intrahepatic portosystemic shunt (TIPS), are performed to decrease the portal venous hypertension that causes variceal hemorrhage. An endovascular procedure typically performed by an interventional radiologist; TIPS is a shunt inserted via the internal jugular vein connecting a hepatic vein (systemic circulation) to a major intrahepatic portal vein (the portal venous circulation). Blood is shunted from the portal venous system (high pressure) into the systemic circulation (lower pressure) which bypasses the liver. A TIPS is illustrated in Figure 38.1. Unfortunately, a consequence of these shunts is an increase in the occurrence of HE due to the accumulation of NH_3 as the liver is responsible for the metabolism of NH_3 to urea.

Increased Intracranial Pressure

Increased intracranial pressure (ICP) is predominantly seen in ALF and is an ominous sign (3). A sustained increase in serum NH_3 levels to ≥150 μmol/L (≥255 μg/dL) is associated with a high risk of intracranial hypertension (3) and can be used as an indication to monitor ICP.

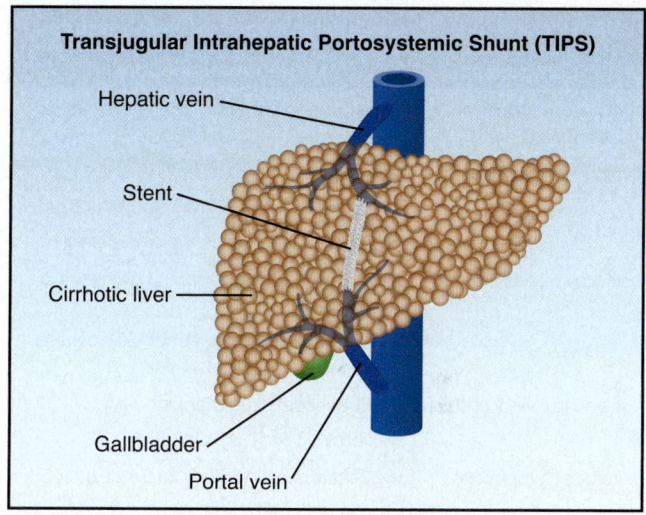

FIGURE 38.1. Transjugular intrahepatic portosystemic shunt (TIPS).

VARICEAL HEMORRHAGE (VH)

Esophageal and/or gastric varices develop as a consequence of portal hypertension (20,37). The risk of hemorrhage increases as portal pressure increases. Variceal hemorrhage can be a trigger for ACLF, can be profound, and is life-threatening. Components of the management of variceal hemorrhage are outlined in Table 38.6 (20,35,37).

For refractory or recurrent variceal hemorrhage, TIPS (Figure 38.1) can be employed as a rescue for failed medical and endoscopic interventions. A Sengstaken-Blakemore (SBTube) or Minnesota tube can also be deployed in refractory bleeding and as a bridge to a TIPS. Inserted nasally or orally, the components of the SBTube are shown in Figure 38.2.

TABLE 38.6	Management of Variceal Hemorrhage
Component	Recommendations
Endoscopy (potential banding/ligation)	• Perform within 12 h.
Volume resuscitation	• MAP goal of 65 mm Hg • Use 5% albumin if serum albumin <3 g/dL. • Balanced crystalloids, avoid normal saline
Blood products	• Transfuse RBCs, plasma, and platelets in a 1:1:1 ratio. • Use thromboelastography (TEG) to guide correction of coagulopathy.
Splanchnic vasoconstrictor	• Octreotide: 50 µg IV bolus • Followed by 50 µg/h infusion
Antibiotic prophylaxis	• Ceftriaxone, 1 g IV daily for 5-7 days • Initiate before endoscopy.

Adapted from Liver Failure. In: Marino PL. *Marino's The ICU Book*. 5th ed. Wolters Kluwer; 2025:605-17.

The tube is inserted into the stomach and the gastric balloon is inflated with 250-500 mL air. Gentle traction is then applied (250-500 g tension) to secure the inflated balloon in the stomach at the gastroesophageal junction. The face mask of a football helmet is commonly used to secure the tube and maintain the traction. The esophageal balloon is inflated to 22-40 mm Hg (using a manometer) to apply tamponade to the esophageal varices. The lowest pressure accomplishing hemostasis is recommended as higher pressures can be associated with tissue necrosis. Gastric decompression is accomplished using the gastric aspiration port. A Minnesota tube has the addition of an esophageal aspiration port.

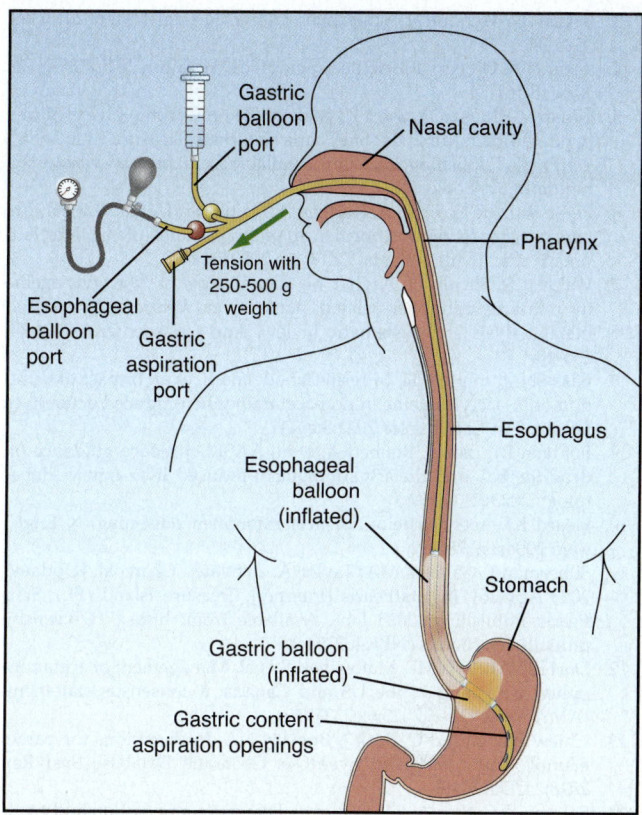

FIGURE 38.2. Sengstaken-Blakemore Tube.

References

1. Rubin JB, Hameed B, Gottfried M, et al. Acetaminophen-induced acute liver failure is more common and more severe in women. Clin Gastroenterol Hepatol 2018;16:936-46.
2. Shah NJ, Royer A, John S. Acute Liver Failure. [Updated 2023 Apr 7]. In: StatPearls [Internet]. Treasure Island (FL): StatPearls Publishing; 2025 Jan-. Available from: https://www.ncbi.nlm.nih.gov/books/NBK482374/

3. Bernal W, Wendon J. Acute liver failure. N Engl J Med 2013;369: 2525-34.
4. Asrani SK, O'Leary JG. Acute-on-chronic liver failure. Clin Liver Dis 2014;18:561-74.
5. Girish V, Mousa OY, Syed K, et al. Acute on Chronic Liver Failure. [Updated 2025 Jun 2]. In: StatPearls [Internet]. Treasure Island (FL): StatPearls Publishing; 2025 Jan-. Available from: https://www.ncbi.nlm.nih.gov/books/NBK499902/
6. Perez Ruiz de Garibay A, Kortgen A, Leonhardt J, et al. Critical care hepatology: definitions, incidence, prognosis and role of liver failure in critically ill patients. Crit Care 2022;26:289.
7. Walayat S, Shoaib H, Asghar M, Kiet al. Role of N-acetylcysteine in non-acetaminophen-related acute liver failure: an updated meta-analysis and systematic review. Ann Gastroenterol 2021;34: 235-40.
8. Bass SN, Lumpkin M, Mireles-Cabodevila E, et al. Impact of duration of N-acetylcysteine in non-acetaminophen-induced acute liver failure. Crit Care Explor 2021;3:e0411.
9. Fontana RJ, Liou I, Reuben A, et al. AASLD practice guidance on drug, herbal, and dietary supplement-induced liver injury. Hepatology 2023;77:1036-65.
10. Heard KJ. Acetylcysteine for acetaminophen poisoning. N Engl J Med 2008;359:285-92.
11. Silberman J, Galuska MA, Taylor A. Activated Charcoal. [Updated 2023 Apr 26]. In: StatPearls [Internet]. Treasure Island (FL): StatPearls Publishing; 2025 Jan-. Available from: https://www.ncbi.nlm.nih.gov/books/NBK482294/
12. Dart RC, Mullins ME, Matoushek T, et al. Management of acetaminophen poisoning in the US and Canada: a consensus statement. JAMA Netw Open 2023;6:e2327739.
13. Chiew AL, Gluud C, Brok J, Buckley NA. Interventions for paracetamol (acetaminophen) overdose. Cochrane Database Syst Rev 2018;2:CD003328.
14. Salerno F, Gerbes A, Gines P, et al. Diagnosis, prevention and treatment of hepatorenal syndrome in cirrhosis. Gut 2007;56:1310-8.
15. Ranasinghe IR, Sharma B, Bashir K. Hepatorenal Syndrome. [Updated 2023 Aug 8]. In: StatPearls [Internet]. Treasure Island (FL): StatPearls Publishing; 2025 Jan-. Available from: https://www.ncbi.nlm.nih.gov/books/NBK430856/
16. Simonetto DA, Gines P, Kamath PS. Hepatorenal syndrome: pathophysiology, diagnosis, and management. BMJ 2020;370:m2687.
17. Wong F. The evolving concept of acute kidney injury in patients with cirrhosis. Nat Rev Gastroenterol Hepatol 2015;12:711-9.
18. American Liver Foundation. Hepatorenal syndrome. Updated June 4, 2024. Accessed May 1, 2025. https://liverfoundation.org/

liver-diseases/complications-of-liver-disease/hepatorenal-syndrome/#:~:text=There%20used%20to%20be%20a,term%20is%20no%20longer%20used]
19. Duong N, Kakadiya P, Bajaj JS. Current pharmacologic therapies for hepatorenal syndrome-acute kidney injury. Clin Gastroenterol Hepatol 2023;21:S27-S34.
20. Van Eldere A, Pirani T. Liver intensive care for the general intensivist. Anaesthesia 2023;78:884-901.
21. Ameer MA, Foris LA, Mandiga P, Haseeb M. Spontaneous Bacterial Peritonitis (Archived). [Updated 2023 Aug 8]. In: StatPearls [Internet]. Treasure Island (FL): StatPearls Publishing; 2025 Jan–.
22. Koulaouzidis A, Bhat S, Karagiannidis A, et al. Spontaneous bacterial peritonitis. Postgrad Med J 2007;83:379-83.
23. Gilbert JA, Kamath PS. Spontaneous bacterial peritonitis: an update. Mayo Clin Proc 1995;70:365-70.
24. Biggins SW, Angeli P, Garcia-Tsao G, et al. Diagnosis, evaluation, and management of ascites, spontaneous bacterial peritonitis and hepatorenal syndrome: 2021 practice guidance by the American Association for the Study of Liver Diseases. Hepatology 2021;74:1014-48.
25. Runyon BA. Management of adult patients with ascites caused by cirrhosis. Hepatology 1998;27:264-72.
26. Moore CM, Van Thiel DH. Cirrhotic ascites review: pathophysiology, diagnosis and management. World J Hepatol 2013;5:251-63.
27. Clay AS, Hainline BE. Hyperammonemia in the ICU. Chest 2007; 132:1368-78.
28. Ferenci P, Lockwood A, Mullen K, et al. Hepatic encephalopathy—definition, nomenclature, diagnosis, and quantification: final report of the working party at the 11th World Congresses of Gastroenterology, Vienna, 1998. Hepatology 2002;35:716-21.
29. Kundra A, Jain A, Banga A, et al. Evaluation of plasma ammonia levels in patients with acute liver failure and chronic liver disease and its correlation with the severity of hepatic encephalopathy and clinical features of raised intracranial tension. Clin Biochem 2005;38:696-9.
30. Vilstrup H, Amodio P, Bajaj J, et al. Hepatic encephalopathy in chronic liver disease: 2014 practice guideline by the American Association for the Study of Liver Diseases and the European Association for the Study of the Liver. Hepatology 2014;60:715-35.
31. Mandiga P, Kommu S, Bollu PC. Hepatic Encephalopathy. [Updated 2025 Jan 20]. In: StatPearls [Internet]. Treasure Island (FL): StatPearls Publishing; 2025 Jan–. Available from: https://www.ncbi.nlm.nih.gov/books/NBK430869/
32. Ballester MP, Durmazer EN, Qi T, Jalan R. The value of ammonia as a biomarker in patients with cirrhosis. Semin Liver Dis 2024;44:356-68.

33. Leise MD, Poterucha JJ, Kamath PS, Kim WR. Management of hepatic encephalopathy in the hospital. Mayo Clin Proc 2014;89:241-53.
34. Mukherjee S, Patel P, John S. Lactulose. [Updated 2024 Feb 28]. In: StatPearls [Internet]. Treasure Island (FL): StatPearls Publishing; 2025 Jan-. Available from: https://www.ncbi.nlm.nih.gov/books/NBK536930/
35. Nanchal R, Subramanian R, Alhazzani W, et al. Guidelines for the management of adult acute and acute-on-chronic liver failure in the ICU: Neurology, peri-transplant medicine, infectious disease, and gastroenterology considerations. Crit Care Med 2023;51:657-76.
36. Warrillow S, Bellomo R. Intensive care management of severe acute liver failure. In: Vincent JL, ed. *Annual Update in Intensive Care and Emergency Medicine 2015*. Springer; 2015:415-30.
37. Zuckerman MJ, Elhanafi S, Mendoza Ladd A. Endoscopic treatment of esophageal varices. Clin Liver Dis 2022;26:21-37.

Acute Pancreatitis

Chapter 39

OVERVIEW

The worldwide incidence of acute pancreatitis (AP) is 7-134.9 per 100,000 person-years with an overall mortality of 1%. However, those with organ failure or necrosis (severe), mortality can reach 40% (1). This chapter will focus on severe pancreatitis requiring ICU admission.

Classification

AP can be divided into two types (2):

1. *Interstitial edematous pancreatitis* is the most common form of pancreatitis and is characterized by inflammatory infiltration of the pancreas without involvement of other organs.
2. *Necrotizing pancreatitis* occurs in 10-15% of cases (3) and is characterized by areas of pancreatic necrosis and peri-pancreatic tissue, usually accompanied by a progressive systemic inflammatory response. The mortality rate can be as high as 40% (4), and management requires ICU-level care.

Etiology and Diagnosis

There is a diversity of mechanisms causing AP with over two-thirds as a result of gallstones or alcohol consumption (1-2,5). Other causes are shown in Table 39.1 (2,5-7).

The diagnostic and severity criteria for AP using the revised Atlanta classification are shown in Table 39.2 (8).

TABLE 39.1 Etiologies of Acute Pancreatitis

- Gallstones (39-44%)
- Alcohol consumption (17-25%)
- Idiopathic (15-22%)
- Hypertriglyceridemia (2.3-10%)
- Trauma (blunt or penetrating)
- Endoscopic retrograde cholangiopancreatography (ERCP)
- Infections
  - Viral: cytomegalovirus, mumps, coxsackie-B, Epstein-Barr
  - Parasitic: ascaris, clonorchis
- Ischemia/reperfusion
- Drugs
  - E.g., furosemide, immunosuppressants, sulfonamides, estrogens
- Other associated risk factors:
  - Diabetes
  - Obesity
  - Smoking

TABLE 39.2 Diagnostic and Severity of Illness Criteria for Acute Pancreatitis

Diagnostic*
- Abdominal pain consistent with (severe, acute persistent epigastric pain, often radiating to back)
- Increase in amylase or lipase to >3 times upper limit of normal
- Imaging evidence of acute pancreatitis (typically contrast-enhanced computed tomography)

Severity of Illness
- Mild: no organ failure, and no local or systemic complications
- Moderate: transient organ failure (<48 h), or local or systemic complications without persistent organ failure
- Severe: persistent organ failure (>48 h), single or multiple

*Two or more criteria.

Laboratory Evaluation

Pancreatic Enzyme

The pancreatic enzymes amylase and lipase are used in the diagnosis of AP, but levels are *not* associated with severity of disease.

Amylase. An enzyme that cleaves starch into smaller polysaccharides. The principal sources of amylase are the pancreas, salivary glands, and fallopian tubes. Serum amylase levels begin to rise 6-12 h after the onset of AP, and they return to normal in 3-5 days. Elevated serum amylase levels to three times the upper limit of normal has a high sensitivity (>90%) but a low specificity (as low as 70%) for the diagnosis of AP (9). This low specificity of serum amylase reflects the numerous conditions that can elevate serum amylase levels (10).

Lipase. An enzyme that hydrolyses triglycerides to form glycerol and free fatty acids. The principal sources of lipase are the tongue, pancreas, liver, intestine, and circulating lipoproteins. Serum lipase levels begin to rise 4-8 h after the onset of AP (earlier than the rise in serum amylase), and the serum levels remain elevated for 8-14 days (longer than the rise in serum amylase). Unlike amylase, nonpancreatic conditions rarely raise serum lipase levels high enough to overlap with the levels seen in AP (11). An increase in serum lipase to three times the upper limit of normal has a sensitivity and specificity of 80-100% for AP (9). Therefore, serum lipase is more specific than serum amylase for the diagnosis of AP.

> RECOMMENDATION: *The serum lipase alone can be used for the diagnostic evaluation of pancreatitis. Adding the serum amylase does not improve diagnostic accuracy (9).*

Other Laboratory Testing (specific points)

Complete Blood Count (CBC)
- Leukocytosis is a result of the inflammatory response to AP and not necessarily infection.
- Hemoconcentration (hematocrit >44% is an independent risk factor for pancreatic necrosis) (12).

Basic Metabolic Panel. Assessment of renal function, acid-base status, and glycemia status.

Liver Function Testing. Elevations in total bilirubin and enzymes such as the AST, ALT, and alkaline phosphatase strongly implicate a biliary cause of AP.

Arterial Blood Gas. Assessment of acid-base status and pulmonary function.

Serum Triglycerides
- Should be obtained in absence of biliary disease or alcohol use history.
- Level >1,000 mg/dL indicates hypertriglyceridemia as the etiology of AP.

Serum Lactate. Predictive of ICU admission and mortality but is nonspecific and should be used in conjunction with other markers (12-13).

C-Reactive Protein. An acute phase reactant, nonspecific to AP. It has been described as predictive of AP severity (12,14) but this outcome is not consistent (15).

Procalcitonin. A sensitive test for pancreatic infection. A low value is a negative predictor of infection (12). A threshold >1.0 nanogram/mL to initiate or continue antibiotics decreased antibiotic use by 16% without increasing harm (16).

Computed Tomography

The most reliable test for diagnosing AP is contrast-enhanced computed tomography (CT), which can determine the type of pancreatitis (edematous vs. necrotizing), its severity, localized complications (e.g., infection), and pancreatic complications like necrosis, fluid collections, and the presence of pneumoperitoneum and retroperitoneal air (2,12). A contrast-enhanced CT image of edematous pancreatitis is shown in Figure 39.1. The pancreas is thickened and enhanced completely, and the border of the pancreas is blurred, which is characteristic of pancreatic edema.

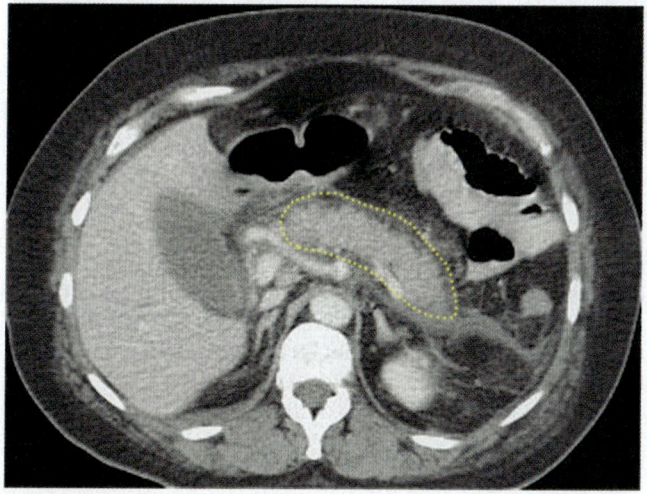

FIGURE 39.1. Contrast-enhanced CT image showing edematous pancreatitis. The pancreas (outlined by the dotted line) is enlarged and enhances completely. There is also blurring of the pancreatic border, which is characteristic of edema formation. (From Acute Pancreatitis. In: Marino PL. *Marino's The ICU Book*. 5th ed. Wolters Kluwer; 2025:618-26. Figure 40.1.)

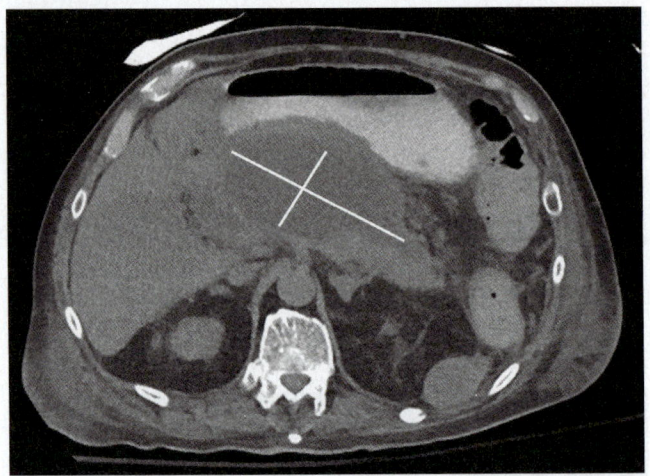

FIGURE 39.2. Contrast-enhanced CT image of pancreatic necrosis. The necrosis if central (crosshairs) often appears with a rim of perfused pancreatic tissue. (Image courtesy of Erin Baker, MD.)

A contrast-enhanced CT image of necrotizing pancreatitis is shown in Figure 39.2. Note the large area that is not contrast-enhanced in the region of the neck and body of the pancreas. This represents pancreatic necrosis. The full extent of pancreatic necrosis may not be evident on CT imaging for the first week after the onset of symptoms (1).

A non-contrast CT scan is of little value.

Biliary Evaluation

Ultrasonography is non-invasive and useful in evaluating for a biliary cause of AP (i.e., gallstones, choledocholithiasis, and a dilated common bile duct [CBD]). A dilated CBD is not always present but is indicative of CBD stones.

Magnetic Resonance Cholangio-Pancreatography (MRCP) can be used in lieu of contract-enhanced CT in patients with severe contrast allergies, acute renal failure, and pregnancy. MRCP demonstrating CBD stones is shown in Figure 39.3.

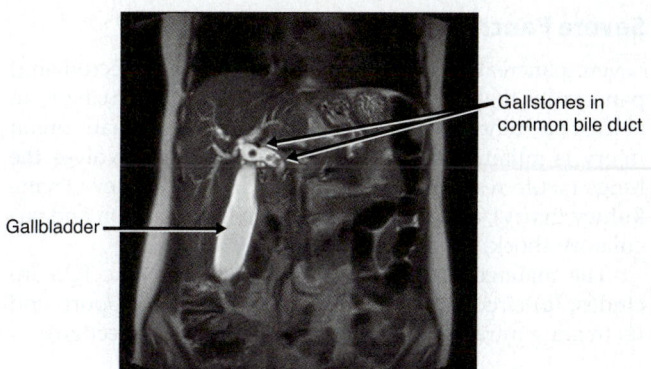

FIGURE 39.3. Magnetic resonance cholangiopancreatography of choledocholithiasis. (Image courtesy of Erin Baker, MD.)

TREATMENT

Gallstone Pancreatitis

Management of gallstone pancreatitis requires surgical and/or gastroenterology input. Timing of surgery or endoscopic retrograde cholangiopancreatography (ERCP) is case dependent. Coexistent cholangitis requires emergent drainage and antibiotics (2,17).

Hypertriglyceridemic Pancreatitis

Reduction of hypertriglyceridemia can be accomplished with plasma pheresis (18-19), insulin infusion (6,19), or combination of insulin infusion heparin (20). Literature describes insulin infusion dosing range from 0.1 units to 0.4 units/kg/h with concurrent 5% dextrose infusion (6,19,21). An insulin/heparin combination appears to have a more dramatic response, but risk of hemorrhagic conversion is present.

Severe Pancreatitis

Severe pancreatitis is defined as acute (usually necrotizing) pancreatitis that is associated with persistent (>48 h) injury in at least one other organ system (5). The extrapancreatic organ injury is inflammatory in origin and typically involves the lungs (acute respiratory distress syndrome), kidneys (acute kidney injury), and circulatory system (hypotension and circulatory shock).

The management of severe pancreatitis in the ICU includes: (a) circulatory support, (b) nutritional support, and (c) treating intraabdominal complications (e.g., infection).

Circulatory Support

Circulatory support includes volume resuscitation and vasopressor drugs, if necessary.

Fluid Resuscitation

Severe pancreatitis is accompanied by loss of intravascular fluid through leaky systemic capillaries, and the resulting hypovolemia and poor perfusion which can produce additional pancreatic necrosis. As a result, early fluid resuscitation should be targeted at perfusion goals guided by frequent assessment of hemodynamic status. Balanced crystalloids, e.g., lactated Ringers and PlasmaLyte are preferred over normal saline (22-23). See Chapter 11: Fluid Management.

> CAUTION: *Existing evidence appears to show that aggressive volume infusion does not improve clinical outcomes (5,24), can contribute to the development of abdominal compartment syndrome (see section that follows) (25), and may increase the mortality (26). Therefore, after the initial 24-48 h of aggressive volume infusion, the infusion rate of IV fluids should be guided by hemodynamic assessments and urine output (12).*

Vasopressor Therapy

There are no official recommendations regarding vasopressor therapy in severe pancreatitis, but *norepinephrine*

(2-20 µg/min) is an appropriate choice targeting a mean blood pressure of 65 mm Hg. All vasoconstrictor drugs can reduce splanchnic blood flow (especially epinephrine) and could aggravate pancreatic necrosis, so careful titration of infusion rates (and avoiding epinephrine) is advised.

Nutrition Support

Patients who are unable to tolerate oral intake through a nasogastric tube should begin enteral nutrition support within 24-48 h of being admitted to the ICU (12,27). There is no advantage to nasojejunal feedings unless there is intolerance to nasogastric feeds (e.g., delayed gastric emptying). Despite the multitude of available feeding formulas, the current guidelines on nutrition support recommend standard (non-specialized) feeding formulas for most ICU patients (27-28). The clinical benefits of early enteral nutrition are discussed in Chapter 47: Enteral Nutrition. Total parenteral nutrition should be avoided unless there is contraindication to enteral feedings.

Pancreatic Infections

About one-third of patients with necrotizing pancreatitis develop infections in the necrotic areas of the pancreas (5). Gram-negative enteric organisms and less frequently *Staphylococcus aureus* and *Enterococcus* spp. are the responsible pathogens (29).

The diagnosis is confirmed by either of the following:

1. A contrast-enhanced CT scan showing gas bubbles in the necrotic areas of the pancreas.
2. A positive culture from necrotic areas of the pancreas (using CT-guided needle aspiration)

Antibiotic prophylaxis does not reduce the incidence of pancreatic infections (30). As a result, *prophylactic antibiotics are not recommended in AP, including necrotizing pancreatitis* (2,8,12). Considering the similarities of the inflammatory response of AP to sepsis, antibiotic decisions are challenging. Prophylactic antibiotic use may show benefit in biliary causes (31). Antibiotic options should cover enteric aerobic gram negative and anaerobic organisms. Meropenem, piperacillin/tazobactam, or combination of cefepime and metronidazole are appropriate empiric choices (5,12,32).

Abdominal Compartment Syndrome

Abdominal compartment syndrome (ACS) is defined as an intra-abdominal pressure of >20 mm Hg with associated organ dysfunction such as acute oliguric renal failure and elevated airway pressures on mechanical ventilation (25) and is reported in about half of patients with severe pancreatitis (33). Since ACS can cause organ failure, abdominal pressure should be measured in any patient with AP who develops oliguric renal failure. ACS requires emergent surgical decompression. An open abdomen is not a contraindication to enteral feedings (27).

The Multi-Disciplinary Team

Multiple subspecialties, including gastroenterology, surgery, interventional radiology, and endocrinology, are often involved due to the complexity of etiologies, complications, and sequelae. For management to be successful, early involvement is crucial.

References

1. Iannuzzi JP, King JA, Leong JH, et al. Global incidence of acute pancreatitis is increasing over time: a systematic review and meta-analysis. Gastroenterology 2022;162:122-34.
2. MacGoey P, Dickson EJ, Puxty K. Management of the patient with acute pancreatitis. BJA Educ 2019;19:240-5.
3. Banks PA, Bollen TL, Dervenis C, et al. Classification of acute pancreatitis—2012: revision of the Atlanta classification and definitions by international consensus. Gut 2013;62:102-11.
4. Cavallini G, Frulloni L, Bassi C, et al. Prospective multicentre survey on acute pancreatitis in Italy (ProInf-AISP): results on 1005 patients. Dig Liver Dis 2004;36:205-11.

5. Gapp J, Tariq A, Chandra S. Acute Pancreatitis. In: StatPearls. Treasure Island (FL): StatPearls Publishing; 2025.
6. Garg R, Rustagi T. Management of hypertriglyceridemia induced acute pancreatitis. Biomed Res Int 2018;2018:4721357.
7. Zilio MB, Eyff TF, Azeredo-Da-Silva ALF, et al. A systematic review and meta-analysis of the aetiology of acute pancreatitis. HPB (Oxford) 2019;21:259-67.
8. Banks PA, Freeman ML; Practice Parameters Committee of the American College of Gastroenterology. Practice guidelines in acute pancreatitis. Am J Gastroenterol 2006;101:2379-400.
9. Yadav D, Agarwal N, Pitchumoni CS. A critical evaluation of laboratory tests in acute pancreatitis. Am J Gastroenterol 2002;97:1309-18.
10. Verge SS. Approach to the patient with elevated serum amylase or lipase. In: Adler DG, editor. *UpToDate*. Wolters Kluwer; 2025.
11. Gumaste VV, Roditis N, Mehta D, Dave PB. Serum lipase levels in nonpancreatic abdominal pain versus acute pancreatitis. Am J Gastroenterol 1993;88:2051-5.
12. Leppaniemi A, Tolonen M, Tarasconi A, et al. 2019 WSES guidelines for the management of severe acute pancreatitis. World J Emerg Surg 2019;14:27.
13. Zeng J, Wan J, He W, et al. Prognostic value of arterial lactate metabolic clearance rate in moderate and severe acute pancreatitis. Dis Markers 2022;2022:9233199.
14. Stirling AD, Moran NR, Kelly ME, et al. The predictive value of C-reactive protein (CRP) in acute pancreatitis—is interval change in CRP an additional indicator of severity? HPB (Oxford) 2017;19:874-80.
15. Ahmad R, Bhatti KM, Ahmed M, et al. C-reactive protein as a predictor of complicated acute pancreatitis: reality or a myth? Cureus 2021;13:e19265.
16. Siriwardena AK, Jegatheeswaran S, Mason JM, et al. A procalcitonin-based algorithm to guide antibiotic use in patients with acute pancreatitis (PROCAP): a single-centre, patient-blinded, randomised controlled trial. Lancet Gastroenterol Hepatol 2022;7:913-21.
17. Kabaria S, Mutneja H, Makar M, et al. Timing of endoscopic retrograde cholangiopancreatography in acute biliary pancreatitis without cholangitis: a nationwide inpatient cohort study. Ann Gastroenterol 2021;34:575-81.
18. Munoh Kenne F, Cimpeanu E, Al-Zakhari R, et al. Plasmapheresis treatment of hypertriglyceridemia-induced acute pancreatitis: a case report. Cureus 2020;12:e8360.
19. White BN, Carter BL, Bradford JL. Analysis of intravenous insulin dosing requirements for treatment of severe hypertriglyceridemia. Hosp Pharm 2023;58:79-83.
20. Kuchay MS, Farooqui KJ, Bano T, et al. Heparin and insulin in the management of hypertriglyceridemia-associated pancreatitis: case series and literature review. Arch Endocrinol Metab 2017;61:198-201.

21. Inayat F, Zafar F, Baig AS, et al. Hypertriglyceridemic pancreatitis treated with insulin therapy: a comparative review of 34 cases. Cureus 2018;10:e3501.
22. Semler MW, Kellum JA. Balanced crystalloid solutions. Am J Respir Crit Care Med 2019;199:952-60.
23. Yaowmaneerat T, Sirinawasatien A. Update on the strategy for intravenous fluid treatment in acute pancreatitis. World J Gastrointest Pharmacol Ther 2023;14:22-32.
24. de-Madaria E, Buxbaum JL, Maisonneuve P, et al. Aggressive or moderate fluid resuscitation in acute pancreatitis. N Engl J Med 2022;387:989-1000.
25. Zarnescu NO, Dumitrascu I, Zarnescu EC, et al. Abdominal compartment syndrome in acute pancreatitis: a narrative review. Diagnostics (Basel) 2022;13.
26. Long B, Gottlieb M. Aggressive intravenous fluid resuscitation for acute pancreatitis. Acad Emerg Med 2023;30:880-1.
27. Arvanitakis M, Ockenga J, Bezmarevic M, et al. ESPEN guideline on clinical nutrition in acute and chronic pancreatitis. Clin Nutr 2020;39:612-31.
28. McClave SA, Taylor BE, Martindale RG, et al. Guidelines for the provision and assessment of nutrition support therapy in the adult critically ill patient: Society of Critical Care Medicine (SCCM) and American Society for Parenteral and Enteral Nutrition (A.S.P.E.N.). JPEN J Parenter Enteral Nutr 2016;40:159-211.
29. Severino A, Varca S, Airola C, et al. Antibiotic utilization in acute pancreatitis: a narrative review. Antibiotics (Basel). 2023;12:1120.
30. Hart PA, Bechtold ML, Marshall JB, et al. Prophylactic antibiotics in necrotizing pancreatitis: a meta-analysis. South Med J 2008;101:1126-31.
31. Wen Y, Xu L, Zhang D, et al. Effect of early antibiotic treatment strategy on prognosis of acute pancreatitis. BMC Gastroenterol 2023;23:431.
32. Racketa S, Gandhi K, Lambie M. Meropenem versus piperacillin-tazobactam for the treatment of pancreatic necrosis. Diagn Microbiol Infect Dis 2024;109:116209.
33. Al-Bahrani AZ, Abid GH, Holt A, et al. Clinical relevance of intra-abdominal hypertension in patients with severe acute pancreatitis. Pancreas 2008;36:39-43.

Abdominal Infections — Chapter 40

Abdominal infections encountered in the ICU may include the reason for ICU admission, such as sepsis from diverticulitis, or may arise as complications of critical illness, e.g., acalculous cholecystitis and ischemic bowel due to vasopressors.

ACALCULOUS CHOLECYSTITIS

Acalculous cholecystitis accounts for <15% of cases of acute cholecystitis (1), but it is more common in critically ill patients, and it has a mortality rate (up to 50%) that rivals septic shock (1-3).

Predisposing Conditions

Common conditions associated with acalculous cholecystitis include the postoperative period, trauma, circulatory shock, critical illness, prolonged bowel rest, and prolonged total parenteral nutrition (1-3).

Clinical Features

Right upper quadrant pain and tenderness are common but can be *absent in one-third of patients with acalculous cholecystitis*. Moreover, physical exam findings may be limited in ICU patients with altered mental status, continuous sedation, and/or analgesia (4).

Diagnosis

Right upper quadrant ultrasonography is the preferred initial diagnostic test for acalculous cholecystitis (5). Ultrasound has multiple advantages such as being noninvasive, portable for bedside evaluation in the ICU, and greater diagnostic accuracy compared with computed tomography. Sonographic features include distension of the gallbladder (diameter >40 mm in the short-axis view), wall thickening (>3 mm), and the presence of sludge (a mixture of particulate matter that has precipitated from bile) (6). The diagnostic yield from ultrasound varies widely due to operator proficiency and patient characteristics (e.g., obesity). A meta-analysis of 26 studies demonstrated a sensitivity of 81% and a specificity of 83% (7). Even the classic, "sonographic Murphy sign" has sensitivity as low as 63% and a specificity as low as 35% (8). Finally, critically ill patients commonly display sonographic abnormalities unrelated to cholecystitis. If ultrasound is not diagnostic, *the gold standard test for acalculous cholecystitis is the hepatobiliary iminodiacetic acid (HIDA) scan* (9); however, this may not be logistically possible in critically ill patients. HIDA cannot be performed at bedside and may take several hours to perform (8).

Management

Broad-spectrum antibiotic therapy should be started as soon as the diagnosis is confirmed, but treatment is drainage. Although laparoscopic or open cholecystectomy is the best definitive treatment, percutaneous cholecystostomy is the safest and most effective option for critically ill patients who cannot tolerate surgery (2). Due to diagnostic challenges, percutaneous cholecystostomy may be appropriate in ICU patients with unexplained sepsis (8).

CLOSTRIDIUM DIFFICILE INFECTION

The most important risk factor for *Clostridium difficile* infection (CDI) is antibiotic exposure lending credence to the importance of antibiotic stewardship (10-11). Gastric acid suppression (e.g., stress ulcer prophylaxis) may also contribute to an increased risk for CDI (12-13).

Pathogenesis

C. difficile is a ubiquitous, spore-forming, toxin-producing, gram-positive, anaerobic bacillus that can colonize the intestines of healthy individuals without causing infection (10). Rates of colonization are shown in Table 40.1 (14).

TABLE 40.1 Rates of Colonization with *Clostridium difficile*

- 3-7% of healthy adults
- 4-15% of hospitalized adults
- Up to 50% of long-term care adults

Data from Dubberke ER, Burnham CA. Diagnosis of *Clostridium difficile* infection: treat the patient, not the test. JAMA Intern Med 2015;175:1801-2.

By altering the natural colonic microbiome and disrupting the colon's homeostasis, antibiotic use permits *C. difficile* to proliferate and release toxins that injure the colon. The severe inflammation that is produced causes raised, plaque-like lesions on the mucosal surface of the bowel. These are called "pseudomembranes," and the condition is called *pseudomembranous colitis*.

Clinical Features

The principal manifestation of CDI is watery diarrhea that can be associated with nausea, emesis, abdominal pain, and fever. Fulminant *C. difficile* colitis (FCDC) is characterized by the development of severe acute inflammation of the colon, associated with systemic sepsis. *Toxic megacolon* is a life-threatening complication of CDI characterized by a nonobstructive dilatation of the colon with systemic toxicity and risk for perforation. Early surgical consultation should occur in patients who do not respond to medical therapy as a rapid deterioration to FCDC and/or toxic megacolon can occur requiring immediate surgery. Surgical management is discussed in the following text.

Diagnostic Evaluation

CDI is a clinical diagnosis supported by laboratory testing (14). Patients with three or more loose stools within 24 h, especially with recent antibiotic exposure, warrants consideration of CDI (10). A two-step approach to diagnosis is recommended (10,15) where polymerase chain reaction (PCR) testing is used as a screening test and an enzyme-linked immunosorbent assay (ELISA) is used to confirm the diagnosis (15).

Colonoscopy

Direct visualization of pseudomembranes on the mucosal surface of the large bowel can provide confirmatory evidence of CDI, but this is rarely necessary.

Treatment

Medical

Medical treatment for CDI is shown in Table 40.2 (10,16). A favorable antibiotic response is characterized by resolution of fever (if present) in 24-48 h and resolution of the diarrhea in 4-5 days (17).

Fidaxomicin. Fidaxomicin (200 mg PO twice a day for 10 days) is the preferred regimen of the Infectious Diseases Society of America (IDSA) and the Society for Healthcare Epidemiology of America (SHEA) for the treatment of the initial CDI (16).

Vancomycin. Vancomycin is an acceptable alternative to fidaxomicin and can also be instilled as an enema as adjuvant therapy for fulminant CDI. Dosage varies contingent on clinical scenario (Table 40.2). Use as an antegrade colonic lavage is discussed below under surgical considerations.

Metronidazole. Metronidazole has been replaced by fidaxomicin and vancomycin as first-line therapy due to efficacy. A dose of 500 mg three times daily for 10-14 days is acceptable for *nonsevere* CDI if fidaxomicin and vancomycin are not available. Intravenous metronidazole is used in conjunction with vancomycin for fulminant CDI (16).

Rifaximin. Rifaximin, a nonabsorbable antibiotic with activity against *C. difficile,* has been found to be useful in reducing recurrence in CDI (16,18).

Bezlotoxumab. Bezlotoxumab is an U.S. Food and Drug Administration (FDA)-approved monoclonal antibody active against *C. difficile* toxin B and is used as adjunctive therapy for recurrent CDI (10,16).

TABLE 40.2 Medical Treatment for CDI

Type	Treatment
Initial episode	• *Preferred*: fidaxomicin: 200 mg PO or via NGT BID for 10 days *or* • *Vancomycin*: 125 mg PO or via NGT every 6 h for 10 days
Fulminant CDI	• *Vancomycin*: 500 mg (PO or via NGT) every 6 h; consider rectal vancomycin enema (500 mg in 100 mL normal saline) every 6 h. • *Metronidazole*: 500 mg IV every 8 h should be administered together with vancomycin.
First recurrence	• *Preferred*: fidaxomicin 200 mg given twice daily for 10 days, *or* twice daily for 5 days followed by once every other day for 20 days • *Alternative*: vancomycin by mouth in a tapered and pulsed regimen • *Adjunctive treatment*: bezlotoxumab 10 mg/kg given intravenously once during administration of SOC antibiotics
Second or subsequent recurrence	• *Fidaxomicin*: 200 mg given twice daily for 10 days, *or* twice daily for 5 days followed by once every other day for 20 days • *Vancomycin*: 125 mg 4 times daily by mouth for 10 days followed by rifaximin 400 mg 3 times daily for 20 days • Fecal microbiota transplantation • *Adjunctive treatment*: bezlotoxumab 10 mg/kg given intravenously once during administration of SOC antibiotics

BID = twice daily; CDI = *Clostridium difficile* infection; IV = intravenous; NGT = nasogastric tube; PO = orally; SOC = standard of care.

From References 10 and 16.

Antimotility Agents. The use of agents to control diarrhea may afford symptomatic relief along with appropriate antimicrobial agents (19) but should be avoided in cases of severe CDI.

Surgical Treatment

Surgical consultation should occur early in severe CDI, especially when ICU admission is required to facilitate decisions regarding possibility and timing decisions for surgical intervention. Surgical options include total abdominal colectomy and diverting loop ileostomy with antegrade colonic lavage with warmed polyethylene glycol followed by scheduled vancomycin lavage via the loop ileostomy (20-22).

Recolonization

Recolonization of the bowel with normal microflora is used primarily to prevent recurrent episodes of CDI.

Probiotics and Prebiotics

Probiotics are "nonpathogenic" organisms that purportedly aid to restore the normal microbiome of the colon. Prebiotics, such as fermentable fiber, are plant-derived polysaccharides that are not digested by humans. They are broken down by anaerobic colonic bacteria into short-chain fatty acids (SCFA), which not only promotes sodium and water absorption but also serve as a crucial energy source for the large bowel mucosa. This process is essential for maintaining intestinal barrier integrity and immune homeostasis. Some evidence has shown a benefit to SCFA impairing the ability of *C. difficile* to colonize or grow (23). There have been occasional reports of a decrease in recurrences with probiotic therapy, but a meta-analysis of the accumulated experience with probiotics found no convincing evidence of definitive treatment effects. In addition, adverse events have been reported. As a result, *the use of probiotics is not supported* in the current American College of Gastroenterology guidelines for CDI (24). Prebiotic use is promising, however its role, whether preventative or therapeutic, remains obscure.

Fecal Microbiota Transplantation (FMT)

Instillation of liquid preparations of stool from healthy donors (via nasogastric tubes, retention enemas, or colonoscopy) can prevent recurrent episodes of CDI in 90% of cases (24). FMT is currently recommended for patients with three or more recurrences of CDI.

Prevention of Spread

CDI is a nosocomial infection that is transmitted via the fecal-oral route. Patient-to-patient transmission occurs through contact, mostly via the hands of hospital personnel. Patients with CDI and even *C. difficile* exposure should have clear identification of their risk to staff with appropriate isolation precautions (25). (See Figure 40.1.) Personal protective equipment such as gloves and gowns are used for patient contact. Eye protection and masks should be used if there is a risk for splashes. Spores can attach to equipment; thus, disposable, single-patient use equipment such as stethoscopes should be used. Detailed environmental cleaning procedures to prevent CDI can be viewed at https://www.cdc.gov/c-diff/hcp/clinical-guidance/index.html.

Hand Hygiene

The use of disposable gloves and handwashing with soap and water is critical in preventing the spread of *C. difficile*. Alcohol-based sanitizers are not effective against *C. difficile* spores.

COMPLICATED INTRA-ABDOMINAL INFECTIONS

Complicated intra-abdominal infections are defined as infections that involve the peritoneal cavity and can be generalized peritonitis, phlegmon, or a localized abscess (26). They are often the result of a perforation somewhere along the gastrointestinal tract, or an anastomotic leak following abdominal surgery. These infections can be difficult to treat and

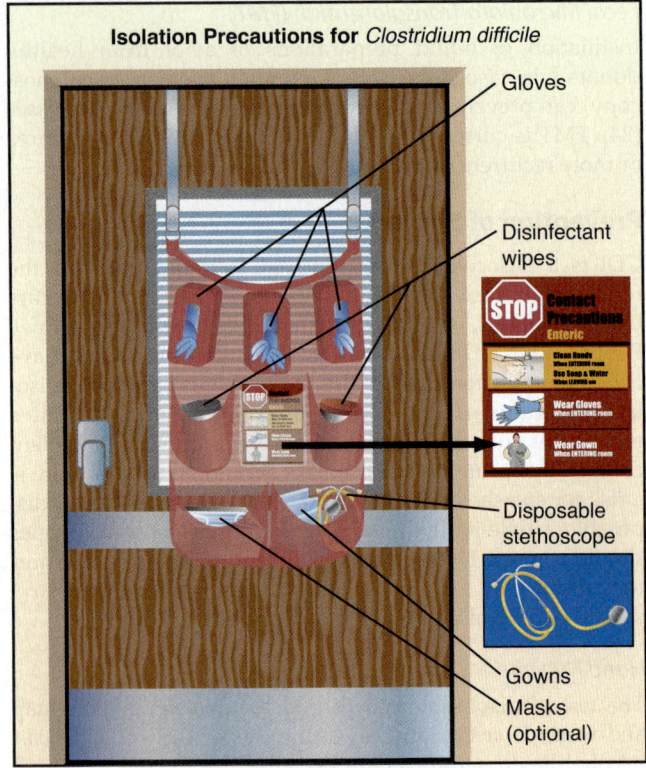

FIGURE 40.1. Isolation precautions for *Clostridium difficile*.

require prompt source control and appropriate empiric antibiotics. Postoperative infection risk is shown in Table 40.3.

Diagnostics

History and Physical

The basic history and physical (H&P) cannot be overstressed regarding the evaluation of a potential intra-abdominal infection. Appropriate diagnostic algorithms and initial therapies are guided by this assessment. For example, a recent colon

TABLE 40.3 Infection Risk Based on Wound Classification

Classification	Description	Infection Risk
Class 1 Clean wound	Wounds are not infected, do not exhibit any signs of inflammation, and are typically closed. If drainage is required, a closed draining approach is recommended. It is worth noting that Class 1 wounds do not involve the respiratory, alimentary, genital, or urinary tracts. *Example: inguinal hernia repair*	1-5%
Class 2 Clean-contaminated	Low level of contamination. These types of wounds involve entry into the respiratory, alimentary, genital, or urinary tracts but only under controlled circumstances.	3-11%
Class 3 Contaminated	Contaminated and typically result from a breach in sterile techniques or leakage from the gastrointestinal tract. Incisions resulting from acute or nonpurulent inflammation are also considered Class 3 wounds.	10-17%
Class 4 Dirty or infected	These injuries usually occur from inadequate treatment of traumatic wounds, gross purulence, and evident infections. When tissues lose vitality, it can lead to Class 4 wounds. This is often caused by surgery or microorganisms found in perforated organs.	>27%

resection may prompt computed tomography (CT) scanning whereas acute right upper quadrant pain may indicate right upper quadrant ultrasound as initial imaging.

Peritonitis. Diffuse peritonitis warrants emergent surgical exploration. The lack of peritonitis, however, does not exclude a surgical emergency such as mesenteric ischemia which presents as "pain out of proportion to exam" (27). Thus, surgical consultation should be obtained early with concerns for an intra-abdominal infection.

Radiologic Imaging

CT of the abdomen is the preferred method for detecting most abdominal processes (5,26). However, CT imaging in the early postoperative period can be misleading because collections of blood or irrigant solutions in the peritoneal cavity can be misread as an abscess. The use of intravenous and oral contrast significantly adds to the diagnostic accuracy of CT scans. The concerns regarding the use of intravenous contrast in the face of acute kidney injury are overstated (28). The use of IV contrast needs to be balanced against the importance of an accurate diagnosis.

Plain Film Radiography

Plain film radiography can be diagnostic for the presence of pneumoperitoneum suggesting intestinal perforation. Figure 40.2 demonstrates a large pneumoperitoneum.

Although radiographic pneumoperitoneum can persist for 7 days after laparotomy, interpretation as "benign" should be made with caution (29). "Large" pneumoperitoneum is atypical, and pneumoperitoneum in the context of clinical changes such as tachycardia, increased leukocytosis, and abdominal pain should prompt further (and aggressive) investigation.

Management

Antibiotics

Presumptive antibiotic therapy should begin as soon as possible using antibiotics that are active against enteric organisms,

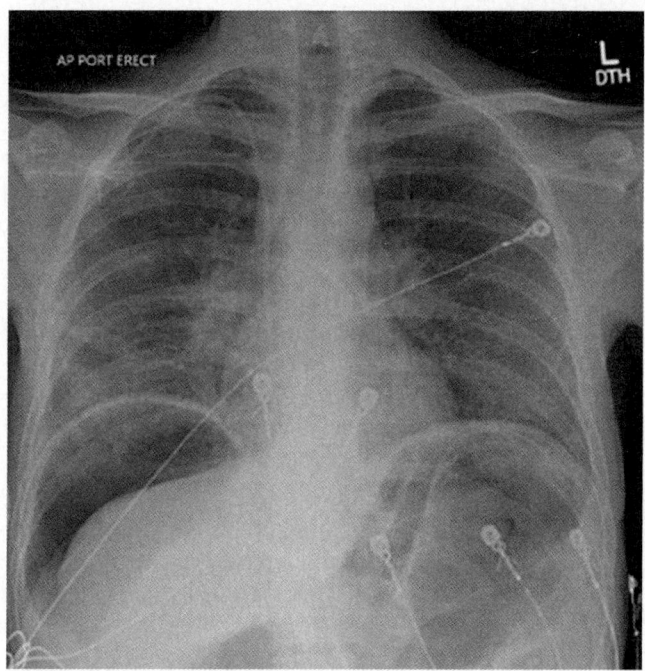

FIGURE 40.2. Large pneumoperitoneum on chest radiograph.

both aerobic and anaerobic. If no resistant organisms are suspected, *piperacillin-tazobactam* is suitable for single agent coverage (26). The combination of *ceftriaxone* and *metronidazole* is an alternative recommendation for patients that are not seriously ill, but the coverage is far inferior to piperacillin-tazobactam. Organisms that produce extended-spectrum beta-lactamases (ESBLs) are resistant to penicillins and third-generation cephalosporins. If these organisms are suspected (e.g., from prior colonization or infection), the antibiotic options are *meropenem*, *tigecycline*, and *ceftazidime/avibactam*.

Candidal Coverage

Candida albicans and related species can be prominent inhabitants of the bowel (especially in patients who have recently received antibiotics), and perforation in the upper GI tract has been identified as a major risk factor for *Candida* peritonitis (30). Empiric antifungal coverage should consider covering all *Candida* species, such as one of the echinocandins (i.e., *micafungin*, *anidulafungin*, or *caspofungin*).

Source Control

The inability to control the infectious (septic) source is associated with a high mortality (5,26). Most intra-abdominal processes require surgical intervention; thus, the importance of early surgical consultation. Focal processes, such as acalculous cholecystitis and abscesses can be controlled and sometimes cured with percutaneous drainage (PC). Limitations to PC include lack of a safe access route (risk to intervening structure such as bowel), bleeding risk, and complex (e.g., multiloculated) abscesses.

References

1. McChesney JA, Northup PG, Bickston SJ. Acute acalculous cholecystitis associated with systemic sepsis and visceral arterial hypoperfusion: a case series and review of pathophysiology. Dig Dis Sci 2003;48:1960-7.
2. Jones MW, Ferguson T. Acalculous cholecystitis. [Updated 2023 Apr 24]. In: StatPearls [Internet]. Treasure Island (FL): StatPearls Publishing; 2025 Jan-. Available from: https://www.ncbi.nlm.nih.gov/books/NBK459182/
3. Laurila J, Syrjala H, Laurila PA, et al. Acute acalculous cholecystitis in critically ill patients. Acta Anaesthesiol Scand 2004;48:986-91.
4. Solomkin JS, Mazuski JE, Bradley JS, et al. Diagnosis and management of complicated intra-abdominal infection in adults and children: guidelines by the Surgical Infection Society and the Infectious Diseases Society of America. Surg Infect (Larchmt) 2010;11:79-109.
5. Bonomo RA, Chow AW, Edwards MS, et al. 2024 clinical practice guideline update by the Infectious Diseases Society of America on complicated intra-abdominal infections: risk assessment, diagnostic imaging, and microbiological evaluation in adults, children, and pregnant people. Clin Infect Dis 2024;79:S81-7.
6. Frankel HL, Kirkpatrick AW, Elbarbary M, et al. Guidelines for the appropriate use of bedside general and cardiac ultrasonography in the evaluation of critically ill patients—part I: general ultrasonography. Crit Care Med 2015;43:2479-502.

7. Kiewiet JJ, Leeuwenburgh MM, Bipat S, et al. A systematic review and meta-analysis of diagnostic performance of imaging in acute cholecystitis. Radiology 2012;264:708-20.
8. Brook OR, Kane RA, Tyagi G, et al. Lessons learned from quality assurance: errors in the diagnosis of acute cholecystitis on ultrasound and CT. AJR Am J Roentgenol 2011;196:597-604.
9. Pisano M, Allievi N, Gurusamy K, et al. 2020 World Society of Emergency Surgery updated guidelines for the diagnosis and treatment of acute calculus cholecystitis. World J Emerg Surg 2020;15:61.
10. Mada PK, Alam MU. Clostridioides difficile infection. [Updated 2024 Apr 10]. In: StatPearls [Internet]. Treasure Island (FL): StatPearls Publishing; 2025 Jan-. Available from: https://www.ncbi.nlm.nih.gov/books/NBK431054/
11. Rohde JM, Jones K, Padron N, et al. A tiered approach for preventing *Clostridioides difficile* infection. Ann Intern Med 2019;171:S45-S51.
12. Aseeri M, Schroeder T, Kramer J, Zackula R. Gastric acid suppression by proton pump inhibitors as a risk factor for *Clostridium difficile*-associated diarrhea in hospitalized patients. Am J Gastroenterol 2008;103:2308-13.
13. Dial S, Delaney JA, Barkun AN, Suissa S. Use of gastric acid-suppressive agents and the risk of community-acquired *Clostridium difficile*-associated disease. JAMA 2005;294:2989-95.
14. Dubberke ER, Burnham CA. Diagnosis of *Clostridium difficile* infection: treat the patient, not the test. JAMA Intern Med 2015;175:1801-2.
15. American College of Gastroenterology. *Clostridium difficile* (*C. difficile*) infection (CDI). Accessed May 1 2025. https://gi.org/topics/c-difficile-infection/
16. Johnson S, Lavergne V, Skinner AM, et al. Clinical practice guideline by the Infectious Diseases Society of America (IDSA) and Society for Healthcare Epidemiology of America (SHEA): 2021 focused update guidelines on management of *Clostridioides difficile* infection in adults. Clin Infect Dis 2021;73:755-7.
17. Bartlett JG. Clinical practice. Antibiotic-associated diarrhea. N Engl J Med 2002;346:334-9.
18. Ng QX, Loke W, Foo NX, et al. A systematic review of the use of rifaximin for *Clostridium difficile* infections. Anaerobe 2019;55:35-9.
19. Koo HL, Koo DC, Musher DM, DuPont HL. Antimotility agents for the treatment of *Clostridium difficile* diarrhea and colitis. Clin Infect Dis 2009;48:598-605.
20. Forrester JD, Colling KP, Diaz JJ, et al. Surgical Infection Society guidelines for total abdominal colectomy versus diverting loop ileostomy with antegrade intra-colonic lavage for the surgical management of severe or fulminant, non-perforated *Clostridioides difficile* colitis. Surg Infect (Larchmt) 2022;23:97-104.

21. McKechnie T, Khamar J, Lee Y, et al. Total abdominal colectomy versus diverting loop ileostomy and antegrade colonic lavage for fulminant clostridioides colitis: analysis of the national inpatient sample 2016-2019. J Gastrointest Surg 2023;27:1412-22.
22. Morgan M, Farrell T, Ndubizu GU, Farrell TJ. Colonic lavage in treatment of refractory *Clostridium difficile* infection: an adaptation of the Pittsburgh protocol. J Surg Case Rep 2020;2020:rjaa159.
23. Gregory AL, Pensinger DA, Hryckowian AJ. A short chain fatty acid-centric view of *Clostridioides difficile* pathogenesis. PLoS Pathog 2021;17:e1009959.
24. Kelly CR, Fischer M, Allegretti JR, et al. ACG clinical guidelines: prevention, diagnosis, and treatment of *Clostridioides difficile* infections. Am J Gastroenterol 2021;116:1124-47.
25. U.S. Centers for Disease Control and Prevention. Clinical guidance for C. Diff prevention in acute care facilities. March 8, 2024. Accessed May 12, 2005. https://www.cdc.gov/c-diff/hcp/clinical-guidance/index.html
26. Sartelli M, Coccolini F, Kluger Y, et al. WSES/GAIS/SIS-E/WSIS/AAST global clinical pathways for patients with intra-abdominal infections. World J Emerg Surg 2021;16:49.
27. Martin SJ, Stephen VS. Pitfalls in medicine: pain out of proportion to examination findings. Br J Hosp Med (Lond) 2022;83:1-8.
28. Davenport MS, Perazella MA, Yee J, et al. Use of intravenous iodinated contrast media in patients with kidney disease: consensus statements from the American College of Radiology and the National Kidney Foundation. Radiology 2020;294:660-8.
29. Quadir MA, Mirza R, Beg MO, et al. Study of days required resolving of pneumoperitoneum after laparoscopic cholecystectomy. Int J Surg Sci 2024;8:53-6.
30. Hasibeder W, Halabi M. Candida peritonitis. Minerva Anestesiol 2014;80:470-81.

Urinary Tract Infections

Chapter 41

ASYMPTOMATIC BACTERIURIA

Hospital-acquired urinary tract infections (UTIs) are among the most common nosocomial infections (1-3). However, asymptomatic bacteriuria (ASB), even at high quantitative colony counts, does not necessarily confer infection. The Infectious Diseases Society of America defines ASB as *the presence of one or more species of bacteria growing in the urine at specified quantitative counts ($\geq 10^5$ colony-forming units [CFU]/mL or $\geq 10^8$ CFU/L), irrespective of the presence of pyuria, in the absence of signs or symptoms attributable to urinary tract infection (UTI)* (4).

Treatment

ASB does not require treatment with antibiotics in the majority of cases. Exceptions include the following (4-5):

1. Pregnancy
2. Planned urologic procedures
3. Recent (<3 months renal transplant). Please note: The 2018 Cochran Review had mixed results regarding a clinical benefit in renal transplant recipients (6).

Antimicrobial impregnated urinary catheters (silver alloy or nitrofurazone) can reduce the incidence of ASB in short-term catheterization (<1 week) (7), but the benefit in preventing symptomatic UTIs is not clear (8-9).

CATHETER-ASSOCIATED URINARY TRACT INFECTIONS

Etiology

Approximately 15% of all hospital admissions will have an indwelling urinary catheter (IUC) at some point during their hospitalization. IUCs increase the risk of urinary tract infections (UTIs) by 3-7% per day (10). UTIs, as a result of an IUC, are known as a catheter-associated urinary tract infections or CAUTI. Urinary catheterization is thus responsible for as many as 20% of hospital-acquired bacteremia (11).

The insertion of an IUC can introduce bacteria (despite sterile technique) and the catheters themselves can facilitate colonization via biofilms produced by the bacteria (9).

Microbiology

Pathogens isolated in CAUTI are shown in Table 41.1 (3,11-12).

TABLE 41.1 Most Common Bacterial Pathogens Isolated from CAUTI

Escherichia coli	*20-32%*
Enterococci	11.9-15.5%
Klebsiella pneumoniae	*7.5-11.1%*
Pseudomonas aeruginosa	10.1-13.3%
Proteus mirabilis	*~5%*
Coagulase negative *staphylococcus*	<5%
Staphylococcus aureus	*<3%*
Klebsiella oxytoca	<3%

CAUTI = catheter-associated urinary tract infections.
From References 3, 11-12.

The predominant organisms are gram-negative aerobic bacilli (especially *Escherichia coli*), enterococci, while staphylococci are infrequent isolates. *Candida* species will be discussed below.

Prevention

The primary risk of catheter-associated infection is the duration of catheterization (13-14). *Clearly removing catheters when they are no longer necessary is the single most effective prophylactic measure for catheter-associated infections.* Catheters should only be inserted for appropriate indications and the continued need for an IUC should be addressed daily. Examples of appropriate indications for IUC use are shown in Table 41.2. Nurse-driven protocols have effectively decreased unnecessary catheter days (15-16).

TABLE 41.2 Examples of Appropriate Indications for Indwelling Urethral Catheter Use

- Patient has acute urinary retention or bladder outlet obstruction.
- Need for accurate measurements of urinary output intraoperatively or in critically ill patients
- Perioperative use for selected surgical procedures:
  - Patients undergoing urologic surgery or other surgery on contiguous structures of the genitourinary tract
  - Anticipated prolonged duration of surgery (catheters inserted for this reason should be removed in PACU)
  - Patients anticipated to receive large-volume infusions or diuretics during surgery
- To assist in healing of open sacral or perineal wounds in incontinent patients
- Patient requires prolonged immobilization (e.g., potentially unstable thoracic or lumbar spine, multiple traumatic injuries such as pelvic fractures).
- To improve comfort for end-of-life care, e.g., urinary incontinence

PACU = post-anesthesia care unit.

Urinary incontinence alone is not an appropriate indicator. Alternatives to IUC should be considered in selected patients.

Alternatives to IUC

Intermittent Catheterization (IC). Performed at regular intervals (to avoid overdistention). Portable ultrasound can be performed to assess urinary volume in patients undergoing IC.

Condom Catheters (males). When fitted properly, male condom catheters allow for precise measures of urine production while avoiding the IUC and further instrumentation of the urinary tract.

Negative Pressure "Wick" Systems (male and female). The Pure-Wick Urine Collection system (CR Bard, Inc., Murray Hill, New Jersey) uses negative pressure (wall suction) to pull urine away from the body that is then absorbed using a soft and absorbent fabric. The urine is rapidly "wicked" away through tubing to the connected collection canister leaving skin feeling dry thus averting irritation.

- The male version requires shaving of the pubic hair as the collection system is held in place by an adhesive covering the phallus similar to a condom catheter (Figure 41.1).
- The female version is passively held in place between the labia in the supine or seated position (Figure 41.2).

Prophylaxis with systemic antibiotics are of no benefit in preventing CAUTI (4) and risk the development of resistant organisms (17).

CHAPTER 41 ■ Urinary Tract Infections 659

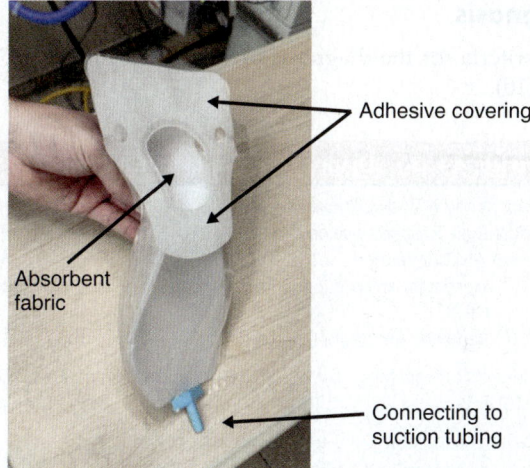

FIGURE 41.1. Male version PureWick Urine Collection system. See text for detailed description.

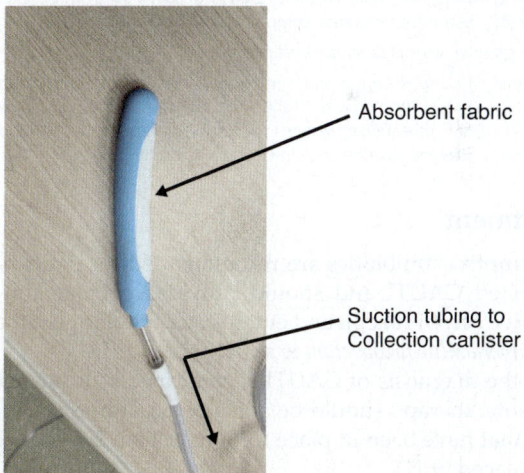

FIGURE 41.2. Female version of PureWick Urine Collection system. See text for detailed description.

Diagnosis

The criteria for the diagnosis of CAUTI are shown in Table 41.3 (10).

TABLE 41.3 Diagnostic Criteria for CAUTI

1	Patient had an indwelling urinary catheter that had been in place for more than 2 consecutive days in an inpatient location on the date of event AND was either: • Present for any portion of the calendar day on the date of event, OR • Removed the day before the date of event
2	Urine culture growing no more than 2 organisms, 1 with growth of ≥10^5 cfu/mL
3	Patient has at least 1 of the following signs or symptoms[†]: • Fever (>38°C or >100.4°F) • Suprapubic pain or tenderness • Costovertebral pain or tenderness

[†]Frequency, urgency, and dysuria are not included for patients with indwelling urinary catheter (IUC) as these are common complaints of the IUC itself.

CAUTI = catheter-associated urinary tract infections.

From Centers for Disease Control and Prevention. Urinary tract infection (catheter-associated urinary tract infection [CAUTI] and non-catheter-associated urinary tract infection [UTI]) and other urinary system infection [USI]) events. Accessed March 6, 2025. https://www.cdc.gov/nhsn/pdfs/pscmanual/7psccauticurrent.pdf

Treatment

Presumptive antibiotics are recommended for patients with suspected CAUTI and should provide coverage for gram negative aerobic bacilli and enterococci. Single agent therapy, e.g., *piperacillin-tazobactam* is appropriate (9,11).

If the diagnosis of CAUTI is confirmed by urine culture, antibiotic therapy should be adjusted accordingly, and catheters that have been in place for longer than 2 weeks should be replaced (9,11).

The duration of antibiotic therapy for CAUTI should be 7 days for patients who respond promptly, and 10-14 days for patients with a delayed response. A three-day duration is appropriate for patients ≤65 years of age (11).

CANDIDURIA

The presence of *Candida* species in urine is reported in 3-32% of patients with IUC (9). This usually represents colonization, but candiduria can also be a sign of disseminated candidiasis (i.e., the candiduria being the result, not the cause, of the disseminated candidiasis).

Microbiology

The most frequent isolate is *Candida albicans* (about 50% of cases), followed by *Candida glabrata* (about 15% of cases) (18). The latter organism is resistant to the antifungal agent fluconazole. In cases of candiduria, the colony count has no predictive value for identifying renal or disseminated candidiasis (18).

Asymptomatic Candiduria

Asymptomatic candiduria does not require treatment unless the patient is neutropenic or will undergo urologic manipulation (19).

Patients with neutropenia should receive the recommended course of treatment for candidemia (19). The "strong recommendations" of the Infectious Diseases Society of America include the following:

- Echinocandins
  - Caspofungin: loading dose 70 mg, then 50 mg daily
  - Micafungin: 100 mg daily
  - Anidulafungin: loading dose 200 mg, then 100 mg daily is recommended as initial therapy
- Lipid formulation amphotericin B
  - 3-5 mg/kg daily, is an effective but less attractive alternative because of the potential for toxicity

Chronic candiduria in neutropenic patients should be investigated using blood cultures, kidney imaging studies, and repeat urine cultures. Removal of the catheter is advised, when possible (19-20). *Patients undergoing urologic procedures should receive oral fluconazole, 400 mg daily, or amphotericin B, 0.3-0.6 mg/kg IV daily, for several days before and after the procedure* (19).

Symptomatic Candiduria

Symptomatic candiduria (i.e., associated with fever, suprapubic tenderness, etc.) requires blood cultures and imaging studies of the kidneys (ultrasound or computed tomography) to search for renal abscesses or urinary tract obstruction. The following recommendations for antifungal therapy are from the 2016 Infectious Diseases Society of America guidelines on treating candidiasis (19):

Cystitis
- For fluconazole-susceptible organisms, give oral fluconazole, 200 mg daily, for 2 weeks.
- For fluconazole-resistant *C. glabrata*, give oral flucytosine, 25 mg/kg, 4 times daily, for 7-10 days.
- For *C. krusei*, give amphotericin B, 0.3-0.6 mg/kg daily, for up to 7 days.

Pyelonephritis
- For fluconazole-susceptible organisms, give oral fluconazole, 200-400 mg daily, for 2 weeks.
- For fluconazole-resistant *C. glabrata*, give amphotericin B, 0.3-0.6 mg/kg daily, for up to 7 days, with or without oral flucytosine, 25 mg/kg, 4 times daily.
- For *C. krusei*, give amphotericin B, 0.3-0.6 mg/kg daily, for up to 7 days.

Fluconazole
Fluconazole is concentrated in the urine and is well suited for treating *Candida* UTIs caused by susceptible organisms.

However, the incidence of non-albicans *Candida* with fluconazole resistance has increased by 7% as reported by the Centers for Disease Control (21-23). Decreasing the dose of fluconazole for a creatinine clearance <50 mL/min (which is normally recommended) is not advised for *Candida* UTIs because this decreases the urinary concentration of fluconazole to subtherapeutic levels (24).

References

1. Dalen DM, Zvonar RK, Jessamine PG. An evaluation of the management of asymptomatic catheter-associated bacteriuria and candiduria at The Ottawa Hospital. Can J Infect Dis Med Microbiol 2005;16:166-70.
2. Podkovik S, Toor H, Gattupalli M, et al. Prevalence of catheter-associated urinary tract infections in neurosurgical intensive care patients—the overdiagnosis of urinary tract infections. Cureus 2019;11:e5494.
3. Rubi H, Mudey G, Kunjalwar R. Catheter-associated urinary tract infection (CAUTI). Cureus 2022;14:e30385.
4. Nicolle LE, Gupta K, Bradley SF, et al. Clinical practice guideline for the management of asymptomatic bacteriuria: 2019 update by the Infectious Diseases Society of America. Clin Infect Dis 2019;68:e83-e110.
5. Givler DN, Givler A. Asymptomatic Bacteriuria. [Updated 2023 Jul 17]. In: StatPearls [Internet]. Treasure Island (FL): StatPearls Publishing; 2025 Jan-. Available from: https://www.ncbi.nlm.nih.gov/books/NBK441848/
6. Coussement J, Scemla A, Abramowicz D, et al. Antibiotics for asymptomatic bacteriuria in kidney transplant recipients. Cochrane Database Syst Rev 2018;2:CD011357.
7. Schumm K, Lam TB. Types of urethral catheters for management of short-term voiding problems in hospitalised adults. Cochrane Database Syst Rev 2008:CD004013.
8. Gould CV, Umscheid CA, Agarwal RK, et al. Guideline for prevention of catheter-associated urinary tract infections 2009. Infect Control Hosp Epidemiol 2010;31:319-26.
9. Hooton TM, Bradley SF, Cardenas DD, et al. Diagnosis, prevention, and treatment of catheter-associated urinary tract infection in adults: 2009 International Clinical Practice Guidelines from the Infectious Diseases Society of America. Clin Infect Dis 2010;50:625-63.

10. Centers for Disease Control and Prevention. Urinary tract infection (catheter-associated urinary tract infection [CAUTI] and non-catheter-associated urinary tract infection [UTI]) and other urinary system infection [USI]) events. Accessed March 6, 2025. https://www.cdc.gov/nhsn/pdfs/pscmanual/7psccauticurrent.pdf
11. Sabih A, Leslie SW. Complicated Urinary Tract Infections. [Updated 2024 Dec 7]. In: StatPearls [Internet]. Treasure Island (FL): StatPearls Publishing; 2025 Jan-. Available from: https://www.ncbi.nlm.nih.gov/books/NBK436013/
12. D'Incau S, Atkinson A, Leitner L, et al. Bacterial species and antimicrobial resistance differ between catheter and non-catheter-associated urinary tract infections: data from a national surveillance network. Antimicrob Steward Healthc Epidemiol 2023;3:e55.
13. Letica-Kriegel AS, Salmasian H, Vawdrey DK, et al. Identifying the risk factors for catheter-associated urinary tract infections: a large cross-sectional study of six hospitals. BMJ Open 2019;9:e022137.
14. Centers for Disease Control and Prevention. Indwelling urinary catheter culture stewardship: overview. Accessed March 6, 2025. https://www.cdc.gov/uti/hcp/clinical-guidance
15. Durant DJ. Nurse-driven protocols and the prevention of catheter-associated urinary tract infections: a systematic review. Am J Infect Control 2017;45:1331-41.
16. Tyson AF, Campbell EF, Spangler LR, et al. Implementation of a nurse-driven protocol for catheter removal to decrease catheter-associated urinary tract infection rate in a surgical trauma ICU. J Intensive Care Med 2020;35:738-44.
17. Flores-Mireles A, Hreha TN, Hunstad DA. Pathophysiology, treatment, and prevention of catheter-associated urinary tract infection. Top Spinal Cord Inj Rehabil 2019;25:228-40.
18. Hollenbach E. To treat or not to treat—critically ill patients with candiduria. Mycoses. 2008;51 Suppl 2:12-24.
19. Pappas PG, Kauffman CA, Andes DR, et al. Clinical practice guideline for the management of candidiasis: 2016 update by the Infectious Diseases Society of America. Clin Infect Dis 2016;62:e1-50.
20. Rajni E, Jorwal A, Jain T. Candiduria in the critically ill: a gray zone for the microbiologist and clinician alike! Arch Med Health Sci 2024;12:134-6.
21. Abdel-Hamid RM, El-Mahallawy HA, Abdelfattah NE, Wassef MA. The impact of increasing non-albicans Candida trends on diagnostics in immunocompromised patients. Braz J Microbiol 2023;54:2879-92.
22. Centers for Disease Control and Prevention. Data and Statistics on Candidemia. Accessed March 6, 2025. https://www.cdc.gov/candidiasis/data-research/facts-stats/index.html

23. Vallabhaneni S, Cleveland AA, Farley MM, et al. Epidemiology and risk factors for echinocandin nonsusceptible Candida glabrata bloodstream infections: data from a large multisite population-based candidemia surveillance program, 2008-2014. Open Forum Infect Dis 2015;2:ofv163.
24. Fisher JF, Sobel JD, Kauffman CA, Newman CA. Candida urinary tract infections—treatment. Clin Infect Dis 2011;52 Suppl 6:S457-66.

SECTION XI
NERVOUS SYSTEM DISORDERS

Chapter 42
Disorders of Consciousness

This chapter describes the major disorders of consciousness encountered in the intensive care unit (ICU), with an emphasis on delirium, coma, and brain death.

ALTERED CONSCIOUSNESS

Definitions

Consciousness is defined by two components: arousal and awareness (1-4).

1. *Arousal* is the ability to experience one's surroundings and is also known as *wakefulness*.
2. *Awareness* is the ability to understand one's relationship to one's surroundings and is also known as *responsiveness*.

Altered states of consciousness can be classified using these two components, as described in Table 42.1.

TABLE 42.1	Altered States of Consciousness	
Can Be Awakened and Is Aware	Can Be Awakened but Is Not Aware	Cannot Be Awakened and Is Not Aware
Anxiety	Delirium	Coma
Lethargy	Dementia	Brain death
Locked-in state	Psychosis	
	Stupor	
	Vegetative state	

From Disorders of Consciousness. In: Marino PL. *Marino's The ICU Book*. 5th ed. Wolters Kluwer; 2025:677-92. Table 45.1.

Predisposing Conditions

Predisposing conditions are illustrated in Figure 42.1.

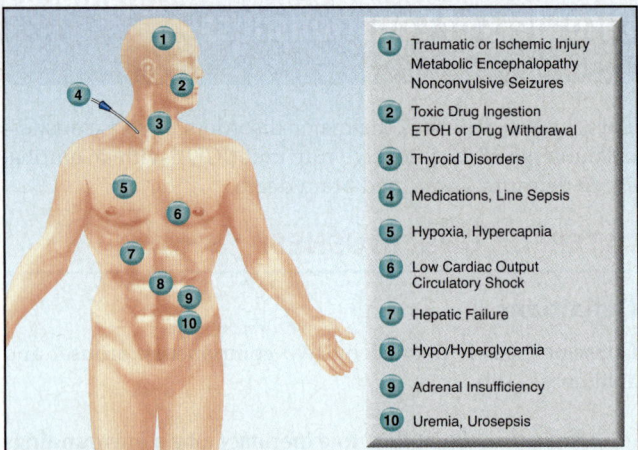

FIGURE 42.1. Common sources of altered consciousness in ICU patients. (From Disorders of Consciousness. In: Marino PL. *Marino's The ICU Book*. 5th ed. Wolters Kluwer; 2025:677-92. Figure 45.1.)

DELIRIUM

Clinical Features

The clinical features of delirium are summarized in Figure 42.2.

The hallmark of delirium is a state of *inattentiveness* (i.e., inability to focus) that has a rapid onset or a rapidly fluctuating course and is accompanied by either disordered thinking or an altered level of consciousness (5). *Hypoactive delirium is the most common form* (5).

Predisposing Conditions

Any condition that can precipitate an encephalopathy is a source for delirium. Common causes in the ICU include

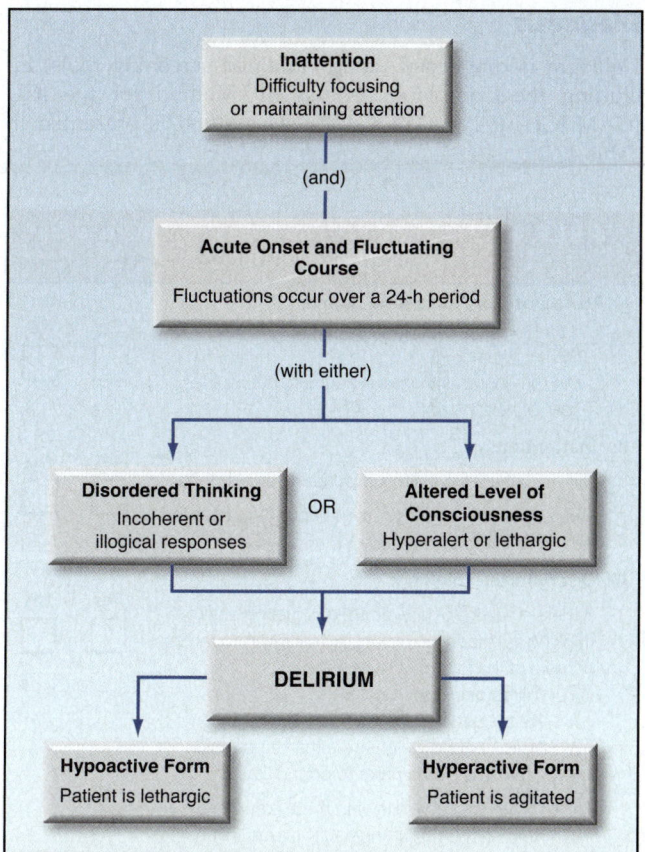

FIGURE 42.2. The clinical features of delirium in critically ill patients. (From Disorders of Consciousness. In: Marino PL. *Marino's The ICU Book*. 5th ed. Wolters Kluwer; 2025:677-92. Figure 45.2.)

sepsis, liver failure, uremia, and the use of sedative-hypnotic drugs (5). The prolonged use of sedatives is a major risk factor for delirium (6), and benzodiazepines have been identified as the principal class of sedatives that promote delirium (7-9).

Diagnosis

Delirium is diagnosed using validated screening tools, including the Confusion Assessment Method for the ICU (CAM-ICU) (5,7,9). The CAM-ICU method is presented in Table 42.2.

TABLE 42.2 The Confusion Assessment Method for the ICU (CAM-ICU)

I: Acute Onset or Fluctuating Course: A. Is there evidence of an acute change in metal status? OR B. Did the abnormal behavior fluctuate during the past 24 h?	Yes ☐	No ☐
II: Inattention: Did the patient have difficulty focusing attention? (The patient can be shown five simple items as asked to recall the items in succession.)	Yes ☐	No ☐
III: Disorganized Thinking: Is there evidence of disorganized or incoherent thinking as evidenced by incorrect answers to three or more of the following questions? 1. Will a stone float in water? 2. Are there fish in the sea? 3. Does 1 pound weigh more than 2 pounds? 4. Can you use a hammer to pound a nail? AND is there difficulty following these commands? 1. Hold up this many fingers. (The examiner holds two fingers in front of the patient.) 2. Now do the same thing with the other hand (without holding the two fingers in front of the patient).	Yes ☐	No ☐
IV: Altered Level of Consciousness: Is the patient's level of consciousness anything other than alert, such as being hyperalert or lethargic?	Yes ☐	No ☐
A Yes answer to I and II, and either III or IV = Delirium.		

From References 7 and 9.

Delirium versus Dementia

Delirium and dementia are distinct mental disorders that can be confused because they have overlapping clinical features, including attention deficits and disordered thinking. However, delirium is distinguished from dementia based on two features: i.e., the acute onset and fluctuating course.

Delirium versus Psychosis

Delirium can be difficult to distinguish from psychosis. Over 40% of hospitalized patients with delirium have psychotic symptoms (e.g., visual hallucinations) (10), and delirium has been given the misnomer of "ICU psychosis" (10).

Management

No drug has proven effective in preventing or correcting ICU-related delirium, and drugs are recommended only to restore calm in severely agitated patients (5,11). The drugs that can be used for this purpose are included in Table 42.3 (see Chapter 5: Analgesia and Sedation).

Prevention

Current guidelines recommend the "ABCDEF bundle" for the prevention of ICU delirium (12-13). This bundle includes:

(A) *assessing*, preventing, and treating pain
(B) promoting *both* spontaneous awakening and breathing trials
(C) *choosing* analgesics and sedatives judiciously
(D) assessing, preventing and managing *delirium*
(E) encouraging *early* mobilization and *exercise*
(F) engaging and empowering *family* members

ALCOHOL WITHDRAWAL

Chronic alcohol intake predisposes patients to an excitatory state (i.e., alcohol withdrawal syndrome) because the density of inhibitory γ-aminobutyric acid (GABA) receptors in the

TABLE 42.3	Drugs for Severe Agitation in ICU Delirium
Drug	**Recommendations**
Dexmedetomidine	Dosing: Loading dose (optional) is 1 µg/kg IV over 10 min followed by an infusion of 0.2-1.5 µg/kg/h. Comment: Can produce bradycardia and hypotension. A withdrawal syndrome (with hyperexcitability) has been reported.
Haloperidol	Dosing: Start with 5 mg IV as a bolus dose. If no effect after 15 min, double the dose (10 mg IV) or switch to another agent. For maintenance dosing, use 25% of the initial effective dose every 6 h. Comment: Has a relatively slow onset of action. Not advised if the corrected QT interval is >500 msec.
Ziprasidone	Dosing: 10 mg IM every 2 h, or 20 mg IM every 4 h, to a total daily dose of 40 mg Comment: The IM route can be useful if IV access is problematic.

From Disorders of Consciousness. In: Marino PL. *Marino's The ICU Book*. 5th ed. Wolters Kluwer; 2025:677-92. Table 45.2.

brain is increased (14). Alcohol is a potent stimulant for the neuronal release of GABA, and when stopped abruptly, alcohol withdrawal syndrome can develop.

Clinical Features

The clinical features of alcohol withdrawal are described in Table 42.4 (15).

The Clinical Institute Withdrawal Assessment of Alcohol Scale, Revised (CIWA-AR) (Table 42.5) is the most popular method for monitoring the severity of alcohol withdrawal, but the CAM-ICU instrument is recommended for patients with *alcohol withdrawal delirium* (see Table 42.2) (16-18). Both instruments are used to assess the response to treatment.

TABLE 42.4 Clinical Features of Alcohol Withdrawal

Features	Onset after Last Drink	Duration
Early Withdrawal	6-8 h	1-2 days
Anxiety, nausea, tremulousness		
Generalized Seizures	6-48 h	2-3 days
One or two		
Hallucinations	12-48 h	1-2 days
Visual, auditory, or tactile		
Delirium Tremens	48-96 h	3-5 days
Fever, tachycardia hypertension, delirium (hyperactive), autonomic instability		

From Tetrault JM, O'Connor PG. Substance abuse and withdrawal in the critical care setting. Crit Care Clin 2008;24:767-88.

Seizures

Generalized seizures can appear as early as 6-8 h after the last drink (the risk of seizures peaks at 24 h), and they can appear in isolation, without other signs of withdrawal (16). The recommended treatment is lorazepam (2 mg IV push), which prevents recurrent seizures (19). Phenytoin is not recommended for alcohol-withdrawal seizures (16).

Delirium Tremens

About 5% of patients develop a severe form of alcohol withdrawal known as delirium tremens (DTs) (16-17), which appears about 2-3 days after the last drink and is characterized by *hyperactive* delirium, hallucinations, and signs of autonomic hyperactivity (e.g., fever, tachycardia, hypertension) that can progress to hemodynamic instability. This condition typically lasts 3-5 days (16), and delirium that persists for longer than 5 days should prompt consideration of other causes.

TABLE 42.5 Clinical Institute Withdrawal Assessment for Alcohol, Revised (CIWA-Ar)

Nausea and Vomiting	Headache
0: No nausea or vomiting	0: Not present
1	1: Very mild
2	2: Mild
3	3: Moderate
4: Intermittent nausea with dry heaves	4: Moderately severe
5	5: Severe
6	6: Very severe
7: Constant nausea, frequent dry heaves and vomiting	7: Extremely severe

Paroxysmal Sweats	Auditory Disturbances
0: No sweats visible	0: Not present
1: Barely perceptible sweating, palms moist	1: Very mild harshness or ability to frighten
2	2: Mild harshness or ability to frighten
3	3: Moderate harshness or ability to frighten
4: Beads of sweat obvious on forehead	4: Moderately severe hallucination
5	5: Severe hallucinations
6	6: Extremely severe hallucinations
7: Drenching sweats	7: Continuous hallucinations

Anxiety	Visual Disturbances
0: No anxiety, at ease	0: Not present
1	1: Very mild photosensitivity
2	2: Mild photosensitivity
3	3: Moderate photosensitivity
4: Moderately anxious, guarded	4: Moderately severe visual hallucinations
5	5: Severe visual hallucinations
6	6: Extremely severe visual hallucinations
7: Acute panic state, consistent with severe delirium or acute schizophrenia	7: Continuous visual hallucinations

TABLE 42.5 (continued)

Agitation	Tactile Disturbances
0: Normal activity	0: None
1: Somewhat more than normal activity	1: Very mild paresthesias
2	2: Mild paresthesias
3	3: Moderate paresthesias
4: Moderately fidgety and restless	4: Moderately severe hallucinations
5	5: Severe hallucinations
6	6: Extremely severe hallucinations
7: Paces back and forth during most of the interview or constantly thrashes about	7: Continuous hallucinations

Tremor	Orientation and Clouding of Sensorium
0: No tremor	0: Oriented and can do serial additions
1: Not visible, but can be felt at fingertips	1: Cannot do serial additions
2	2: Disoriented for date by no more than 2 calendar days
3	3: Disoriented for date by more than 2 calendar days
4: Moderate when patient's hands extended	4: Disoriented for place and/or patient
5	**Total Score Is a Simple Sum of Each Item Score (maximum score is 67)**
6	Score:
7: Severe, even with arms not extended	<10: Very mild withdrawal
	10 to 15: Mild withdrawal
	16 to 20: Modest Withdrawal
	>20: Severe withdrawal

Adapted from Sullivan JT, Sykora K, Schneiderman J, et al. Assessment of alcohol withdrawal: the revised Clinical Institute Withdrawal Assessment for Alcohol Scale (CIWA-Ar). Br J Addict 1989;84(11):1353-7.

Management

Symptom-Triggered Management

Benzodiazepines are the drugs of choice for treating alcohol withdrawal delirium, and lorazepam (Ativan) is frequently preferred due to its short half-life (16). Although there are only moderate strength data to support a *symptom-triggered approach* (i.e., waiting until symptoms manifest before administering sedatives), several small studies suggest that lower benzodiazepine doses can be achieved with equivalent or better clinical outcomes (20-21). A symptom-triggered algorithm for the management of alcohol withdrawal delirium is presented in Figure 42.3 (16,18-22).

Alternative Agents

Midazolam is an alternative to lorazepam and diazepam, although midazolam has a higher hepatic extraction ratio, which may result in prolonged effects in patients with liver disease (which is common in many chronic alcoholics). Midazolam may be given at a dose of 2-5 mg IV every 5 min, then 4-10 mg IV until either a CIWA-Ar score <8 or Richmond Agitation Sedation Scale (RASS) of 0 to −1 is achieved (21,23). Chlordiazepoxide (Librium) can also be given at a dose of 25-100 mg if the patient can tolerate oral dosing and repeated every hour until the CIWA-Ar or RASS goal is achieved. Chlordiazepoxide is rarely used in ICU patients because most cannot safely tolerate oral medications and the drug has a longer half-life and may lead excessive sedation in patients with hepatic insufficiency.

Other Considerations

Wernicke Encephalopathy

Wernicke encephalopathy can occur patients with alcohol use disorder and is the result of thiamine deficiency. This syndrome presents as an acute deterioration in mental status several days after admission. Nystagmus and oculomotor palsies (e.g., lateral gaze paralysis) may be present. Thiamine replacement at a dose of 500 mg over 30 min, three times

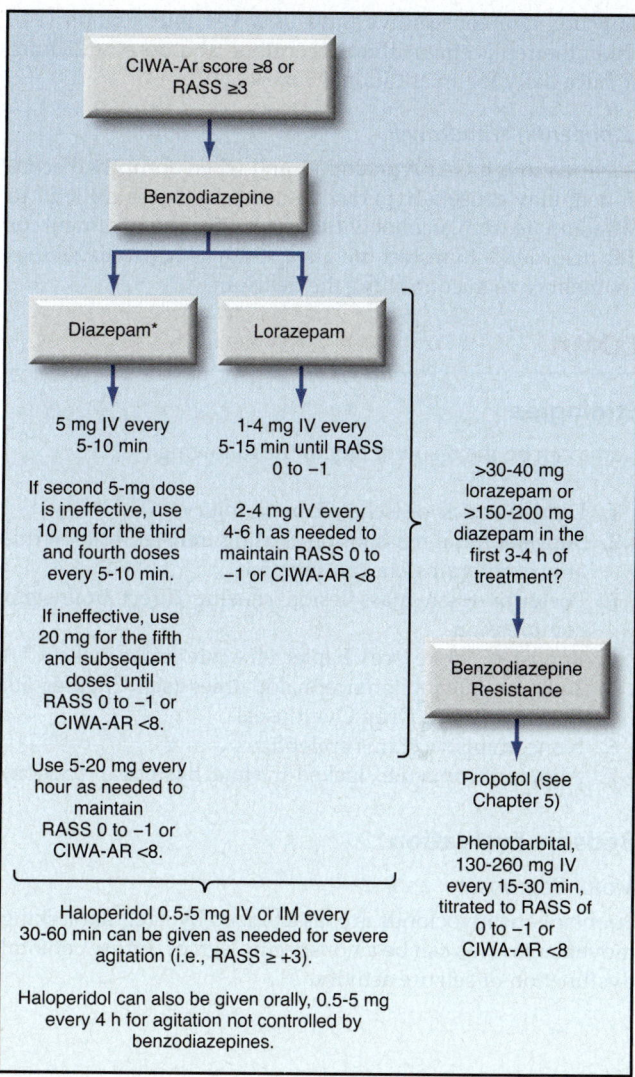

FIGURE 42.3. Symptom-triggered approach to alcohol withdrawal delirium. (From References 16, 18-22.)

daily for two consecutive days, is a key intervention (24). Thiamine replacement should continue at a dose of 250 mg IV once daily for an additional 5 days (24).

Gabapentin Withdrawal

Gabapentin is a GABA analogue, and when abruptly discontinued, may cause a hyperactive delirium that is difficult to differentiate from alcohol withdrawal (25). The treatment for this disorder is to restart the gabapentin as benzodiazepines are ineffective in controlling the delirium.

COMA

Etiologies

Coma can be the result of any of the following:

1. Diffuse anoxic or ischemic brain injury
2. Supratentorial mass lesion causing transtentorial herniation and brainstem compression
3. Posterior fossa mass lesion causing direct brainstem compression
4. Brainstem stroke (see Chapter 44: Acute Stroke in the ICU)
5. Toxic or metabolic encephalopathies (see Chapter 50: Pharmaceutical Drug Overdoses)
6. Nonconvulsive status epilepticus
7. Apparent coma (i.e., locked-in state, hysterical reaction)

Bedside Evaluation

Motor Responses

Spontaneous myoclonus is characterized by irregular jerking movements. This can be a nonspecific sign of diffuse cerebral dysfunction or seizure activity.

Responses to Pain

A purposeful response to pain is not a feature of the comatose state. The following responses are determined by specific areas of brain injury (26):

1. *Thalamic injury*: Painful stimuli provide flexion of the upper extremities (*decorticate posturing*).
2. *Midbrain and upper pons*: The arms and legs extend and pronate in response to pain (*decerebrate posturing*).
3. *Lower brainstem*: The extremities remain flaccid during painful stimulation.

Pupillary Findings

Spontaneous eye opening indicates arousal, not coma, although spontaneous eye opening without a lack of awareness may be associated with a vegetative state (26). Conditions that affect pupillary size and light reactivity are shown in Table 42.6 (27–29).

Ocular Motility and Reflexes

Spontaneous eye movements (conjugate or disconjugate) are a nonspecific sign of a toxic or metabolic encephalopathy (28). The ocular reflexes are used to evaluate the functional integrity of the lower brainstem (28). These reflexes are illustrated in Figure 42.4.

Oculocephalic Reflex. The oculocephalic reflex is assessed by briskly rotating the head from side to side. When the lower brainstem is damaged, the eyes will follow the direction of head rotation.

Oculovestibular Reflex. The oculovestibular reflex is assessed by injecting 50 mL of cold saline in the external auditory canal of each ear (using a 50-mL syringe attached to a 2-inch-

TABLE 42.6 Conditions that Affect Pupillary Size and Reactivity	
Pupil Size and Reactivity	**Associated Conditions**
Large, both reactive (+)(+)	Atropine, anticholinergic toxicity, adrenergic agonists (e.g., dopamine), stimulant drugs (e.g., amphetamines), or nonconvulsive seizures
Large, both nonreactive (−)(−)	Diffuse brain injury, hypothermia (<28° C), or brainstem compression from an expanding intracranial mass or intracranial hypertension
Unequal, one nonreactive (−)(+)	Expanding intracranial mass (e.g., uncal herniation), ocular trauma or surgery, or focal seizure
Midsize, both reactive (+)(+)	Toxic/metabolic encephalopathy, sedative overdose, or neuromuscular blockade
Midsize, both nonreactive (−)(−)	Acute liver failure, postanoxic encephalopathy, or brain death
Unequal, both reactive (+)(+)	Horner syndrome
Pinpoint (+/−)(+/−)	Opiate overdose, toxic/metabolic encephalopathy, hypercapnia, or pontine injury

From References 27-29.

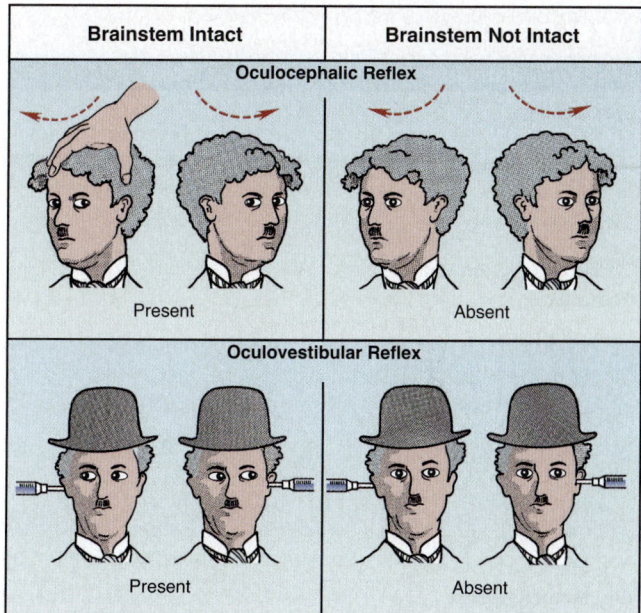

FIGURE 42.4. The ocular reflexes in the evaluation of coma. See text for explanation. (From Disorders of Consciousness. In: Marino PL. *Marino's The ICU Book*. 5th ed. Wolters Kluwer; 2025:677-92. Figure 45.3.)

long plastic intravenous catheter). Prior to performing this test, the tympanic membrane should be checked to ensure that it is intact and that the ear canal is unobstructed. With an intact brainstem, both eyes deviate slowly toward the irrigated ear. This reflex is lost when the lower brainstem is damaged. After testing one side, the opposite side should not be tested until 5 min later.

The Glasgow Coma Scale Score

The Glasgow Coma Scale (GCS) score is shown in Table 42.7.

The GCS is not reliable in patients who are paralyzed, heavily sedated, or hypotensive. Intubated patients cannot

TABLE 42.7 The Glasgow Coma Scale Score

Rating	Score
Eye Opening	
Spontaneous	4
To sound	3
To pressure	2
None	1
Non testable	NT
Verbal Response	
Oriented	5
Confused	4
Words	3
Sounds	2
None	1
Non testable	NT
Best Motor Response	
Obeys commands	6
Localizes (to stimulation)[1]	5
Flexes (to stimulation)[1,2]	4
Abnormal flexion[1,2]	3
Extension (to stimulation)[1]	2
None	1
Non testable	NT

[1]Sites for physical stimulation include fingertip pressure, trapezius pinch, and pressure over the supraorbital notch.

[2]Abnormal flexion is slow, stereotyped, and includes forearm rotation or movement of the arm across the chest, with the thumb clenched and the lower extremity often simultaneously extended. Normal flexion is rapid and usually involves movement away from the body.

From References 30-31.

provide a verbal response; hence, the maximum score an intubated patient can achieve is "11-NT." Coma is generally defined as a score of ≤8; a score of ≤8 is generally accepted as an indication for endotracheal intubation.

BRAIN DEATH

The Uniform Determination of Death Act states that "an individual who has sustained either (1) irreversible cessation of circulatory and respiratory functions, or (2) irreversible cessation of all functions of the entire brain, including the brainstem, is dead" (32-33).

Determination

A checklist for the diagnosis of brain death/death by neurologic criteria (BD/DNC) in adults is shown in Table 42.8 (33).

BD/DNC testing should not be done until a minimum of 24 h has transpired, although many clinicians employ more conservative observation periods to ensure that elevated intracranial pressure has been maximally treated (33). It should be noted that the mean arterial pressure goal of ≥75 mm Hg is higher than the usual target (65 mm Hg) because a higher pressure is required to maintain cerebral perfusion when intracranial pressure is elevated. A minimum of one examination is required for BD/DNC, although performance of two independent BD/DNC examinations may decrease the risk of a false-positive determination (33).

Apneal Testing

Brain death is confirmed by the absence of a spontaneous respiratory response to a hypercarbic ($PaCO_2$ >60 mm Hg or 20 mm Hg above baseline) and acidemic (pH of <7.28) challenge (33). The apnea test proceeds as follows:

1. Prior to the test, the patient is preoxygenated with 100% oxygen O_2 for at least 10 min (to prevent profound hypoxemia) and an arterial blood gas is obtained to establish the baseline $PaCO_2$.

TABLE 42.8 Checklist for Brain Death Determination in Adults

Step 1: Prerequisites

1. The patient must have sustained a catastrophic, permanent brain injury caused by an identified mechanism that is known to lead to BD/BDN.
2. Neuroimaging must be consistent with the mechanism and severity of brain injury.
3. A sufficient amount of time after brain injury must transpire to ensure there is no potential for recovery of brain function. In hypoxic ischemic brain injury, this is ≥24 h.
4. Core body temperature must be ≥36°C for >24 h.
5. Systolic blood pressure must be ≥100 mm Hg and mean arterial pressure ≥75 mm Hg.
6. Residual pharmacological paralysis must be ruled out (with either a train-of-four stimulator or demonstration of deep tendon reflexes).
7. Drug levels for medications that suppress the central nervous system must be therapeutic or subtherapeutic.
    a. The pentobarbital level must be <5 μg/mL (if this drug was used) and at least 5 half-lives must transpire for all other drugs (or longer if the patient has renal/hepatic dysfunction).
8. Alcohol blood levels must be ≤80 mg/dL (if clinically indicated).
9. Toxicology screen (urine and blood) must be negative.
10. Severe metabolic, acid-base, and endocrine derangements must not be present.
11. A reasonable attempt to inform the patient's family that a BD/DNC examination will take place.

- Proceed to step 2 if all prerequisites met.

If not met, proceed to ancillary testing.

TABLE 42.8	(continued)
Step 2. Clinical Exam	
1. Coma with unresponsiveness to visual, auditory, and tactile stimulation	
2. Absent motor responses to noxious stimuli to the head, face, trunk, and limbs (other than spinally mediated reflexes)	• Proceed to Step 3 if all prerequisites met.
3. Absent pupillary responses to bright light bilaterally	*If there is a concern for s spinal cord injury, oculocephalic testing is deferred and ancillary testing is indicated.*
4. Absent oculocephalic reflex bilaterally	
5. Absent oculovestibular reflex bilaterally	
6. Absent corneal reflexes bilaterally	
7. Absent gag reflex	
8. Absent cough reflex	
Step 3. Apnea Test	

From Greer DM, Kirschen MP, Lewis A, et al. Pediatric and adult brain death/death by neurologic criteria Consensus Guideline. Neurolog 2023;101(24):1112-32.

2. The patient is removed from the ventilator and O_2 is insufflated into the endotracheal tube (via a tracheal cannula, T-piece system, or continuous positive airway pressure) to prevent O_2 desaturation during the period of apnea.
3. The patient is observed for observable respiratory efforts for 8-10 min (the $PaCO_2$ rises about 3 mm Hg /min during apnea). A repeat arterial blood gas is obtained prior to reconnection to the ventilator to confirm that the target $PaCO_2$ is achieved.
4. In patients who do not have chronic CO_2 retention, the apnea test is positive if no respirations occur, the arterial pH level is <7.30, and the $PaCO_2$ is ≥60 and/or ≥20 mm Hg above the patient's pretest baseline (33). In patients known to have chronic CO_2 retention, the same criteria apply, but the key indicator is a *$PaCO_2$ that is 20 mm Hg*

above the baseline. If the patient's pretest baseline CO_2 is not clear, ancillary testing should be performed (33).
5. The time of death is recorded as the time that the confirmatory blood gas result becomes available.

Ancillary Testing

BD/DNC is a clinical evaluation, and ancillary tests to confirm BD/DNC are only indicated when clinical criteria cannot be fully or accurately evaluated. Conventional four-vessel catheter angiography is the preferred ancillary test to aid in the diagnosis of BD/DNC (33). Radionuclide cerebral perfusion scintigraphy, planar radionuclide angiography, and transcranial doppler ultrasonography can also be used as alternative tests if catheter angiography is not available. Electroencephalogram (EEG), somatosensory evoked potentials, and auditory evoked potentials *should not be used* because these tests do not provide complete information about brainstem function (33). CT angiography, MRI, or MR angiography should not be used as ancillary tests due to the lack of validation and potential for false positives (33).

References

1. Young GB, Wijdicks EFM. Consciousness: its neurologic relevance. Handb Clin Neurol 2008;90:33-6.
2. Howard RS. Stupor and coma. Handb Clin Neurol 2008;90:57-78.
3. Leon-Carrion J, van Eeckhout P, Dominguez-Morales Mdel R. The locked-in syndrome: a syndrome looking for a therapy. Brain Inj 2002;16:555-69.
4. The Multi-Society Task Force on PVS. Medical aspects of the persistent vegetative state (part 1). N Engl J Med 1994;330:1499-508.
5. Stollings JL, Kotfis K, Chanques G, et al. Delirium in critical illness: clinical manifestations, outcomes, and management. Intensive Care Med 2021;47:1089-103.
6. Reade MC, Finfer S. Sedation and delirium in the ICU. N Engl J Med 2014;370:444-54.
7. Ely EW, Margolin R, Francis J, et al. Evaluation of delirium in critically ill patients: Validation of the Confusion Assessment Method for the Intensive Care Unit (CAM-ICU). Crit Care Med 2001;29:1370-9.

8. Fraser GL, Devlin JW, Worby CP, et al. Benzodiazepine versus non-benzodiazepine-based sedation for mechanically ventilated, critically ill adults: a systematic review and meta-analysis of randomized trials. Crit Care Med 2013;41(9 suppl 1):S30-8.
9. Ely EW, Inouye SK, Bernard GR, et al. Delirium in mechanically ventilated patients. Validity and reliability of the Confusion Assessment Method for the intensive care unit. JAMA 2001;286:2703-10.
10. Webster R, Holroyd S. Prevalence of psychotic symptoms in delirium. Psychosomatics 2000;41:519-22.
11. Devlin JW, Skrobik Y, Gélinas C, et al. Clinical practice guidelines for prevention and management of pain, agitation/sedation, delirium, immobility, and sleep disruption in adult patients in the ICU. Crit Care Med 2018;46:e825-e873.
12. Marra A, Ely EW, Pandharipande PP, Patel MB. The ABCDEF bundle in critical care. Crit Care Clin 2017;33(2):225-43.
13. Bannon L, McGaughey J, Verghis R, et al. The effectiveness of non-pharmacological interventions in reducing the incidence and duration of delirium in critically ill patients: a systematic review and meta-analysis. Intensive Care Med 2019;45:1-12.
14. Krystal JH, Staley J, Mason G, et al. Gamma-aminobutyric acid type A receptors and alcoholism: intoxication, dependence, vulnerability, and treatment. Arch Gen Psychiatry 2006;63:957-68.
15. Tetrault JM, O'Connor PG. Substance abuse and withdrawal in the critical care setting. Crit Care Clin 2008;24:767-88.
16. American Society of Addiction Medicine. *The ASAM Clinical Practice Guideline on Alcohol Withdrawal Management*. Rockville, MD: American Society of Addiction Medicine; 2020. Accessed March 14, 2025. https://www.asam.org/quality-care/clinical-guidelines/alcohol-withdrawal-management-guideline
17. Sullivan JT, Sykora K, Schneiderman J, et al. Assessment of alcohol withdrawal: the revised Clinical Institute Withdrawal Assessment for Alcohol Scale (CIWA-Ar). Br J Addict 1989;84(11):1353-7.
18. Pribék IK, Kovács I, Kádár BK, et al. Evaluation of the course and treatment of alcohol withdrawal syndrome with the Clinical Institute Withdrawal Assessment for Alcohol - Revised: a systematic review-based meta-analysis. Drug Alcohol Depend 2021;220:108536.
19. D'Onofrio G, Rathlev N, Ulrich A, et al. Lorazepam for the prevention of recurrent seizures related to alcohol. N Engl J Med 1999;340:915-9.
20. Saitz R, Mayo-Smith MF, Roberts MS, et al. Individualized treatment for alcohol withdrawal. A randomized double-blind controlled trial. JAMA 1994;272(7):519-23.
21. Holleck JL, Merchant N, Gunderson CG. Symptom-triggered therapy for alcohol withdrawal syndrome: a systematic review and meta-analysis of randomized controlled trials. J Gen Intern Med 2019;34(6):1018-24. doi:10.1007/s11606-019-04899-7

22. Mayo-Smith MF, Beecher LH, Fischer TL, et al. Management of alcohol withdrawal delirium. An evidence-based practice guideline. Arch Intern Med 2004;164(13):1405-12.
23. Bird RD, Makela EH. Alcohol withdrawal: what is the benzodiazepine of choice? Ann Pharmacother 1994;28(1):67-71.
24. Cook CC, Hallwood PM, Thomson AD. B Vitamin deficiency and neuropsychiatric syndromes in alcohol misuse. Alcohol Alcohol 1998;33(4):317-36.
25. Mersfelder TL, Nichols WH. Gabapentin: abuse, dependence, and withdrawal. Ann Pharmacother 2016;50:229-33.
26. Zakaria Z, Abdullah MM, Halim SA, et al. The neurological exam of a comatose patient: an essential practical guide. Malays J Med Sci 2020;27(5):108-23.
27. Stevens RD, Bhardwaj A. Approach to the comatose patient. Crit Care Med 2006;34:31-41.
28. Bateman DE. Neurological assessment of coma. J Neurol Neurosurg Psychiatry 2001;71:i13-17.
29. Wijdicks EFM. Neurologic manifestations of pharmacologic agents commonly used in the intensive care unit. In: *Neurology of Critical Illness*. F.A. Davis; 1995:3-17.
30. The Royal College of Physicians and Surgeons of Glasgow. The Glasgow structured approach to assessment of the Glasgow Coma Scale. Accessed March 15, 2025. https://www.glasgowcomascale.org/gcs-aid/
31. Teasdale G, Allen D, Brennan P, et al. The Glasgow Coma Scale: an update after 40 years. Nursing Times 2014;110:12-6.
32. Uniform Determination of Death Act, 12 uniform laws annotated (U.L.A.) 589 (West 1993 and West suppl 1997).
33. Greer DM, Kirschen MP, Lewis A, et al. Pediatric and adult brain death/death by neurologic criteria Consensus Guideline. Neurolog 2023;101(24):1112-32.

Disorders of Movement — Chapter 43

This chapter summarizes three movement disorders that are commonly encountered in the ICU: seizures (involuntary movement), neuromuscular weakness (weak or ineffective movement), and drug-induced paralysis (no movements).

SEIZURES

Conditions that cause new-onset seizures in the ICU are listed in Table 43.1 (1-3).

TABLE 43.1	Reported Occurrence Rates of Seizures	
Condition	Seizures	Status Epilepticus
Traumatic brain injury	20-50%	15-25%
Ischemic brain injury	40%	30%
Encephalitis*	35-45%	20%
Intracerebral hemorrhage	20-30%	10-20%
Subarachnoid hemorrhage	10-20%	15%
No neurologic illness	4-15%	<1%
Acute ischemic stroke[†]	2-5%	—

*Includes infectious and autoimmune encephalitis.
[†]Includes only the early period (one week) after acute stroke.
From References 1-3.

Types of Seizures

Seizures are classified by the presence or absence of abnormal movements (i.e., convulsive vs. nonconvulsive), the type of movement (i.e., tonic-clonic, myoclonic), and extent of involvement (generalized vs. focal).

Abnormal Movements

The movements associated with seizures can be *tonic* (caused by sustained muscle contraction), *clonic* (rhythmic movements with a regular amplitude and frequency), or *myoclonic* (irregular, jerky movements that vary in amplitude and frequency). The abnormal movements can also be familiar but repetitive (e.g., chewing or lip smacking); these are called *automatisms*.

Generalized vs. Focal Seizures

Generalized seizures arise from synchronous, rhythmic electrical discharges that involve most of the cerebral cortex, and they are always associated with loss of consciousness, but not always associated with abnormal (convulsive) movements. Focal seizures arise from discrete areas of the brain and may or may not be accompanied by loss of consciousness; however, focal seizures frequently progress to generalized seizures (1).

Complex Partial Seizures

Complex partial seizures are focal seizures with impaired awareness. These seizures are nonconvulsive but are associated with behavioral changes. The usual presentation is a patient who is awake but not aware of the surroundings (similar to *absence* seizures). These seizures are often preceded by an *aura* (e.g., a particular smell) and can be accompanied by automatisms.

Status Epilepticus

Status epilepticus (SE) is defined as ≥5 min of continuous clinical and/or electrographic seizure activity and recurrent seizure activity without an intervening return to baseline consciousness (4-6). The most common types of SE observed in the ICU are (a) generalized convulsive and nonconvulsive SE, (b) myoclonic SE, and (c) focal motor SE (with and without loss of consciousness). Refractory status epilepticus (RSE) occurs in approximately 20-25% of all cases of

SE and is defined as SE that fails to cease when at least two appropriately dosed anti-seizure medications (ASM) are administered (4,7). Super-refractory status epilepticus (SRSE) is defined as SE that persists or recurs after more than 24 h of intravenous anesthetics (e.g., midazolam, propofol) or highly sedating ASM (e.g., pentobarbital) (8).

Nonconvulsive Status Epilepticus

Nonconvulsive SE is difficult to diagnose because the clinical manifestations are atypical and variable, as described in Table 43.2 (9).

TABLE 43.2 Clinical Manifestations of Nonconvulsive Status Epilepticus	
Impaired Consciousness	**Others**
Confusion (49%)	Speech disturbances (15%)
Coma (22%)	Myoclonus (13%)
Lethargy (21%)	Bizarre behavior (11%)
	Agitation or delirium (8%)
	Hallucinations (6%)

From Sutter R, Rüegg S, Kaplan PW. Epidemiology, diagnosis, and management of nonconvulsive status epilepticus. Neurol Clin Pract 2012;2:275-86.

The diagnosis of nonconvulsive SE is essential because most seizures in ICU patients are nonconvulsive (10) and the prevalence of nonconvulsive SE has been reported to be as high as 30% in ICU patients with impaired consciousness (9-12). Given these observations, *continuous electroencephalogram (EEG) monitoring should be strongly considered in ICU patients with undifferentiated impaired consciousness* (13).

Treatment

The initial pharmacotherapy for SE is described in Tables 43.3 and applies to both convulsive SE and nonconvulsive SE (1,4,8,14-19).

TABLE 43.3	Drug Regimens for Status Epilepticus
Drug	**Recommendations**
Step 1: Benzodiazepines	
Lorazepam	Dosing: 0.1 mg/kg (up to 4 mg per dose) IV over 2 min; repeat in 5 min, if needed.
	Comment: The preferred drug regimen for terminating SE. Onset of action is <2 min, and effect lasts 6-12 h.
Midazolam	Dosing: 0.2 mg/kg (up to 10 mg max dose) IV, or by intramuscular (IM) injection
	Comment: IM midazolam is as effective as IV lorazepam, and the IM route is advantageous when IV access is problematic (e.g., in the field).
Step 2: Anticonvulsants	
Levetiracetam	Dosing: 60 mg/kg IV over 5-10 min; max single dose is 4,500 mg.
	Comment: Levetiracetam is often preferred to the other anticonvulsants because it has few side effects and is not hepatically metabolized.
Valproic acid	Dosing: 40 mg/kg IV over 5-10 min; may give an additional 20 mg/kg 10 min after loading infusion; max single dose is 3,000 mg.
	Comment: Valproic acid is as effective as the other anticonvulsants. Only side effect of concern is hyperammonemia, which creates a risk of encephalopathy.
Fosphenytoin	Dosing: 20 mg PE.kg IV at ≤150 mg/min; max single dose is 1,500 mg PE.
	Comment: Fosphenytoin is a water-soluble prodrug with less risk of hypotension than phenytoin because it does not contain the solvent propylene glycol.

From References 1, 4, 8, 14-19.

Step 1: Benzodiazepines. Benzodiazepines are the first-line drugs of choice for the rapid termination of generalized SE (4,14). Intravenous lorazepam is the preferred agent, and intramuscular midazolam is effective when IV access is not available (16).

Step 2: Antiseizure Medications (ASM). Approximately one-third of generalized SE cases do not respond to benzodiazepines (17), and the next step is the administration of an ASM: i.e., levetiracetam, valproic acid, or fosphenytoin. Levetiracetam has the fewest side effects and is the preferred ASM, although all three ASMs have equivalent effectiveness (18). Valproic acid also has relatively few side effects except for a 40% risk of hyperammonemia which can contribute to encephalopathy (19).

Step 3: Refractory Status Epilepticus. Generalized SE persists in about 10-15% of patients who receive step 1 and step 2 drugs (4,6-8). Drugs for the management of RSE are described in Table 43.4 (see also Chapter 5: Analgesia and Sedation).

TABLE 43.4 Drug Regiments for Refractory Status Epilepticus

Drug	Dosing Regimens
Propofol	Start with an IV bolus dose of 1-2 mg/kg, and begin infusion at 1 mg/kg/h (30-200 µg/kg/min). Titrate upward as needed to max dose rate of 15 mg/kg/h (or 5 mg/kg/h if infusion longer than 48 h) use caution with high doses (see Chapter 5: Analgesia and Sedation).
Midazolam	Load with 0.2 mg/kg IV, then infuse at 0.2 mg/kg/h, and titrate upward as needed to a max dose rate of 4 mg/kg/h.
Pentobarbital	Load with 5-15 mg/kg IV over 1 h, then begin infusion at 1 mg/kg/h. Titrate upward, if needed, to a max dose rate of 5 mg/kg/h. An IV bolus dose of 5 mg/kg can be given for breakthrough SE.

From References 1, 4, 8, 14-19.

Drugs other than those listed in Table 43.4 may also be effective for the management of RSE (i.e., ketamine, thiopental, phenobarbital) (1,8).

Prognosis

SE and RSE are associated with substantial in-hospital mortality; the mortality for generalized SE is 21%, nearly 50% for nonconvulsive SE, and over 60% for RSE (13).

NEUROMUSCULAR WEAKNESS SYNDROMES

Myasthenia Gravis

Myasthenia gravis (MG) is caused by antibody-mediated destruction of acetylcholine (ACh) receptors on the postsynaptic side of neuromuscular junctions (20). MG can be triggered by physiological stressors, including major surgery or a concurrent illness. Thymomas are responsible for 10% of cases of MG (20-21). Drugs that can exacerbate MG are listed in Table 43.5 (22).

TABLE 43.5 Drugs that Can Exacerbate Myasthenia Gravis

1. *Antibiotics*: aminoglycosides, fluoroquinolones, macrolides, penicillins
2. *Cardiovascular Drugs*: β-blockers, calcium channel blockers, class Ia antiarrhythmics (procainamide, quinidine, disopyramide)
3. *Neuromuscular Blockers*: both depolarizing and non-depolarizing agents
4. *Others*: high-dose steroids, inhalational anesthetics, magnesium, lithium

From Sheikh S, Alvi U, Soliven B, Rezania K. Drugs that can induce or cause deterioration of myasthenia gravis: an update. J Clin Med 2021;10:1537.

It should be noted that corticosteroids, which are a primary treatment for MG, may paradoxically aggravate MG initially (possibly due to impaired neuromuscular junction function) (21,23).

Clinical Features

Skeletal muscles are affected by MG and the weakness has the following characteristics (20,24):

1. The eye muscles are always involved, with the earliest signs being diplopia and ptosis (due to oculomotor and eyelid weakness). Symmetrical limb weakness usually follows eye weakness.
2. The muscle weakness worsens with muscle activity (fatigable) and improves with rest.
3. Deep tendon reflexes are preserved. The neurological deficit is purely motor.
4. As the disease progresses, the diaphragm and chest wall muscles weaken, with rapid progression to respiratory failure (i.e., *myasthenic crisis*) (24).

Diagnosis

MG is suspected in patients who present with ptosis, diplopia, and fatigable muscle weakness as dominant features. Confirmatory diagnostic testing is done with ACh receptor antibody testing, but 10-15% of patients with MG will not have ACh antibodies in the blood (20), and for these cases, a muscle-specific kinase (MuSK) antibody should be assayed. Nerve conduction testing is reserved for atypical clinical presentations, when antibody tests are negative.

Respiratory Failure Prediction

Patients with rapidly worsening muscle weakness are at increased risk for respiratory failure. No single clinical sign or scoring assessment has sufficient sensitivity and specificity for the prediction of respiratory failure, but multimodal assessments, as listed in Table 43.6, can aid with risk stratification to evaluate the need for endotracheal intubation (24-25).

TABLE 43.6 Multimodal Assessment of Warning Signs Indicating the Need for Endotracheal Intubation in Patients with Neuromuscular Weakness

Signs and Symptoms	Measures of Respiratory Muscle Weakness	Scoring Instruments
• Dyspnea • Bulbar features (e.g., dysarthria, dysphagia, weak cough, pooling secretions) • Hypophonia • Poor respiratory effort (i.e., paradoxical breathing) • Tachypnea (with shallow respirations) • Single breath count ≤13 (≤5 has higher sensitivity and specificity) • Neck flexion strength (≤3 on MRC scale)	• Vital capacity (VC) <20 mL/kg (or <60% predicted) • Maximum inspiratory force (MIF) ≤30 cm H_2O • Maximum expiratory force (MEF) ≤40 cm H_2O	• Higher EGRIS score (score range is 0-7). See https://qxmd.com/calculate/calculator_527/erasmus-gbs-respiratory-insufficiency-score-egris

MRC = Medical Research Council scale (5 = full power; 3 = antigravity; 1 = trace contraction). EGRIS = Erasmus Guillan-Barré Syndrome Respiratory Insufficiency Score.

From References 24 and 25.

Management

There are two principal treatment options for the management of myasthenic crisis:

1. *Intravenous immunoglobulin (IVIG)* to neutralize pathologic antibodies. The dose is 2 g/kg in divided doses over 2-5 days (26).
2. *Plasmapheresis* (to remove the pathologic antibodies from the bloodstream), which typically involves 5 sessions over 7-10 days, with each session exchanging 1.0-1.5 plasma volumes.

Although both therapeutic options are considered equivalent in terms of long-term outcomes (27), plasmapheresis has a faster onset of action and is preferred by many MG experts (28).

Pyridostigmine and Chronic Immunotherapy. The acetylcholinesterase inhibitor pyridostigmine (Mestinon) is used for patients with mild-to-moderate MG. This drug is discontinued temporarily during a myasthenic crisis because the cholinergic effect of this drug can induce problematic secretions. Glucocorticoids (i.e., prednisone 60-80 mg daily) are used for long-term treatment of MG, but transient worsening of weakness can occur within 5-10 days of treatment and may last about 5 days (21-22). Other immunotherapies (e.g., rituximab, tacrolimus, mycophenolate) may also be considered for long-term control of MG but should only be prescribed after consultation with a neurologist who specializes in MG management (26,28).

Additional Considerations

1. MG patients are at high risk for venous thromboembolism due to immobility. Thromboprophylaxis should be initiated quickly and maintained (see Chapter 4: Prophylaxis for VTE).

2. MG patients are at risk for aspiration due to bulbar weakness. Prior to initiation of oral intake, a swallow evaluation should be performed.
3. A contrast-enhanced computed tomography of the chest should be obtained in all patients with new-onset MG to search for a thymoma. If one is present, a thymectomy may be appropriate to reduce the need for immunotherapy.

Prognosis

The vast majority (approximately 95%) of patients hospitalized with a myasthenic crisis will survive the hospitalization, but few recover completely (20,24).

ACUTE IMMUNE-MEDIATIED POLYNEUROPATHY

Acute immune-mediated polyneuropathy, more commonly known by the eponym *Guillain-Barré syndrome* (GBS; henceforth, the terminology used in this section), is an *inflammatory demyelinating polyneuropathy* that often follows an acute infectious illness by 1-3 weeks. Infectious organisms most implicated with precipitating GBS include *Campylobacter jejuni*, Zika virus, and SARS Coronavirus-2 (29).

Clinical Features

The features of GBS are often confused with MG, although several features distinguish the two diseases, as listed in Table 43.7.

GBS is characterized by progressive and symmetrical muscle weakness (in upper and lower limbs) with *absent deep tendon reflexes* (29-30). Oculomotor weakness in GBS is *rare* with the exception of the *Miller Fisher syndrome*, which is a GBS variant associated with ophthalmoplegia and ataxia (31). Respiratory failure occurs in GBS in approximately 25% of cases (30) and autonomic instability may occur in advanced cases (32).

TABLE 43.7 Features that Distinguish Guillain-Barré Syndrome from Myasthenia Gravis

Feature	Guillain-Barré Syndrome	Myasthenia Gravis
Oculomotor weakness	No	Yes
Fatigable weakness	No	Yes
Deep tendon reflexes	Diminished	Intact
Autonomic instability	Yes	No
Cerebrospinal fluid	↑ Protein	Normal

From Disorders of Movement. In: Marino PL. *Marino's The ICU Book*. 5th ed. Wolters Kluwer;2025:693-707. Table 46.6.

Diagnosis

The diagnosis of GBS is established using clinical and electrophysiological criteria (i.e., nerve conduction studies) (33-34). Lumbar puncture is often performed to rule out other conditions, and the cerebrospinal fluid typically reveals elevated protein levels in patients with GBS (34). The risk for respiratory failure can be assessed using the criteria listed in Table 43.6.

Management

Patients with GBS who require ICU-level care are managed in a very similar fashion to the management described for MG. Patients who are unable to walk unaided, or have respiratory failure, should be treated with *IVIG or plasmapheresis* (33-34), using the same regimens described for MG. Both IVIG and plasmapheresis are considered equivalent, and no preference is endorsed in the most recent GBS guidelines (33-34).

Pain Management

A neuropathic pain pattern may occur in the acute and resolving stages of GBS. *Gabapentin* (Neurontin) in a dose of

300 mg three times daily is recommended (34), although supplemental opioids may also be required for more immediate pain relief (35).

Prognosis

According to US-based data, about 97% of patients who are hospitalized for GBS will survive the hospital stay (36), but 10-15% of these patients will be severely disabled (37).

CRITICAL ILLNESS NEUROMYOPATHY

Critical illness polyneuropathy (CIP) and *critical illness myopathy* (CIM) are secondary disorders that may occur in severe systemic inflammatory diseases (38-39).

Pathogenesis

1. The common denominator in both CIP and CIM is *severe or progressive inflammation* (39-41).
2. CIP is the most common peripheral neuropathy in critically ill patients (42). CIP is a diffuse sensory and motor axonal neuropathy that occurs more often in patients with sepsis and septic shock (41). Both limb and truncal muscles are affected.
3. CIM is a diffuse inflammatory myopathy that also affects limb and truncal muscles (41). Predisposing conditions are similar as for CIP but also include prolonged immobility and hyperglycemia (39-40). High-dose steroids have been implicated as a potential contributor to CIP and CIM in earlier studies (43), although other studies have found no effect (44).

Clinical Features

Both CIP and CIM produce a flaccid paralysis in limb and truncal muscles, associated with hyporeflexia or areflexia (36). These disorders often coexist in the same patient and manifest as difficulty encountered when attempting to liberate patients from mechanical ventilation.

1. The diagnosis of CIP is confirmed by *nerve conduction studies*, which demonstrate slowed conduction in sensory and motor fibers (45).
2. The diagnosis of CIM is confirmed by *electromyography* (EMG) and by muscle biopsy (41).

Management

Management of both CIP and CIM is supportive with interventions directed at resolving the underlying pathophysiologic conditions (i.e., sepsis). Measures such as early ambulation and improved nutrition have been proposed as interventions, but none have been definitively shown to accelerate recovery.

Prognosis

Both CIP and CIM complicate the ICU stay for critically ill patients because both involve prolonged mechanical ventilation. Approximately half of all patients affected by CIP or CIM are expected to have a complete recovery but only after months of rigorous rehabilitative therapy (45).

DRUG INDUCED PARALYSIS

Neuromuscular blocking (NMB) drugs produce a flaccid paralysis that is required in the following situations: (a) to facilitate endotracheal intubation (see Chapter 2: Airway Management), (b) to prevent shivering during induced hypothermia, and (c) to promote synchronous mechanical ventilation in patients who are severely agitated (46).

Neuromuscular Blocking Agents

Commonly used NMB agents are listed in Table 43.8 (see Chapter 2: Airway Management for additional information regarding *succinylcholine* and *rocuronium*) (46-47).

TABLE 43.8 Properties of Commonly Used Neuromuscular Blocking Agents

	Succinylcholine	Rocuronium	Cisatracurium
Intubating dose (IV)	1-1.5 mg/kg	1.0 mg/kg	0.15-0.2 mg/kg
Onset time	1-1.5 min	1.5-3 min	5-7 min
Clinical duration	7-12 min	50-70 min	35-50 min
Infusion dose	—	5-12 µg/kg/min	1-3 µg/kg/min
Cardiovascular effects	Bradycardia	None	None
Contraindications	Multiple[†]	None	None
Influence of renal or hepatic dysfunction	None	Prolonged effect with liver failure	None

[†]Contraindications to succinylcholine include hyperkalemia, malignant hyperthermia, rhabdomyolysis, burns, and immobility from spinal cord injury.

Most experts recommend using ideal body weight (IBW) for dosing.

From References 46 and 47.

Cisatracurium

Cisatracurium is a nondepolarizing agent with an onset of action up to 2-3 min and an intermediate duration of effect (35-50 min). Cisatracurium is degraded by a non-biological pathway (i.e., Hofmann degradation and plasma esterases); thus, clearance is not influenced by renal or hepatic failure, making this an appealing NMB drug for use in ICU patients (but *not* for rapid sequence induction and intubation due to a longer onset of action).

Monitoring

The standard method of monitoring for patients who receive NMB agents is train-of-four (TOF) monitoring (46,48). This technique applies a series of four low-frequency (2 Hz) electrical pulses to the ulnar nerve at the forearm, and adduction of the thumb is observed. Total absence of thumb adduction is evidence of a complete block. The desired goal is one or two perceptible twitches, and the drug infusion is adjusted to achieve that endpoint (46,48). Observation of thumb adduction is highly observer-dependent and current guidelines recommend the use of *quantitative* monitors to more precisely assess the degree of neuromuscular blockade (49).

Reversal Agents

Neostigmine

Neostigmine blocks the breakdown of ACh by inhibiting the acetylcholinesterase enzyme, and the subsequent increase in ACh is enough to overcome the competitive blockade by the nondepolarizing agents.

Dosage. The dose of neostigmine needed to reverse neuromuscular paralysis is dependent on several factors, including the NMB agent, the depth of paralysis, and the anesthetic agent that is used. An intravenous neostigmine dose of 70 µg/kg can reverse a moderate level of paralysis, but the recovery time can vary from 8-45 min (47). The dose of neostigmine should not exceed 70 µg/kg because of the risk of parasympathomimetic side effects (47). Glycopyrrolate is often administered prior to neostigmine to prevent parasympathomimetic-associated bradycardia. A dose of 0.2 mg of glycopyrrolate for every 1 mg of neostigmine, given concomitantly (i.e., maximum 1 mg glycopyrrolate and 5 mg neostigmine), has been shown to provide the greatest efficacy for prevention of bradycardia with the lowest incidence of adverse effects (50).

Sugammadex

Sugammadex (Bridion) is a reversal agent that binds directly to the aminosteroid class of neuromuscular blockers (i.e., rocuronium, vecuronium, and pancuronium). It binds most tightly to rocuronium but is equally effective for vecuronium (51). Sugammadex may be rarely associated with bradycardia and anaphylaxis (52). A theoretical decrease in the effectiveness of oral contraceptives is reported, but this is rarely an immediate consideration for critically ill women (52).

Dosage. The dose of sugammadex depends on the depth of paralysis and timing and dosing of NMB drug administration. To reverse rocuronium within minutes after it is administered (i.e., after an intubation dose is given), the sugammadex dose is 16 mg/kg, and the reversal time is only 2-3 min (which is less than the recovery time for succinylcholine) (47,51). With deep paralysis (zero TOF twitches), the dose of sugammadex is 4 mg/kg; with moderate paralysis (at least 2 TOF twitches), the dose is 2 mg/kg, with a time for reversal of 2-3 min (43). Compared to neostigmine, the reversal of NMB drugs with sugammadex is significantly faster, and there are no cholinergic side effects (53-54).

References

1. Rosetti AO, Claasen J, Gaspard N. Status epilepticus in the ICU. Intensive Care Med 2024;50:1-16.
2. Sutter R. Are we prepared to detect subtle and nonconvulsive status epilepticus in critically ill patients? J Clin Neurophysiol 2016;33:25-31.
3. Camilo O, Goldstein LB. Seizures and epilepsy after acute ischemic stroke. Stroke 2004;36:1769-75.

4. Brophy GM, Bell R, Claassen J, et al. Guidelines for the evaluation and management of status epilepticus. Neurocrit Care 2012;17(1):3-23.
5. Meierkord H, Boon P, Engelsen B, et al. EFNS guideline on the management of status epilepticus in adults. Eur J Neurol 2010;17:348-55.
6. Trinka E, Cock H, Hesdorffer D, et al. A definition and classification of status epilepticus—report of the ILAE Task Force on classification of status epilepticus. Epilepsia 2015;56:1515-23.
7. Novy J, Logroscino G, Rossetti AO. Refractory status epilepticus: a prospective observational study. Epilepsia 2010;51(2):251-6.
8. Shorvon S, Ferlisi M. The treatment of super-refractory status epilepticus: a critical review of available therapies and a clinical treatment protocol. Brain 2011;134(Pt 10):2802-18.
9. Sutter R, Rüegg S, Kaplan PW. Epidemiology, diagnosis, and management of nonconvulsive status epilepticus. Neurol Clin Pract 2012;2:275-86.
10. Wang X, Yang F, Chen B, Jiang W. Non-convulsive seizures and non-convulsive status epilepticus in neuro-intensive care unit. Acta Neurol Scand 2022;146(6):752-60.
11. Zafar A. Prevalence, electroclinical spectrum and effect on the outcome of non-convulsive status epilepticus in critically ill patients; the utility of routine electroencephalogram. Epilepsy Behav 2023;141:109144.
12. Towne AR, Waterhouse EJ, Boggs JG, et al. Prevalence of nonconvulsive status epilepticus in comatose patients. Neurology 2000;54:340-5.
13. Rossetti AO, Schindler K, Sutter R, et al. Continuous vs routine electroencephalogram in critically ill adults with altered consciousness and no recent seizure: a multicenter randomized clinical trial. JAMA Neurol 2020; 77:1225-32.
14. Glauser T, Shinnar S, Gloss D, et al. Evidence-based guidelines: treatment of convulsive status epilepticus in children and adults: report of the Guideline Committee of the American Epilepsy Society. Epilepsy Curr 2016;16:48-61.
15. Kienitz R, Kay L, Beuchat I, et al. Benzodiazepines in the management of seizures and status epilepticus: a review of routes of delivery, pharmacokinetics, efficacy, and tolerability. CNS Drugs 2022;36:951-75.
16. Silbergleit R, Durkalski V, Lowenstein D, et al. Intramuscular versus intravenous therapy for prehospital status epilepticus. N Engl J Med 2012;366:591-600.
17. Treiman DM, Meyers PD, Walton NY, et al. A comparison of four treatments for generalized convulsive status epilepticus. N Engl J Med 1998;339:792-8.
18. Kapur J, Elm J, Chamberlain JM, et al. Randomized trial of three anticonvulsant medications for status epilepticus. N Engl J Med 2019;381:2103-13.

19. Nordlund LJ. Intravenous use of valproic acid in status epilepticus is associated with a high risk of hyperammonemia. Seizure 2019;69:20-4.
20. Gilhus NE. Myasthenia gravis. N Engl J Med 2016;375:2570-81.
21. Lotan I, Hellmann MA, Wilf-Yarkoni A, Steiner I. Exacerbation of myasthenia gravis following corticosteroid treatment: What is the evidence? A systematic review. J Neurol 2021;268(12):4573-86.
22. Sheikh S, Alvi U, Soliven B, Rezania K. Drugs that can induce or cause deterioration of myasthenia gravis: an update. J Clin Med 2021;10:1537.
23. Gilhus NE, Andersen H, Andersen LK, et al. Generalized myasthenia gravis with acetylcholine receptor antibodies: a guidance for treatment. Eur J Neurol 2024;31(5):e16229.
24. Claytor B, Cho S-M, Li Y. Myasthenic crisis. Muscle Nerve 2023;68: 8-19.
25. McKenzie ED, Kromm JA, Mobach T, et al. Risk stratification and management of acute respiratory failure in patients with neuromuscular disease. Crit Care Med 2024;52(11):1781-9.
26. Sussman J, Farrugia ME, Maddison P, et al. Myasthenia gravis: Association of British Neurologists' management guidelines. Pract Neurol 2015;15(3):199-206.
27. Gajdos P, Chevret S, Toyka KV. Intravenous immunoglobulin for myasthenia gravis. Cochrane Database Syst Rev 2012;12(12): CD002277.
28. Sanders DB, Wolfe GI, Benatar M, et al. International consensus guidance for management of myasthenia gravis: executive summary. Neurology 2016;87(4):419-25.
29. Shahrizaila N, Lehmann HC, Kuwabara S. Guillain-Barré syndrome. Lancet 2021;397:1214-28.
30. Hughes RA, Cornblath DR. Guillain-Barré syndrome. Lancet 2005; 366:1653-66.
31. Teener JW. Miller Fisher's syndrome. Semin Neurol 2012; 32:512-6.
32. Pfeiffer G, Schiller B, Kruse J, et al. Indicators of dysautonomia in severe Guillain-Barré syndrome. J Neurol 1999;246:1015-22.
33. Leonhard SE, Mandarakas MR, Gondim FAA, et al. Diagnosis and management of Guillain-Barré syndrome in ten steps. Nat Rev Neurol 2019;15(11):671-83.
34. van Doorn PA, Van den Bergh PYK, Hadden RDM, et al. European Academy of Neurology/Peripheral Nerve Society guideline on diagnosis and treatment of Guillain-Barré syndrome. Eur J Neurol 2023;30:3646-74.
35. Eisenberg E, McNicol ED, Carr DB. Efficacy and safety of opioid agonists in the treatment of neuropathic pain of nonmalignant origin: systematic review and meta-analysis of randomized controlled trials. JAMA 2005; 293:3043-52.

36. Alshekhlee A, Hussain Z, Sultan B, Katiriji B. Guillain-Barré syndrome: incidence and mortality rates in US hospitals. Neurology 2008;70:1608-13.
37. Jasti AK, Selmi C, Sarmiento-Monroy JC, et al. Guillain-Barré syndrome: causes, immuno-pathogenic mechanisms and treatment. Expert Rev Clin Immunol 2016;12:1175-80.
38. Vanhorebeek I, Latronico N, Van den Berghe G. ICU-acquired weakness. Intensive Care Med 2020;46:637-53.
39. Chueng K, Rathbone A, Melanson M, et al. Pathophysiology and management of critical illness polyneuropathy and myopathy. J Appl Physiol 2021;130:1479-89.
40. Hund E. Neurological complications of sepsis: critical illness polyneuropathy and myopathy. J Neurol 2001;248:929-34.
41. Lacomis D. Critical illness myopathy. Curr Rheumatol Rep 2002; 4:403-8.
42. Malaiyandi D, James E. Neuromuscular weakness in intensive care. Crit Care Clin 2023;39(1):123-38.
43. Griffin D, Fairman N, Coursin D, et al. Acute myopathy during treatment of status asthmaticus with corticosteroids and steroidal muscle relaxants. Chest 1992;102:510-4.
44. Hermans G, De Jonghe B, Bruyninckx F, Van den Berghe G. Interventions for preventing critical illness polyneuropathy and critical illness myopathy. Cochrane Database Syst Rev 2014;2014(1):CD006832.
45. van Mook WN, Hulsewe-Evers RP. Critical illness polyneuropathy. Curr Opin Crit Care 2002;8:302-10.
46. Murray MJ, DeBlock H, Erstad B, et al. Clinical practice guidelines for sustained neuromuscular blockade in the adult critically ill patient. Crit Care Med 2016;40:2079-103.
47. Weigel WA, Grant SA, Thilen SR. Neuromuscular Blocking Drugs. In: Barash PG, Cullen BF, Stoelting RK, et al, eds. *Barash, Cullen, and Stoelting's Clinical Anesthesia*. 9th ed. Wolters Kluwer, 2024:505-28.
48. Ortega R, Brull SJ, Prielipp R, et al. Monitoring neuromuscular function. N Engl J Med 2018;378(4):e6.
49. Thilen SR, Weigel WA, Todd MM, et al. 2023 American Society of Anesthesiologists practice guidelines for monitoring and antagonism of neuromuscular blockade: a report by the American Society of Anesthesiologists Task Force on neuromuscular blockade. Anesthesiology 2023;138(1):13-41.
50. Howard J, Wigley J, Rosen G, D'mello J. Glycopyrrolate: It's time to review. J Clin Anesth 2017;36:51-3.
51. Bridion (sugammadex) injection. Prescribing Information. Merck Sharp & Dohme LLC; 2024.
52. Liang WM, Nguyen D, Anche G, et al. Potential adverse effects of sugammadex administration: a scoping review. Cureus 2025;17(1):e77666.

53. Maqusood S, Bele A, Verma N, et al. Sugammadex vs neostigmine, a comparison in reversing neuromuscular blockade: a narrative review. Cureus 2024;16(7): e65656.
54. Chhabra R, Gupta R, Gupta LK. Sugammadex versus neostigmine for reversal of neuromuscular blockade in adults and children: a systematic review and meta-analysis of randomized controlled trials. Curr Drug Saf 2024;19(1):33-43.

Acute Stroke in the ICU

Chapter 44

This chapter describes the management of ischemic stroke as well as strokes caused by spontaneous intracerebral hemorrhage and subarachnoid hemorrhage. The focus is on immediate management in the ICU.

ISCHEMIC STROKE

Ischemic strokes account for about 85% of all strokes (1). Most are the result of atherosclerotic plaques that rupture and trigger a thrombotic occlusion (like the pathogenesis of myocardial infarctions), but about 20% are *embolic strokes* (1). Emboli more commonly arise from the left side of the heart, but a small fraction of emboli begin as deep vein thrombosis in the legs and reach the brain through a patent foramen ovale.

Management

The general support measures for stroke are summarized in Table 44.1.

Respiratory Support

Oxygen. Guidelines for stroke management recommend supplemental O_2 only in patients who are hypoxemic (2). However, the same guidelines also state that the SaO_2 should be kept >94% (2), which is above the hypoxemic level (i.e., <90%), but higher SaO_2 levels have been shown to decrease cerebral blood flow (3) and promote the formation of reactive oxygen species (4). Therefore, it seems wise to *maintain the SaO_2 at 90-92% and no higher*.

TABLE 44.1	General Support Measures for Acute Ischemic Stroke
Concern	Recommendations
Oxygen	• Use supplemental O_2 only for patients who are hypoxemic (SaO_2 <90%).
Hypertension	• After thrombolytic Rx or mechanical thrombectomy, keep BP <180/105 mm Hg for 24 h. • Otherwise, lower BP only if >220/120 mm Hg for the first 72 h after admission (unless there is heart failure, etc.).
Hyperglycemia	• Lower the blood glucose if >180 mg/dL and maintain the level at 140-180 mg/dL for 24-48 h after admission. • Avoid dextrose-containing IV fluids.
Fever	• Aggressively treat fever for the first 24-48 h. • Search for infection as source of fever.
Antiplatelet therapy	• Start aspirin, 325 mg daily, on day 1 (to prevent early recurrence). • Following thrombolytic Rx, wait 24 h before starting aspirin.
Thromboprophylaxis	• All patients should receive prophylaxis for deep vein thrombosis using low-molecular-weight heparin. • Following thrombolytic therapy, use sequential compression devices for the first 24 h.

From Acute Stroke in the ICU. In: Marino PL. *Marino's The ICU Book*. 5th ed. Wolters Kluwer; 2025:708-24. Table 47.1.

Mechanical Ventilation

Intubation and mechanical ventilation are indicated for (*a*) patients with impaired consciousness who are unable to protect their airways from aspiration of mouth or gastric secretions and (*b*) patients with acute respiratory failure (hypoxemic and/or hypercapnic) who cannot be managed otherwise.

Hemodynamic Management

Hypertension. Guidelines recommend the following goals for blood pressure (BP) control in patients with acute ischemic stroke (2):

1. For patients who do not receive thrombolytic therapy, BP reduction is advised only at pressures >220/120 mm Hg for the first 72 h after the stroke unless there is a condition like left heart failure that requires a more aggressive approach. Any decrease in BP should not exceed 15% in the first 24 h after the stroke.
2. For patients who receive thrombolytic therapy, the BP should be <180/105 mm Hg for 24 h.
3. Consensus has not been reached regarding the optimal BP following mechanical thrombectomy with successful reperfusion. Some guidelines recommend a BP <180/105 mm Hg for 24 h (2), whereas other protocols aim for a normal BP (<140/90) after revascularization (5).

Antihypertensive drugs that are used to achieve BP targets in acute ischemic stroke are listed in Table 44.2.

TABLE 44.2 Antihypertensive Drugs for Use in Acute Ischemic Stroke

Drug	Dosage and Comments
Labetalol	Dosage: 10 mg as IV bolus, and then infuse at 2-8 mg/min; titrate to desired BP.
	Comment: equivalent to nicardipine in efficacy and safety
Nicardipine	Dosage: Infuse at 5 mg/h, and increase in increments of 2.5 mg/h, if needed, to 15 mg/h.
	Comment: equivalent to labetalol in efficacy and safety
Clevidipine	Dosage: Infuse at 1-2 mg/h, and double the dose rate every 2-5 min, if needed, to 21 mg/h.
	Comment: equivalent to nicardipine in efficacy and safety

From References 2, 5, 6.

Hypotension. Prompt correction of hypotension is mandatory in acute ischemic stroke because cerebral autoregulation is impaired. Hypotension can be managed according to the following guideline recommendations (2):

1. Isotonic saline is recommended for volume resuscitation (2), based on studies showing no difference in outcomes between colloid and crystalloid fluids in acute stroke (7).
2. For vasopressors, phenylephrine (a pure α-1 receptor agonist) is appropriate for patients with rapid atrial fibrillation; otherwise, norepinephrine is an appropriate choice.
3. There is no recommendation concerning the minimum target BP in acute stroke, but considering that cerebral autoregulation is impaired, a target pressure that is higher than usual (i.e., greater than a mean arterial pressure of 65 mm Hg) seems warranted.

Echocardiography

A transthoracic echocardiogram (TTE) should be obtained for patients with acute ischemic stroke in the following circumstances:

1. When embolic stroke is suspected (e.g., neuroimaging shows multiple areas of infarction)
2. Atrial fibrillation (past or present)
3. History of transmural myocardial infarction (for possible mural thrombus)
4. Positive blood cultures (for possible endocarditis; a transesophageal echocardiogram [TEE] is often required because transthoracic echocardiography can miss up to 25% of vegetations [8])
5. History of venous thromboembolism (for possible patent foramen ovale)
6. Cryptogenic stroke (i.e., when the cause remains unknown)

Bubble Test. A patent foramen ovale (PFO) has been reported to exist in up to 24% of adults based on autopsy studies (9). Ischemic stroke may result when a thrombus originating in leg veins passes through a PFO and embolizes into the cerebral circulation. A bubble study can be performed with either TTE or TEE. With TTE, the four-chamber view is obtained (Chapter 7: Bedside Echocardiography) and 10 mL of saline is first agitated to create microbubbles (i.e., by rapidly filling and emptying two syringes attached by a three-way stopcock). The saline is then rapidly injected intravenously. In the presence of a PFO, bubbles will appear in the left side of the heart after a few cardiac cycles, as demonstrated in Figure 44.1 (10).

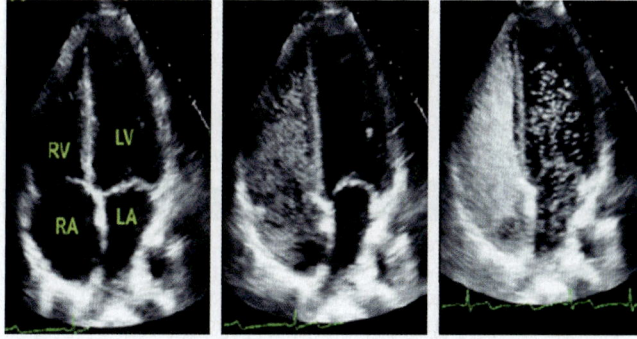

FIGURE 44.1. Transesophageal echocardiography in a patient with acute ischemic stroke, showing microbubbles (from the injection of agitated saline) moving from the right to left side of the heart. This is evidence of a right-to-left shunt from a patent foramen ovale. (From Wade E, Robinson M, Singla A, et al. PFO, push-ups and heavy lifting; Valsalva provocation before cryptogenic stroke. Interv Cardiol 2021;13:273-8.)

The presence of a PFO in the setting of an acute ischemic stroke does not necessarily support causality but should prompt consideration for elective PFO closure following neurologic recovery.

Complications

Intracerebral Hemorrhage

Figure 44.2 shows an intracerebral hemorrhage (i.e., hemorrhagic conversion)—a devastating complication of stroke management (11).

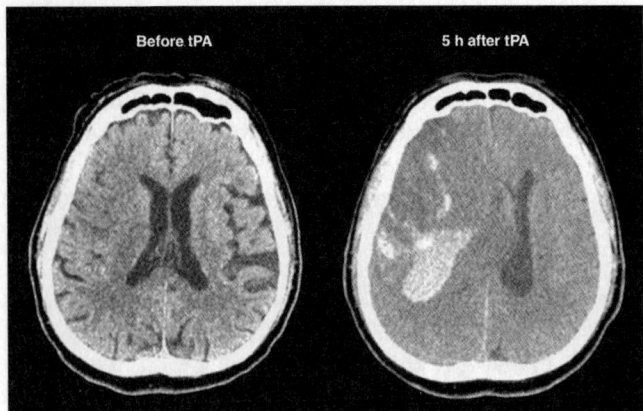

FIGURE 44.2. Noncontrast CT images of the brain from a patient who experienced an abrupt deterioration in mental status 5 h after receiving thrombolytic therapy with tissue plasminogen activator (tPA). The CT scan on the right shows a massive intracerebral hemorrhage (hyperdense areas) with midline shift. (From Ko S-B, Yoon B-W. Blood pressure management for acute ischemic and hemorrhagic stroke: the evidence. Semin Resp Crit Care Med 2017;38:718-25.)

The incidence of symptomatic intracerebral hemorrhage following thrombolytic therapy for acute stroke is 6.4-8.8% (12-13). Risk factors include advanced age, BP >180/105 mm Hg, and a stroke that involves more than one-third of a cerebral hemisphere. The risk of hemorrhage is the reason that patients who receive thrombolytic therapy are often admitted to an ICU or stroke unit for 24 h, where it is possible to closely monitor neurologic status and BP. Anticoagulants and antiplatelet agents are also withheld for the first 24 h after thrombolytic therapy.

Management. The following measures are recommended for management of acute stroke with hemorrhagic conversion (2).

1. Cryoprecipitate (10 U) is recommended as a source of fibrinogen, and the dose can be repeated if the serum fibrinogen is <200 mg/dL (2). *Fibrinogen concentrates* are an alternative with two advantages over cryoprecipitate (14): (*a*) thawing is not necessary, so treatment can be started immediately, and (*b*) the concentration of fibrinogen is more consistent (at 20 g/L).
2. If cryoprecipitate is not immediately available, tranexamic acid (an antifibrinolytic agent) can be given in a dose of 1,000 mg IV over 10 min (2).
3. A neurosurgery consultation is warranted (to consider decompressive hemicraniectomy).

Cerebral Edema

There are two types of cerebral edema: *cytotoxic edema*, which is the result of cell necrosis, and *vasogenic edema*, which involves loss of vascular control mechanisms, and results in disruption of the blood-brain barrier. The larger the ischemic area, the more extensive the cerebral edema. Hemorrhage and cerebral edema are the principal determinants of poor outcomes after acute stroke.

Management. Intracranial pressure (ICP) monitoring is *not* recommended for acute ischemic stroke that is complicated by cerebral edema (2). Instead, monitoring neurologic symptoms and signs is acceptable. *Hypertonic saline* can be used to lower the ICP when cerebral edema causes a deterioration in neurologic status (15-16). Mannitol is also capable of lowering the ICP, but it is not as effective as hypertonic saline in patients with an elevated ICP after stroke (17). Table 44.3 lists the doses and characteristics of hypertonic saline solutions (16).

Seizures

Poststroke seizures are relatively rare, occurring in about 5% of patients <7 days after a stroke (i.e., early) and in 7% of stroke patients a week or more after the stroke (i.e., late)

TABLE 44.3 Hypertonic Saline Solutions for Treating Cerebral Edema

	3% NaCL	5% NaCL	7.5% NaCL	14.6% NaCL	23.4% NaCL
[Na⁺] (mEq/L)	513	856	1,293	2,500	4,000
Osmolality (mOsm/L)	1,027	1,711	2,566	5,000	8,008
Commercially available	Yes	Yes	No	Yes	Yes
Bolus dose for cerebral edema	250 mL or 5 mL/kg	100 mL	100 mL or 2-4 mL/kg	24-48 mL	30 mL or 0.68-2 mL/kg

NaCL = sodium chloride.

From Holden DN, Mucksavage JJ, Cokley JA, et al. Hypertonic saline use in neurocritical care for treating cerebral edema: a review of optimal formulation, dosing, safety, administration and storage. Am J Health Syst Pharm 2023;80:331-42.

(18-19). Antiseizure medication (e.g., levetiracetam) is not recommended for prophylaxis; however, if a poststroke seizure occurs, antiseizure medication is used for 1-4 weeks following an *early* stroke, and long term following a *late* stroke (20-21).

SPONTANEOUS INTRACEREBRAL HEMORRHAGE

Spontaneous (nontraumatic) intracerebral hemorrhage (ICH) accounts for roughly 10-15% of acute strokes, with hypertension and systemic anticoagulation as the two principal predisposing conditions. ICH has a less favorable prognosis than ischemic strokes: i.e., about half of the patients do not survive for 30 days, and two-thirds of the survivors have significant neurologic deficits (22-23).

Management

Table 44.4 lists general ICU supportive measures for patients with spontaneous ICH (24-26).

TABLE 44.4	General Support Measures for Patients with Spontaneous Intracerebral Hemorrhage
Component	**Measures**
Airway / oxygenation	• O$_2$ to maintain SaO$_2$ >92% • Intubation if unable to protect airway (i.e., GCS <8) • PaO$_2$ >100 mm Hg, PaCO$_2$ 35-35 mm Hg
BP management	• Titrate vasoactives (i.e., nicardipine or clevidipine) to SBP <140-160 mm Hg
Hemostasis	• Reverse anticoagulation (see Tables 44.5 and 44.6)
ICP monitoring	• Consider for GCS <8, hydrocephalus, intraventricular hemorrhage, or signs of transtentorial herniation • ICP <20 mm Hg, cerebral perfusion pressure 50-70 mm Hg
ICP management	• Osmotherapy with hypertonic saline (see Table 44.3) • Neurosurgical consultation • Pentobarbital (per institutional guideline) • Temperature control (per institutional guideline)
Seizure prophylaxis	• Not indicated unless high suspicion for seizures or if seizure activity noted on EEG (EEG indicated for 24-48 h in patients with GCS <8)
VTE prophylaxis	• Subcutaneous enoxaparin or heparin 24 h after head CT demonstrates stability/lack of hematoma expansion
Other ICU considerations	• Progressive mobilization, as tolerated • Avoid hyperglycemia or hypoglycemia • Sodium: 135-145 mEq/L • Maintain normothermia (avoid fever). • Initiate nutrition 24 h after admission.

CT = computed tomography; EEG = electroencephalogram; GCS = Glasgow Coma Scale; ICP = intracranial pressure; SBP = systolic blood pressure.

From References 24-26.

Anticoagulant Reversal

Arresting hematoma expansion is a primary concern after an ICH is diagnosed. For patients on anticoagulants, prompt reversal is imperative (24-28). The reversal agents and dosing regimens for commonly used anticoagulants are presented in Tables 44.5 and 44.6 (27-28).

Warfarin reversal is discussed in Chapter 14: Coagulopathy Management. Four-factor prothrombin complex concentrate (PCC) at a dose of 50 IU/kg is an effective option

TABLE 44.5 Reversal of Anticoagulants in Intracerebral Hemorrhage

Antithrombotics	Reversal Agents and Dosage
Warfarin	• Vitamin K: 10 mg IV, plus • Four-factor PCC, dosing as follows: 　INR　　　　　　　Dose 　2-4 .... 25 U/kg 　4-6 .... 35 U/kg 　>6 .... 50 U/kg
Dabigatran (Pradaxa®)	• Idarucizumab 2.5 mg IV bolus and repeat within 15 min. • Consider high-dose four-factor PCC (50 IU/kg) if idarucizumab is not available.
Apixaban (Eliquis®) or Rivaroxaban (Xarelto®)	• Andexanet alfa—see Table 47.5 for dosing. • Consider high-dose four-factor PCC (50 IU/kg) if andexanet is not available.
Unfractionated heparin	• Protamine sulfate: 1 mg/100 U of heparin given at last dose.
Enoxaparin (Lovenox®)	• Protamine sulfate: 1 mg/1 mg of enoxaparin at last dose; less effective than against unfractionated heparin.
Aspirin, clopidogrel	• Desmopressin: 3 μg/kg subQ or IV. Can repeat once.

IV = intravenous; PCC = prothrombin complex concentrate.

From References 27-28.

TABLE 44.6 Dosing Recommendations for Andexanet Alfa

Regimen	Criteria	Dosage
Low-dose regimen	Last apixaban dose ≤5 mg or rivaroxaban dose ≤10 mg or time since last dose ≥8 h.	Start with IV bolus of 400 mg (at 30 mg/min) and then infuse at 4 mg/min for up to 120 min.
High-dose regimen	Last apixaban dose >5 mg or rivaroxaban dose >10 mg or time since last dose <8 h or unknown.	Start with IV bolus of 800 mg (at 30 mg/min) and then infuse at 8 mg/min for up to 120 min.

From Frontera JA, Lewin JJ III, Rabinstein AA, et al. Guideline for reversal of antithrombotics in intracranial hemorrhage: A statement for healthcare professionals from the Neurocritical Care Society and Society of Critical Care Medicine. Neurocrit Care 2016;24:6-46.

for reversal of factor Xa inhibitors (e.g., apixaban, rivaroxaban) when andexanet alfa is not available (26,28). The anticoagulant effect of the direct thrombin inhibitor dabigatran can be reversed rapidly with the monoclonal antibody idarucizumab (Praxbind), but four-factor PCC can also be used (50 IU/kg) (26,28-29). Heparin and enoxaparin are reversed with protamine sulfate (1 mg/100 U of heparin or enoxaparin), although protamine is less effective reversing the effect of enoxaparin. Desmopressin (see Chapter 14: Coagulopathy Management) may be used to help reverse the effect of antiplatelet agents (i.e., aspirin or clopidogrel).

SUBARACHNOID HEMORRHAGE

Subarachnoid hemorrhage (SAH) is a severe form of stroke and is caused by rupture of a saccular aneurysm within the cerebral arteries in >85% of cases (Figure 44.3) (30-32).

SAH affects a younger age group than other types of strokes (i.e., mean age of 55 years) (33-34). Women are affected more frequently than men, and hypertension and smoking are independent risk factors (34).

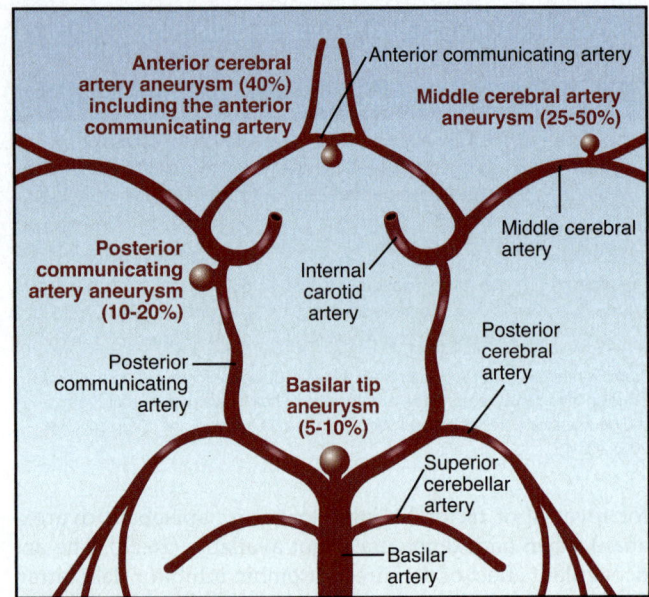

FIGURE 44.3. Common sites of intracerebral aneurysms.

Pathophysiology

The poor outcomes in aneurysmal SAH are explained by multiple pathophysiologic changes, as summarized:

1. The presence of blood in the subarachnoid space triggers an intense inflammatory response that damages the blood brain barrier (which promotes vasogenic cerebral edema) and produces oxidative damage in neurons and glial cells (which produces cytotoxic cerebral edema) (35).
2. Blood in the subarachnoid space blocks the flow of cerebrospinal fluid, which often leads to an obstructive hydrocephalus and increased ICP.
3. In about one-third of patients, there is a second phase of tissue injury referred to as *delayed cerebral ischemia* (DCI)

that occurs between days 4 and 14 (34). DCI is a major source of morbidity and mortality and is attributed to vasospasm and thrombotic occlusion of cerebral arteries and arterioles (36).
4. SAH is often associated with inflammatory injury in organs other than the brain. Commonly associated conditions include the acute respiratory distress syndrome (ARDS), myocardial dysfunction, and acute kidney injury (AKI) (33-34).

Management

Management priorities in the ICU are similar to ICH and summarized in Table 44.7 (33-34,37-38).

Some supportive measures that deserve special mention include the following:

1. The incidence of venous thromboembolism in SAH is as high as 25% (33), so thromboprophylaxis is required and should be started 24 h after the aneurysm is secured.
2. Normothermia should be maintained. Fever is common after SAH and has a negative influence on outcomes (39).
3. Normoglycemia should be maintained. Hyperglycemia in the first 72 h after SAH is associated with worse neurologic outcomes (33).
4. Hyponatremia is reported in 35% of patients with SAH (40) and may be the result of cerebral salt wasting (see Chapter 34: Sodium and Chloride). Treatment involves administration of crystalloids and hypertonic saline to prevent hypovolemia and correct the serum sodium.

Aneurysm Management

Once the patient is stabilized, the aneurysm should be secured (preferably within 24 h) either with neurosurgery (i.e., surgical clipping) or an interventional radiology procedure (i.e., endovascular coiling) (33-34).

TABLE 44.7 General Support Measures for Patients with Subarachnoid Hemorrhage

Component	Measures
Airway / oxygenation	• O_2 to maintain SaO_2 >92% • Intubation if unable to protect airway (i.e., GCS <8) • PaO_2 >100 mm Hg, $PaCO_2$ 35-35 mm Hg
BP management	• Titrate vasoactives (i.e., nicardipine or clevidipine) to SBP <160 mm Hg
Hemostasis	• Reverse anticoagulation (see Tables 44.5 and 44.6)
ICP monitoring	• External ventricular device for monitoring and CSF diversion (performed by neurosurgery) • ICP <20 mm Hg, cerebral perfusion pressure 50-70 mm Hg
ICP management	• Osmotherapy if required (see Table 44.3) • Neurosurgical consultation • Pentobarbital (per institutional guideline) • Temperature control (per institutional guideline)
Seizure prophylaxis	• Hunt-Hess grade 1-3 without prior seizure: levetiracetam IV loading dose 40-60 mg/kg up to 4.5 g followed by 750 mg PO/IV BID • Hunt-Hess grade 4-5 and/or seizure at ictus (regardless of grade): levetiracetam IV loading dose 40-60 mg/kg up to 4.5 g followed by 1500 mg PO/IV BID
Calcium channel blocker	• Nimodipine 60 mg PO/NGT q 4 h × 21 days or while hospitalized (should be started within 4 h of hospital arrival)
Other ICU considerations	• Document the Hunt-Hess grade (clinically based) and modified Fisher score (CT based) and obtain baseline GCS. • Avoid hyperglycemia or hypoglycemia • Sodium: 135-145 mEq/L • Maintain normothermia (avoid fever) • Initiate nutrition 24 h after admission • Start VTE prophylaxis with enoxaparin or heparin 24 h after aneurysm secured

CT = computed tomography; GCS = Glasgow Coma Scale; PO/IV BID = per os [by mouth] or intravenously twice a day (BID); PO/NGT = per os (by mouth) nasogastric tube; ICP = intracranial pressure; SBP = systolic blood pressure; VTE = venous thromboembolism.

From References 33-34, 37-38.

Delayed Cerebral Ischemia

DCI can appear 4-14 days after SAH and is considered a major cause of morbidity and mortality. The following measures are recommended to reduce the risk of DCI (33-34).

1. The calcium channel blocker *nimodipine* is recommended orally in a dose of 60 mg every 4 h, starting as soon as possible (i.e., <4 h after hospital arrival) and continued for 21 days (33-34,37). Mechanisms thought to contribute to its beneficial effect include reduced microvasospasms and neuroprotection (possibly from prevention of intraneuronal calcium overload) (38).
2. Clinical signs of DCI can include a new focal deficit, or a change in mental status. CT angiography (CTA) and transcranial Doppler ultrasound are both helpful, with sensitivities of about 90% for the detection of cerebral vasospasm (33). *A CTA with perfusion is the best noninvasive test for the radiographic detection of vasospasm.*
3. Interventional neuroradiology should be consulted for severe cases of vasospasm because intra-arterial vasodilators or angioplasty may be helpful.
4. If vasospasm is radiologically confirmed, hemodynamic augmentation with vasopressors (i.e., norepinephrine) for a higher mean arterial pressure (MAP) goal (i.e., ~85 mm Hg) may be attempted to maintain perfusion (34). Euvolemia should be established and maintained prior to initiation of vasopressors (see Chapter 11: Fluid Management).

References

1. Tsao CW, Aday AW, Almarzooq ZI, et al. Heart disease and stroke statistics—2023 update: a report from the American Heart Association. Circulation 2023;147:e93-e621.
2. Powers WJ, Rabinstein AA, Ackerson T, et al. Guidelines for the early management of patients with acute ischemic stroke. A guideline for healthcare professionals from the American Heart Association/American Stroke Association. Stroke 2018; 49:e46-e99.

3. Watson NA, Beards SC, Altaf N, et al. The effect of hyperoxia on cerebral blood flow: a study in healthy volunteers using magnetic resonance phase-contrast angiography. Eur J Anaesthesiol 2000;17:152-9.
4. Lopez HV, Vivas MF, Ruiz RN, et al. Association between post-procedural hyperoxia and poor functional outcome after mechanical thrombectomy for ischemic stroke: an observational study. Ann Intensive Care 2019;9:59.
5. El-Ghoroury H, Sudekum DM, Hecht JP. Blood pressure control in acute stroke: labetalol or nicardipine? J Stroke Cerebrovasc Dis 2021;30:105959.
6. Rosenfeldt Z, Conlen K, Jones B, et al. Comparison of nicardipine with clevidipine in the management of hypertension in acute cerebrovascular diseases. J Stroke Cerebrovasc Dis 2018;27:2067-73.
7. Visvanathan A, Dennis M, Whiteley W. Parenteral fluid regimens for improving functional outcome in people with acute stroke. Cochrane Database Syst Rev 2015:CD011138.
8. Habib G, Badano L, Tribouilloy C, et al. Recommendations for the practice of echocardiography in infective endocarditis. Eur J Echocardiogr 2010;11(2):202-19.
9. Koutroulou I, Tsivgoulis G, Tsalikakis D, et al. Epidemiology of patent foramen ovale in general population and in stroke patients: a narrative review. Front Neurol 2020;11:281.
10. Wade E, Robinson M, Singla A, et al. PFO, push-ups and heavy lifting; Valsalva provocation before cryptogenic stroke. Interv Cardiol 2021;13:273-8.
11. Ko S-B, Yoon B-W. Blood pressure management for acute ischemic and hemorrhagic stroke: the evidence. Semin Resp Crit Care Med 2017;38:718-25.
12. Cucchiara B, Kasner SE, Tanne D, et al. Factors associated with intracerebral hemorrhage after thrombolytic therapy for ischemic stroke: pooled analysis of placebo data from the Stroke-Acute Ischemic NXY Treatment (SAINT) I and SAINT II trials. Stroke 2009;40:3067-72.
13. Whiteley WN, Emberson J, Lees KR, et al. Risk of intracerebral hemorrhage with alteplase after acute ischemic stroke: a secondary analysis of an individual patient data meta-analysis. Lancet Neurol 2016;15:925-33.
14. Grottke O, Mallaiah S, Karkouti K, et al. Fibrinogen supplementation and its indications. Semin Thromb Hemost 2020;46:38-49.
15. Cook AM, Jones M, Hawryluk GW, et al. Guidelines for the acute treatment of cerebral edema in neurocritical care. Neurocrit Care2020;32:647-66.
16. Holden DN, Mucksavage JJ, Cokley JA, et al. Hypertonic saline use in neurocritical care for treating cerebral edema: a review of optimal formulation, dosing, safety, administration and storage. Am J Health Syst Pharm 2023;80:331-42.

17. Schwarz S, Schwab S, Bertram M, et al. Effects of hypertonic saline, hydroxyethyl starch solution and mannitol in patients with increased intracranial pressure after stroke. Stroke 1998;29:1550-5.
18. Leung T, Leung H, Soo YOY, et al. The prognosis of symptomatic seizures after ischaemic stroke. J Neurol Neurosurg Psychiatry 2017;88:86-94.
19. Nandan A, Zhou YM, Demoe L, et al. Incidence and risk factors of post-stroke seizures and epilepsy: systematic review and meta-analysis. J Int Med Res 2023;51(11):3000605231213231.
20. Ryu HU, Kim HJ, Shin BS, Kang HG. Clinical approaches for post-stroke seizure: a review. Front Neurol 2024;15:1337960.
21. Holtkamp M, Beghi E, Benninger F, et al. European Stroke Organisation guidelines for the management of post-stroke seizures and epilepsy. Eur Stroke J 2017;2(2):103-15.
22. Sacco S, Marini C, Toni D, et al. Incidence and 10-year survival of intracerebral hemorrhage in a population-based registry. Stroke 2009;40:394-9.
23. Kuramatsu JB, Sembill JA, Hyttner HB. Reversal of oral anticoagulation in patients with acute intra-cerebral hemorrhage. Crit Care 2019;23:206.
24. Kim JY, Bae HJ. Spontaneous intracerebral hemorrhage: management. J Stroke 2017;19(1):28-39.
25. Law ZK, Appleton JP, Bath PM, Sprigg N. Management of acute intracerebral haemorrhage—an update. Clin Med (Lond) 2017;17(2):166-72.
26. Hemphill JC III, Greenberg SM, Anderson CS, et al. Guidelines for the management of spontaneous intracerebral hemorrhage: a guideline for healthcare professionals from the American Heart Association/American Stroke Association. Stroke 2015;46(7):2032-60.
27. Kuramatsu JB, Sembill JA, Hyttner HB. Reversal of oral anticoagulation in patients with acute intra-cerebral hemorrhage. Crit Care 2019;23:206.
28. Frontera JA, Lewin JJ III, Rabinstein AA, et al. Guideline for reversal of antithrombotics in intracranial hemorrhage: a statement for healthcare professionals from the Neurocritical Care Society and Society of Critical Care Medicine. Neurocrit Care 2016;24:6-46.
29. Sarode R, Milling TJ Jr, Refaai MA, et al. Efficacy and safety of a 4-factor prothrombin complex concentrate in patients on vitamin K antagonists presenting with major bleeding: a randomized, plasma-controlled, phase IIIb study. Circulation 2013;128:1234-43.
30. Inagawa T. Site of ruptured intracranial saccular aneurysms in patients in Izumo City, Japan. Cerebrovasc Dis 2010;30(1):72-84.
31. Chalouhi N, Hoh BL, Hasan D. Review of cerebral aneurysm formation, growth, and rupture. Stroke 2013;44(12):3613-22.
32. Moss C, Wilson SR. Subarachnoid haemorrhage and anaesthesia for neurovascular surgery. Anesthesia and Intensive Care Medicine 2011;204-7.

33. Hoh BL, Ko NU, Amin-Hankani S, et al. 2023 guideline for the management of patients with aneurysmal subarachnoid hemorrhage: a guideline from the American Heart Association/American Stroke Association. Stroke 2023;54:e314-379.
34. Robba C, Busl KM, Claassen J, et al. Contemporary management of aneurysmal subarachnoid haemorrhage. An update for the intensivist. Intensive Care Med 2024;50(5):646-64.
35. Lauzier DC, Jayaraman K, Yuam JY, et al. Early brain injury after subarachnoid hemorrhage: incidence and mechanisms. Stroke 2023;54:1426-40.
36. Macdonald RL. Delayed neurological deterioration after subarachnoid haemorrhage. Nat Rev Neurol 2014;10:44-58.
37. Connolly Jr ES, Rabinstein AA, Carhuapoma JR, et al. Guidelines for the management of aneurysmal subarachnoid hemorrhage: a guideline for healthcare professionals from the American Heart Association/American Stroke Association. Stroke 2012;43:1711-37.
38. Carlson AP, Hänggi D, Macdonald RL, Shuttleworth CW. Nimodipine reappraised: an old drug with a future. Curr Neuropharmacol 2020;18(1):65-82.
39. Naidech AM, Bendok BR, Bernstein RA, et al. Fever burden and functional recovery after subarachnoid hemorrhage. Neurosurgery 2008;63:212-7.
40. Mapa B, Taylor BES, Appelboom G, et al. Impact of hyponatremia on morbidity, mortality, and complications after aneurysmal subarachnoid hemorrhage: a systematic review. World Neurosurg 2016;85:305-14.

Traumatic Brain Injury — Chapter 45

Traumatic brain injury (TBI) constitutes a serious public health threat, affecting millions of patients worldwide (1). Patients with severe TBI have a mortality rate of 25-40%, and for those who survive, 80% have some degree of lifelong disability (2-3)." In this chapter, ICU management of patients with severe TBI is summarized.

DEFINITION

The Glasgow Coma Scale (GCS) score (see Chapter 42: Disorders of Consciousness, Table 42.7) is used to classify TBI (4-5). *Moderate* TBI is defined as a GCS 9-12 and *severe* TBI is defined as a GCS ≤8 (2-5).

PATHOPHYSIOLOGY

TBI is caused by an external force that results in damage to intracranial structures. Causes of TBI are listed in Table 45.1.

TABLE 45.1 Types of Structural TBI

Focal	Diffuse
• Concussion	• Epidural hematoma
• Diffuse axonal injury	• Subdural hematoma
• Blast injury	• Subarachnoid hemorrhage
• Skull fracture	• Intraventricular hemorrhage
• BCVI	• Intracerebral hemorrhage
	• Intraparenchymal hematoma
	• Contusion
	• Penetrating*

*May be diffuse or focal.
BCVI = blunt cerebrovascular injury; TBI = traumatic brain injury.

TBI elicits a complex pathophysiological response and is associated with hypoxia, CBF limitation (<70% of normal in many cases), and secondary injuries due to activation of coagulation and innate immunological pathways (Figure 45.1) (6-10).

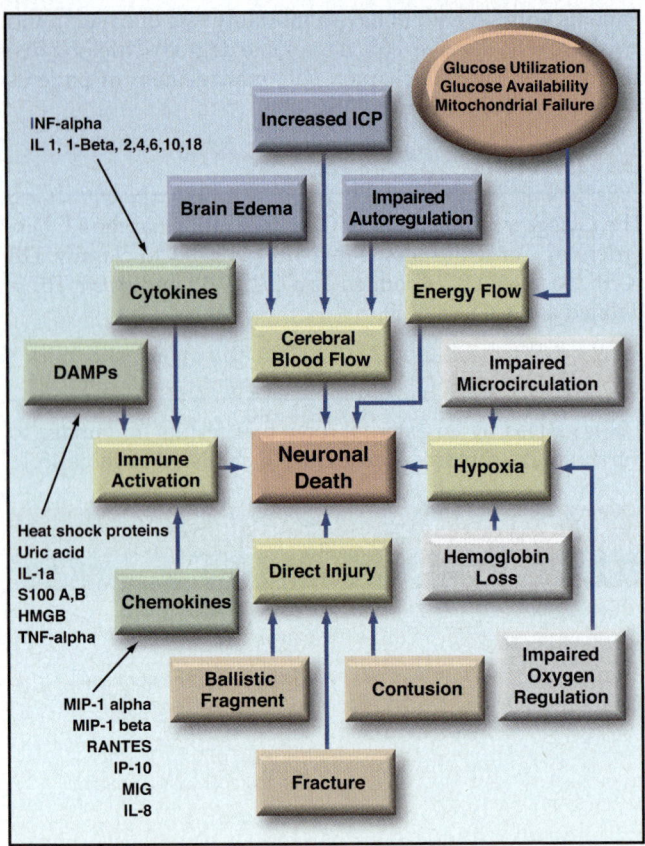

FIGURE 45.1. Pathophysiological mechanisms contributing to neuronal death in TBI. Hypoxia and cerebral blood flow are two of the principle pathophysiological mechanisms that may be most amenable to ICU interventions. DAMPs = damage-associated molecular patterns.

NEUROCRITICAL CARE MANAGEMENT

Neurocritical Care Interventions

The Brain Trauma Foundation and American College of Surgeons recommendations for severe TBI management are described in Table 45.2 (4-5).

Table 45.3 lists physiological thresholds that should prompt interventions to prevent secondary neurological damage (4-5).

Intracranial Pressure Monitoring

TBI patients are at increased risk for dysregulation of cerebral autoregulation, which may result in decreased cerebral blood flow (CBF) and ischemia (11-12). CBF is best estimated clinically by measuring the cerebral perfusion pressure (CPP) using the following equation:

$$\text{CPP} = \text{Mean Arterial Pressure (MAP)} - \text{Intracranial Pressure (ICP)} \quad (45.1)$$

Current guidelines recommend monitoring ICP and targeting a CPP of 60-70 mm Hg in patients meeting the criteria listed in Table 45.4 (2,5). The preferred technique for measuring ICP involves placement of an external ventricular drain (EVD). An EVD offers the dual advantage of ICP monitoring and cerebrospinal fluid (CSF) drainage (Figure 45.2). Other techniques for monitoring ICP include a subarachnoid bolt, epidural sensor, and intraparenchymal pressure monitor (13).

EVD Management

The EVD collecting chamber can be adjusted (i.e., raised or lowered) so that CSF will only drain at a specified pressure (i.e., 0-20 mm Hg); some EVD systems use cm H_2O (1 mm Hg = 1.359 cm H_2O). *It is imperative that the correct units being used—and EVD settings— are clearly understood by the ICU team because errors in EVD settings can lead to serious complications*

TABLE 45.2 Summary of ICU Management Considerations for Severe TBI

Intervention	Recommendation	Additional Considerations
Hyperosmolar therapy	• Hyperosmolar therapy with mannitol or hypertonic saline may lower intracranial pressure, but there is insufficient evidence to support the use of one rather than the other.	See Chapter 44, Table 44.3
CSF drainage	• The use of an EVD to lower ICP in patients with an initial GCS <6 during the first 12 h of injury may be considered. • An EVD zeroed at the midbrain with continuous drainage of CSF may be considered to lower ICP; this may be more effective than intermittent use.	*Continuous monitoring requires constant vigilance*; excessive drainage can lead to brain herniation.
Anesthetics, analgesics, sedatives	• High-dose barbiturate administration is recommended only if required to control elevated ICP refractory to maximum standard medical and surgical treatment. • Propofol is recommended to help control ICP, but caution is required as high-dose propofol is associated with significant morbidity (see Chapter 5).	Barbiturates are believed to be effective in refractory cases of elevated ICP by suppressing cerebral metabolism. High-dose propofol is only used for severe, refractory elevations in ICP (see Figure 45.3)
Steroids	• Steroids are not recommended.	High-dose methylprednisolone is associated with increased mortality in TBI patients.

TABLE 45.2 (continued)

Intervention	Recommendation	Additional Considerations
Seizure prophylaxis	• Early (within 7 days of injury) administration of phenytoin is recommended to decrease the incidence of posttraumatic seizures. • There is insufficient evidence to recommend levetiracetam (Keppra) over phenytoin regarding efficacy in preventing posttraumatic seizures.	Active seizures should be treated according to the standard of care (i.e., midazolam or lorazepam; see Chapter 43).

CSF = cerebrospinal fluid; EVD = external ventricular device; GCS = Glasgow Coma Scale; ICP = intracranial pressure; TBI = traumatic brain injury.

From References 4-5.

TABLE 45.3 Treatment Thresholds for TBI in the ICU

Blood pressure	• Maintaining SBP ≥100 mm Hg for patients 50-69 years old or ≥110 m Hg for patients 15-49 or >70 years old may be considered to decrease mortality and improve outcomes. • Hypotension is strongly associated with poor neurological outcomes.
ICP	• Treatment for ICP >22 mm Hg is recommended because values above this level are associated with increased mortality. • In practice, a combination of ICP values, serial neurological examinations, and brain CT findings are required to make management decisions.
CPP	• The recommended CPP target is between 60 and 70 mm Hg. • The exact CPP threshold is unclear and depends on the patient's autoregulatory status.
Advanced monitoring	• A jugular venous saturation <50% may be a threshold to avoid in order to reduce mortality and improve outcomes.

TBI = traumatic brain injury; CPP = cerebral perfusion pressure; ICP = intracranial pressure; SBP = systolic blood pressure; CT = computed tomography.

From References 4-5.

TABLE 45.4 Indications for Invasive ICP Monitoring*

- GCS score of ≤8
- Abnormal CT scan of the head
- Two or more of the following:
  - Age >40 years
  - Unilateral or bilateral motor posturing
  - SBP <90 mm Hg

*ICP monitoring may also be considered in patients with a GCS ≥9 who have structural brain damage with a high risk for progression (e.g., large or multiple cerebral contusions, coagulopathy).

CT = computed tomography; GCS = Glasgow Coma Scale; ICP = intracranial pressure; SBP = systolic blood pressure.

From References 4-5, 13.

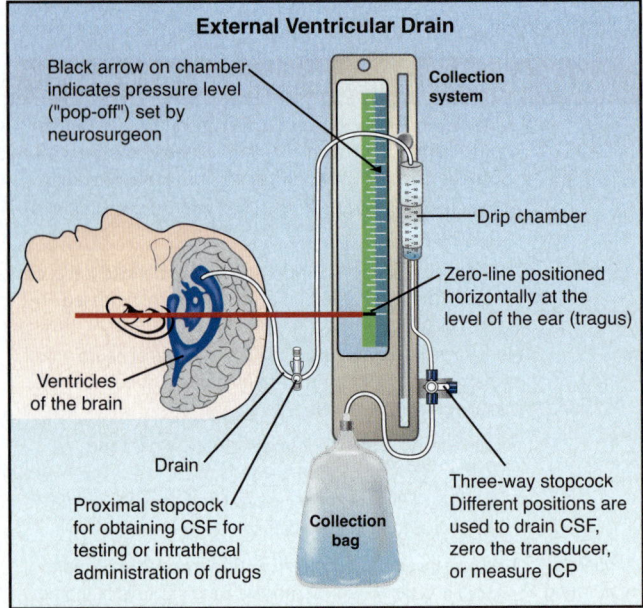

FIGURE 45.2. An external ventricular drain (EVD) system.

(i.e., over-drainage and brain herniation). Patients with a higher ICP and lower CPP are expected to have lower drain levels initially (0-5 mm Hg) to allow CSF to be drained, but as the patient improves, the following procedure can be followed to "wean" and eventually remove the EVD (14):

1. The following conditions must be met before the EVD is weaned:
   a. TBI should be stable or resolving (e.g., stable ICP and CPP, stable computed tomography [CT] scan).
   b. The CSF output should be <250 mL over 24 h and nonbloody.
   c. The ICP should be within normal limits (i.e., <15 mm Hg).
   d. The patient should be neurologically stable.

2. If all conditions are satisfied, EVD weaning may commence by increasing drain height 5 mm Hg every 24 h until reaching 20 mm Hg, at which point the EVD can be clamped.
3. If a head CT obtained 24 h after clamping shows a stable ventricular system (i.e., no evidence of hydrocephalus), the EVD can be removed.

Management of Elevated ICP

A tiered approach to elevated ICP is presented in Figure 45.3 (15).

Although central venous access is preferred, hypertonic saline, including 23.4%, may be given safely through a properly functioning peripheral IV (16).

Impending Herniation

For patients with impending herniation (i.e., pupillary asymmetry, respiratory depression, decorticate or decerebrate posturing, or "Cushing's triad" [hypertension, bradycardia,

Tier 1
- Elevate the head of the bed to 30 degrees (reverse Trendelenburg, to improve cerebral venous outflow) and ensure neck is midline (to optimize venous drainage)
- Sedation and analgesia using recommended short-acting agents (see Chapter 5)
- Intermittent ventricular drainage (continuous drainage is not recommended unless an additional ICP monitor is placed because when the drain is open, it does not accurately reflect the actual ICP)

If ICP remains 20-25 mm Hg, proceed to Tier 2.

Tier 2
- Place an EVD (if not already done)
- Intermittent osmotherapy
- Administer mannitol (0.25-1 gm/kg body weight) in intermittent boluses
  - Use with caution in hypovolemic patients
  - Monitor serum sodium and osmolality every 6 h
- Administer hypertonic saline 3%, in intermittent boluses (250 mL over 1 h) or use other concentrations (e.g., 30 mL of 23.4%); consider a 3% saline infusion at 0.1 to 1 mL/kg/h
  - Monitor serum sodium and osmolality every 6 h
  - Consider holding doses if serum sodium >160 mEq/L
- Augment MAP to achieve CPP of 60-70 mm Hg
- Adjust ventilation for $PaCO_2$ of 30-35 mm Hg
- Consider neuromuscular blockade (i.e., test dose, then if ICP decreases, continuous infusion)

If ICP remains 20-25 mm Hg, proceed to Tier 3.

Tier 3
- Neurosurgery consultation for decompressive craniectomy or craniotomy
- Use a continuous neuromuscular blocker infusion (i.e., cisatracurium), titrated to a train-of-four of at least two twitches (if ICP decreased in response to an initial bolus)
- Consider high-dose propofol infusion or barbiturate coma (note: hypotension is common with higher doses of these agents)
- Hypothermia (<36°C) is not currently recommended as an initial TBI treatment but may be considered as a "salvage" therapy if all other attempts to decrease ICP fail

FIGURE 45.3. A three-tiered approach for managing increased ICP.

irregular respirations]) more aggressive management is indicated, as described in Table 45.5 (17-19).

Emergent neurosurgical consultation should be considered for decompressive craniectomy or craniotomy (4-5,20).

TABLE 45.5 Additional Interventions for the Management of Elevated ICP with Impending Herniation

High-Dose Osmotherapy
- 23.4% sodium 30-60 mL or 0.5-1 mL/kg administered over 10 min
- 3% saline: 2-5 mL/kg
- Mannitol 1-1.5 g/kg

Temporary Hyperventilation while Awaiting a Definitive Neurosurgical Procedure
(i.e., decompressive hemicraniectomy or hemicraniotomy)
- $PaCO_2$ 25-35 mm Hg

Blood Pressure Augmentation (to maintain CPP)
- MAP of 80-100 mm Hg

CPP = cerebral perfusion pressure; ICP = intracranial pressure; MAP = mean arterial pressure.

From References 17-19.

Advanced Neuromonitoring

Advanced neuromonitoring techniques may be helpful for tailoring individualized approaches in TBI patients. These techniques are summarized in Table 45.6.

Some TBI trials have correlated lower values of $SjVO_2$ and $PbtO_2$ with worse neurological outcomes (5,21), and others have shown trends toward lower mortality when PbO_2 values were used to guide management (22), but other trials have failed to demonstrate a change in outcomes when these techniques are used (23).

TABLE 45.6 Advanced Neuromonitoring Techniques

Technique	Technique	Normal Value	Comment / Limitations
$PbtO_2$	An electrode is placed into the intraparenchymal white matter of the brain	>20 mm Hg (<15 mm Hg associated with worse outcomes)	Only detects focal ischemia where the electrode is placed
PRx	Calculated by correlating mean ICP and MAP	PRx = 0; autoregulation intact PRx~ +1.0, indicates near absence of cerebral autoregulation	Subject to signal noise May help determine optimal CPP in an individual patient
$SjVO_2$	A catheter is placed in a retrograde manner in the internal jugular vein	$SjVO_2$ >60%*	Not supported by robust randomized trials
Cerebral microdialysis	An intraparenchymal catheter is placed for the extracellular measurement of glucose, glutamate, lactate, and pyruvate	A lactate-to-pyruvate ratio >25-40 suggests anaerobic metabolism (i.e., worse neurological outcomes)	Requires specialized equipment, including the catheter and analyzer
Thermal diffusion flowmetry	An intraparenchymal probe is placed in the white matter of the brain	Measures CBF	Not widely available Less studied compared to other tools

*$SjVO_2$ <50% for 10 min indicates cerebral hypoxemia.

CBF = cerebral blood flow; CPP = cerebral perfusion pressure; ICP = intracranial pressure; MAP = mean arterial pressure; PRx = pressure reactivity index; $PbtO_2$ = brain tissue oxygen tension monitoring; $SjVO_2$ = jugular venous oximetry.

From References 4-5, 21-23.

General ICU Management

ICU management of the TBI patient follows standard ICU practices with a few caveats. General critical care management goals are summarized in Table 45.7 (24-27).

TABLE 45.7	General ICU Management Goals for TBI Patients
Airway management	Patients with severe TBI initially require intubation and mechanical ventilation with the following goals: • SpO_2 >95% • $PaCO_2$ 35-45 mm Hg • PaO_2 >100 mm Hg • Lung protective ventilation whenever possible (tidal volume = 6-8 mL/kg predicted body weight) • pH 7.35-7.45
Hemodynamic management	• Hypotension should be avoided (see Table 45.3). • MAP augmentation may be required to preserve CPP.
Temperature management	Hypothermia is not recommended. Normothermia (36-38°C) should be maintained.
Electrolyte management	• Sodium should be maintained between 135-145 mEq/L (unless receiving osmotherapy). • The serum OG (OG = $Osm_{CALCULATED}$ − $Osm_{MEASURED}$) may be used to guide mannitol therapy (renal failure is rare when the OG is <55 mOsm/L).
Hematological management	In general, the following goals are applicable for TBI patients: • INR <1.4 • Platelets >75 × 10^3/mm^3 • Hemoglobin >7 mg/dL • Normalization of viscoelastic test parameters (see Chapter 14) TBI patients are a high risk for VTE (up to 30%); prophylaxis should be started within 72 h of admission. An IVC filter should be placed in patients for whom anticoagulation is contraindicated.

TABLE 45.7	(continued)
Antibiotics	A single dose of ceftriaxone (2 g IV) within 12 h of intubation and mechanical ventilation has been shown to prevent ventilator-associated pneumonia.
Tracheostomy timing	Tracheostomy performed within 7 days of admission may decrease ICU length of stay and duration of mechanical ventilation.
Antiseizure medications	Although high level evidence is lacking, antiseizure medications (phenytoin or levetiracetam, given for 7 days) may prevent posttraumatic seizures, especially in patients with depressed skull fracture, penetrating skull injury, cortical contusion, or epidural/subdural/intracerebral hematoma.

CPP = cerebral perfusion pressure; IV = intravenous; IVC = inferior vena cava; MAP = mean arterial pressure; OG = osmolal gap; TBI = traumatic brain injury; VTE = venous thromboembolism.

From References 4-5, 24-27.

References

1. Centers for Disease Control and Prevention. Get the facts: TBI data. October 2024. Accessed May 5, 2025. https://www.cdc.gov/traumatic-brain-injury/data-research/index.html
2. Roozenbeek B, Maas AI, Menon DK. Changing patterns in the epidemiology of traumatic brain injury. Nat Rev Neurol 2013;9(4):231-6.
3. Maas AIR, Menon DK, Manley GT, et al. Traumatic brain injury: progress and challenges in prevention, clinical care, and research. Lancet Neurol 2022;21(11):1004-60.
4. American College of Surgeons Trauma Quality Improvement Program (TQIP) Expert Panel. *Best Practices in the Management of Traumatic Brain Injury*. American College of Surgeons Committee on Trauma; 2015.
5. Carney N, Totten AM, O'Reilly C, et al. Guidelines for the management of severe traumatic brain injury, Fourth edition. Neurosurgery 2017;80(1):6-15.
6. Sillesen M. Coagulation changes following traumatic brain injury and shock. Dan Med J 2014;61(12):B4974.
7. Genét GF, Bentzer P, Ostrowski SR, Johansson PI. Resuscitation with pooled and pathogen-reduced plasma attenuates the increase in brain water content following traumatic brain injury and hemorrhagic shock in rats. J Neurotrauma 2017;34(5):1054-62.

8. Bambakidis T, Dekker SE, Sillesen M, et al. Resuscitation with valproic acid alters inflammatory genes in a porcine model of combined traumatic brain injury and hemorrhagic shock. J Neurotrauma 2016;33(16):1514-21.
9. Bouzat P, Sala N, Payen JF, Oddo M. Beyond intracranial pressure: optimization of cerebral blood flow, oxygen, and substrate delivery after traumatic brain injury. Ann Intensive Care 2013;3(1):23.
10. Karri J, Cardenas JC, Matijevic N, et al. Early fibrinolysis associated with hemorrhagic progression following traumatic brain injury. Shock 2017;48(6):644-50.
11. Bouma GJ, Muizelaar JP. Cerebral blood flow, cerebral blood volume, and cerebrovascular reactivity after severe head injury. J Neurotrauma 1992;9 Suppl 1:S333-48.
12. Bouma GJ, Muizelaar JP, Bandoh K, Marmarou A. Blood pressure and intracranial pressure-volume dynamics in severe head injury: relationship with cerebral blood flow. J Neurosurg 1992;77(1):15-9.
13. Bertuccio A, Marasco S, Longhitano Y, et al. External ventricular drainage: a practical guide for neuro-anesthesiologists. Clin Pract 2023;13(1):219-29.
14. Kothari SA, Siddiq MS, Rahimi S, et al. Standardized criteria to initiate external ventricular drain (EVD) weaning in a neurological intensive care unit to increase the safety of EVD discontinuation and reduce the need for a shunt. Cureus 2024;16(4):e58362.
15. Grande PO. The "Lund Concept" for the treatment of severe head trauma—physiological principles and clinical application Intensive Care Med 2006;32(10):1475-84.
16. Faiver L, Hensler D, Rush SC, et al. Safety and efficacy of 23.4% sodium chloride administered via peripheral venous access for the treatment of cerebral herniation and intracranial pressure elevation. Neurocrit Care 2021;35(3):845-52.
17. Cadena R, Shoykhet M, Ratcliff JJ. Emergency Neurological Life Support: intracranial hypertension and herniation. Neurocrit Care 2017;27(Suppl 1):82-8.
18. Koenig MA, Bryan M, Lewin JL III, et al. Reversal of transtentorial herniation with hypertonic saline. Neurology 2008;70(13):1023-9.
19. Qureshi AI, Geocadin RG, Suarez JI, Ulatowski JA. Long-term outcome after medical reversal of transtentorial herniation in patients with supratentorial mass lesions. Crit Care Med 2000;28(5):1556-64.
20. Decompressive craniectomy versus craniotomy for acute subdural hematoma. N Engl J Med 2023;388(24):2219-29.
21. White H, Baker A. Continuous jugular venous oximetry in the neurointensive care unit—a brief review. Can J Anaesth 2002;49(6):623-9.
22. Okonkwo DO, Shutter LA, Moore C, et al. Brain oxygen optimization in severe traumatic brain injury phase-II: a phase II randomized trial. Crit Care Med 2017;45(11):1907-14.

23. Payen JF, Launey Y, Chabanne R, et al. Intracranial pressure monitoring with and without brain tissue oxygen pressure monitoring for severe traumatic brain injury in France (OXY-TC): an open-label, randomised controlled superiority trial. Lancet Neurol 2023;22(11):1005-14.
24. Ziaka M, Exadaktylos A. Brain-lung interactions and mechanical ventilation in patients with isolated brain injury. Crit Care 2021;25(1):358.
25. Dahyot-Fizelier C, Lasocki S, Kerforne T, et al. Ceftriaxone to prevent early ventilator-associated pneumonia in patients with acute brain injury: a multicentre, randomised, double-blind, placebo-controlled, assessor-masked superiority trial. Lancet Respir Med 2024;12(5):375-85.
26. de Franca SA, Tavares WM, Salinet ASM, et al. Early tracheostomy in severe traumatic brain injury patients: a meta-analysis and comparison with late tracheostomy. Crit Care Med 2020;48(4):e325-31.
27. Schierhout G, Roberts I. Anti-epileptic drugs for preventing seizures following acute traumatic brain injury. Cochrane Database Syst Rev 2001;(4):CD000173.

SECTION XII
NUTRITION AND METABOLISM

Chapter 46
Nutritional Requirements

The goal of nutritional support is to provide substrates for daily cellular growth and maintenance and wound healing and to provide the energy needs for metabolic processes. Reducing the catabolic reaction to the inflammatory response of critical illness is the aim for the critically ill patient. This chapter describes how to determine those needs in critically ill patients.

INITIAL NUTRITIONAL ASSESSMENT

An assessment of nutritional risk should be performed on patients whose ability for oral intake is compromised, e.g., mechanical ventilation, impaired mental status, etc., or has a contraindication to enteral nutrition. The Nutrition Risk in Critically Ill (NUTRIC) or Nutritional Risk Screening (NRS) 2002 assessments have been endorsed by the Society of Critical Care Medicine (SCCM) and the American Society for Parenteral and Enteral Nutrition (ASPEN) (1). These assessments have been shown to be predictive of days on mechanical ventilation, intensive care unit (ICU) length of stay, and mortality (1-4).

Nutritional Risk

An NRS 2002 score of >3 or a modified NUTRIC score of >6 places a patient in a high-risk category. (See Figure 46.1 for NRS 2002 score variables.) The "modified" NUTRIC score is assessed without an IL-6 measurement which is not readily available in many institutions. An assessment of 482 patients with sepsis found the NUTRIC and modified NUTRIC scores

Pre-Screening	
Is the BMI of the patient < 20.5 kg/m² ?	Yes
Did the patient lose weight in the past 3 months?	Yes
Was the patient's food intake reduced in the past week?	Yes
Is the patient critically ill?	Yes
If yes to one of those questions, proceed to screening If no for all answers, the patient should be re-screened weekly	

Screening			
Nutritional status	score	**Stress metabolism (severity of the disease)**	score
None	0	None	0
Mild Weight loss >5% in 3 months OR 50-75% of the normal food intake in the last week	1	Mild stress metabolism Patient is mobile Increased protein requirement can be covered with oral nutrition *Hip fracture, chronic disease especially with complications, e.g., liver cirrhosis, COPD, diabetes, cancer, chronic hemodialysis*	1
Moderate Weight loss >5% in 2 months OR BMI 18.5-20.5 kg/m² AND reduced general condition OR 25-50% of the normal food intake in the last week	2	Moderate stress metabolism Patient is bedridden due to illness Highly increased protein requirement, may be covered with ONS *Stroke, hematologic cancer, severe pneumonia, extended abdominal surgery*	2
Severe Weight loss >5% in 1 month OR BMI <18.5 kg/m² AND reduced general condition OR 0-25% of the normal food intake in the last week	2	Severe stress metabolism Patient is critically ill (intensive care unit) Very strongly Increased protein requirement, can only be achieved with (par)enteral nutrition *APACHE-II >10, bone marrow transplantation, head traumas*	2
Total (A)		**Total (B)**	
Age <70 years: 0 pt ≥70 years: 1 pt			
TOTAL = (A) + (B) + Age			
3 points: patient is at nutritional risk. Nutritional care plan should be set up. <3 points: repeat screening weekly			

FIGURE 46.1. Nutritional Risk Screening (NRS) 2002. APACHE = acute physiology and chronic health evaluation; BMI = body mass index; COPD = chronic obstructive pulmonary disease; ONS = oral nutritional supplement. (From Reber E, Gomes F, Vasiloglou MF, et al. Nutritional Risk Screening and Assessment. J Clin Med 2019;8[7]:1065. Table 1.)

to be equivalent in predicting 28-day mortality (2). (See Figure 46.2 for modified NUTRIC score variables.)

Variable	Range	Points
Age	<50	0
	50 – <75	1
	>75	2
APACHE II	<15	0
	15 – <20	1
	20 – 28	2
	>28	3
SOFA	<6	0
	6 – <10	1
	>10	2
Number of Co-morbidities	0 – 1	0
	2	1
Days from hospital to ICU admission	0 – <1	0
	1	1

Sum of points	Category	Explanation
5 – 9	High Score	• Associated with worse clinical outcomes (mortality, ventilation). • These patients are the most likely to benefit from aggressive nutrition therapy
0 – 4	Low Score	• These patients have a low malnutrition risk

FIGURE 46.2. Modified NUTRIC score variables. NUTRIC = nutrition risk in critically ill; SOFA = sequential organ failure assessment. (From Rahman A, Hasan RM, Agarwala R, et al. Identifying critically-ill patients who will benefit most from nutritional therapy: further validation of the "modified NUTRIC" nutritional risk assessment tool. Clin Nutr 2016;35[1]:158-62.)

CALORIC REQUIREMENTS

Oxidation of Nutrient Fuels

Cellular respiration or oxidative metabolism is the mechanism for energy production for life with final the step in this process being the uptake of oxygen (O_2). Oxidative metabolism captures the energy stored in nutrient fuels (carbohydrates, lipids, and proteins), and uses this energy to sustain life. This process consumes O_2 and generates carbon dioxide (CO_2), water (H_2O), and heat. The ratio of CO_2 produced over O_2 consumed varies among the substrates. This ratio is called the "Respiratory Quotient." Knowing the amount of

CO_2 produced, the amount of O_2 consumed, and amount of heat produced per substrate can be used to calculate the resting energy expenditure (REE) of patients through a process called, "Indirect Calorimetry" (5). (See Table 46.1.)

TABLE 46.1	Energy Yield from Each Nutrient Fuel	
Substrate	R/Q	Heat Production
Glucose	1.0	3.7 kcal/g
Lipid	0.7	9.1 kcal/g
Protein	0.8	4.0 kcal/g

The heat generated by the complete oxidation of a nutrient fuel is the energy yield (in kcal/g) of that fuel. Lipids have the highest energy yield (9.1 kcal/g), followed by protein (4.3 kcal/g), whereas glucose has the lowest energy yield (3.7 kcal/g).

The summed oxidation of all three nutrient fuels determines the whole-body O_2 consumption (VO_2), CO_2 production (VCO_2), and heat production for any given time period. *The 24-h heat production (daily energy expenditure) in kilocalories determines how many calories to provide each day in nutritional support.* The daily energy expenditure can be measured (indirectly) or estimated.

Indirect Calorimetry

The Principle

It is not possible to measure metabolic heat production in hospitalized patients, so the daily energy expenditure is determined indirectly using the whole-body O_2 consumption (VO_2) and CO_2 production (VCO_2) and the relationships in Table 46.1. This is the principle of *indirect calorimetry*, which measures the REE in kcal/min, using the following relationships (6):

$$REE = (3.6 \times VO_2) + (1.1 \times VCO_2) - 61 \text{ (kcal/min)} \quad (46.1)$$

The Method

Indirect calorimetry is performed with "metabolic carts" that measure whole-body VO_2 and VCO_2 at the bedside by measuring the concentrations of O_2 and CO_2 in inhaled and exhaled gas (usually in intubated patients). Steady-state measurements are required for 15-30 min to determine the REE (kcal/min) and are challenging in the critically ill patient. The REE is then multiplied by 1,440 (the number of minutes in 24 h) to derive the daily energy expenditure (kcal/24 h) (7).

Indirect calorimetry is not readily available in many ICUs, is costly, and is supported by a low quality of evidence (1). Daily energy requirements are typically estimated, as described next.

The Simple Way

More than 200 cumbersome equations are available for estimating daily energy requirements (1), but none is more accurate than the following simple relationship (8):

$$REE \text{ (kcal/day)} = 25 \times \text{body weight (kg)} \quad (46.2)$$

Body weight adjustments have been proposed for obese patients (9), but such adjustments are not recommended in the current guidelines on nutrition support (1).

CALORIE RESTRICTION

Calorie restriction has several potential advantages, including a decrease in O_2 consumption (which creates less demand on the cardiac output), a decrease in respiratory quotient (RQ) and CO_2 production (which is advantageous in ventilator-dependent patients, especially those with chronic obstructive pulmonary disease [COPD]), and improved glycemic control.

At least six clinical trials have shown no apparent harm when the daily caloric intake is reduced by about 50% (*while protein intake is maintained*) (10). The current guidelines for nutrition support in the ICU includes a recommendation for *calorie restriction in obese patients* (11-12) (see Table 46.2).

TABLE 46.2 Calorie-Restricted, High-Protein Feeding Regimen for Obese ICU Patients

If indirect calorimetry (IC) is available, measure REE and provide 70% of the daily caloric requirement.

If IC not available, use BMI and actual body weight.
- BMI 30-50: 11-14 kcal/kg actual body weight
- BMI >50: 22-25 kcal/kg actual body weight

Daily protein intake
- BMI 30-40: 2 g/kg ideal body weight
- BMI >40: 2.5 g/kg

BMI = body mass index; ICU = intensive care unit; REE = resting energy expenditure.

From McClave SA, Martindale RG, Vanek VW, et al. Guidelines for the provision and assessment of nutrition support therapy in the adult critically ill patient: Society of Critical Care Medicine (SCCM) and American Society for Parenteral and Enteral Nutrition (A.S.P.E.N.). JPEN J Parenter Enteral Nutr 2009;33(3):277-316.

SUBSTRATE REQUIREMENTS

The daily energy requirement is provided by nonprotein calories (from carbohydrates and lipids), whereas protein intake is used to maintain lean body mass (among other things).

Protein

Protein is the most important nutrient substrate for healing wounds, supporting immune function, and maintaining lean body mass (1). The normal daily protein intake is 0.8-1 g/kg (actual body weight), but in ICU patients, the daily protein intake is higher at 1.2-2 g/kg (1) to compensate for the hypercatabolism in critically ill patients.

Monitoring the adequacy of protein intake with the nitrogen balance (the difference between intake and excretion of protein-derived nitrogen) or plasma protein levels (e.g., albumin, prealbumin) is more of a manifestation of the acute phase response, is unreliable in critically ill patients, and is not recommended (1,13).

Carbohydrates

Standard nutrition regimens use carbohydrates (dextrose) to provide about *70% of the nonprotein calories*. The human body has limited carbohydrate stores (see glycogen stores in Table 46.3), and daily intake of carbohydrates is essential for proper functioning of the brain, which relies heavily on glucose as a nutritive fuel.

Lipids

Lipids are used to provide about *30% of the nonprotein calories*. As mentioned, lipids have the highest energy yield of the three nutrient fuels (see Table 46.1), and lipid stores in adipose tissues represent the major endogenous fuel source in healthy adults (see Table 46.3).

TABLE 46.3	Endogenous Fuel Stores in Healthy Adults	
Fuel Source	Amount (kg)	Energy Yield (kcal)
Adipose Tissue Fat	15.0	141,000
Muscle Protein	6.0	24,000
Total Glycogen	0.09	900
		Total: 165,900

Data from Cahill GF Jr. Starvation in man. N Eng J Med 1970;282:668-75.

Linoleic Acid

Dietary lipids are triglycerides, which are composed of a glycerol molecule linked to three fatty acids. The only dietary fatty acid that is essential (i.e., must be provided in the diet) is *linoleic acid*, a long chain, polyunsaturated fatty acid.

A deficient intake of linoleic acid produces a clinical disorder characterized by a scaly dermopathy, cardiac dysfunction, and increased susceptibility to infections (14). This disorder is prevented by providing 0.5% of the dietary fatty acids as linoleic acid.

The source of the lipids (e.g., fish oil, olive oil, soybean oil, or mixed lipid injectable emulsions has not demonstrated any impact on clinical outcomes (11).

Propofol

Propofol (a prevalent agent for short-term sedation in the ICU) is mixed in a 10% lipid emulsion that provides 1.1 kcal/mL. As a result, *the calories provided by propofol infusions must be considered when determining the nonprotein calories in a nutrition support regimen* (15). Monitoring of serum triglycerides is required as hypertriglyceridemia is potential complication of propofol therapy (16-17).

VITAMIN REQUIREMENTS

Thirteen vitamins are considered an essential part of the daily diet. Daily requirements for these vitamins varies with age (18). The vitamin requirements in critically ill patients are not defined and probably cannot be defined (because the clinical condition of these patients is constantly changing). Vitamin deficiencies are likely to occur in critically ill patients, and the following deficiencies deserve mention.

Thiamine Deficiency

Thiamine (vitamin B1) is a cofactor for four (8) enzymes involved in ATP production and the synthesis of essential cellular molecules (19). Thiamine deficiency can adversely affect cellular energy metabolism, particularly in the central nervous system, which relies heavily on glucose metabolism.

Predisposing Factors

Several conditions promote thiamine deficiency that are also prevalent in ICU patients. These include alcoholism, hypermetabolic states like trauma (20), increased urinary excretion of thiamine by furosemide (21), and magnesium depletion (22). Thiamine is also degraded by sulfites, which are used as preservatives in parenteral nutrition solutions (23).

Clinical Features

There are four manifestations of thiamine deficiency (24): cardiomyopathy (wet beriberi), Wernicke encephalopathy (nystagmus, lateral gaze palsy, ataxia, and confusion), lactic acidosis, and peripheral neuropathy.

Diagnosis

The plasma thiamine level can be measured: The reference range is 5.3-7.9 µg/dL. Plasma levels can correct within 24 h after starting thiamine replacement.

The most reliable measure of thiamine stores is the *erythrocyte transketolase assay* (25), which measures the activity of a thiamine pyrophosphate (TPP)-dependent transketolase enzyme in the patient's red blood cells in response to the addition of TPP. An increase in enzyme activity >25% evidence of thiamine depletion.

Treatment

A minimum thiamine intake of 1 mg daily is recommended for adults. The treatment of symptomatic thiamine deficiency is 50-100 mg by intravenous or intramuscular injection daily for 7-14 days, followed by an oral dose of 10 mg daily until the condition resolves.

Vitamin D Deficiency

Vitamin D deficiency is found in as many as 50% of the general adult population (26), and it is so common in ICU patients that one study found normal blood levels of vitamin D in only 5% of the patients tested (27). The problem here may not be vitamin D deficiency, but the diagnostic criteria.

The diagnosis of vitamin D deficiency is based solely on a plasma level of 25-hydroxyvitamin D (a metabolite of vitamin D) that is below 50 nmol/L (20 ng/mL) (28). Evidence of adverse consequences are not required, and virtually all patients are asymptomatic. Therefore, *vitamin D deficiency in ICU patients is a laboratory value that is outside the expected range for healthy adults*. The clinical significance of this condition is unclear. Routine monitoring of 25(OH) vitamin D levels is not recommended (the assay is costly), and because vitamin D deficiency is asymptomatic in ICU patients, there are no real indications for pursuing the diagnosis of vitamin D deficiency.

Furthermore, there is no consensus on a definition of vitamin D deficiency in critical illness (29). There is some evidence that vitamin D deficiency is associated with an increased risk of infection in ICU patients, but the risk ratios (1.4-1.5) are not convincing (30).

Nevertheless, if confronted with a low plasma level of 25(OH) vitamin D, a single intramuscular injection of 150,000 IU of cholecalciferol can correct the blood levels in 80% of patients.

The recommended daily intake of vitamin D in adults is 600 IU up to age 70, and 800 IU after age 70.

TABLE 46.4	Daily Allowances for Essential Trace Elements	
Trace Element	Recommended Daily Intake	Maximum Daily Intake
Chromium	30 µg	ND
Copper	900 µg	10,000 µg
Iodine	150 µg	1,100 µg
Iron	8 mg	45 mg
Manganese	2.3 mg	11 mg
Selenium	55 µg	200 µg
Zinc	11 mg	40 mg

Recommendations for adult males, ages 51-79 years.

Doses rounded off to nearest whole number. ND = not determined.

From Food & Nutrition Board, Institute of Medicine. Available at the Food and Nutrition Information Center (http://fnic.nal.usda.gov).

ESSENTIAL TRACE ELEMENTS

A trace element is a substance that is present in the body in amounts <50 mg per gram of body tissue (31). Seven trace elements are considered essential in humans (i.e., are associated with deficiency syndromes), and these are listed in Table 46.4, along with the daily requirement for each in healthy adults. As mentioned for vitamins, the daily requirement for trace

Iron

The normal adult has approximately 4.5 g of iron, yet there is virtually no free iron in plasma. Most of the iron is bound to hemoglobin, and the remainder is bound to ferritin in tissues and transferrin in plasma. The absence of free iron can be viewed as a defense mechanism that protects the tissues from oxidant injury. The understanding of iron metabolism in critical illness is evolving. Iron metabolism is greatly affected by critical illness, affecting infections, cardiopulmonary dysfunction, cognitive, and neuromuscular dysfunction. Further confounding are the use of ferritin and transferrin saturations which are not able to identify iron deficiency in critical illness. Serum hepcidin appears to be more reliable but not readily available (32).

Iron and Oxidant Injury

The metabolism of oxygen to water, which is depicted in Figure 46.3, occurs in a series of single-electron reduction reactions that generate highly reactive intermediates. These are identified in Figure 46.3 as the *superoxide radical*, *hydrogen peroxide*, and the *hydroxyl radical*. (A radical is an atom or molecule with an unpaired electron in its outer orbital.) These oxygen metabolites are powerful oxidizing agents, capable of damaging cell membranes and fracturing nuclear DNA. The most reactive metabolite (and the most powerful oxidant known in biochemistry) is the hydroxyl radical, and iron (in the reduced state) is essential for the formation of hydroxyl radicals, as indicated in Figure 46.3. The following statements deserve emphasis.

- Iron represents a major risk for oxidant cell injury, especially when transferrin levels in blood are reduced (e.g., in critically ill patients).

- Iron supplementation in the ICU should be balanced against the risk of oxidant injury and infection risk. Iron supplementation has not shown a mortality benefit and can result in increased infectious complications.

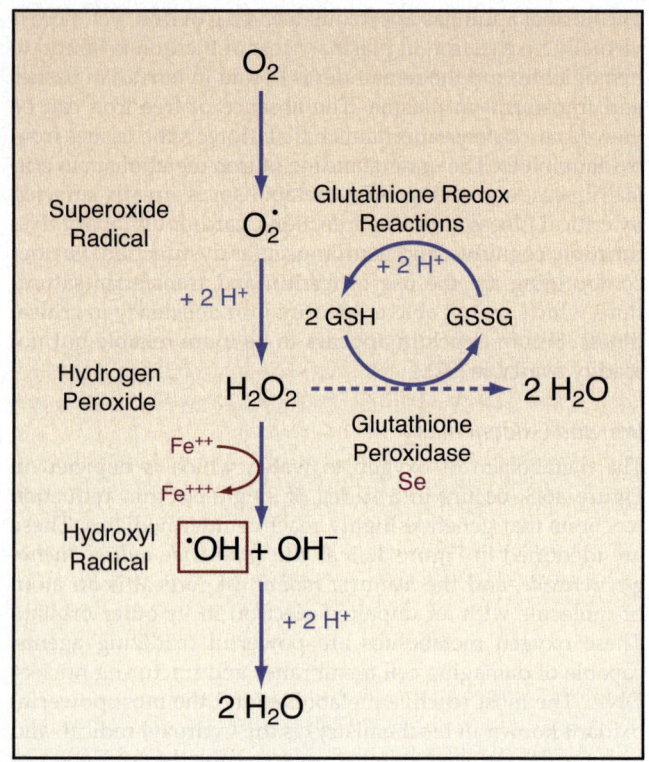

FIGURE 46.3. The metabolism of molecular oxygen to water and the actions of the glutathione redox reactions. Symbols with a dot are free radicals. See text for explanation. Fe^{++} = reduced iron; Fe^{+++} = oxidized iron; Se = selenium; GSH = reduced glutathione; GSSG = oxidized glutathione (a dipeptide connected by a disulfide bridge).

Selenium

Selenium has gotten a lot of attention in recent years due to its antioxidant properties. It has a recommended daily allowance of 55 µg in healthy adults. Selenium utilization is increased in acute illness (23), so daily requirements are likely to be higher in critically ill patients.

Selenium as an Antioxidant

Figure 46.3 shows that hydrogen peroxide can be reduced directly to water (thus bypassing the formation of hydroxyl radicals) with the aid of reduced glutathione (GSH) and the enzyme glutathione peroxidase, which uses selenium as a cofactor. The glutathione redox reactions represent the major intracellular antioxidant system, and thus, selenium has a significant role in promoting endogenous antioxidant protection.

Selenium in Sepsis

Reduced plasma levels of selenium are common in patients with severe sepsis. Data is currently conflicting, with some low-level evidence of selenium supplementation that is associated with a lower mortality rate and acute kidney injury (1). Therefore, monitoring plasma selenium levels in patients with severe sepsis seems justified. The normal plasma selenium concentration is 89-113 µg/L (25). Selenium can be replaced intravenously, and the maximum daily dose is 200 µg.

References

1. McClave SA, Taylor BE, Martindale RG, et al. Guidelines for the provision and assessment of nutrition support therapy in the adult critically ill patient: Society of Critical Care Medicine (SCCM) and American Society for Parenteral and Enteral Nutrition (A.S.P.E.N.). JPEN J Parenter Enteral Nutr 2016;40:159-211.
2. Jeong DH, Hong SB, Lim CM, et al. Comparison of accuracy of NUTRIC and modified NUTRIC scores in predicting 28-day

mortality in patients with sepsis: a single center retrospective study. Nutrients 2018;10.
3. Kumar S, Gattani SC, Baheti AH, Dubey A. Comparison of the performance of APACHE II, SOFA, and mNUTRIC scoring systems in critically ill patients: a 2-year cross-sectional study. Indian J Crit Care Med 2020;24:1057-61.
4. Reber E, Gomes F, Vasiloglou MF, et al. Nutritional risk screening and assessment. J Clin Med 2019;8(7):1065.
5. Patel H, Kerndt CC, Bhardwaj A. Physiology, Respiratory Quotient. In: StatPearls. Treasure Island (FL): StatPearls Publishing; 2023.
6. Bursztein S, Saphar P, Singer P, Elwyn DH. A mathematical analysis of indirect calorimetry measurements in acutely ill patients. Am J Clin Nutr 1989;50:227-30.
7. Lev S, Cohen J, Singer P. Indirect calorimetry measurements in the ventilated critically ill patient: facts and controversies—the heat is on. Crit Care Clin 2010;26:e1-9.
8. Paauw JD, McCamish MA, Dean RE, Ouellette TR. Assessment of caloric needs in stressed patients. J Am Coll Nutr 1984;3:51-9.
9. Krenitsky J. Adjusted body weight, pro: evidence to support the use of adjusted body weight in calculating calorie requirements. Nutr Clin Pract 2005;20:468-73.
10. Marik PE, Hooper MH. Normocaloric versus hypocaloric feeding on the outcomes of ICU patients: a systematic review and meta-analysis. Intensive Care Med 2016;42:316-23.
11. Compher C, Bingham AL, McCall M, et al. Guidelines for the provision of nutrition support therapy in the adult critically ill patient: The American Society for Parenteral and Enteral Nutrition. JPEN J Parenter Enteral Nutr 2022;46:12-41.
12. Mogensen KM, Andrew BY, Corona JC, Robinson MK. Validation of the Society of Critical Care Medicine and American Society for Parenteral and Enteral Nutrition recommendations for caloric provision to critically ill obese patients: a pilot study. JPEN J Parenter Enteral Nutr 2016;40:713-21.
13. Davis CJ, Sowa D, Keim KS, et al. The use of prealbumin and C-reactive protein for monitoring nutrition support in adult patients receiving enteral nutrition in an urban medical center. JPEN J Parenter Enteral Nutr 2012;36:197-204.
14. Jones PJH, Kubow S. Lipids, sterols, and their metabolites. In: Shils M, Shike M, Ross A, et al., editors. *Modern Nutrition in Health and Disease*. 10th ed. Lippincott Williams & Wilkins; 2006:92-122.
15. Dickerson RN, Buckley CT. Impact of propofol sedation upon caloric overfeeding and protein inadequacy in critically ill patients receiving nutrition support. Pharmacy (Basel) 2021;9.

16. Corrado MJ, Kovacevic MP, Dube KM, et al. The incidence of propofol-induced hypertriglyceridemia and identification of associated risk factors. Crit Care Explor 2020;2:e0282.
17. Witenko CJ, Littlefield AJ, Abedian S, et al. The safety of continuous infusion propofol in mechanically ventilated adults with coronavirus disease 2019. Ann Pharmacother 2022;56:5-15.
18. Institute of Medicine (US) Committee to Review Dietary Reference Intakes for Vitamin D and Calcium; Ross AC, Taylor CL, Yaktine AL, et al., editors. *Dietary Reference Intakes for Calcium and Vitamin D.* Washington, DC: National Academies Press; 2011. https://www.ncbi.nlm.nih.gov/books/NBK56070/
19. Attaluri P, Castillo A, Edriss H, Nugent K. Thiamine deficiency: an important consideration in critically ill patients. Am J Med Sci 2018;356:382-90.
20. McConachie I, Haskew A. Thiamine status after major trauma. Intensive Care Med 1988;14:628-31.
21. Seligmann H, Halkin H, Rauchfleisch S, et al. Thiamine deficiency in patients with congestive heart failure receiving long-term furosemide therapy: a pilot study. Am J Med 1991;91:151-5.
22. Dyckner T, Ek B, Nyhlin H, Wester PO. Aggravation of thiamine deficiency by magnesium depletion. A case report. Acta Med Scand 1985;218:129-31.
23. Scheiner JM, Araujo MM, DeRitter E. Thiamine destruction by sodium bisulfite in infusion solutions. Am J Hosp Pharm 1981;38:1911-3.
24. Butterworth RF. Thiamine. In: Shils M, Shike M, Ross A, et al., editors. *Modern Nutrition in Health and Disease.* 10th ed. Lippincott Williams & Wilkins; 2006:426-33.
25. Boni L, Kieckens L, Hendrikx A. An evaluation of a modified erythrocyte transketolase assay for assessing thiamine nutritional adequacy. J Nutr Sci Vitaminol (Tokyo) 1980;26:507-14.
26. Kennel KA, Drake MT, Hurley DL. Vitamin D deficiency in adults: when to test and how to treat. Mayo Clin Proc 2010;85:752-7; quiz 7-8.
27. Venkatram S, Chilimuri S, Adrish M, et al. Vitamin D deficiency is associated with mortality in the medical intensive care unit. Crit Care 2011;15:R292.
28. Holick MF, Binkley NC, Bischoff-Ferrari HA, et al. Evaluation, treatment, and prevention of vitamin D deficiency: an Endocrine Society clinical practice guideline. J Clin Endocrinol Metab 2011;96:1911-30.
29. Menger J, Lee ZY, Notz Q, et al. Administration of vitamin D and its metabolites in critically ill adult patients: an updated systematic review with meta-analysis of randomized controlled trials. Crit Care 2022;26:268.

30. Singh S, Sarkar S, Gupta K, Rout A. Vitamin D supplementation in critically ill patients: a meta-analysis of randomized controlled trials. Cureus 2022;14:e24625.
31. Fleming CR. Trace element metabolism in adult patients requiring total parenteral nutrition. Am J Clin Nutr 1989;49:573-9.
32. Litton E, Lim J. Iron metabolism: an emerging therapeutic target in critical illness. Crit Care 2019;23:81.

Enteral Nutrition

Chapter 47

When oral intake is not possible, the preferred method of nutrition support is the infusion of liquid feeding formulas into the stomach or small bowel (enteral tube feedings). Enteral nutrition should be initiated within 24-48 h of intensive care unit (ICU) admission (1).

GENERAL CONSIDERATIONS

Trophic Effects

The benefits of early *enteral* nutrition have been known for years (2-3). The preference for enteral over parenteral nutrition is based on numerous studies showing that enteral nutrition is associated with fewer infections of bowel origin (1-2,4). This is related to the trophic effects of enteral feeding (Table 47.1).

TABLE 47.1 Benefits of Early Enteral Nutrition
Maintains mucosal integrity
Stimulates endogenous trophic hormones and growth factors such as • Cholecystokinin • Gastrin • Secretin • Somatostatin

Immunologic impact
• Maintains villous height and gut-associated lymphoid tissue (GALT)
  » Lung
  » Liver
  » Kidneys

Promotes mesenteric blood flow
Attenuates catabolic protein losses

1. The presence of food or tube feedings in the lumen of the bowel stimulates mesenteric blood flow, which has several trophic effects and immunologic benefits. A number of trophic gastrointestinal (GI) hormones are stimulated, e.g., cholecystokinin, gastrin. This also supports the integrity of the gut-associated lymphoid tissue that preserves the structural integrity of the mucosa and supports the immune defenses in the bowel (such as the production of immunoglobulin A, which blocks the attachment of pathogens to the bowel mucosa) (1,5-7).
2. These trophic effects maintain the barrier function of the bowel, which protects against invasion from enteric pathogens; a phenomenon known as *translocation* (8).
3. Periods of bowel rest are associated with progressive atrophy of the bowel mucosa (5), which can lead to translocation and the systemic spread of enteric pathogens. Parenteral nutrition does not prevent the deleterious effects of bowel rest (9).

Indications and Contraindications

Patients who are unable to eat and have no contraindications are candidates for enteral tube feeding:

1. Tube feedings should be started within 24-48 h of admission to the ICU (10) to take advantage of the protective effects of tube feedings just described. There is evidence that early institution of enteral nutrition is associated with fewer infectious complications, a shorter hospital stay, and decreased mortality (1,3).
2. Contraindications to enteral tube feedings (listed in Table 47.2) include complete bowel obstruction, bowel ischemia, ileus, unstable hemodynamics, or circulatory shock requiring high-dose vasopressors (10).

Slow advancement of tube feedings can be attempted in stable patients on low doses of vasopressors typically beginning with trophic volumes (10), but any signs of intolerance should prompt immediate termination of feedings.

TABLE 47.2 Contraindications to Enteral Tube Feeds

- Complete bowel obstruction
- Mesenteric ischemia
- Ileus
- Unstable hemodynamics
- Circulatory shock requiring high-dose vasopressors
- Active gastrointestinal bleeding
- High-output intestinal fistula

From Adeyinka A, Rouster AS, Valentine M. Enteric Feedings. In: StatPearls. Treasure Island (FL): StatPearls Publishing; 2024 and Doley J. Enteral nutrition overview. Nutrients 2022;14(11):2180.

Trophic versus Full Feedings

1. *Trophic feedings* (10-20 kcal/h, or up to 500 kcal/day) can be used for the first week in patients who are not malnourished (NRS 2002 <3 or modified NUTRIC <4) and are not seriously ill (e.g., post-op patients) (1).
2. For patients who are malnourished, or seriously ill, calculated goals (full nutritional support) should be achieved within hours of starting tube feedings (1).

FEEDING FORMULAS

There are numerous enteral feeding formulas and modular supplements. Formulas are complete nutrition, whereas modulars contain specific nutrients typically added as supplements (Table 47.3).

Caloric Density

Feeding formulas are available with caloric densities of 1 kcal/mL, 1.5 kcal/mL, and 2 kcal/mL. Standard tube feeding regimens use formulas with 1 kcal/mL. High-calorie formulas (2 kcal/mL) are intended for patients with severe physiological stress and are often used when volume restriction is a priority (11).

TABLE 47.3	Types of Enteral Formulations
Standard	Intact nutrients; caloric concentration 1-2 kcal/mL; +/− fiber
Peptide-based	Proteins hydrolyzed into peptides; fat sources include medium chain triglycerides; formula used for gastrointestinal intolerance to tube feeds of malabsorption
Immune modulating	Additional antioxidant components with arginine and glutamine
Disease Specific	
Hyperglycemia/diabetes	Specialized carbohydrate blends that blunt glycemic spikes
Hepatic failure	Lower protein content with high branched chain amino acid to aromatic amino acid ratios
Standard	Lower content of potassium, phosphates, and magnesium; higher caloric density (fluid restriction); not necessary with renal replacement therapy

Nonprotein Calories

The caloric density of feeding formulas includes both protein and nonprotein calories, but *daily caloric requirements should be provided by nonprotein calories*. In standard feeding formulas, nonprotein calories account for about 85% of the total calories.

Osmolality

The osmolality of feeding formulas is determined primarily by the caloric density. Standard feeding formulas with 1 kcal/mL have an osmolality similar to plasma (280-300 mOsm/kg). Hypertonic feedings can promote diarrhea, but this risk is minimized by intragastric feeding, where the large volume of gastric secretions attenuates the osmolality.

Protein Content

Standard feeding formulas provide 35-40 g of protein per liter. High-protein formulas provide about 20% more protein than the standard formulas (Table 47.4) and are typically used to promote wound healing (11).

TABLE 47.4 Examples of Enteral Formulations

Per 1,000 mL	Standard		Peptide-Based	Immuno-Modulating	Disease-Specific	
	Jevity 1.5	Osmolyte 1.5	Promote	Impact	Glucerna 1.5 (Hyperglycemia)	Nepro (CKD)
Calories	1,500	1,500	1,000	1,000	1,500	1,770
Protein (g)	63.8	62.7	63	56	82.5	81
Carbohydrate (% cal)	54.4	54.3	52	53	33	33
Fat (% cal)	28.6	29	23	25	45	49
Osmolality (mOsm/kg H_2O)	525	525	405	N/A	875	745
Potassium (mg)	2,180	2,180	2,667	1,340	2,520	717
Phosphorus (mg)	1,250	1,250	833	720	1,000	1,050
Arginine (g/L)	N/A	N/A	N/A	13	N/A	N/A
ω-3 Fatty acids (g/L)	N/A	N/A	N/A	3.3	N/A	N/A
Comment					Mixed carbohydrates	*

CKD = chronic kidney disease; N/A = not available.
*Decreased potassium.

Intact versus Hydrolyzed Protein

Most enteral formulas contain intact proteins that are broken down into amino acids in the upper GI tract. These are called *polymeric* formulas. Feeding formulas are also available that contain small peptides (*polymeric* formulas) and individual amino acids (*semi-elemental* formulas) that are absorbed more readily than intact protein. These formulas promote water reabsorption from the bowel and could be of benefit. Polymeric formulas include *Peptamen* and *Vivonex*.

Carbohydrate Content

Carbohydrates (usually polysaccharides) provide 40-70% of the total calories in most feeding formulas. Reduced carbohydrate formulas, in which carbohydrates provide 30-40% of the calories, are available for diabetics (see Tables 47.3 and 47.4); these formulas typically contain fiber.

MODULAR SUPPLEMENTS

Examples of modular supplements can be found in Table 47.5.

TABLE 47.5	Examples of Enteral Modular Supplements		
	Banatrol	ProSource	Juven
Clinical Use	*Diarrhea*	*Protein*	*Wound healing*
Nutritional value per	1 pkt (10.75 g)	1 pkt (45 mL)	1 pkt (27.5 g)
Calories	40	40	90
Protein (g)	0	11	2.5
Arginine	N/A	N/A	7 g
Glutamine	N/A	N/A	7 g
Comment	Two sources of soluble fiber		

Fiber

The term *fiber* refers to polysaccharides from plants that are not digested by humans. There are two types of fiber: fermentable and nonfermentable.

1. Fermentable fiber, a "prebiotic" being broken down by anaerobic colonic bacteria into short-chain fatty acids (SCFA), not only promotes sodium and water absorption but also is an important energy source for the large bowel mucosa, critical to the maintenance of intestinal

barrier integrity and immune homeostasis (12). There is evidence of the benefit of SCFA impairing the ability of *Clostridium difficile* to colonize or grow (13).

2. *Nonfermentable fiber* is not broken down by gut bacteria. This type of fiber draws water into the bowel.

The fiber in most feeding formulas is a mixture of fermentable and nonfermentable fiber, so it is no surprise that the effects of mixed-fiber formulas on diarrhea have been inconsistent (10). The current guidelines on nutrition support recommend the following(10):

- For patients with diarrhea, a source of fermentable fiber (e.g., fructo-oligosaccharides) should be added to the feeding regimen in a dose of 10-20 g daily. This is preferred to the use of mixed-fiber formulas.
- Mixed-fiber feeding formulas should *not* be used in patients with a risk of bowel ischemia, or with severe bowel dysmotility (because of reports of bowel obstruction in such patients).

Lipid Content

Standard feeding formulas contain polyunsaturated fatty acids (PUFAs) from vegetable oils, which can serve as precursors for inflammatory mediators (eicosanoids) that are capable of promoting inflammatory cell injury.

PUFAs from fish oils (ω-*3 fatty acids*) do not produce inflammatory mediators. Feeding formulas that contain nutrients that may influence the inflammatory response (e.g., omega-3 fatty acids, arginine, and glutamine) are known as *immune modulating nutrition* (14).

Clinical studies have shown that patients with acute respiratory distress syndrome (ARDS) derive some benefit (fewer days on the ventilator) from feeding formulas enriched with omega-3 fatty acids and antioxidants (15). However, the benefits are marginal, and there is a general reluctance to adopt these feeding formulas for patients with ARDS (10).

Arginine and Glutamine

Arginine and glutamine are essential amino acids that are quickly depleted in the critically ill (1,16-17). Both are implicated in the response to inflammation and oxidative stress. Arginine promotes wound healing and is a precursor of nitric oxide (16).

These formulas are recommended for postoperative patients (10,14) and for patients with severe trauma or traumatic brain injury (10).

Caveat: There are reports of increased mortality associated with arginine-enriched feeding formulas in patients with severe sepsis (10,18). The presumed mechanism is arginine-induced formation of nitric oxide, with subsequent vasodilation and hypotension.

Recommendation

Despite the multitude of available feeding formulas, the current guidelines on nutrition support (1) recommend standard (nonspecialized) feeding formulas for most ICU patients.

Immunomodulating formulas containing arginine, glutamine, and fish oils may have a (low-level evidence) benefit to the postoperative, trauma, and traumatic brain-injured population (1-3).

CREATING A FEEDING REGIMEN

This section describes a simple method for creating a tube feeding regimen, which is summarized in Table 47.6. There are four steps in this method.

Step 1. Estimate Daily Energy and Protein Requirements

1. The daily requirement for calories and protein is first estimated with the simple formulas in Table 47.6 (10). Actual body weight is used.
2. For obese patients (body mass index of 30 kg/m^2 or higher), use the calorie-restricted, high-protein estimates in Table 46.2.

Step 2. Select a Feeding Formula

As mentioned earlier, standard feeding formulas with a caloric density of 1 kcal/mL should be sufficient for most patients (1).

Step 3. Calculate the Desired Infusion Rate

For mechanically ventilated patients, continuous enteral tube feeds achieve target nutritional goals more rapidly as compared to intermittent bolus feeds (19).

To determine the desired infusion rate for feeding,

1. First calculate the volume of the feeding formula that must be infused to meet the daily requirement for calories, as indicated in Table 47.6.
2. Then divide the feeding volume by the number of hours each day that the feeding formula will be infused.
3. If propofol is being infused, subtract the calories provided by propofol (1 kcal/mL) from the daily calorie requirement.
4. Although nonprotein calories are recommended for providing the daily energy needs, tube feeding regimens often use the total caloric yield of the feeding formula to determine the desired volume and infusion rate. (Nonprotein calories account for about 85% of the total calories in standard feeding formulas.)

Step 4. Adjust the Protein Intake, If Necessary

The final step in the process is to determine if the feeding regimen will provide enough protein to satisfy the daily protein requirement (from *Step 1*). The projected protein intake is simply the daily feeding volume multiplied by the protein concentration in the feeding formula. If the projected protein intake is less than the desired protein intake, powdered protein is added to the tube feedings to correct the discrepancy.

TABLE 47.6 Creating an Enteral Feeding Regimen

Step 1: Estimate daily calorie and protein requirements.

$$\text{Calories (kcal/day)} = 25 \times \text{wt (kg)}$$

$$\text{Protein (g/day)} = (1.2\text{-}2.0) \times \text{wt (kg)}$$

Step 2: Select feeding formula.

Step 3: Calculate desired infusion rate.

$$\text{Feeding volume (mL)} = \frac{\text{kcal/day required}}{\text{kcal/mL in feeding formula}}$$

$$\text{Infusion rate (mL/h)} = \frac{\text{Feeding volume (mL)}}{\text{Feeding time (h)}}$$

Step 4: Adjust protein intake, if necessary.

a. Calculate the projected protein intake (g/day) as follows:

   Feeding volume (L/day) × protein (g/L) in feeding

b. If the projected intake is less than desired intake, add protein powder to the feeding regimen to correct the discrepancy.

INITIATING TUBE FEEDINGS

Feeding Tube Placement

1. Feeding tubes are inserted through the nares or orally in endotracheally intubated patients and advanced blindly into the stomach or duodenum. The distance required to reach the stomach can be estimated by measuring the distance from the tip of the nose to the earlobe and then to the xiphoid process (typically 50-60 cm) (20).

2. Advancing the tip of the feeding tube into the duodenum is not necessary in most patients (1) because *there is no difference in the risk of aspiration with gastric versus duodenal feedings* (21).

3. *A portable chest x-ray is required to verify proper tube position* before the feeding formula is infused. The common practice of *evaluating tube placement by pushing air through the tube and listening for bowel sounds is not reliable* because sounds emanating from a misplaced tube in the

distal airways or pleural space can be transmitted into the upper abdomen (22-23). Figure 47.1 demonstrates appropriate positioning of the Dobhoff feeding tube positioned in the duodenum.

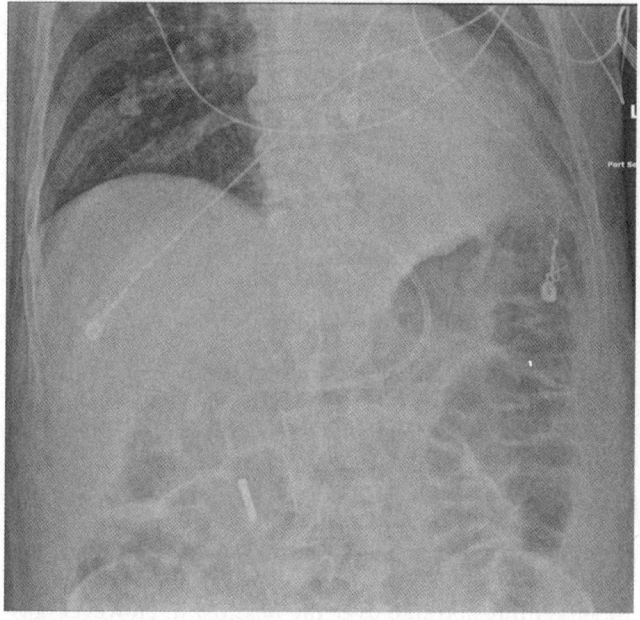

FIGURE 47.1. Dobhoff feeding tube positioned in the duodenum.

4. Feeding tubes end up in the trachea during 1% of insertions (24). Intubated patients often do not cough when feeding tubes enter the trachea (unlike healthy subjects); as a result, feeding tubes can be advanced deep into the lungs without any warning signs and can puncture the visceral pleura and create a pneumothorax (22-23). Massive aspiration can occur with the infusion of tube feeds into the lung in sedated and/or encephalopathic patients. The portable chest x-ray in Figure 47.2 shows a nasogastric tube that has been advanced deep into the right mainstem bronchus.

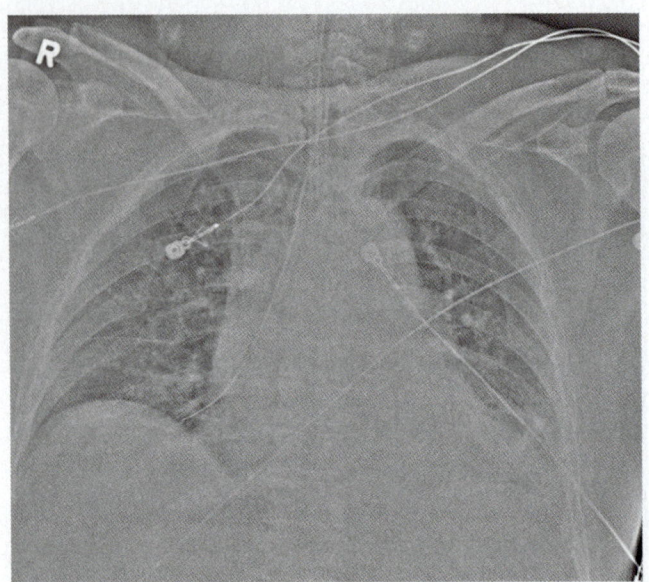

FIGURE 47.2. Nasogastric tube in the right mainstem bronchus.

Feeding Regimens

The traditional practice is to begin tube feedings at a low infusion rate (10-20 ml/h) and then gradually advance to the target infusion rate over the next 6-8 h. However, gastric feedings can begin at the desired (target) rate in most patients without the risk of vomiting or aspiration (25). Although the continuous infusion of enteral tube feeds compared with bolus feeds has not shown a clinical outcome difference, it offers a number of advantages in the critical care (1). Continuous enteral feeding is associated with better tolerance and improved achievement of target nutritional requirements (19).

For critically ill trauma and surgical patients, it is advised to adopt a comprehensive approach by implementing a volume-based feeding protocol within a multidisciplinary nutrition enhancement framework. This strategy, integrating revised non-oral guidelines and volume-based feeding, not only compensates for feeding interruptions but also significantly elevates the delivery of enteral nutrition by up to 10%, aligning with national standards. Proven to enhance nutritional support without increasing the incidence of feeding-related complications, it offers a more efficient and safe method for nutritional delivery in the ICU setting (26).

PROBLEMS AND COMPLICATIONS

Problems associated with enteral tube feedings include occlusion of the feeding tube, regurgitation of the feeding formula into the mouth and airways, and diarrhea.

Occlusion of Feeding Tubes

Narrow-bore feeding tubes can become occluded by protein precipitates that form when acidic gastric secretions reflux into the feeding tubes (27). Standard preventive measures include flushing the feeding tubes with 30 mL of water every 4 h, and a 10-mL water flush after medications are instilled.

Restoring Patency

If flow through the feeding tube is sluggish, flushing the tube with warm water can restore flow in 30% of cases (27). If this is ineffective, *pancreatic enzyme* (Viokase) can be used as follows (28):

- *Regimen:* Dissolve 1 tablet of Viokase and 1 tablet of sodium carbonate (324 mg) in 5 mL of water. Inject this mixture into the feeding tube and clamp for 5 min. Follow with a warm water flush. This should relieve the obstruction in about 75% of cases (28).
- If the tube is completely occluded, advance a flexible wire or a drum cartridge catheter through the feeding tube in an attempt to clear the obstruction. If this is unsuccessful, replace the feeding tube without delay.

Regurgitation/Aspiration

The most feared complication of enteral tube feeding is regurgitation of feeding formula and subsequent pulmonary aspiration.

The following measures are recommended for reducing the risk of regurgitation and pulmonary aspiration (10):

- Elevation of the head of the bed to 30-45° above the horizontal plane
- Oral care with chlorhexidine
- Reducing the level of sedation, when possible
- Post-pyloric feedings and prokinetic agents should be considered in patients who have an increased risk of aspiration (e.g., those who are comatose or have abnormal swallowing function).

Monitoring gastric residual volumes is not recommended (10) because residual volumes do not correlate with the incidence of pneumonia (29), regurgitation, or aspiration (30).

Gastroparesis

Gastroparesis is multifactorial in the ICU setting. Factors such as cytokines released during sepsis, bowel wall edema, medications, bowel perfusion, and electrolyte abnormalities can all negatively impact gastric motility (31) and risk regurgitation and aspiration. The available prokinetic agents and recommended dosing regimens are shown in Table 47.7.

Of these options, only metoclopramide is FDA-approved for this indication (Isola). Prokinetic therapy is associated with short-term improvement in gastric motility, but drug shortages and overall clinical significance of this effect has been difficult to demonstrate (32).

Erythromycin and Azithromycin

Erythromycin and azithromycin are used as antibiotics. These drugs have also been shown to promote gastric emptying by stimulating motilin receptors in the GI tract (33-34) and can be administered PO, IV, IM, or PR. Erythromycin is more effective in combination with metoclopramide (1,35).

Adverse Reactions. Erythromycin is associated with cardiac toxicity, tachyphylaxis, diarrhea, and bacterial resistance (1,31,36).

TABLE 47.7 Prokinetic Agents

Agent	Dosing
Metoclopramide[1]	Dosing: 5-10 mg before meals and sleep; or 5 mg IV before meal; Q 6 h IV with continuous tube feeding Comment: reduce dose for both hepatic and renal impairment; effect decreases over time; can be combined with erythromycin or azithromycin
Erythromycin[2]	Dosing: 200 mg IV Q 8 h Comment: QT prolongation; effects decreases over time; can be combined with metoclopramide
Azithromycin[3]	Dosing: 250 mg IV daily Comment: less adverse reactions than erythromycin; can be combined with metoclopramide

[1]Isola S, Hussain A, Dua A, et al. Metoclopramide. In: StatPearls. Treasure Island (FL): StatPearls Publishing; 2024.

[2]Stojek M, Jasinski T. Gastroparesis in the intensive care unit. Anaesthesiol Intensive Ther 2021;53:450-5.

[3]Potter TG, Snider KR. Azithromycin for the treatment of gastroparesis. Ann Pharmacother 2013;47(3):411-5.

Metoclopramide

Metoclopramide promotes gastric emptying by antagonizing the actions of dopamine in the GI tract. At a dose of 10 mg PO, IV, or IM every 6 h, gastric residual volumes decrease by 30% after 24 h, but the effect wanes rapidly (37). Metoclopramide is more effective in combination with erythromycin (1,35).

Adverse Reactions. Adverse reactions to metoclopramide include QT prolongation, laryngospasm, trismus, torticollis, and extrapyramidal effects, including tardive dyskinesia and even neuroleptic malignant syndrome (31,38).

Diarrhea

Diarrhea is common in tube-fed patients and is often attributed to the hyperosmolality of many feeding formulas. However, other factors may have an important role; i.e., antibiotic-associated diarrhea (altered normal flora), *Clostridium difficile* infection, and liquid drug preparations (which may be the culprit in a majority of cases) (39). Liquid drug preparations (which are favored for drug delivery through feeding tubes) have two features that create a risk for diarrhea (40):

1. They can be extremely hyperosmolar (≥3,000 mOsm/kg).
2. They can contain sorbitol, a well-known laxative that draws water into the bowel lumen.

References

1. McClave SA, Taylor BE, Martindale RG, et al. Guidelines for the provision and assessment of nutrition support therapy in the adult critically ill patient: Society of Critical Care Medicine (SCCM) and American Society for Parenteral and Enteral Nutrition (A.S.P.E.N.). JPEN J Parenter Enteral Nutr 2016;40:159-211.
2. Heyland DK, Stephens KE, Day AG, McClave SA. The success of enteral nutrition and ICU-acquired infections: a multicenter observational study. Clin Nutr 2011;30:148-55.
3. Marik PE, Zaloga GP. Early enteral nutrition in acutely ill patients: a systematic review. Crit Care Med 2001;29:2264-70.
4. Quiroz-Olguin G, Gutierrez-Salmean G, Posadas-Calleja JG, et al. The effect of enteral stimulation on the immune response of the intestinal mucosa and its application in nutritional support. Eur J Clin Nutr 2021;75:1533-9.
5. Alpers DH. Enteral feeding and gut atrophy. Curr Opin Clin Nutr Metab Care 2002;5:679-83.
6. Jabbar A, Chang WK, Dryden GW, McClave SA. Gut immunology and the differential response to feeding and starvation. Nutr Clin Pract 2003;18:461-82.

7. Ohta K, Omura K, Hirano K, et al. The effects of an additive small amount of a low residual diet against total parenteral nutrition-induced gut mucosal barrier. Am J Surg 2003;185:79-85.
8. Wiest R, Rath HC. Gastrointestinal disorders of the critically ill. Bacterial translocation in the gut. Best Pract Res Clin Gastroenterol 2003;17:397-425.
9. Alverdy JC, Aoys E, Moss GS. Total parenteral nutrition promotes bacterial translocation from the gut. Surgery 1988;104:185-90.
10. Taylor BE, McClave SA, Martindale RG, et al. Guidelines for the provision and assessment of nutrition support therapy in the adult critically ill patient: Society of Critical Care Medicine (SCCM) and American Society for Parenteral and Enteral Nutrition (A.S.P.E.N.). Crit Care Med 2016;44:390-438.
11. Lefton J, Esper DH, Kochevar M. Enteral formulations. In: Gottschlich MM, ed. *The ASPEN Nutrition Support Core Curriculum*. American Society for Parenteral and Enteral Nutrition; 2017: 209-32.
12. Vinelli V, Biscotti P, Martini D, et al. Effects of dietary fibers on short-chain fatty acids and gut microbiota composition in healthy adults: a systematic review. Nutrients 2022;14.
13. Gregory AL, Pensinger DA, Hryckowian AJ. A short chain fatty acid-centric view of *Clostridioides difficile* pathogenesis. PLoS Pathog 2021;17:e1009959.
14. Heyland DK, Novak F, Drover JW, et al. Should immunonutrition become routine in critically ill patients? A systematic review of the evidence. JAMA 2001;286:944-53.
15. Karlic H, Lohninger A. Supplementation of L-carnitine in athletes: does it make sense? Nutrition 2004;20:709-15.
16. Kirk SJ, Barbul A. Role of arginine in trauma, sepsis, and immunity. JPEN J Parenter Enteral Nutr 1990;14:226S-9S.
17. van Zanten AR, Dhaliwal R, Garrel D, Heyland DK. Enteral glutamine supplementation in critically ill patients: a systematic review and meta-analysis. Crit Care 2015;19:294.
18. Bertolini G, Iapichino G, Radrizzani D, et al. Early enteral immunonutrition in patients with severe sepsis: results of an interim analysis of a randomized multicentre clinical trial. Intensive Care Med 2003;29:834-40.
19. Lee HY, Lee JK, Kim HJ, et al. Continuous versus intermittent enteral tube feeding for critically ill patients: a prospective, randomized controlled trial. Nutrients 2022;14.
20. Stroud M, Duncan H, Nightingale J, for the British Society of Gastroenterology. Guidelines for enteral feeding in adult hospital patients. Gut 2003;52 suppl 7:vii1-vii12.
21. Marik PE, Zaloga GP. Gastric versus post-pyloric feeding: a systematic review. Crit Care 2003;7:R46-51.

22. Fisman DN, Ward ME. Intrapleural placement of a nasogastric tube: an unusual complication of nasotracheal intubation. Can J Anaesth 1996;43:1252-6.
23. Kolbitsch C, Pomaroli A, Lorenz I, et al. Pneumothorax following nasogastric feeding tube insertion in a tracheostomized patient after bilateral lung transplantation. Intensive Care Med 1997;23:440-2.
24. Baskin WN. Acute complications associated with bedside placement of feeding tubes. Nutr Clin Pract 2006;21:40-55.
25. Mizock BA. Avoiding common errors in nutritional management. Journal of Critical Illness 1993;8:1116.
26. McCartt J, Loszko A, Backes K, et al. Improving enteral nutrition delivery in the critically ill trauma and surgical population. JPEN J Parenter Enteral Nutr 2022;46:1191-7.
27. Marcuard SP, Perkins AM. Clogging of feeding tubes. JPEN J Parenter Enteral Nutr 1988;12:403-5.
28. Marcuard SP, Stegall KS. Unclogging feeding tubes with pancreatic enzyme. JPEN J Parenter Enteral Nutr 1990;14:198-200.
29. Reignier J, Mercier E, Le Gouge A, et al. Effect of not monitoring residual gastric volume on risk of ventilator-associated pneumonia in adults receiving mechanical ventilation and early enteral feeding: a randomized controlled trial. JAMA 2013;309:249-56.
30. McClave SA, DeMeo MT, DeLegge MH, et al. North American Summit on Aspiration in the Critically Ill Patient: consensus statement. JPEN J Parenter Enteral Nutr 2002;26:S80-5.
31. Stojek M, Jasinski T. Gastroparesis in the intensive care unit. Anaesthesiol Intensive Ther 2021;53:450-5.
32. Booth CM, Heyland DK, Paterson WG. Gastrointestinal promotility drugs in the critical care setting: a systematic review of the evidence. Crit Care Med 2002;30:1429-35.
33. Hawkyard CV, Koerner RJ. The use of erythromycin as a gastrointestinal prokinetic agent in adult critical care: benefits versus risks. J Antimicrob Chemother 2007;59:347-58.
34. Saljoughian M. A new approach to managing gastroparesis. US Pharm 2019;44:32-4.
35. Nguyen NQ, Chapman M, Fraser RJ, et al. Prokinetic therapy for feed intolerance in critical illness: one drug or two? Crit Care Med 2007;35:2561-7.
36. Shaikh N, Nainthramveetil MM, Nawaz S, et al. Optimal dose and duration of enteral erythromycin as a prokinetic: a surgical intensive care experience. Qatar Med J 2020;2020:36.
37. Nguyen NQ, Chapman MJ, Fraser RJ, et al. Erythromycin is more effective than metoclopramide in the treatment of feed intolerance in critical illness. Crit Care Med 2007;35:483-9.

38. Isola S, Hussain A, Dua A, et al. Metoclopramide. In: StatPearls. Treasure Island (FL): StatPearls Publishing; 2024.
39. Edes TE, Walk BE, Austin JL. Diarrhea in tube-fed patients: feeding formula not necessarily the cause. Am J Med 1990;88:91-3.
40. Williams NT. Medication administration through enteral feeding tubes. Am J Health Syst Pharm 2008;65:2347-57.

Parenteral Nutrition

Chapter 48

Fundamentally, the indication for parenteral nutrition (PN) is the inability to support the nutritional needs of a patient using the gastrointestinal (GI) tract (1-2). This inability can be due to a variety of causes, a few examples being bowel in discontinuity, anastomotic leak, prolonged ileus, short bowel syndrome, enteric fistulas, and high-dose vasopressors. This chapter describes the basic features of intravenous nutritional support and discusses total parenteral nutrition (TPN), peripheral parenteral nutrition (PPN), and supplemental parenteral nutrition (SPN).

MACRONUTRIENT SOLUTIONS

Dextrose Solutions

Carbohydrates are the main source of nonprotein calories of PN, and dextrose (glucose) is the carbohydrate source in PN. Typical dextrose solutions are shown in Table 48.1. Osmolarity will become important in the discussion of PPN later.

Because the energy yield from dextrose is relatively low (3.4 kcal/g), the dextrose solutions must be concentrated to provide enough calories to satisfy daily requirements.

Five percent dextrose in water (D_5W) is typically used for hypoglycemia, dehydration, and as "free water" for hypernatremia. It also aids in minimizing hepatic glycogen depletion and has a protein-sparing effect in patients who are not receiving nutritional support (3).

D_5W can be combined with other standard common crystalloids, e.g., lactated ringers, normal saline, or half normal saline in maintenance fluids.

$D_{10}W$ is also a source of dextrose and free water and is frequently used as a "bridge" to prevent hypoglycemia when TPN is temporarily paused. $D_{50}W$ is packaged in a prefilled

TABLE 48.1 Intravenous Dextrose Solutions

Solution	Strength	Concentration (g/L)	Energy Yield* (kcal/L)	Osmolarity (mOsm/L)
D_5W	5%	50	170	253
$D_{10}W$	10%	100	340	505
$D_{50}W$	50%	500	1,700	2,525
$D_{70}W$	70%	700	2,380	3,530

*Based on an oxidative energy yield of 3.4 kcal/g for dextrose.

syringe (25 g/50 mL) and is used for rapid infusion for the treatment of symptomatic hypoglycemia.

$D_{70}W$ is a very hyperosmolar solution and must be infused into the central venous circulation. It is typically mixed with electrolytes, lipid emulsions, and amino acid solutions for "total" nutritional support: carbohydrates, protein, and micronutrients

Amino Acid Solutions

Protein is provided as amino acid solutions that contain varying mixtures of essential (N = 9), semi-essential (N = 4), and nonessential (N = 10) amino acids. These solutions are mixed with dextrose solutions to balance caloric and protein needs.

Standard and specialized amino acid solutions are available, e.g., high branched-chain amino acid mixtures; however, there is no evidence to support these products over standard amino acid solutions (1).

Standard Solutions

Standard amino acid solutions (e.g., 20% ProSol [Baxter Healthcare Corp, Deerfield, IL]) are balanced mixtures of 50% essential amino acids and 50% nonessential and semi-essential amino acids. These can be combined with dextrose solutions and electrolytes to create a custom parenteral infusion based on a patient's individual needs.

Specialty Solutions

Specially designed amino acid solutions have been formulated for patients with severe metabolic stress (e.g., multisystem trauma or burns) and for patients with renal or liver failure. Solutions with enriched branch-chained amino acids have not been shown to improve outcomes in critically ill patients with liver disease (1,4). Renal failure solutions are rich in essential amino acids because the nitrogen in essential amino acids is partially recycled to produce nonessential amino acids, which results in smaller increments in blood urea nitrogen (BUN) than seen with the breakdown of nonessential amino acids. Similarly, renal failure solutions have not improved outcomes (1,4).

Renal insufficiency/failure does have an impact on the clearance of the breakdown products of amino acid metabolism and should be dosed accordingly (1,5). See Table 48.2.

TABLE 48.2   Amino Acid Dosing in Renal Failure

Patient Status	Dosage
Unstressed healthy patient	1 g/kg/day
Acute kidney injury	0.6-0.8 g/kg/day
Chronic renal failure	0.8-1 g/kg/day
Hemodialysis	1.2-1.5 g/kg/day
CRRT	1.3-2 g/kg/day

CRRT = continuous renal replacement therapy.

Glutamine

Glutamine is the principal metabolic fuel for rapidly dividing cells like intestinal epithelial cells and vascular endothelial cells (6). However, several meta-analyses showed increased mortality in patients receiving intravenous glutamine (2,7). Current guidelines on nutrition support do *not* recommend IV glutamine for PN regimens (2).

Lipid Emulsions

Lipids are provided as emulsions composed of cholesterol, phospholipids, and triglycerides (8). The triglycerides are derived from vegetable oils (safflower or soybean oils) and are rich in linoleic acid, an essential fatty acid (9).

Lipids are used to provide 30% of daily calorie requirements, and 4% of the daily calories should be provided as linoleic acid to prevent essential fatty acid deficiency (10). The 10% emulsions provide about 1 kcal/mL, and the 20% emulsions provide 2 kcal/mL. Unlike the hypertonic dextrose solutions, lipid emulsions are roughly isotonic to plasma and *can be infused through peripheral veins.*

Lipid emulsions are available in unit volumes of 50 to 500 mL and can be infused separately (at a maximum rate of 50 mL/h) or added to the dextrose–amino acid mixtures.

The infused triglycerides are not cleared for 8-10 h, and lipid infusions often produce a transient lipemic appearance in plasma. Lipids were commonly added directly to TPN admixtures (multi-compounding); however, some nutrients have a destabilizing effect on lipid emulsion, thus lipids are infused separately for custom parenteral regimens (1). Similar to the specialized "anti-inflammatory" enteral regimens, specialized anti-inflammatory lipid emulsions, e.g., containing omega-3 fatty acids, have not demonstrated clinical outcome improvement and are not currently recommended (2).

MICRONUTRIENTS

Commercially available mixtures of electrolytes, vitamins, and trace elements are added directly to the dextrose–amino acid mixtures.

Electrolytes

Typical daily parenteral electrolyte requirements are listed in Table 48.3.

TABLE 48.3 Typical Daily Parenteral Electrolyte Requirements

Electrolyte	Parenteral Requirement
Sodium	60-100 mEq/day
Potassium	60-100 mEq/day
Chloride/acetate	Adjusted to maintain acid-base balance
Calcium	10-15 mEq/day
Phosphorus	20-40 mmol/day
Magnesium	8-20 mEq/day

PN ultimately will be tailored based on individual patient needs. In addition, the chloride-to-acetate ratio can affect the acid/base status of a patient. Clinical monitoring of fluid status along with laboratory monitoring of electrolytes and acid/base status will help guide day-to-day fluid volume, electrolyte, and acid/base needs of the PN. For example, GI fluid losses, i.e., high nasogastric tube output, enteric fistulas, diarrhea, refeeding syndrome can lead to alterations requiring adjustments in the daily PN orders. Laboratory monitoring is essential for the appropriate administration of PN. The frequency should be daily in critical illness and lessened based on the stability of clinical circumstances.

Recommended laboratory monitoring for PN is listed in Table 48.4.

Vitamins

Aqueous multivitamin preparations are added to the dextrose–amino acid mixtures. One vial of a standard multivitamin preparation will provide the normal daily requirements for most vitamins in healthy adults. The daily vitamin requirement in intensive care unit (ICU) patients is not known (and probably varies with each patient), but vitamin deficiencies can be common in ICU patients despite the provision of normal daily requirements.

TABLE 48.4 Recommended Laboratory Monitoring for PN

Parameter	Baseline	Initiation	Critically Ill Patients	Stable Patients
CBC with differential	Yes		Weekly	
Na, K, Cl, CO_2, Mg, Ca, Phos	Yes	Daily × 3	Daily	Weekly
BUN, creatinine	Yes	Daily × 3	Daily	Weekly
Serum glucose	Yes	Daily × 3	Daily	Weekly
ALT, AST, ALP, total bilirubin	Yes	Day 1	Weekly	Monthly
Serum triglycerides	Yes	Day 1	Weekly	Monthly

ALP = alkaline phosphatase; ALT = alanine aminotransferase; AST = aspartate aminotransferase; Ca = calcium; BUN = blood urea nitrogen; Cl = chloride; CO_2, bicarbonate; K = potassium; Mg = magnesium; Na = sodium; Phos = phosphorus; PN = parenteral nutrition.

Trace Elements

Since the second edition, significant advancements in the role and dosages of trace elements have occurred (11). As the name infers, trace elements are present in very small amounts in humans. However, they have diverse and important roles in human physiology and metabolism.

Trace elements are typically added to PN as a fixed-dose combination solution or can be added as single-entity doses.

Single-entity doses can be added in those patients with increased needs, e.g., GI losses and burns.

Of the fixed-dose combination options Tralement® was the first U.S. Food and Drug Administration (FDA)-approved multitrace element injection and was also approved by the American Society for Parenteral and Enteral Nutrition (ASPEN) (11). See Table 48.5.

TABLE 48.5 Tralement Trace Elements Injection*

Tralement Dosage (mL)	Zinc	Copper	Manganese	Selenium
1 mL	3 mg	0.3 mg	55 µg	60 µg

*Recommended daily dosage (at least 50 kg).

Conspicuously, chromium is not included, and selenium has been added, although in the past, selenium was not routinely added to combination trace element injections. It was determined that chromium is a common contaminant in most parenteral solutions and that would satisfy the daily estimated requirement.

Selenium has antioxidant properties through actions with glutathione peroxidase, is an important cofactor in DNA synthesis, and is decreased in inflammatory states. Now ASPEN recommends its routine use in PN (11-12).

WHEN TO START PN

PN does not offer the same benefits described for enteral tube feedings (Chapter 47: Enteral Nutrition) and can be withheld for 7 days in patients who are well nourished (13). In malnourished patients (who are unable to receive tube feedings), it should be started within 24 h of ICU admission, see Chapter 32: Lactic Acidosis and Ketoacidosis.

Creating a PN Regimen for the Critically Ill Patient

PN is the formulation combining the macronutrients and micronutrients with consideration of volume into an injectable solution. The components of PN can be found in Table 48.6.

TABLE 48.6 Components of PN

Macronutrients	Micronutrients
Intravenous dextrose solution	Electrolytes
Amino acid solutions	Vitamins
Lipid emulsions	Trace elements

PN = parenteral nutrition.

The following is a stepwise approach to creating a standard PN regimen.

Step 1

The initial task is to determine the daily requirement for calories and protein. The following simple approximations can be used:

$$\text{Daily Calories} = 25 \times \text{weight (kg)} \quad (48.1)$$

$$\text{Daily Protein} = 1.2\text{-}2 \text{ g/kg} \quad (48.2)$$

Actual or dry body weight is used in these estimates.

Example: For an adult with a dry body weight of 70 kg, the daily requirement for calories is $25 \times 70 = 1,750$ kcal/day. Using a protein requirement of 1.4 g/kg/day, the daily protein requirement is $1.4 \times 70 = 98$ g/day. *Note:* If propofol is being used for sedation, the daily caloric requirement should be adjusted because propofol is infused in a lipid emulsion with a caloric density of about 1 kcal/mL.

Step 2

Determine micronutrient needs. The initial electrolytes are added based on typical daily requirements. These can be modified based on the patient's current electrolyte and acid/base condition. Aqueous vitamins and trace elements are added in standardized combination preparations. Specific additional vitamins and/or trace elements are added based on individual needs.

Step 3

The next step is to determine how much lipid emulsion to infuse daily. Lipids should provide 20-30% of *total* daily caloric needs but should not exceed 1 g/kg/day (1). Again, lipid calories need to include any propofol intake.

Step 4

The final consideration for PN is the contribution to the overall fluid balance of the patient. Typical PN volumes are approximately 2,000 mL/day to provide daily maintenance fluid volume. Critically ill patients, however, can have a wide range of fluid intake and losses (Table 48.7) that need to be considered in the final concentration (osmolarity) and total volume of the daily PN.

TABLE 48.7 Volume Considerations for PN

Intake	Output
IV meds *Example: antibiotics* IV infusions *Examples: vasopressors, inotropes, analgesics, sedatives, antiarrhythmics*	• Oliguria/anuria • Fistulas • Emesis • Drains • Chest tubes • Blood loss

PN = parenteral nutrition.

PN regimens are compounded in the pharmacy and commonly overseen by nutrition support services. Oversight by the clinical ICU service is paramount to ensure appropriate monitoring of not only the laboratories but also the clinical progress of the patient.

COMPLICATIONS

Catheter-Related Complications

The hyperosmolarity of TPN requires infusion into the central venous circulation, so central venous cannulation, or a peripherally inserted central catheter (PICC), is required. Complications related to the insertion of these catheters are described in Chapter 9: The Pulmonary Artery Catheter.

Specific to TPN, the most common catheter-related complications are catheter occlusion and central line-associated blood stream infections (CLABSI) (14-15).

Precipitation of electrolytes and de-emulsification of lipids (clumping) are likely culprits to nonthrombotic occlusion owing to the importance of pharmacy oversight in compounding TPN.

Restoration of flow due to thrombotic catheter occlusion is done with the instillation of 2 mg of tissue plasminogen activator (TPA). Cathflo® Activase® (Genetech, San Francisco, CA) is the only TPA product approved by the FDA for the restoration of flow in occluded central venous catheters. Several prospective studies have demonstrated a >80% success rate with return of flow (14,16). If unsuccessful, further investigation to evaluate the central venous patency is warranted.

MACRONUTRIENT/MICRONUTRIENT COMPLICATIONS

Hyperglycemia

Hyperglycemia is common during PN, but tight glycemic control is not recommended in critically ill patients because of the risk of hypoglycemia, which is more deleterious than hyperglycemia (17-18). *The current recommendation of the nutrition support guidelines is a target range of 140-180 mg/dL for plasma glucose in the general ICU population* (19). Tighter glycemic control is recommended for patients with acute brain injury from cardiac arrest, ischemic stroke, or intracranial hemorrhage (17,20) because hyperglycemia can aggravate the brain injury in these patients.

Hypophosphatemia

Phosphorus is the critical substrate of energy (adenosine triphosphate [ATP]) and is rapidly depleted when nutrition is reinstituted in malnourished and catabolic patients (21).

The movement of glucose into cells is associated with a similar movement of phosphate into cells, and plasma phosphate levels typically show a steady decline after PN is initiated.

Hypokalemia

Glucose movement into cells is also accompanied by an intracellular shift of potassium, and continuous infusions of glucose during PN can lead to persistent hypokalemia.

Lipid Complications

Hypertriglyceridemia may contribute to hepatic dysfunction. A frequently overlooked feature of lipid infusions is the potential to *promote inflammation*. The lipid emulsions used in PN regimens are rich in oxidizable lipids (22), and the oxidation of infused lipids will trigger an inflammatory response. In fact, infusions of oleic acid, one of the lipids in PN, are a standard method for producing the acute respiratory distress syndrome (ARDS) in animals (23), and this might explain why *lipid infusions are associated with impaired oxygenation and prolonged respiratory failure* (24-25). Triglyceride levels >400 mg/dL should prompt a reduced dosage or discontinuation (1).

Hepatobiliary Complications

Hepatic Steatosis

Fat accumulation in the liver (hepatic steatosis) is common in patients receiving long-term PN and is believed to be the result of chronic overfeeding with carbohydrates and lipids. This condition is associated with elevated liver enzymes (26), but it may not be a pathological entity.

Cholestasis

The presence of lipids in the proximal small bowel stimulates cholecystokinin-mediated bile flow and contraction of the gallbladder.

PN can lead to bile stasis, elevated liver enzymes, and the accumulation of sludge in the gallbladder. Acalculous cholecystitis can result, and long-term cholestasis from PN can lead to cirrhosis and hepatic failure (27).

PERIPHERAL PARENTERAL NUTRITION

PPN is a limited form of PN infused through peripheral veins. It has limited macronutrient composition to reduce the osmolarity restrictions of peripheral venous access which must be <900 mOsm/L (1,28). PPN is typically used for short-term nutritional support in selected high-risk patient populations without a central venous catheter or is used as "supplemental" PN (SPN) in addition to enteral feedings (29-30). Guidelines by the Society of Critical Care Medicine and ASPEN recommend SPN be considered in patients unable to meet >60% of their energy and protein needs enterally (2). SPN may have reduced nosocomial infections and mortality (29,31-32).

References

1. Berlana D. Parenteral nutrition overview. Nutrients 2022;14:4480.
2. McClave SA, Taylor BE, Martindale RG, et al. Guidelines for the provision and assessment of nutrition support therapy in the adult critically ill patient: Society of Critical Care Medicine (SCCM) and American Society for Parenteral and Enteral Nutrition (A.S.P.E.N.). JPEN J Parenter Enteral Nutr 2016;40:159-211.
3. Thomas DD, Istfan NW, Bistrian BR, Apovian CM. Protein sparing therapies in acute illness and obesity: a review of george blackburn's contributions to nutrition science. Metabolism 2018;79:83-96.
4. Andris DA, Krzywda EA. Nutrition support in specific diseases: back to basics. Nutr Clin Pract 1994;9:28-32.
5. Fiaccadori E, Regolisti G, Maggiore U. Specialized nutritional support interventions in critically ill patients on renal replacement therapy. Curr Opin Clin Nutr Metab Care 2013;16:217-24.
6. Souba WW, Klimberg VS, Plumley DA, et al. The role of glutamine in maintaining a healthy gut and supporting the metabolic response to injury and infection. J Surg Res 1990;48:383-91.
7. Sun Y, Zhu S, Li S, Liu H. Glutamine on critical-ill patients: a systematic review and meta-analysis. Ann Palliat Med 2021;10:1503-20.
8. Driscoll DF. Compounding TPN admixtures: then and now. JPEN J Parenter Enteral Nutr 2003;27:433-8; quiz 9.

9. Warshawsky KY. Intravenous fat emulsions in clinical practice. Nutr Clin Pract 1992;7:187-96.
10. Barr LH, Dunn GD, Brennan MF. Essential fatty acid deficiency during total parenteral nutrition. Ann Surg 1981;193:304-11.
11. Perks P, Huynh E, Kaluza K, Boullata JI. Advances in trace element supplementation for parenteral nutrition. Nutrients 2022;14.
12. American Society for Parenteral and Enteral Nutrition. Important facts about parenteral selenium (selenious acid). Accessed August 11 2024. https://nutritioncare.org/wp-content/uploads/2024/12/Important-Facts-Parenteral-Selenium.pdf
13. Taylor BE, McClave SA, Martindale RG, et al. Guidelines for the provision and assessment of nutrition support therapy in the adult critically ill patient: Society of Critical Care Medicine (SCCM) and American Society for Parenteral and Enteral Nutrition (A.S.P.E.N.). Crit Care Med 2016;44:390-438.
14. Buchman AL. Catheter-related complications of total parenteral nutrition. American Journal of Gastroenterology 2007;102:S97-S101.
15. Fonseca G, Burgermaster M, Larson E, Seres DS. The relationship between parenteral nutrition and central line-associated bloodstream infections: 2009-2014. JPEN J Parenter Enteral Nutr 2018;42:171-5.
16. Jafari N, Seidl E, Dancsecs K. Evaluation of alteplase 1 mg for the restoration of occluded central venous access devices in a tertiary care hospital. J Assoc Vasc Access 2018;23:51-5.
17. Jacobi J, Bircher N, Krinsley J, et al. Guidelines for the use of an insulin infusion for the management of hyperglycemia in critically ill patients. Crit Care Med 2012;40:3251-76.
18. Marik PE, Preiser JC. Toward understanding tight glycemic control in the ICU: a systematic review and metaanalysis. Chest 2010;137:544-51.
19. Chawla R, Gangopadhyay KK, Lathia TB, et al. Management of hyperglycemia in critical care. J Diabetol 2022;13:33-42.
20. American College of Surgeons. Best practices guidelines in the management of traumatic brain injury. Accessed August 15, 2024. https://www.facs.org/media/vgfgjpfk/best-practices-guidelines-traumatic-brain-injury.pdf
21. Wong GJY, Pang JGT, Li YY, Lew CCH. Refeeding hypophosphatemia in patients receiving parenteral nutrition: prevalence, risk factors, and predicting its occurrence. Nutr Clin Pract 2021;36:679-88.
22. Carpentier YA, Dupont IE. Advances in intravenous lipid emulsions. World J Surg 2000;24:1493-7.
23. Schuster DP. ARDS: clinical lessons from the oleic acid model of acute lung injury. Am J Respir Crit Care Med 1994;149:245-60.
24. Boscarino G, Conti MG, De Luca F, et al. Intravenous lipid emulsions affect respiratory outcome in preterm newborn: a case-control study. Nutrients 2021;13.

25. Suchner U, Katz DP, Furst P, et al. Effects of intravenous fat emulsions on lung function in patients with acute respiratory distress syndrome or sepsis. Crit Care Med 2001;29:1569-74.
26. Freund HR. Abnormalities of liver function and hepatic damage associated with total parenteral nutrition. Nutrition 1991;7:1-6.
27. Nowak K. Parenteral nutrition-associated liver disease. Clin Liver Dis (Hoboken) 2020;15:59-62.
28. Hamdan M, Puckett Y. Total parenteral nutrition. [Updated 2023 Jul 4]. In: StatPearls [Internet]. Treasure Island (FL): StatPearls Publishing; 2025 Jan-. Available from: https://www.ncbi.nlm.nih.gov/books/NBK559036/.
29. Alsharif DJ, Alsharif FJ, Aljuraiban GS, Abulmeaty MMA. Effect of supplemental parenteral nutrition versus enteral nutrition alone on clinical outcomes in critically ill adult patients: a systematic review and meta-analysis of randomized controlled trials. Nutrients 2020;12.
30. Russell MK, Wischmeyer PE. Supplemental parenteral nutrition: review of the literature and current nutrition guidelines. Nutr Clin Pract 2018;33:359-69.
31. Inayat-Hussain A, Falck H, Oorschot S, et al. Peripheral parenteral nutrition: an evaluation of its use, safety and cost implications in a tertiary hospital setting. Clin Nutr ESPEN 2023;56:215-21.
32. Sim J, Hong J, Na EM, et al. Early supplemental parenteral nutrition is associated with reduced mortality in critically ill surgical patients with high nutritional risk. Clin Nutr 2021;40:5678-83.

Adrenal and Thyroid Dysfunction

CRITICAL ILLNESS-RELATED CORTICOSTEROID INSUFFICIENCY

Adrenal Suppression in Critical Illness

In 2008, the term *critical illness-related corticosteroid insufficiency* (CIRCI) was coined to describe the hypothalamic-pituitary-adrenal impairment that occurs during critical illness (1). This is differentiated from "adrenal crisis" which is a state of a preexisting intrinsic hypothalamic-pituitary-adrenal axis disease triggered by acute illness (2). The incidence of CIRCI for intensive care unit (ICU) admissions can be as high as 30%, with specific diagnoses such as sepsis and trauma with an incidence of up to 70% (3-5).

CIRCI encompasses three major pathophysiologic mechanisms (6):

1. Dysregulation of the hypothalamic-pituitary-adrenal axis
2. Altered cortisol metabolism
3. Tissue resistance to glucocorticoids

Figure 49.1 depicts some known inciting factors and foci for these mechanisms. Clearly, the ubiquitous systemic inflammatory response of the critically ill patient plays a major role, explaining the prevalence of CIRCI in the ICU.

Drug-Induced Adrenal Insufficiency

A recent review of the Federal Food and Drug Administration Adverse Event Reporting System (FAERS) has uncovered a heterogenous spectrum of drug classes reported as drug-induced adrenal insufficiency adverse events (7). Table 49.1 shows a list

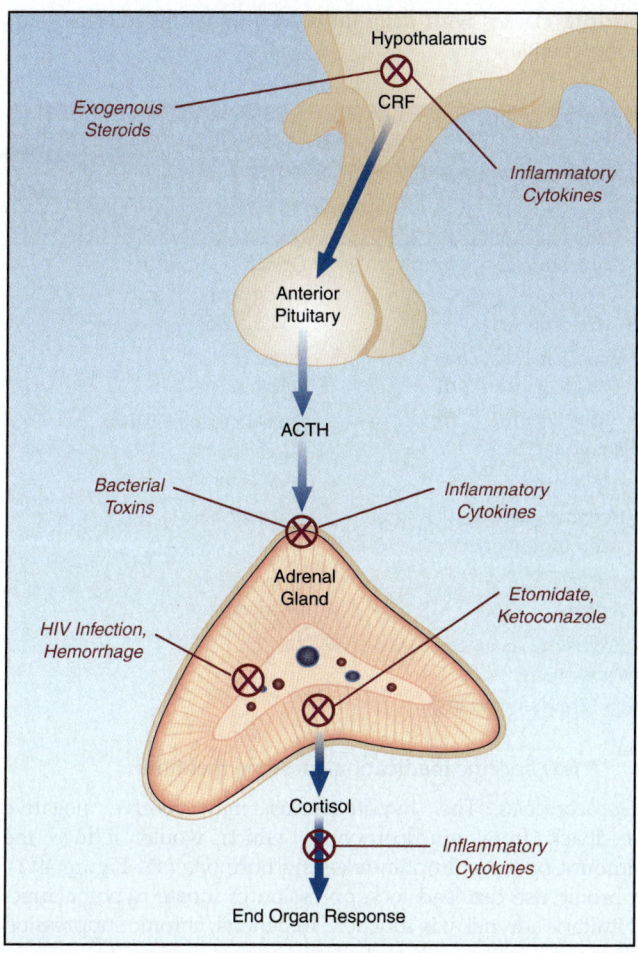

FIGURE 49.1. Mechanisms of adrenal suppression in ICU patients. CRF = corticotrophin-releasing hormone; ACTH = adrenocorticotrophic hormone. (From Adrenal and Thyroid Dysfunction. In: Marino PL. *Marino's The ICU Book*. 5th ed. Wolters Kluwer; 2025:768-78. Figure 51.1.)

of drug classes with drug-induced adrenal insufficiency adverse events.

TABLE 49.1 Drug Classes* Reported to the FAERS with at Least 20 Cases Reported as Primary Suspect for Drug-Induced Adrenal Insufficiency

Glucocorticoids
- Prednisone
- Hydrocortisone

Monoclonal antibodies
- Tocilizumab
- Ipilimumab

β-2 agonist
- Salmeterol

Hormone therapy
- Levothyroxine
- Megestrol

Antivirals
- Ritonavir

Opioids
- Morphine
- Methadone

Antibiotics
- Rifampicin

Protein kinase inhibitors
- Axitinib
- Cabozantinib

Bisphosphates

Triazole antifungals
- Fluconazole
- Voriconazole

*With examples.
From References 7 and 10.

A few specific medications deserve mention:

Glucocorticoids. The hypothalamus may receive negative feedback from glucocorticoids, which would reduce the amount of corticotrophin-releasing hormone (see Figure 49.1). Chronic use can lead to suppression of innate hypothalamic-pituitary-adrenal axis function. In general, chronic suppression does not develop with acute corticosteroid therapy (8).

Patients who take chronic corticosteroids only require maintenance dosing but do not require "stress dose" steroids if asymptomatic (9). A recent study suggests 5 mg/day of prednisolone or equivalent for 4 weeks or longer should be considered a risk for CIRCI (2).

Opioids. Opioid-induced adrenal insufficiency (OIAI) is one of several opioid-induced endocrinopathies occurring in 9-29% of chronic users (10). The potential contribution to the risk of CIRCI should always be taken into account, because 2% of the population fills four or more opioid prescriptions each year (11).

Etomidate. A commonly used sedative in the ICU setting, etomidate can suppress the adrenal production of cortisol, and this has been reported after a single intubation dose (12). Its potential as a contributing risk factor for CIRCI should be suspected (see Figure 49.1).

Clinical Manifestations

Although the majority of the clinical signs and symptoms of CIRCI are nonspecific (Table 49.2), the standout manifestations include hypoxia and *hypotension that is refractory to volume resuscitation* (2,13). Notably, the typical laboratory abnormalities of adrenal insufficiency are rare in acute adrenal insufficiency and easily confounded by crystalloid fluid resuscitation (14).

TABLE 49.2 Clinical Signs and Symptoms of Critical Illness-Related Corticosteroid Insufficiency

General
- Fever
- Fatigue
- Weight loss
- Back and leg cramps

Neurological
- Somnolence
- Delirium
- Coma

Pulmonary
- Persistent hypoxia

Gastrointestinal
- Nausea
- Emesis
- Intolerance to enteral nutrition

Laboratory
- Eosinophilia
- Hyponatremia
- Hyperkalemia
- Hypoglycemia
- Non-gap metabolic acidosis

From References 3, 6, and Hamm LL, Ambühl PM, Alpern RJ. Role of glucocorticoids in acidosis. Am J Kidney Dis 1999;34(5):960-5.

Diagnosis

CIRCI should be suspected in any ICU patient with signs and symptoms consistent with adrenal insufficiency, unexplained hypoxia, refractory hypotension, or septic shock requiring high dose vasopressors (2-3). Unfortunately, the conventional diagnostic tests for adrenal insufficiency are impacted by a variety of physiologic factors (examples below) that occur during critical illness, making interpretation more suggestive than diagnostic.

Physiologic mechanisms for CIRCI

- CIRCI has normal or low plasma cortisol levels (2).
- Plasma corticotropin levels vary throughout critical illness.
- Low incremental cortisol levels are caused by increased cortisol distribution volume due to low plasma binding of cortisol (15).
- Tissue resistance to glucocorticoids (6)

Due to a lack of diagnostic certainty, treatment can be recommended combining clinical findings along with suggestive laboratory findings.

Treatment

Hydrocortisone

The treatment of CIRCI (not septic shock) is *intravenous hydrocortisone, 60 mg daily*, in two divided doses: 40 mg in the early morning and 20 mg in the evening, to replicate normal diurnal variation (2-3). The onset of effect for corticosteroids is 3-8 h (16). Hydrocortisone can be discontinued after satisfactory resolution of the predisposing condition. If the period of hydrocortisone therapy exceeds 7-10 days, a gradual taper of the dosage is recommended (1).

Methylprednisolone

CIRCI in moderate to severe ARDS is treated with *intravenous methylprednisolone* (1 mg/kg/day) (3), whereas refractory shock (unresponsive to fluids and vasopressors) is treated with high-dose hydrocortisone (200-400 mg/day in divided doses) (2-3,13).

Fludrocortisone

Early (retrospective) data regarding the addition of the mineralocorticoid, fludrocortisone (50 µg orally once daily) were promising. However, the multicenter randomized clinical trial, Fludrocortisone Dose–Response Relationships and Vascular Responsiveness in Septic Shock (FluDReSS), did not demonstrate a benefit (17).

EVALUATION OF THYROID FUNCTION

Transient changes in the hypothalamic-pituitary-thyroid (HPT) axis are present in 75% of hospitalized patients (18), resulting in abnormal laboratory tests of thyroid function for up to 90% of critically ill patients (19-21). In most cases, the abnormality is a consequence of nonthyroidal illness (i.e., *euthyroid sick syndrome*) and is not a sign of thyroid disease (21-22). This section describes the laboratory evaluation of thyroid function and how to distinguish nonthyroidal illness from thyroid disease.

Thyroxine and Triiodothyronine

Thyroxine (T_4) is the principal hormone secreted by the thyroid gland, but the active form is triiodothyronine (T_3), which is formed by deiodination of T_4 in extrathyroidal tissues.

T_3 and T_4 are extensively bound to plasma proteins, and <1% of either hormone is present in the free or biologically active form (20-23).

Because of the potential for alterations in plasma proteins and protein binding in acute illness, *free T_4 levels are used to evaluate thyroid function in acutely ill patients*. (Free T_3 levels are not routinely available.)

Thyroid-Stimulating Hormone

The plasma level of thyroid-stimulating hormone (TSH) is considered *the first-line test of thyroid function*; it is useful for identifying nonthyroidal illness and for distinguishing between primary and secondary thyroid disorders (20).

Plasma TSH levels are normal in a majority of patients with euthyroid sick syndrome (21). However, TSH secretion can be depressed by sepsis, corticosteroids, and dopamine infusions (24). In patients with hypothyroidism, an elevated plasma TSH level is evidence of primary hypothyroidism, while a reduced TSH level is evidence of secondary hypothyroidism (from hypothalamic–pituitary dysfunction).

Plasma TSH levels have a diurnal variation (with the lowest values in late afternoon and the highest values around the hour of sleep), and TSH levels can vary by as much as 40% over a 24-h period (25). This diurnal variation must be considered when interpreting plasma TSH levels.

Abnormal Thyroid Function Tests

Table 49.3 shows the expected changes in plasma free T_4 and TSH levels in specific conditions.

TABLE 49.3 Patterns of Abnormal Thyroid Function Tests

Condition	Free T_4	TSH
Normal range	0.8-1.8 ng/dL	0.3-4.5 mU/mL
Primary hyperthyroidism	↑	↑
T_3-toxicosis	NL	↓
Euthyroid hyperthyroxinemia	↑	NL
Primary hyperthyroidism	↓	↑
Secondary hypothyroidism	↓	↓
Euthyroid sick	↓	↓

NL = normal.

From Adrenal and Thyroid Dysfunction. In: Marino PL. *Marino's The ICU Book*. 5th ed. Wolters Kluwer; 2025:768-78. Table 51.2.

Acute, nonthyroidal illness is associated with low plasma levels of free T_3, which is the result of impaired conversion of T_4 to T_3 in nonthyroidal tissue (21). With increasing severity of illness, both free T_3 and free T_4 levels are depressed, which is the pattern reported in 30-50% of ICU patients (21-22). As mentioned earlier, plasma TSH levels are normal in a majority of patients with euthyroid sick syndrome.

Primary hypothyroidism is characterized by reciprocal changes in free T_4 and TSH levels, whereas in secondary hypothyroidism (from hypothalamic-pituitary dysfunction), both free T_4 and TSH levels are depressed.

THYROTOXICOSIS AND THYROID STORM

Thyrotoxicosis is a state of excessive T_4 and T_3 resulting in derangements across the spectrum of organ systems, whereas *thyroid storm* represents the extreme end of the spectrum of thyrotoxicosis, involving life-threatening organ-system involvement (26-27).

Clinical Manifestations

The clinical manifestations of thyrotoxicosis can affect all organ systems (27-28).

Elderly patients with hyperthyroidism can demonstrate depression rather than agitation; along with weight loss and signs of heart failure, this condition is called *apathetic thyrotoxicosis* (29). Table 49.4 shows signs and symptoms of thyrotoxicosis. The mortality rate for thyroid storm is 10-20% (26,30).

Diagnosis

Except for an enlarged gland, palpable anterior cervical nodule, or the classic proptosis of Graves syndrome, the majority of signs and symptoms are nonspecific. There are a number of scoring systems available (e.g., the Japanese Thyroid

Association and the Burch-Wartofsky Point Scale); however, these are functionally guidelines, and the diagnosis is based on laboratory analysis and clinical judgment (27).

- Free T_3 and free T_4 (serum levels) are elevated with suppressed TSH levels, with the rare exception of a TSH-secreting pituitary adenoma (26).
- A normal TSH level excludes the diagnosis of hyperthyroidism (31)

TABLE 49.4 Signs and Symptoms of Thyrotoxicosis

Symptoms		Signs	
Constitutional			
• Hyperthermia	• Weight loss	• Muscle wasting	
Neurological/psychological			
• Weakness	• Anxiety	• Tremors	• Psychosis
• Poor concentration	• Confusion	• Hyperreflexia	• Agitation
Cardiovascular			
• Palpitations	• Edema	• Atrial fibrillation	• High output heart failure
• Decreased appetite		• Tachyarrhythmias	
Gastrointestinal			
• Decreased appetite	• Diarrhea		
• Hyperdefecation			
Reproductive			
• Decreased libido	• Oligomenorrhea	• Gynecomastia	
Dermatologic			
• Hair loss		• Palmar erythema	• Vitiligo
		• Pretibial myxedema	
Adrenergic			
• Heat intolerance	• Hyperhidrosis	• Hyperthermia	
Ophthalmologic			
• Eye irritation	• Diplopia	• Exophthalmos	

Treatment

There are four major objectives in the acute pharmacologic management of thyrotoxicosis:

1. Control of the peripheral adrenergic effects of excess thyroid hormone
2. Inhibition of thyroid hormone synthesis
3. Inhibition of hormone release
4. Inhibition of peripheral conversion of T_4 to T_3

Table 49.5 shows the drug therapies for each objective. Note that several drugs affect more than one objective.

TABLE 49.5	Drug Therapy for Thyrotoxicosis and Thyroid Storm	
Objective	Drug	Dose
Control of peripheral adrenergic effects	Propranolol	10-40 mg PO TID for thyrotoxicosis; 60-80 mg IV or PO for thyroid storm
	Metoprolol	25-50 mg PO or IV TID
	Esmolol	Loading dose 500 µg/kg followed by 50 µg/kg/min titrating to effect
Inhibition of hormone synthesis	Propylthiouracil (PTU)	50-150 mg PO TID for thyrotoxicosis; 500-1000 mg PO loading dose followed by 250 mg PO Q4 h for thyroid storm
	Methimazole	20 mg PO Q6 h
Inhibition of hormone release	Iodine	5 drops saturated solution of potassium iodide (SSKI) PO Q6 h
		Should be administered 30 minutes after starting PTU
Inhibition of conversion of T_4 to T_3	Hydrocortisone	100 mg IV Q8 h

Aspirin is contraindicated due to the potential risk of increasing free T$_4$ by interfering with thyroid-binding protein (27).

Surgery may be required in selected cases but typically 5-7 days after treatment (27-28).

Special Concerns in Thyroid Storm

Aggressive volume resuscitation is often required in thyroid storm because of vomiting, diarrhea, and heightened insensible fluid loss.

Thyroid storm has been associated with relative adrenal insufficiency, further supporting empiric stress-dose hydrocortisone (28). However, the outcomes of hydrocortisone therapy have been mixed (28,32).

HYPOTHYROIDISM

Symptomatic hypothyroidism is uncommon, with a prevalence of only 0.3% in the general population (33). Most cases are the result of chronic autoimmune thyroiditis (Hashimoto thyroiditis), whereas less common causes include radioiodine or surgical treatment of hyperthyroidism, hypothalamic-pituitary dysfunction from tumors and hemorrhagic necrosis (Sheehan syndrome), and drugs (lithium, amiodarone).

Myxedema Coma

Myxedema coma is a life-threatening presentation of hypothyroidism initiated by a precipitating event such as infection, trauma, surgery, certain drugs (e.g., lithium, amiodarone), and many other clinical conditions (34). The name itself is a misnomer as the most common presentation is hypothermia, depressed level of consciousness, and cardiac instability. The process can progress to coma, but the typical presentation is lethargy. The nonpitting edema is a clinical sign of chronic hypothyroidism caused by buildup of mucopolysaccharides in the skin. Even with early diagnosis and treatment mortality is reported as high as 60% (34).

Clinical Manifestations

Table 49.6 demonstrates examples of the clinical manifestations of myxedema coma.

TABLE 49.6	Clinical Manifestations of Myxedema Coma	
System		
Neurologic	• Depression • Paranoia • Decreased deep tendon reflexes	• Lethargy • Psychosis • Seizures • Coma
Cardiovascular	• Bradycardia • Hypotension	• Heart block • Reduced cardiac output
Respiratory	• Hypoventilation • Decreased response to hypercapnia	• Sleep apnea (aggravated by macroglossia)
Gastrointestinal	• Nausea • Emesis	• Constipation • Ascites
Renal and electrolytes	• Hyponatremia	
Musculoskeletal	• Weight gain	• Myxedema

Contrary to popular perception, *obesity is not a consequence of hypothyroidism* (33).

Diagnosis

The changes in free T_4 and TSH levels in hypothyroidism are shown in Table 49.3. Serum T_3 levels can be normal in hypothyroidism, but free T_4 levels are always reduced (33). Serum TSH levels are increased (often >10 mU/dL) in primary hypothyroidism and are depressed in hypothyroidism from hypothalamic-pituitary dysfunction.

Treatment

Hydrocortisone

To avoid an acute adrenal crisis, 100 mg is administered intravenously prior to initiating thyroid replacement treatment. This is followed by 200-400 mg/day (in divided doses) (34).

Levothyroxine

The American Thyroid Association guidelines offer two options for initial replacement hormones (35):

1. Large-dose levothyroxine (300-500 µg IV); if no response, add T_3.
2. Initial IV dose 200-300 µg levothyroxine plus 10-25 mµ T_3

Because the conversion of T_4 to T_3 (the active form of thyroid hormone) can be depressed in critically ill patients (36), oral therapy with T_3 (25 µg every 12 h) can be used to supplement T_4 replacement in seriously ill patients (37). (T_3 can be given via nasogastric tube, if necessary.) Studies evaluating the benefits of T_3 supplementation have shown mixed results (33).

Treatment Caveat

The identification of an inciting event, such as sepsis is essential for a positive outcome.

References

1. Marik PE, Pastores SM, Annane D, et al. Recommendations for the diagnosis and management of corticosteroid insufficiency in critically ill adult patients: consensus statements from an international task force by the American College of Critical Care Medicine. Crit Care Med 2008;36:1937-49.
2. Teblick A, Gunst J, Van den Berghe G. Critical illness-induced corticosteroid insufficiency: what it is not and what it could be. J Clin Endocrinol Metab 2022;107:2057-64.
3. Fredrick FC, Meda AKR, Singh B, Jain R. Critical illness-related corticosteroid insufficiency: latest pathophysiology and management guidelines. Acute Crit Care 2024;39:331-40.

4. Haberlach M, Cedar C, McCague A. Empiric stress dose steroids in trauma patients: a case report of hypopituitarism in traumatic hemorrhage. J Emerg Trauma Shock 2019;12:61-3.
5. Marik PE. Adrenal insufficiency and CIRCI. In: *Handbook of Evidence-Based Critical Care*. Springer; 2010:427-34.
6. Annane D, Pastores SM, Arlt W, et al. Critical illness-related corticosteroid insufficiency (CIRCI): a narrative review from a Multispecialty Task Force of the Society of Critical Care Medicine (SCCM) and the European Society of Intensive Care Medicine (ESICM). Crit Care Med 2017;45(12):2089-98.
7. Raschi E, Fusaroli M, Massari F, et al. The changing face of drug-induced adrenal insufficiency in the Food and Drug Administration Adverse Event Reporting System. J Clin Endocrinol Metab 2022;107:e3107-e14.
8. Yasir M, Goyal A, Sonthalia S. Corticosteroid Adverse Effects. In: StatPearls. Treasure Island (FL): StatPearls Publishing; 2025.
9. Chilkoti GT, Singh A, Mohta M, Saxena AK. Perioperative "stress dose" of corticosteroid: pharmacological and clinical perspective. J Anaesthesiol Clin Pharmacol 2019;35:147-52.
10. Coluzzi F, LeQuang JAK, Sciacchitano S, et al. A closer look at opioid-induced adrenal insufficiency: a narrative review. Int J Mol Sci 2023;24.
11. Moriya AS, Fang Z. Any Use and "Frequent Use" of Opioids among Adults Aged 18–64 in 2020–2021, by Socioeconomic Characteristics. Statistical Brief (Medical Expenditure Panel Survey (US). Agency for Healthcare Research and Quality (US); 2001.
12. Thompson Bastin ML, Baker SN, Weant KA. Effects of etomidate on adrenal suppression: a review of intubated septic patients. Hosp Pharm 2014;49:177-83.
13. Annane D, Pastores SM, Rochwerg B, et al. Guidelines for the diagnosis and management of critical illness-related corticosteroid insufficiency (CIRCI) in critically ill patients (part I): Society of Critical Care Medicine (SCCM) and European Society of Intensive Care Medicine (ESICM) 2017. Crit Care Med 2017;45:2078-88.
14. Sobolewska J, Dzialach L, Kuca P, Witek P. Critical illness-related corticosteroid insufficiency (CIRCI)—an overview of pathogenesis, clinical presentation and management. Front Endocrinol (Lausanne) 2024;15:1473151.
15. Peeters B, Meersseman P, Vander Perre S, et al. Adrenocortical function during prolonged critical illness and beyond: a prospective observational study. Intensive Care Med 2018;44:1720-9.
16. Williams DM. Clinical pharmacology of corticosteroids. Respir Care 2018;63:655-70.
17. Walsham J, Hammond N, Blumenthal A, et al. Fludrocortisone dose-response relationship in septic shock: a randomised phase II trial. Intensive Care Med 2024;50:2050-60.

18. Ganesan K, Anastasopoulou C, Wadud K. Euthyroid Sick Syndrome. In: StatPearls. Treasure Island (FL): StatPearls Publishing; 2025.
19. Fliers E, Bianco AC, Langouche L, Boelen A. Thyroid function in critically ill patients. Lancet Diabetes Endocrinol 2015;3:816-25.
20. Soh SB, Aw TC. Laboratory testing in thyroid conditions --pitfalls and clinical utility. Ann Lab Med 2019;39:3-14.
21. Umpierrez GE. Euthyroid sick syndrome. South Med J 2002;95:506-13.
22. Peeters RP, Debaveye Y, Fliers E, Visser TJ. Changes within the thyroid axis during critical illness. Crit Care Clin 2006;22:41-55, vi.
23. Dayan CM. Interpretation of thyroid function tests. Lancet 2001;357:619-24.
24. Burman KD, Wartofsky L. Thyroid function in the intensive care unit setting. Crit Care Clin 2001;17:43-57.
25. Karmisholt J, Andersen S, Laurberg P. Variation in thyroid function tests in patients with stable untreated subclinical hypothyroidism. Thyroid 2008;18:303-8.
26. Carroll R, Matfin G. Endocrine and metabolic emergencies: thyroid storm. Ther Adv Endocrinol Metab 2010;1:139-45.
27. Pokhrel B, Aiman W, Bhusal K. Thyroid Storm. In: StatPearls. Treasure Island (FL): StatPearls Publishing; 2025.
28. Nayak B, Burman K. Thyrotoxicosis and thyroid storm. Endocrinol Metab Clin North Am 2006;35:663-86, vii.
29. Akivis Y, Kurnick A, Castro-Auvet P, McFarlane SI. Apathetic thyrotoxicosis presenting with new-onset pulmonary hypertension. Ann Intern Med Clin Cases 2023;2:e220946.
30. Furukawa Y, Tanaka K, Isozaki O, et al. Prospective multicenter registry-based study on thyroid storm: the guidelines for management from Japan are useful. J Clin Endocrinol Metab 2024;110:e87-e96.
31. Bahn Chair RS, Burch HB, Cooper DS, et al. Hyperthyroidism and other causes of thyrotoxicosis: management guidelines of the American Thyroid Association and American Association of Clinical Endocrinologists. Thyroid 2011;21:593-646.
32. Senda A, Endo A, Tachimori H, et al. Early administration of glucocorticoid for thyroid storm: analysis of a national administrative database. Crit Care 2020;24:470.
33. Garber JR, Cobin RH, Gharib H, et al. Clinical practice guidelines for hypothyroidism in adults: cosponsored by the American Association of Clinical Endocrinologists and the American Thyroid Association. Endocr Pract 2012;18:988-1028.
34. Elshimy G, Chippa V, Correa R. Myxedema. In: StatPearls. Treasure Island (FL): StatPearls Publishing; 2025.

35. Wiersinga WM. Myxedema and coma (severe hypothyroidism). In: Feingold KR, Anawalt B, Blackman MR, et al., editors. *Endotext*. MDText.com, Inc.; 2000.
36. Myers L, Hays J. Myxedema coma. Crit Care Clin 1991;7:43-56.
37. McCulloch W, Price P, Hinds CJ, Wass JA. Effects of low dose oral triiodothyronine in myxoedema coma. Intensive Care Med 1985;11:259-62.

SECTION XIII
OVERDOSES AND POISONS

Chapter 50
Pharmaceutical Drug Overdoses

This chapter addresses some of the most frequent and problematic pharmaceutical drug overdoses encountered in the ICU.

ACETAMINOPHEN

Acetaminophen is a ubiquitous analgesic-antipyretic agent that is also a hepatotoxin and is *the leading cause of acute liver failure in North America, Europe, and Australia* (1).

Toxic Mechanisms

The toxicity of acetaminophen is related to its metabolism in the liver, as shown in Figure 50.1. When the daily dose of acetaminophen is excessive, the conjugation pathway can become saturated (i.e., glutathione is depleted), and metabolism shifts to the pathway with toxic cysteine metabolites (2).

Toxic Dose

The toxic dose of acetaminophen varies in each individual patient but is usually between 7.5 and 15 g in most adults (3-4). Most poison centers use 10 g as a threshold dose that requires further investigation (5). The FDA advises that adults should not exceed 4 g/d (6), although some clinical practice guidelines recommend a lower total daily dose of 3 g/d (7).

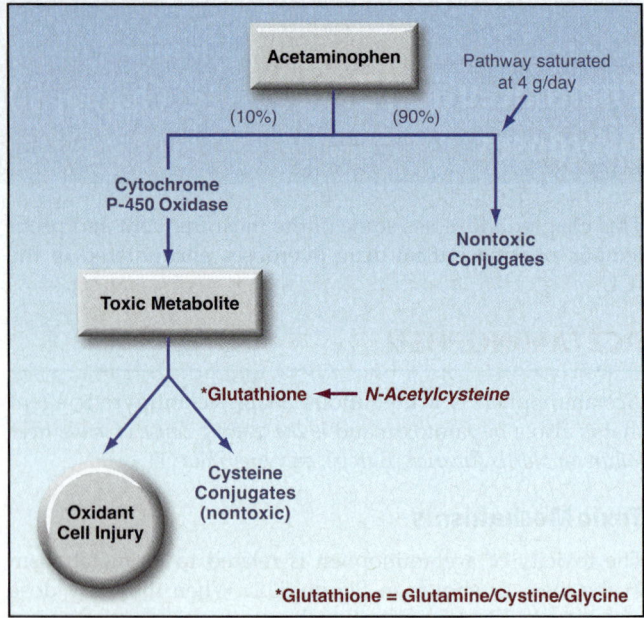

FIGURE 50.1. The hepatic metabolism of acetaminophen. (From Pharmaceutical Drug Overdoses. In: Marino PL. *Marino's The ICU Book,* 5e. Wolters Kluwer; 2025:781-95. Figure 52.2.)

Predisposing Conditions

The following conditions can increase the risk of liver damage from acetaminophen (5,8):

1. Malnutrition or prolonged periods of fasting, due to potential depletion of glutathione stores.
2. Chronic alcohol use disorder, even when daily acetaminophen doses are <4 g/d. This is likely due to the ability of alcohol to increase the activity of the cytochrome P450 enzyme, which is responsible for about 10% of acetaminophen metabolism. Chronic malnutrition is also frequently contributory with this disorder.

3. Drugs that stimulate cytochrome P450 activity (e.g., carbamazepine, phenytoin, isoniazid, rifampin). Opioids can also increase the risk by competing for the conjugation pathway (see Figure 50.1).

Clinical Presentation

Acetaminophen toxicity clinically manifests in three stages:

1. *Stage 1 (First 24 h)* : Symptoms are absent or nonspecific. There may be no laboratory evidence of hepatic injury.
2. *Stage 2 (24-72 h)*: Hepatic aminotransferases (aspartate aminotransferase [AST], alanine aminotransferase, [ALT]) begin to rise at 24 h, and can reach levels of 10,000 IU/L (9). Signs of progressive hepatic injury (e.g., jaundice and prolonged INR) begin to appear, and there may be signs of renal impairment.
3. *Stage 3 (72-96 h)*: The hepatic injury peaks. Hepatic encephalopathy is likely at this juncture, along with progressive lactic acidosis and acute, oliguric renal failure. Death from multiorgan failure can occur.

Risk Assessment

The evaluation of acetaminophen overdoses must include the following:

- Time and dose ingested
- Type of ingestion (acute overdose versus unintentional supratherapeutic dosing)
- Drug preparation (immediate vs. extended release)
- Presence of predisposing conditions
- Evidence of hepatic injury

If an overdose presents within 24 h of ingestion of an immediate-release preparation, the plasma acetaminophen level can be used to identify the need for N-acetylcysteine (NAC) therapy.

Predictive Nomogram

Plasma acetaminophen levels obtained from 4-24 h after an acute drug ingestion can be used to predict the risk of hepatotoxicity using the nomogram in Figure 50.2 (10).

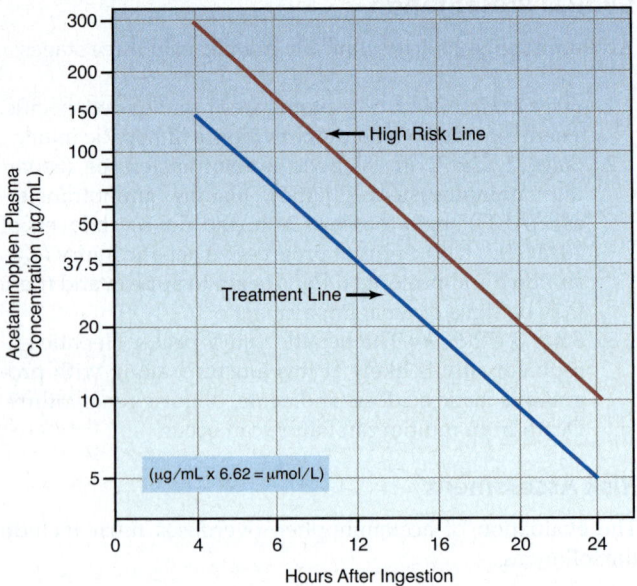

FIGURE 50.2. Nomogram for predicting the risk of hepatotoxicity according to the plasma acetaminophen level between 4 and 24 h after ingestion. (From Dart RC, Mullins ME, Matoushek T, et al. Management of acetaminophen poisoning in the US and Canada: a consensus statement. JAMA Netw Open 2023; 6:e2327739.)

If the plasma level is *above the treatment line* (which extends from 150 µg/mL at 4 h to 5 µg/mL at 24 h), the risk of hepatotoxicity is high enough to warrant antidotal therapy with NAC. If the plasma level is *above the high-risk line* (from 300 µg/mL at 4 h to 10 µg/mL at 24 h), there is a 90% chance of developing hepatotoxicity, and these cases may require extended treatment with NAC. The nomogram is only useful for acute ingestions that can be accurately timed. For overdoses with extended-release preparations, if the initial level is not above the treatment line at 4-12 h after ingestion, a repeat level should be obtained after another 4-6 h (10).

N-Acetylcysteine (NAC)

NAC is a cysteine surrogate that helps clear the toxic acetaminophen metabolite, as displayed in Figure 50.1. Treatment with NAC is indicated for any patient with a plasma acetaminophen level above the treatment line in the predictive nomogram. *NAC is also recommended for any case of potential acetaminophen toxicity when the hepatic aminotransferase levels are increased* (10).

Intravenous Regimen

Although NAC can be given via intravenous (IV) or oral route, the IV route is preferred. Table 50.1 lists an IV regimen that proceeds in two stages. The first stage involves a 21-h infusion of NAC given in three different aliquots. The second stage proceeds with an evaluation of "NAC stopping criteria."

Oral Regimen

An oral regimen is as effective as the IV regimen (11), but it is rarely used because NAC is not easily palatable (due to the sulfur content). Moreover, the stopping criteria or instructions for continuing the NAC treatment period are not as well-defined compared to the IV NAC regimen. A sample oral regimen is as follows (11):

1. Use 10% NAC and dilute 2:1 in water to make a 5% solution (50 mg/mL).
2. Start with a dose of 140 mg/kg and follow with a maintenance dose of 70 mg/kg every 4 h for 72 h.
3. The total dose is 1,330 mg/kg, administered over 72 h.

> **TABLE 50.1 Intravenous N-Acetylcysteine for Acetaminophen Hepatotoxicity**
>
> **1. Regimen:**
> Use 20% NAC (200 mg/mL) for each of the doses below and infuse in sequence.
> 1. 150 mg/kg in 200 mL D_5W over 1 h
> 2. 50 mg/kg in 500 mL D_5W over 4 h
> 3. 100 mg/kg in 1,000 mL D_5W over 16 h
>
> Total Dose: 300 mg/kg over 21 h
>
> **2. NAC Stopping Criteria:**
> 1. Plasma acetaminophen < 10 µg/mL
> 2. AST/ALT normal for patient, or decreased by 25-50%
> 3. INR < 2.0
> 4. Patient feeling well
> a. If NAC stopping criteria are not satisfied, continue IV NAC at a rate of at least 6.25 mg/kg/h.
> b. Recheck criteria every 12-24 h, and continue NAC until criteria are satisfied.

From References 1 and 10.

Adverse Reactions

Adverse reactions to IV NAC include nausea, vomiting, and cutaneous hypersensitivity reactions (e.g., rash, angioedema), which are more common in the first hour (when the NAC dose is the largest), and have a reported incidence that varies from 9-77% (12).

Hemodialysis

Hemodialysis enhances the elimination of acetaminophen. Therefore, hemodialysis, in addition to NAC, is recommended when the plasma acetaminophen concentration exceeds 900 µg/mL and there is evidence of hepatic encephalopathy (10).

Prognosis

Most patients respond favorably to NAC, and the reported mortality from acetaminophen hepatotoxicity is 0.4% (1). Some patients will have progressive hepatic injury despite timely NAC treatment, and these patients should be considered for liver transplantation (see Chapter 38: Liver Failure).

BENZODIAZEPINES

Benzodiazepines are second only to opioids as the drugs most frequently implicated in medication-related deaths (13).

Clinical Features

The clinical presentation of a benzodiazepine overdose is often confounded by the presence of other drugs. Pure benzodiazepine overdoses produce deep sedation but rarely result in coma (14). Respiratory depression (2-12% of cases), bradycardia (1-2% of cases), and hypotension (5-7% of cases) are also uncommon in pure overdoses (14). Benzodiazepine intoxication can also produce an agitated confusional state with hallucinations that can be mistaken for alcohol withdrawal (14). The diagnosis is usually based on the clinical history because urine screening tests may miss some common benzodiazepines such as lorazepam (15).

Management

Benzodiazepine overdoses are managed with supportive care (i.e., blood pressure support and mechanical ventilation if required) and, occasionally, flumazenil.

Flumazenil

Flumazenil (Romazicon) is a benzodiazepine antagonist that works by binding GABA-A benzodiazepine receptors (16). It is effective in reversing benzodiazepine-induced sedation but is inconsistent in reversing benzodiazepine-induced respiratory depression (17). The major use for this agent is rapid awakening following procedural sedation, when an excessive dose of benzodiazepine is used.

Dosing Regimen. Flumazenil is given as intravenous boluses of 0.2 mg that can be repeated every few minutes to a cumulative dose of 1.0 mg. The response is rapid, with onset in 1-2 min, and peak effect occurs at 6-10 min (16). The effect lasts about one hour. Sedation can return after 30-60 min because flumazenil has a shorter duration of action than benzodiazepines. To reduce the risk of re-sedation, the initial dose of flumazenil can be followed by a continuous infusion at 0.3-0.4 mg/h (18).

Adverse Reactions. Minor adverse reactions include agitation, nausea, and vomiting, and may occur in up to nearly a quarter (23%) of patients who receive flumazenil (16,18-19). Major adverse reactions, such as supraventricular arrhythmias and seizures, occur far less frequently (i.e., in approximately 2.4% of patients) (18-19). Because of these risks, flumazenil is not recommended for patients with undifferentiated coma, a history of seizures, or chronic benzodiazepine dependence.

β-RECEPTOR ANTAGONISTS

Toxic Manifestations

Intentional β-blocker overdoses are uncommon but can be life-threatening (20-21). The typical manifestations of β-blocker overdose are *bradycardia* and *hypotension* (20). The bradycardia is usually sinus in origin and is well tolerated (22). The hypotension can be due to peripheral vasodilation (renin blockade), a decrease in cardiac output (negative inotropic effect), or both.

Membrane Stabilizing Side Effects

Severe β-blocker overdoses can be associated with prolonged atrioventricular conduction and complete heart block, which is attributed to a secondary membrane stabilizing effect that is independent of β-blockade (22). Membrane stabilizing effects can also present as lethargy, depressed consciousness, and seizures, likely due to the high degree of lipophilicity associated with these agents (which facilitates accumulation in the lipid-rich central nervous system) (23).

Glucagon

Glucagon is a regulatory hormone that acts in opposition to insulin by stimulating glycogen breakdown to raise blood glucose levels. Glucagon antagonizes the cardiac depression produced by β-blockers as shown in Figure 50.3, thereby functioning as an antidote for β-blocker overdoses.

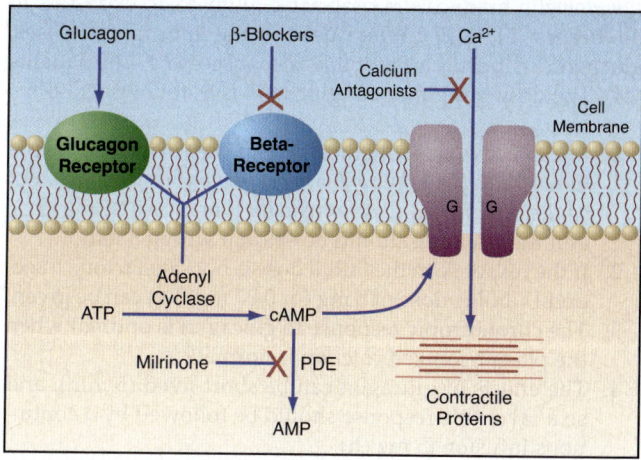

FIGURE 50.3. Mechanisms of drug-induced alterations in cardiac contractile strength. See text for explanation. Abbreviations: ATP = adenosine triphosphate; cAMP = cyclic adenosine monophosphate; PDE = phosphodiesterase; AMP = adenosine monophosphate. (From Pharmaceutical Drug Overdoses. In: Marino PL. *Marino's The ICU Book*, 5e. Wolters Kluwer; 2025:781-95. Figure 52.4.)

Mechanism

Glucagon activates the enzyme adenyl cyclase through an alternative receptor, resulting in the hydrolysis of adenosine triphosphate (ATP) and the formation of cyclic adenosine monophosphate (cyclic AMP). The cyclic AMP then activates a protein kinase that promotes the inward movement of calcium through the cell membrane. The influx of calcium promotes interactions between contractile proteins to enhance the strength of cardiac contraction. This sequence of effects explains the positive inotropic and chronotropic effects caused by activation of the glucagon receptor. Glucagon is also effective for calcium channel blocker overdoses, as shown in Figure 50.3 (21,24-27).

Dosing

Glucagon is indicated for the treatment of hypotension and *symptomatic* bradycardia associated with toxic exposure to β-blockers (21,23-27). When used in the appropriate doses, glucagon will elicit a favorable response in 90% of patients (24). The dosing regimen for glucagon is as follows (26-27):

1. The effective dose of glucagon can vary in individual patients, but *a bolus dose of 3-5 mg IV should be effective in most adults*. The initial dose is usually 3 mg (or 0.05 mg/kg), and the response should be evident within 3 min.
2. If the response to the initial dose is not satisfactory, a second IV bolus dose of 5 mg (or 0.07 mg/kg) can be given.
3. The chronotropic response to glucagon is optimal when the plasma ionized calcium is normal.
4. The effects of glucagon can be short-lived (5 min), and so a favorable response should be followed by a continuous infusion (5 mg/h).

Adverse Effects

Nausea and vomiting that are refractory to ondansetron are common at glucagon doses above 5 mg/h (24). Mild hyperglycemia also frequently occurs (from stimulation of glycogenolysis). The insulin response to the hyperglycemia can drive potassium into cells and promote hypokalemia. Glucagon stimulates catecholamine release from the adrenal medulla, and this can cause unwanted increases in blood pressure in patients with hypertension (24).

Phosphodiesterase Inhibitors

Phosphodiesterase inhibitors (e.g., milrinone) augment cardiac contractile strength by inhibiting the breakdown of cyclic AMP, as illustrated in Figure 50.3. Phosphodiesterase inhibitors can increase cardiac output in the setting of β-blockade (28), but it is unclear if these agents add to the effectiveness of glucagon in β-blocker overdoses. Because these drugs are vasodilators, and can produce unwanted decreases in blood pressure, they are generally reserved for the occasional case of β-blocker toxicity that does not respond to glucagon.

OPIOIDS

Clinical Features

Opioids (discussed in Chapter 5: Analgesia and Sedation) are the leading cause of medication-related deaths (13). The classic description of an opioid overdose is the patient with stupor, pinpoint pupils, and slow breathing (bradypnea). In practice, it is difficult to identify an opioid overdose based solely on the clinical presentation; the diagnosis is most often made by observing the response to the administration of naloxone (29).

Naloxone

Naloxone (Narcan) is a pure opioid antagonist. Naloxone binds to endogenous opioid receptors but does not elicit any opioid-like responses. It is most effective in blocking mu (μ) receptors, which are responsible for analgesia, euphoria, and respiratory depression (29). Naloxone can be given by intranasal (IN) spray or IV injection.

Intranasal Naloxone

IN dosing of naloxone is easy to administer and is as effective as IV naloxone (30). Dosing of IN naloxone proceeds as follows:

1. A single dose (usually 2 mg in 0.1 mL of dilutant) is delivered into one nostril. The recommended dose is either 2 mg or 4 mg, but 2 mg is probably sufficient in most cases, since IN doses of 0.4 mg have been effective in clinical studies (30).

2. If there is no response within 3 min after the initial dose, a second dose can be given in the other nostril. If the 4 mg dose of naloxone is used, it may be more effective if given in two divided (2 mg) doses in each nostril (31).
3. The average response time to IN naloxone is about 3 min, and peak blood levels are reached after about 20 min (30).
4. IN naloxone is effective at reversing both respiratory depression and impaired consciousness caused by an opioid overdose. However, the opioid effects are likely to return after 1-2 h, so a favorable response to naloxone should be followed by a continuous IV infusion (discussed in the section that follows).

Intravenous Naloxone

The IV route for naloxone is the standard method for treating opioid overdoses in the hospital setting. While IN vs. IV naloxone have similar overall clinical effectiveness (30), IV naloxone provides greater bioavailability and a quicker response time (30,32). Dosing for IV naloxone is as follows:

1. The initial IV dose of naloxone for patients with a depressed sensorium but no respiratory depression is 0.4 mg (400 μg). This can be repeated in 2 min, if necessary. A total dose of 0.8 mg (800 μg) should be effective if the mental status changes are caused by an opioid derivative (38).
2. Respiratory depression can be more difficult to reverse than depressed consciousness. The initial naloxone dose for respiratory depression should be 2 mg IV push (29). If there is no response in 2-3 min, double the dose to 4 mg. Further doses, if necessary, can be increased to 15 mg. If there is no response to a dose of 15 mg, then opioids are not the cause of the respiratory depression (29).
3. The reversal by IV naloxone *lasts only about one hour, and opioid effects will return thereafter*. Therefore, a favorable response to IV naloxone should be followed by a continuous infusion, at an hourly dose that is two-thirds of the effective dose (diluted in 250 or 500 mL of isotonic saline) and infused over 6 h (32).

Adverse Effects

Naloxone has few undesirable effects. The most common adverse effect is opioid withdrawal (33,34). There are also case reports of acute pulmonary edema associated with high-dose naloxone, which is attributed to pulmonary venoconstriction from activation of the sympathetic nervous system (34).

SALICYLATES

Salicylate intoxications are second only to acetaminophen as a cause of suicide-related deaths from over-the-counter analgesics (35). Ingestion of 10-30 grams, or 150 mg/kg, of acetylsalicylic acid (aspirin) is often fatal.

Pathogenesis

Acetylsalicylic acid is converted to *salicylic acid* following ingestion. Salicylic acid is readily absorbed from the upper GI tract, and metabolism takes place in the liver. *The hallmark of salicylate intoxication is the combination of a respiratory alkalosis and a metabolic acidosis with an elevated anion gap* (36).

Respiratory Alkalosis

Respiratory alkalosis is caused by direct stimulation of the respiratory centers in the lower brainstem by salicylic acid. This is one of the earliest signs of salicylate poisoning.

Metabolic Acidosis

Salicylic acid is a weak acid that does not readily dissociate and thus does not directly contribute to a metabolic acidosis. However, salicylic acid uncouples oxidative phosphorylation, which results in a compensatory increase in glycolysis (to generate ATP) and an increase in lactate production. The accumulation of lactic acid (and ketoacids) results in a high anion-gap metabolic acidosis. This is a relatively late complication, and an acidemic pH is a poor prognostic sign (37).

Other Pathological Findings

Salicylate-induced uncoupling of oxidative phosphorylation results in an increased metabolic rate, which increases the body temperature and promotes diaphoresis and dehydration.

Clinical Manifestations

The earliest signs of salicylate intoxication are hyperpnea (contributing to respiratory alkalosis), tinnitus, vertigo, nausea and vomiting, which can appear in the first few hours after a toxic ingestion. These signs and symptoms can be followed by agitation and fever, and in severe cases, by coma, cerebral edema, acute respiratory distress syndrome (ARDS), and hemodynamic instability (36). Laboratory studies can reveal hypocapnia and respiratory alkalosis, lactic acidosis, rhabdomyolysis, hypernatremia (from dehydration) and acute kidney injury.

Diagnosis

A plasma salicylate level is required to establish the diagnosis of salicylate intoxication. Levels above 40 mg/dL (2.9 mmol/L) are considered toxic and levels above 75 mg/dL (5.4 mmol/L) are life-threatening (36). In cases of chronic toxicity, levels are often lower.

Management

In addition to general critical care support (i.e., mechanical ventilation, fluids, vasopressors), activated charcoal, urine alkalinization, and hemodialysis are additional interventions for salicylate intoxication.

Activated Charcoal

Salicylates can slow gastric emptying, and enteric-coated or extended-release aspirin preparations can promote retention of the drug in the gastric lumen. Thus, *activated charcoal is recommended for all salicylate intoxications, regardless of the time of drug ingestion*, though activated charcoal is most effective if given within 2 h of the ingestion (36). The dose is 1 g/kg to a maximum dose of 100 g, which is repeated every 4 h until the charcoal appears in the stool or the plasma salicylate levels begin to decrease (36).

Urine Alkalinization

Alkalinization of the urine increases salicylate excretion and is one of the essential interventions for the management of salicylate intoxication (36-38). A protocol for alkalinization of the urine is provided in Table 50.2.

TABLE 50.2 Protocol for Alkalinization of the Urine

1. Create a bicarbonate solution by adding 3 amps NaHCO$_3$ (44 mEq/amp) to 1 L D$_5$W (132 mEq/L). Add 40 mEq KCL.
2. Start with a bicarbonate loading dose of 1-2 mEq/kg.
3. Follow with infusion of the bicarbonate solution at 2-3 mL/kg/h.
4. Maintain a urine output of 1-2 mL/kg/h and a urine pH ≥7.5.

From References 37 and 38.

Potassium is added to the bicarbonate solution because bicarbonate infusions lower serum potassium (see Chapter 35: Potassium).

Hemodialysis

Hemodialysis is the most effective method of clearing salicylates from the body (36-37,39). The indications for hemodialysis include one or more of the following (39):

- Plasma salicylate level >90 mg/dL (>6.5 mmol/L)
- Salicylate level >80 mg/dL (>5.8 mmol/L) *and* impaired renal function
- Evidence of life-threatening intoxication (e.g., cerebral edema, ARDS, multiorgan failure)

References

1. Chiew AL, Buckley NA. Acetaminophen poisoning. Crit Care Clin 2021;37:543-61.
2. Stravitz RT, Lee WM. Acute liver failure. Lancet 2019;394:869-81.
3. Hendrickson RG, Bizovi KE. Acetaminophen. In: Flomenbaum NE, Goldfrank LR, Nelson LS, et al., eds. *Goldfrank's Toxicologic Emergencies*. 8th ed. McGraw-Hill, 2006;523-43.
4. Rumack BH. Acetaminophen hepatotoxicity: the first 35 years. J Toxicol Clin Toxicol 2002;40:3-20.
5. Dart RC, Erdman AR, Olson KR, et al; American Association of Poison Control Centers. Acetaminophen poisoning: an evidence-based consensus guideline for out-of-hospital management. Clin Toxicol (Phila) 2006;44:1-18.
6. U.S. Food and Drug Administration. Consumer Updates. Accessed May 15, 2025. https://www.fda.gov/consumers/consumer-updates
7. Swarm RA, Paice JA, Anghelescu DL, et al. Adult cancer pain, version 3.2019, NCCN clinical practice guidelines in oncology. J Natl Compr Canc Netw 2019;17:977-1007.
8. Zimmerman HJ, Maddrey WC. Acetaminophen (paracetamol) hepatotoxicity with regular intake of alcohol: analysis of instances of therapeutic misadventure. Hepatology 1995;22:767-73.
9. McGovern AJ, Vitkovitsky IV, Jones DL, et al. Can AST/ALT ratio indicate recovery after acute paracetamol poisoning? Clin Toxicol (Phila) 2015;53:164-7.
10. Dart RC, Mullins ME, Matoushek T, et al. Management of acetaminophen poisoning in the US and Canada: a consensus statement. JAMA Netw Open 2023;6:e2327739.
11. Buckley NA, Whyte IM, O'Connell DL, et al. Oral or intravenous N-acetylcysteine: which is the treatment of choice for acetaminophen (paracetamol) poisoning? J Toxicol Clin Toxicol 1999;37:759-67.
12. Chiew AL, Isbister GK, Duffull SB, et al. Evidence for the changing regimens of acetylcysteine. Br J Clin Pharmacol. 2016;81:471-81.
13. Spencer MR, Miniño AM, Warner M. Drug Overdose Deaths in the United States, 2001–2021. NCHS Data Brief, no 457. National Center for Health Statistics; 2022. Accessed May 19, 2025. https://www.cdc.gov/nchs/nvss/drug-overdose-deaths.htm
14. Gaudreault P, Guay J, Thivierge RL, et al. Benzodiazepine poisoning. Drug Saf 1991;6:247-65.
15. Augsburger M, Rivier L, Mangin P. Comparison of different immunoassays and GC-MS screening of benzodiazepines in urine. J Pharm Biomed Anal 1998;18:681-7.
16. Romazicon injection. Package insert. Roche Laboratories; 2007.
17. Shalansky SJ, Naumann TL, Englander FA. Effect of flumazenil on benzodiazepine-induced respiratory depression. Clin Pharm 1993;12:483-7.

18. Penninga EI, Graudal N, Ladekarl MB, et al. Adverse events associated with flumazenil treatment for the management of suspected benzodiazepine intoxication–a systematic review with meta-analyses of randomised trials. Basic Clin Pharmacol Toxicol 2016;118:37-44.
19. An M, Jiang J. Comprehensive evaluation of flumazenil adverse reactions: insights from FAERS data and signal detection algorithms. Medicine (Baltimore) 2025;104(10):e41721.
20. Newton CR, Delgado JH, Gomez HF. Calcium and beta receptor antagonist overdose: a review and update of pharmacological principles and management. Semin Respir Crit Care Med 2002; 23:19-25.
21. Lavonas EJ, Akpunonu PD, Arens AM, et al. 2023 American Heart Association focused update on the management of patients with cardiac arrest or life-threatening toxicity due to poisoning: an update to the American Heart Association guidelines for cardiopulmonary resuscitation and emergency cardiovascular care. Circulation 2023; 148(16):e149-e184.
22. Henry JA, Cassidy SL. Membrane stabilising activity: a major cause of fatal poisoning. Lancet 1986;1:1414-7.
23. Weinstein RS. Recognition and management of poisoning with beta-adrenergic blocking agents. Ann Emerg Med 1984;13:1123-31.
24. Petersen KM, Bøgevig S, Riis T, et al. High-dose glucagon has hemodynamic effects regardless of beta-adrenergic blockade: a randomized clinical trial. J Am Heart Assoc 2020;9:e016828.
25. Kerns W 2nd, Kline J, Ford MD. Beta-blocker and calcium channel blocker toxicity. Emerg Med Clin North Am 1994;12:365-90.
26. Howland MA. Glucagon. In: Flomenbaum NE, Goldfrank LR, Nelson LS, et al., eds. *Goldfrank's Toxicologic Emergencies*. 8th ed. McGraw-Hill, 2006;942-5.
27. Chernow B, Zaloga GP, Malcolm D, et al. Glucagon's chronotropic action is calcium dependent. J Pharmacol Exp Ther 1987;241:833-7.
28. Travill CM, Pugh S, Noblr MI. The inotropic and hemodynamic effects of intravenous milrinone when reflex adrenergic stimulation is suppressed by beta-adrenergic blockade. Clin Ther 1994;16:783-92.
29. Boyer EW. Management of opioid analgesic overdose. N Engl J Med 2012;367:146-55.
30. Sabzghabee AM, Elizadi-Mood N, Yaragh A, et al. Naloxone therapy in opioid overdose patients: intranasal or intravenous? A randomized clinical trial. Arch Med Sci 2014;10:309-14.
31. National Library of Medicine. NARCAN- Naloxone hydrochloride nasal spray. AAccessed May 17, 2025. https://dailymed.nlm.nih.gov/dailymed/
32. Dowling J, Isbister GK, Kirkpatrick CM, et al. Population pharmacokinetics of intravenous, intramuscular, and intranasal naloxone in human volunteers. Ther Drug Monit 2008;30:490-6.
33. Doyon S, Roberts JR. Reappraisal of the "coma cocktail". Dextrose, flumazenil, naloxone, and thiamine. Emerg Med Clin North Am 1994;12:301-16.

34. van Dorp E, Yassen A, Dahan A. Naloxone treatment in opioid addiction: the risks and benefits. Expert Opin Drug Saf 2007;6:125-32.
35. Hopkins AG, Spiller HA, Kistamgari S, et al. Suicide-related over-the-counter analgesic exposures reported to the United States Poison Control Centers, 2000-2018. Pharmacoepidemiol Drug Saf 2020;29:1011-21.
36. Palmer BF, Clegg DJ. Salicylate toxicity. N Engl J Med 2020;382:2544-55.
37. O'Malley GF. Emergency department management of the salicylate-poisoned patient. Emerg Med Clin N Am 2007;25:333-46.
38. Proudfoot AT, Krenzelok EP, Vale JA. Position paper on urine alkalinization. J Toxicol Clin Toxicol 2004;42:1-26.
39. Fertel BS, Nelson LS, Goldfarb DS. The underutilization of hemodialysis in patients with salicylate poisoning. Kidney Int 2009;75:1349-53

Nonpharmaceutical Poisons — Chapter 51

This chapter describes the presentation and management of toxic syndromes produced by exposure to nonpharmaceutical poisons, to include carbon monoxide, cyanide, the toxic alcohols (methanol and ethylene glycol), and organophosphates. Although less common than the drug overdoses presented in the preceding chapter, these syndromes can be lethal if not recognized.

CARBON MONOXIDE

Carbon monoxide (CO) is produced by the incomplete combustion of carbon-based matter. The principal source of CO poisoning is smoke inhalation from house fires, poorly functioning heating systems, and the exhaust from automobile engines (1). CO poisoning affects >50,000 in the United States annually, resulting in >1,000 deaths (1).

Pathogenesis

CO binds to the heme moieties in hemoglobin at the same site that binds oxygen to produce *carboxyhemoglobin* (COHb). The affinity of CO for binding to hemoglobin is over 200 times greater than the affinity of O_2 (2). The effects of COHb on systemic oxygenation are demonstrated by the oxyhemoglobin dissociation curves shown in Figure 51.1 (1).

The curves in Figure 51.1 show how O_2 content is profoundly decreased when COHb comprises 50% of the hemoglobin molecules (2-3). The arterial O_2 content (point A) decreases in proportion to the increase in COHb, reflecting the ability of CO to block O_2 binding to hemoglobin, thereby impairing tissue oxygenation.

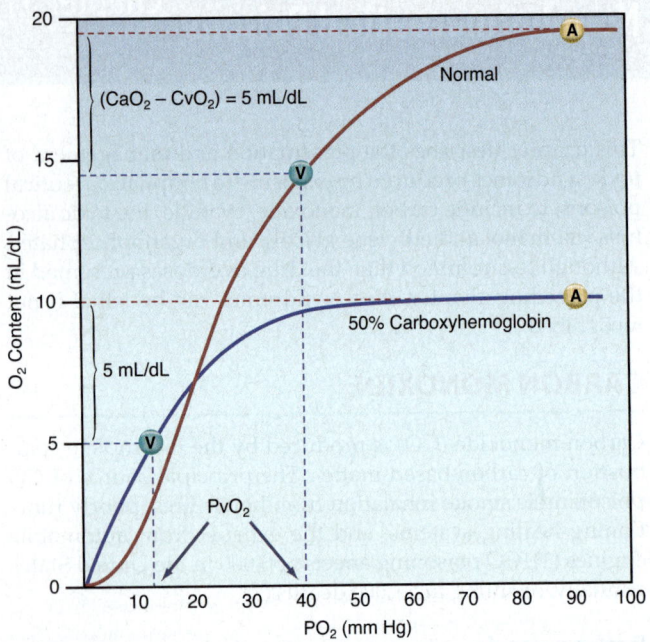

FIGURE 51.1. Influence of 50% carboxyhemoglobin on the oxyhemoglobin dissociation curve (using O_2 content instead of percentage of hemoglobin saturation on the vertical axis). The venous PO_2 (PvO_2) is a reflection of tissue PO and is decreased by the carbon monoxide effect on hemoglobin. A = arterial blood; V = venous blood. (From Nonpharmaceutical Poisons. In: Marino PL. *Marino's The ICU Book*. 5th ed. Wolters Kluwer; 2025:796-806. Figure 53.1.)

Clinical Features

The clinical manifestations of CO poisoning are variable and nonspecific but often correlate with carboxyhemoglobin (COHb) levels as shown in Table 51.1 (1-5). A cherry-red skin color has been described, but this is a rare and unreliable finding (5).

TABLE 51.1	Correlation of Approximate COHb levels (%) and Symptoms
COHb Level (%)	Symptoms
5-10	Headache (usually frontal)
	Dizziness
11-20	Worsening headache
	Drowsiness
	Nausea and vomiting
21-30+	Ataxia
	Obtundation
	Coma
	Generalized seizures
	Respiratory failure

From References 1-5.

Delayed Neurological Sequelae

In 1-4 weeks following CO poisoning, neuropsychiatric manifestations may appear, including impaired judgment, memory loss, cognitive defects, and parkinsonism (1,6).

Cardiac Sequelae

A 12-lead ECG and biomarkers are recommended for all patients with moderate to severe CO poisoning because myocardial injury has been reported in nearly 40% of these patients and is a poor prognostic finding (7).

Diagnosis

The diagnosis of CO poisoning requires evidence of an elevated COHb level in blood (5-6,8). *Pulse oximetry is NOT reliable for the detection of COHb*. The measurement of COHb requires an 8-wavelength oximeter (known as a *CO-oximeter*). This device measures the relative abundance of all forms of hemoglobin in blood, and the abundance of each form is expressed as a percentage of the total hemoglobin in blood.

COHb levels are negligible (<1%) in healthy nonsmokers, but smokers have COHb levels of 3-5% or even higher (5). Therefore, the threshold for elevated COHb levels is 3-4% for nonsmokers and 10% for smokers (5).

Management

The treatment for CO poisoning is inhalation of 100% oxygen. The elimination half-life of COHb is 320 min while breathing room air and 74 min while breathing 100% oxygen (5), so *less than 1 and 1/2 h of breathing 100% oxygen should reduce COHb levels to normal*. To achieve this, high flow, heated, and humidified nasal O_2, which delivers O_2 at rates up to 40 L/min, is a practical option to ensure 100% O_2 inhalation (see Chapter 26: Noninvasive Ventilation).

Hyperbaric Oxygen

Although the sum of evidence concerning the benefit of hyperbaric oxygen (HBO) treatment in CO poisoning has convincingly been shown to be superior to normobaric O_2 therapy (9-10), some guidelines recommend HBO treatment when COHb levels are ≥20% (11). HBO, although more costly than normobaric O_2 therapy, may decrease the incidence of neuropsychiatric and delayed neurological sequelae (9).

CYANIDE POISONING

The most common cause of cyanide poisoning is from domestic household fires, but other sources include oral ingestion, industrial exposure, and some medications (e.g., nitroprusside) (12-15).

Pathogenesis

Cyanide triggers a form of cellular hypoxia by inhibiting the enzyme *cytochrome oxidase* in the mitochondria (Figure 51.2). *Progressive metabolic (lactic) acidosis is a hallmark of cyanide poisoning.* Hyperlactatemia develops as lactate accumulates

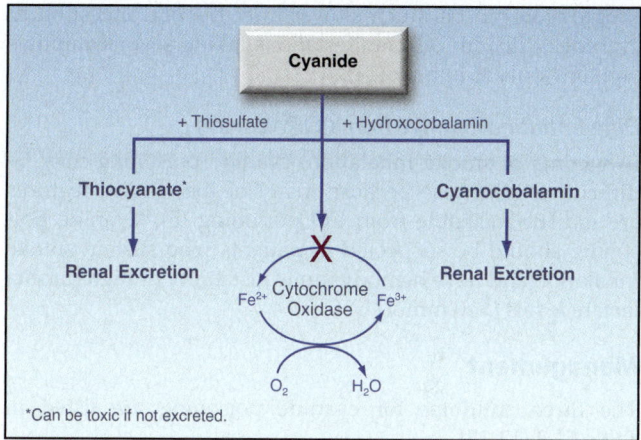

FIGURE 51.2. The actions of cyanide to inhibit cytochrome oxidase, and the clearance of cyanide by hydroxocobalamin and thiocyanate. (From Nonpharmaceutical Poisons. In: Marino PL. *Marino's The ICU Book*. 5th ed. Wolters Kluwer; 2025:796-806. Figure 53.2.)

in plasma, caused by the prevention of pyruvate uptake in the mitochondria.

Clinical Features

Cyanide poisoning is a *clinical diagnosis* because blood cyanide levels are not readily available and waiting for laboratory results will delay the administration of lifesaving antidotes. Early signs of cyanide poisoning include agitation, tachycardia, hypertension, and tachypnea, representing the compensatory stage of metabolic acidosis. This often progresses to loss of consciousness, bradycardia, hypotension, and cardiac arrest. Plasma lactate levels are typically very high (>10 mmol/L), and venous blood can look "arterialized" (and have a high PO_2) because of the marked decrease in tissue O_2 utilization (14). Progression is rapid after smoke inhalation, and the time from onset of symptoms to cardiac arrest can be <5 min (13).

Progression can be much slower after the oral ingestion of cyanide, with clinical manifestations taking several minutes or even hours to appear (14).

Differentiating Cyanide from CO Poisoning

In victims of smoke inhalation, cyanide poisoning may be difficult to diagnose because many of the clinical features are indistinguishable from CO poisoning (5). Cyanide poisoning should be suspected in patients who sustain smoke inhalation and have hemodynamic instability or high plasma lactate levels (>10 mmol/L).

Management

The three antidotes for cyanide poisoning are listed in Table 51.2 (13-15).

TABLE 51.2 Antidotes for Cyanide Poisoning

Antidote	Dosing Regimens and Comments
Hydroxocobalamin	Dosing: 5 g infused IV over 15 min. Give 10 g for cardiac arrest.
	Comment: The antidote of choice for cyanide poisoning; may cause reddish color in urine for a few days
Sodium thiosulfate	Dosing: 12.5 g in 50 mL sterile water, by IV injection
	Comment: Used in combination with hydroxocobalamin; do not use in patients with renal failure.
Amyl nitrite inhalant	Dosing: Inhale for 15 s and then rest for 15 s, and repeat if needed. Use a new ampule (0.3 mL) every 3 min.
	Comment: Used only for temporary relief when IV access not available. Contraindicated in smoke inhalation

From References 13-14, 16.

Thiosulfate is not recommended in patients with renal failure because *thiocyanate is a neurotoxin that undergoes renal elimination and can cause an acute psychosis* (16). Nitrites are *contraindicated in smoke inhalation* because methemoglobin promotes tissue hypoxia (13).

Cyanide Antidote Kits

The CYANOKIT contains 5 g of hydroxocobalamin as a powder, but has no diluent for IV administration, and has no repeat dose of hydroxocobalamin (16). There is also no thiosulfate or amyl nitrite in this kit.

The Cyanide Antidote Kit contains two vials of sodium thiosulfate for injection: each vial contains 12.5 g of sodium thiosulfate in 50 mL of sterile water (17). The kit also contains 12 ampules of 0.3 mL amyl nitrite for inhalation. Each inhalation should be for 15 s, alternating with 15 s of rest, and continued as long as needed. A new ampule should be used every 3 min.

TOXIC ALCOHOLS

Ethylene glycol and methanol are common components of automotive, household, and industrial products, and they both produce toxic syndromes that cause a metabolic acidosis. They are called toxic alcohols (18), but this is a misnomer, because ethanol (see Chapter 42: Disorders of Consciousness) is another alcohol that can be toxic.

ETHYLENE GLYCOL

Ethylene glycol is the main ingredient in automotive antifreeze and deicer products. It is sweet and flavorsome, which makes it a common ingestant in attempted suicide.

Pathogenesis

Ethylene glycol is rapidly absorbed from the gastrointestinal (GI) tract, and 80% of the ingested dose is metabolized by the liver. The metabolism of ethylene glycol involves the formation of a series of acids, ending with the formation of *oxalic acid* (Figure 51.3).

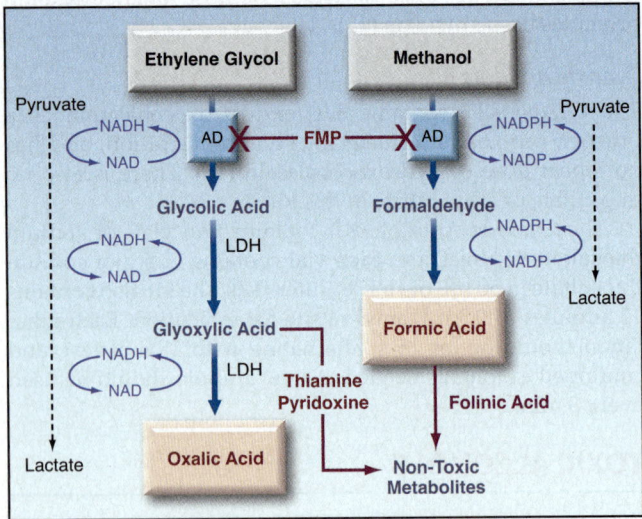

FIGURE 51.3. The metabolism of ethylene glycol and methanol in the liver. AD = alcohol dehydrogenase; LDH = lactate dehydrogenase; FMP = fomepizole; NADH = reduced nicotinamide adenine dinucleotide; NAD = nicotinamide adenine dinucleotide. (From Nonpharmaceutical Poisons. In: Marino PL. *Marino's ICU Book*. 5th ed. Wolters Kluwer; 2025:796-806. Figure 53.3.)

Serum lactate levels are increased in the series of intermediate reactions where NAD is converted to NADH. The oxalic acid forms insoluble crystals that precipitate in tissues including the renal tubules.

Clinical Features

Early signs of ethylene glycol intoxication include nausea, vomiting, and apparent inebriation (altered mental status, slurred speech, and ataxia). Because ethylene glycol is odorless, there is no odor of alcohol on the breath. Severe cases are accompanied by depressed consciousness, coma, generalized seizures, renal failure, pulmonary edema, and cardiovascular collapse (18-20). Renal failure can be a late finding (24 h after ingestion). Laboratory studies reveal a metabolic acidosis with an elevated osmolal gap (see Chapter 31: Acid-Base Analysis) and elevated lactate levels. Plasma assays are available, but results are often delayed, and laboratory results are only obtained for confirmatory purposes. Plasma levels of ethylene glycol that are >20 mg/dL are considered toxic (18), and plasma glycolic acid levels >8 mmol/L are often an indication for hemodialysis (19).

Crystalluria

Calcium oxalate crystals can be visualized in the urine in about 50% of cases, as shown in Figure 51.4 (20). Most hospitals do not routinely inspect for crystals, so a request must be made for the laboratory to search for crystals when the sample is sent.

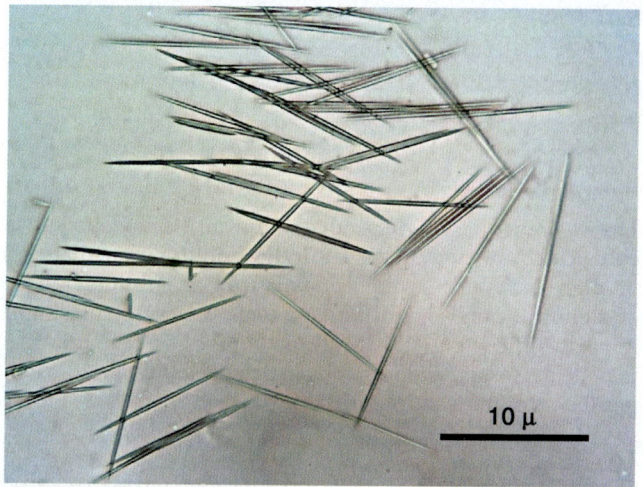

FIGURE 51.4. Microscopic appearance of calcium oxalate monohydrate crystals. The presence of these thin, needle-shaped crystals in urine is highly suggestive of ethylene glycol poisoning. (From Nonpharmaceutical Poisons. In: Marino PL. *Marino's The ICU Book*. 5th ed. Wolters Kluwer; 2025:796-806. Figure 53.4.)

Management

Fomepizole

Fomepizole inhibits alcohol dehydrogenase, the enzyme involved in the initial step of ethylene glycol metabolism (see Figure 51.3). The recommended dosing regimen for both ethylene glycol and methanol poisoning is shown in Table 51.3 (18).

TABLE 51.3 Dosing Regimen for Fomepizole

1. Start with an IV loading dose of 15 mg/kg.
2. Follow with a dose of 10 mg/kg IV every 12 h for 4 doses.
3. If the toxic alcohol level is >20 mg/dL after 4 doses, increase the dose to 15 mg/kg IV every 12 h and continue until the following end points are reached:
   a. The toxic alcohol level is <20 mg/dL.
   b. The plasma pH is normal.
   c. The patient is asymptomatic.
4. If more than one hemodialysis session is required, change the dose to 15 mg/kg IV every 4 h, until dialysis is no longer necessary.

From Ross JA, Borek HA, Holstege CP. Toxic alcohols. Crit Care Clin 2021;37:643-56.

Hemodialysis

The clearance of ethylene glycol and all its metabolites is enhanced by hemodialysis. The indications for immediate hemodialysis include severe acidemia (pH <7.1), and evidence of significant end-organ damage (e.g., coma, seizures, and renal insufficiency) (18). Multiple courses of hemodialysis may be necessary, and fomepizole dosing should be adjusted per the recommendations in Table 51.3.

Adjuncts

Thiamine (100 mg IV daily) and pyridoxine (100 mg IV daily) are recommended to divert glyoxylic acid to the formation of nontoxic metabolites (see Figure 51.3).

METHANOL

Methanol (also known as *wood alcohol*) is a common ingredient in varnish, shellac, paint thinners, windshield washer fluid, and solid cooking fuel.

Pathogenesis

Like ethylene glycol, methanol is readily absorbed from the upper GI tract and is metabolized by alcohol dehydrogenase in the liver. The *principal metabolite is formic acid*, a strong acid that readily dissociates and produces a metabolic acidosis with a high anion gap (18). Formic acid is also a mitochondrial toxin that inhibits cytochrome oxidase and blocks oxidative energy production. Tissues that are predominantly susceptible to damage are the retina, optic nerve, and basal ganglia.

Clinical Features

Early manifestations (within 6 h of ingestion) include signs of apparent inebriation without the odor of ethanol (similar to ethylene glycol intoxication). Later signs (6-24 h after ingestion) include visual disturbances (e.g., scotoma, blurred vision, complete blindness), depressed consciousness, coma, and generalized seizures (20). Examination of the retina can reveal papilledema and generalized retinal edema. Visual disturbances are common with methanol poisoning and *visual signs and symptoms help differentiate methanol from ethylene glycol poisoning*.

Laboratory Studies

Laboratory studies show a metabolic acidosis, high anion gap, and high osmolal gap, like ethylene glycol poisoning. However, *there is no crystalluria in methanol poisoning*. A plasma assay for methanol is available, and a level above 20 mg/dL is considered toxic. However, as with ethylene glycol poisoning, the results of the plasma assay should not delay treatment decisions.

Management

Treatment for methanol poisoning is the same as described for ethylene glycol poisoning, except for the following:

1. Visual impairment is an indication for hemodialysis in methanol poisoning.
2. Folinic acid (leucovorin) is used as adjunctive therapy in methanol poisoning, instead of thiamine and pyridoxine. The recommended dose is 1 mg/kg, up to 50 mg, at 4-h intervals (20). Folic acid can be used as an alternative if folinic acid is not available.

ORGANOPHOSPHATE POISONING

Organophosphates (OP) and carbamates are used as insecticides and biological nerve agents (e.g., sarin). Although the use of these agents has decreased over the past 20 years, >3,000,000 people are still exposed each year with up to 300,000 fatalities worldwide (21-22).

Pathogenesis

OP are cholinesterase inhibitors that inactivate red blood cell acetylcholinesterase (AChE) (23). Inhibition of AChE leads to excessive acetylcholine at the neuronal synapses, as shown in Figure 51.5.

Carbamates are similar to OPs but typically result in shorter durations of intoxication because these agents are *transient* AChE inhibitors. Both OPs and carbamates are readily absorbed through the GI tract, skin, and lungs.

Clinical Features

The cholinergic excess produced by an overabundance of acetylcholine causes a constellation of *muscarinic* (i.e., a type of acetylcholine receptor) physical signs that can be best remembered with the mnemonics listed in Table 51.4 (24).

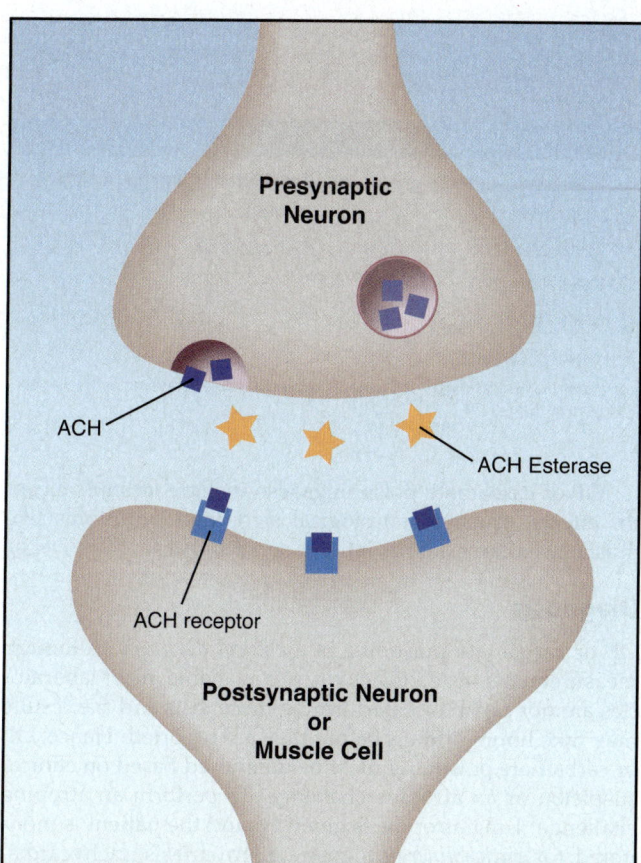

FIGURE 51.5. The mechanism organophosphate or carbamate poisoning. Acetylcholinesterase is inhibited, leading to an overabundance of acetylcholine in the neuromuscular junction. ACH = acetylcholine.

TABLE 51.4	Mnemonics to Assist with Recognition of Muscarinic Signs Associated with OP or Carbamate Poisoning
"SLUDGE"	"3B"
S - Salivation	B - Bronchorrhea
L - Lacrimation	B - Bronchospasm
U - Urination	B - Bradycardia
D - Defecation	
G - Gastric Emesis	

OP = organophosphate.

From Sidell FR. Clinical effects of organophosphorus cholinesterase inhibitors. J Appl Toxicol 1994;14(2):111-3.

OP or carbamate poisonings also include *nicotinic* receptor effects, causing neurological signs and symptoms like muscle weakness, fasciculations, and paralysis.

Diagnosis

OP or carbamate poisoning is a *clinical diagnosis*. Although measurements of AChE activity are available, most laboratories are not capable of performing these tests and the results may take hours or days before they are reported. Hence, OP or carbamate poisoning must be diagnosed based on clinical suspicion or an atropine challenge. To perform an atropine challenge, 1 mg atropine is given IV, and the patient is monitored for *anticholinergic* signs (e.g., mydriasis, tachycardia, dry skin). The presence of anticholinergic signs supports the diagnosis of OP or carbamate poisoning.

Management

Management interventions for OP or carbamate poisoning are summarized in Table 51.5 (21-31).

TABLE 51.5 Management of OP or Carbamate Poisoning

Immediate Antidotes and Decontamination

- Atropine 2-5 mg IV/IM/IO
  - Double the atropine dose every 3-5 min until wheezing and bronchial secretions stop.
  - In severe poisonings, very large doses (>100 mg) of atropine may be required over several days.
  - An infusion using 10-20% of the total cumulative bolus dose as an IV continuous infusion per hour is given, titrated to clinical response (i.e., no wheezing, resolution of signs listed in Table 51.4).
- 2-PAM 30 mg/kg IV over 15-30 min
  - Follow with a continuous infusion at 8-10 mg/kg/h (maximum: 500 mg/h).
  - Must be given with atropine

Neuromuscular Support

- Diazepam 10 mg IV, repeated as needed every 3-5 min for seizures or severe agitation
- Diazepam is also recommended for patients with coma or neuromuscular paralysis.
- Phenytoin is not recommended.

Respiratory Management

- Intubation is required in severe cases due to central nervous system depression (i.e., inability to protect the airway) and nicotinic receptor-mediated diaphragmatic weakness.
- Nondepolarizing neuromuscular blockers (e.g., rocuronium) should be used instead of succinylcholine for rapid sequence induction and intubation (see Chapter 2).
  - Larger doses of nondepolarizing neuromuscular blockers are often needed.
- Nebulized ipratropium (0.5 mg) for bronchospasm

Cardiovascular Support

- Dysrhythmias are treated according to standard guidelines (see Chapter 20).
- For patients who remain bradycardic despite atropine, an epinephrine infusion may be required.

TABLE 51.5 (continued)

Gastrointestinal Management

- If a patient presents within 1 h of *ingesting* an OP or carbamate, activated charcoal *without* sorbitol (50 g orally once) is given.
- Gastric lavage and forced emesis are *not* indicated.

IM/IO = intramuscular/intraosseous; IV = intravenous; OP = organophosphate; 2-PAM = pralidoxime.

From References 21-31.

References

1. Shin M, Bronstein AC, Glidden E, et al. Morbidity and mortality of unintentional carbon monoxide poisoning: United States 2005 to 2018. Ann Emerg Med 2023;81(3):309-17.
2. Guyton AC, Hall JE. *Medical Physiology*. 10th ed. W.B. Saunders, Co; 2000:470.
3. Chenoweth JA, Albertson TE, Greer MR. Carbon monoxide poisoning. Crit Care 2021;37:657-72.
4. Guzman JA. Carbon monoxide poisoning. Crit Care Clin 2012;28: 537-48.
5. Hampson NB, Piantadosi CA, Thom SR, Weaver LK. Practice recommendations in the diagnosis, management, and prevention of carbon monoxide poisoning. Am J Resp Crit Care Med 2012;186: 1095-101.
6. Choi IS. Delayed neurologic sequelae in carbon monoxide intoxication. Arch Neurol 1983;40:433-5.
7. Henry CR, Satran DS, Lindgren B. Myocardial injury and long-term mortality following moderate to severe carbon monoxide poisoning. JAMA 2006;295:398-402.
8. American College of Emergency Physicians Clinical Practice Subcommittee on Carbon Monoxide Poisoning. Clinical policy: critical issues in the evaluation and management of adult patients presenting to the Emergency Department with a carbon monoxide poisoning. Ann Emerg Med 2017;69:98-107.
9. Lin C-H, Su W-H, Chen Y-C, et al. Treatment with normobaric or hyperbaric oxygen and its effect on neuropsychometric dysfunction after carbon monoxide poisoning: a systematic review and meta-analysis of randomized controlled trials. Medicine (Baltimore) 2018;97:e12456.
10. Buckley NA, Juurlick DN, Isbister G, et al. Hyperbaric oxygen for carbon monoxide poisoning. Cochrane Database Syst Rev 4:CD002041.

11. Freytag DL, Schiefer JL, Beier JP, Grieb G. Hyperbaric oxygen treatment in carbon monoxide poisoning–does it really matter? Burns 2023;49(8):1783-7.
12. Mégarbane B, Delahaye A, Goldgran-Tolédano D, Baud FJ. Antidotal treatment of cyanide poisoning. J Chin Med Assoc 2003;66(4):193-203.
13. Anseeuw K, Delvau N, Burill-Putze G, et al. Cyanide poisoning by fire smoke inhalation: a European expert consensus. Eur J Emerg Med 2013;20:2-9.
14. Hendry-Hofer TB, Ng PC, Witeof AE, et al. A review on ingested cyanide: risks, clinical presentation, diagnostics, and treatment challenges. J Med Toxicol 2019;15:128-33.
15. National Library of Medicine. Cyanokit (hydroxocobalamin for injection). Accessed May 23 2025. https://dailymed.nlm.nih.gov/dailymed
16. Hall VA, Guest JM. Sodium nitroprusside induced cyanide intoxication and prevention with sodium thiosulfate prophylaxis. Am J Crit Care 1992;2:19-27.
17. U.S. Department of Health and Human Services: Chemical Hazards Emergency Medical Management. Cyanide antidote kit. Accessed May 23 2025. https://chemm.hhs.gov/antidote_cyanide.htm#sec1
18. Ross JA, Borek HA, Holstege CP. Toxic alcohols. Crit Care Clin 2021;37:643-56.
19. Porter WH, Rutter PW, Bush BA, et al. Ethylene glycol toxicity: the role of serum glycolic acid in hemodialysis. J Toxicol Clin. 2001;39:607-15.
20. Kruse PA. Methanol and ethylene glycol intoxication. Crit Care Clin 2012;28:661-711.
21. Karunarathne A, Gunnell D, Konradsen F, Eddleston M. How many premature deaths from pesticide suicide have occurred since the agricultural Green Revolution? Clin Toxicol (Phila) 2020;58(4):227-32.
22. Eyer P. The role of oximes in the management of organophosphorus pesticide poisoning. Toxicol Rev 2003;22(3):165-90.
23. Khurana D, Prabhakar S. Organophosphorus intoxication. Arch Neurol 2000;57(4):600-2.
24. Sidell FR. Clinical effects of organophosphorus cholinesterase inhibitors. J Appl Toxicol 1994;14(2):111-3.
25. Tuovinen K. Organophosphate-induced convulsions and prevention of neuropathological damages. Toxicology 2004;196(1–2):31-9.
26. Dickson EW, Bird SB, Gaspari RJ, et al. Diazepam inhibits organophosphate-induced central respiratory depression. Acad Emerg Med 2003;10(12):1303-6.
27. Shih T, McDonough JH Jr, Koplovitz I. Anticonvulsants for soman-induced seizure activity. J Biomed Sci 1999;6(2):86-96.
28. Eddleston M, Buckley NA, Eyer P, Dawson AH. Management of acute organophosphorus pesticide poisoning. Lancet 2008;371(9612): 597-607.

29. Eddleston M, Roberts D, Buckley N. Management of severe organophosphorus pesticide poisoning. Crit Care 2002;6(3):259.
30. Newmark J. Therapy for nerve agent poisoning. Arch Neurol 2004;61(5):649-52.
31. Samprathi A, Chacko B, D'sa SR, et al. Adrenaline is effective in reversing the inadequate heart rate response in atropine treated organophosphorus and carbamate poisoning. Clin Toxicol (Phila) 2021;59(7):604-10.

Appendix 1

Units, Conversions, and Ventilator Tidal Volumes

UNITS AND CONVERSIONS

Units of Measurement in the Système Internationale (SI)		
Parameter	**Basic SI Unit (Symbol)**	**Useful Conversions**
Length	Meter (m)	1 m = 3.28 feet 2.54 cm = 1 inch
Area	Square meter (m^2)	1 m^2 = 10.76 square feet
Volume	Cubic meter (m^3)	1 m^3 = 1,000 L 1 cm^3 = 1 mL
Mass	Kilogram (kg)	1 kg = 2.2 lb
Density	Kilogram per cubic meter (kg/m^3)	1 kg/m^3 = density of H_2O
Velocity	Meters per second (m/s)	1 m/s = 3.28 feet/s = 2.23 miles/h
Force	Newton (N) = kg × (m/s^2)	1 dyne = 10^{-5} N
Pressure	Pascal (Pa) = N/m^2	1 kPa = 7.5 mm Hg = 10.2 cm H_2O
Heat	Joule (J) = N × m	1 kcal = 4,184 J
Viscosity	Newton × second per square meter (N · s/m^2)	1 N · s/m^2 = 10^{-3} Centipoise (cP)
Amount of a substance	Mole (mol) = molecular weight in grams	mol × valence = Equivalent (Eq)

PREDICTED BODY WEIGHT (PBW)/ TIDAL VOLUME CHART FOR MALES

Height		PBW	mL/kg				
Feet	Inches		4	5	6	7	8
4'10"	58	45.4	180	230	270	320	360
4'11"	59	47.7	190	240	290	330	380
5'0"	60	50.0	200	250	300	350	400
5'1"	61	52.3	210	260	310	370	420
5'2"	62	54.6	220	270	330	380	440
5'3"	63	56.9	230	280	340	400	460
5'4"	64	59.2	240	300	360	410	470
5'5"	65	61.5	250	310	370	430	490
5'6"	66	63.8	260	320	380	450	510
5'7"	67	66.1	260	330	400	460	530
5'8"	68	68.4	270	340	410	480	550
5'9"	69	70.7	280	350	420	490	570
5'10"	70	73.0	290	370	440	510	580
5'11"	71	75.3	300	380	450	530	600
6'0"	72	77.6	310	390	470	540	620
6'1"	73	79.9	320	400	480	560	640
6'2"	74	82.2	330	410	490	580	660
6'3"	75	84.5	340	420	510	590	680
6'4"	76	86.8	350	430	520	610	690
6'5"	77	89.1	360	450	530	620	710
6'6"	78	91.4	370	460	550	640	730

PREDICTED BODY WEIGHT (PBW)/TIDAL VOLUME CHART FOR FEMALES

Height		PBW	mL/kg				
Feet	Inches		4	5	6	7	8
4'7"	55	34.0	140	170	200	240	270
4'8"	56	36.3	150	180	220	250	290
4'9"	57	38.6	150	190	230	270	310
4'10"	58	40.9	160	200	250	290	330
4'11"	59	43.2	170	220	260	300	350
5'0"	60	45.5	180	230	270	320	360
5'1"	61	47.8	190	240	290	330	380
5'2"	62	50.1	200	250	300	350	400
5'3"	63	52.4	210	260	310	370	420
5'4"	64	54.7	220	270	330	380	440
5'5"	65	57.0	230	290	340	400	460
5'6"	66	59.3	240	300	360	420	470
5'7"	67	61.6	250	310	370	430	490
5'8"	68	63.9	260	320	380	450	510
5'9"	69	66.2	260	330	400	460	530
5'10"	70	68.5	270	340	410	480	550
5'11"	71	70.6	280	350	420	500	570
6'0"	72	73.1	290	370	440	510	580
6'1"	73	75.4	300	380	450	530	600
6'2"	74	77.7	310	390	470	540	620
6'3"	75	80.0	320	400	480	560	640

Appendix 2

Clinical Calculators

SEQUENTIAL ORGAN FAILURE ASSESSMENT (SOFA)

Parameter	Score				
	0	1	2	3	4
PaO_2/FIO_2 (mm Hg)	≥400	<400	<300	<200	<100
				with respiratory support	
Platelets ($10^3/\mu L$)	≥150	<150	<100	<50	<20
Bilirubin (mg/dL)	<1.2	1.2-1.9	2-5.9	6-11.9	>12
MAP (mm Hg)	>70	<70 or dobutamine (any dose)[†]	dopa (<5) or dopa (5-15) or epi (≤0.1) or norepi (≤0.1)[†]	dopa (>15) or epi (>0.1) or norepi (>0.1)[†]	
Glasgow Coma Score	15	13-14	10-12	6-9	<6
Creatinine (mg/dL)	<1.2	1.2-1.9	2-3.4	3.5-4.9	≥5
or Urine Output (mL/d)				or <500	or <200

MAP = mean arterial pressure; dopa = dopamine; epi = epinephrine; norepi = norepinephrine; SOFA= sequential organ failure assessment.

[†]Catecholamine doses are in µg/kg/min.

Adapted from Vincent JL, Moreno R, Takala J, et al. The SOFA (Sepsis-related Organ Failure Assessment) score to describe organ dysfunction/failure. On behalf of the Working Group on Sepsis-Related Problems of the European Society of Intensive Care Medicine. Intensive Care Med 1996;22(7):707-10.

MORTALITY PREDICTION BASED ON SOFA SCORE

SOFA Score	Mortality If Initial Score	Mortality If Highest Score
0-1	0%	0%
2-3	6%	1.5%
4-5	20%	7%
6-7	22%	18%
8-9	33%	26%
10-11	50%	46%
12-14	95%	80%
>14	≥95%	≥88%

SOFA = sequential organ failure assessment.

Adapted from Ferreira FL, Bota DP, Bross A, et al. Serial evaluation of the SOFA score to predict outcome in critically ill patients. JAMA 2001;286(14):1754-8.

THE CHA$_2$DS$_2$-VASc SCORE AND THE RISK OF STROKE IN PATIENTS WITH NONVALVULAR ATRIAL FIBRILLATION

Risk Factor	(Points)	Total Score	Stroke Rate (% per year)
CHF	(1)	0	0.0
Hypertension	(1)	1	1.3
Age ≥75 yr	(2)	2	2.2
Diabetes	(1)	3	3.2
		4	4.0
Stroke/TIA/TE	(2)	5	6.7
Vascular disease	(1)	6	9.8
(Prior MI, PAD)		7	9.6
Age 65-74 yr	(1)	8	6.7
Female sex	(1)	9	15.20

CHA$_2$DS$_2$-VASc = Congestive heart failure, Hypertension, Age >75 yr (doubled), Diabetes mellitus, prior Stroke, TIA or thromboembolism (doubled), Vascular disease, Age 65-74 yr, Sex category (female sex); CHF = congestive heart failure; MI = myocardial infarction; PAD = peripheral artery disease; TE = thromboembolism; TIA = transient ischemic attack.

From January CT, Wann LS, Alpert JS, et al. 2014 AHA/ACC/HRS guideline for the management of patients with atrial fibrillation: a report of the American College of Cardiology/American Heart Association Task Force on practice guidelines and the Heart Rhythm Society. Circulation 2014;130(23):e199-267.

THE SIMPLIFIED ACUTE PHYSIOLOGY SCORE (SAPS) II

Parameter	Value	Score
Age (years)	<40	0
	40-59	+7
	60-69	+12
	70-74	+15
	75-79	+16
	≥80	+18
Heart rate (beats/min) *If patient had cardiac arrest, assign 11 points.*	<40	+11
	40-69	+2
	70-119	0
	120-159	+4
	≥160	+7
Systolic blood pressure (mm Hg) *Worst value in 24 h*	<70	+13
	70-99	+5
	100-199	0
	>200	+2
Temperature >39°C (102.2°F) *Highest temperature in 24 h*	Yes	+3
Lowest GCS score in 24 h (if sedated, lowest GCS before sedation)	14-15	0
	11-13	+5
	9-10	+7
	6-8	+13
	<6	+26
PaO_2/FiO_2 ratio if on mechanical ventilation or CPAP *Lowest value in 24 h*	<100 mm Hg/% (13.3 kPa/%)	+11
	100-199 mm Hg/% (13.3-26.5 kPa/%)	+9
	≥200 mm Hg/% (? 26.6 kPa/%)	+6
	Not on mechanical ventilation or CPAP within the last 24 h	0
BUN (mg/dL)	<28	0
	28-83	+6
	≥84	+10

Parameter	Value	Score
Urine output (mL/d)	<500	+11
	500-999	+4
	≥1,000	0
Sodium (mEq/L) *Worst value in 24 h*	<125	+5
	125-144	0
	≥145	+1
Potassium (mEq/L) *Worst value in 24 h*	<3.0	+3
	3.0-4.9	0
	≥5.0	+3
Bicarbonate (mEq/L) *Lowest value in 24 h*	<15	+6
	15-19	+3
	≥20	0
Bilirubin (mg/dL) *Highest value in 24 h*	<4.0	0
	4.0-5.9	+4
	≥6.0	+9
WBC × 10³/mm³ *Worst value in 24 h*	<1.0	+12
	1.0-19.9	0
	≥20.0	+3
Chronic disease	None	0
	Metastatic cancer	+9
	Hematologic malignancy	+10
	AIDS	+17
Type of admission	Scheduled surgical	0
	Medical	+6
	Unscheduled surgical	+8

Interpretation:

In-hospital mortality, % = ex / 1+ex

where x = 7.7631 + 0.0737 × (SAPS II Score) + 0.9971 × [ln (SAPS II Score + 1)]

BUN = blood urea nitrogen; CPAP = continuous positive airway pressure; GCS = Glasgow Coma score; WBC = white blood cell.

Adapted from Le Gall et al. JAMA 1993;270(24):2957-63 and Beck et al. Intensive Care Med 2003;29(2):249-56.

Index

Note: Page number followed by f or t indicates figure or table, respectively.

A

ABCDEF bundle, 671
Abdominal compartment syndrome (ACS), 541, 638
Abdominal infections, 641–654. *See also specific infections*
ABGs. *See* Arterial blood gases
ABO blood group, 197
Absence seizures, 690
Acalculous cholecystitis, 641–642
   clinical features of, 641
   diagnosis of, 93, 641–642
   fever with, 92–93
   management of, 93, 642
   parenteral nutrition and, 786–787
   risk factors/predisposing conditions for, 93, 641
Acetaminophen (paracetamol), 71–72
   dosing of, 71t, 72
   for fever, 104
   intravenous, 71–72, 71t
   overdoses of, 615–616, 807–813
      clinical presentation of, 809
      hemodialysis for, 812
      liver failure in, 613, 614, 615–616, 615t, 807–812
      N-acetylcysteine for, 615–616, 811–812, 812t
      predisposing conditions for, 808–809
      prognosis of, 812–813
      risk assessment in, 809–811, 810f
      toxic dose in, 807
      toxic mechanisms in, 807, 808f
Acetoacetate, 525–526, 526f
Acetone, 525–526, 526f
Acetylcholine, in myasthenia gravis, 694, 695
Acetylcholinesterase, 836–838, 837f
Acid-base analysis, 505–517
   gaps in, 511–515
   simplified approach (rules of thumb) in, 512t
   step-wise approach to, 510–511
   Stewart approach to, 515–516
Acid-base disorders. *See also specific disorders*
   classification of, 505–509
   diagnosis of, 510–516
   hyperchloremia in, 570t
   hyperkalemia with, 581, 586
   hypochloremia in, 571t
   hypokalemia with, 577
   metabolic, 506
   primary, 505t, 506, 510
   respiratory, 506
   responses to, 505t, 506–509, 507f
   secondary, 510–511
   shock and, 256–257

Acidosis, 505–509. *See also* Lactic acidosis; Metabolic acidosis; Respiratory acidosis
 diagnosis of, 510–516
 gaps in, 511–515
 hyperkalemia with, 581, 586
 responses to, 505t, 506–509, 507f, 508t, 509t
 shock and, 256–257, 262, 267
 strong ion difference in, 516
Acinetobacter, 455t
ACLF. *See* Acute-on-chronic liver failure
ACS. *See* Abdominal compartment syndrome; Acute coronary syndromes; American College of Surgeons
Activated charcoal, 615, 820–821, 840t
Activated prothrombin complex concentrate (aPCC), 236
Acute coronary syndromes (ACS), 352–370
 acute aortic dissection and, 361–367
 anticoagulant therapy for, 361, 362t
 antiplatelet therapy for, 360, 360t
 antithrombotic measures for, 360–361
 cardioprotective measures for, 358–360, 359t
 classification of, 352–353
 clinical presentation of, 354
 diagnostic evaluation of, 354–356
 ECG findings in, 352–353, 354, 355t
 long-term therapies for, 361
 pathogenesis of, 352, 353f
 reperfusion strategies in, 356–358
 thrombolytic therapy for, 356–357, 357t
Acute heart failure, 311–327. *See also* Heart failure
Acute hemolytic reactions, 198–200
Acute immune-mediated polyneuropathy, 698–700. *See also* Guillain-Barré syndrome
Acute kidney injury (AKI), 535–555
 abdominal compartment syndrome and, 541
 amino acid dosing in, 778, 778t
 biomarkers of, 537
 cardiorenal syndrome and, 319, 539
 causes of, 538–545, 539t
 desmopressin use in, 238–240
 diagnostic considerations in, 545–546
 diagnostic criteria for, 535–538, 535t
 fluid challenge in, 547
 hemofiltration for, 547–548, 551–552
 hemolytic uremic syndrome and, 219–220
 hepatorenal syndrome and, 541, 542t, 616–617, 617t, 618t
 hypercalcemia in, 603

hyperchloremia in, 570
hypocalcemia in, 600t, 601
hyponatremia in, 566
hypotension and, 540, 540f
isotonic saline and, 157
management of, 547–552
nephrotoxins and, 541–543, 543t
propofol-related infusion syndrome and, 81–82, 81t
renal replacement therapy for, 547–552, 548f
rhabdomyolysis and, 543–545
selenium in, 753
sepsis and, 538–539
serum creatinine and GFR in, 536, 537f
shock and, 257
subarachnoid hemorrhage and, 721
ultrasound of, 545
urinary indices for, 545–546, 545t
Acute liver failure, 613–614. *See also* Liver failure
Acute myocardial ischemic syndromes (AMIS), 353
Acute-on-chronic liver failure (ACLF), 613–614, 614t. *See also* Liver failure
Acute pancreatitis (AP), 629–640
abdominal compartment syndrome in, 638
biliary evaluation in, 634, 635f
circulatory support in, 636–637
classification of, 629
computed tomography of, 633–634, 634f
diagnostic and severity criteria for, 629, 630t
etiologies of, 629, 630t
infections in, 637–638
laboratory evaluation of, 631–632
nutrition support for, 637
severe, 636
treatment of, 635–638
Acute respiratory distress syndrome (ARDS), 418–430
corticosteroids for, 426–427, 426t
diagnostic criteria for, 419–422, 420t
enteral nutrition in, 763
etiologies of, 418, 418t
extracorporeal membrane oxygenation for, 427
immunopathology of, 418
mechanical ventilation for, 418, 422–427
airway pressure release ventilation in, 425
fluid management in, 425
goals of, 422
lung injury in, 422–423
lung protective protocol for, 423–425, 423t
neuromuscular blockade in, 426
permissive hypercapnia in, 424
plateau pressure in, 424
positive end-expiratory pressure in, 424

Acute respiratory distress syndrome (ARDS) (*Continued*)
  pressure control inverse ratio ventilation in, 425
  prone positioning for, 427
  recruitment maneuvers in, 427
  noninvasive ventilation for, 435f
  pulmonary artery wedge pressure in, 420–422
  radiographic appearance of, 419–420, 421f
  subarachnoid hemorrhage and, 721
Adenosine, 339, 340t, 341f
ADH. *See* Antidiuretic hormone
Adrenal crisis, 790
Adrenal insufficiency
  clinical manifestations of, 793, 793t
  critical illness-related, 790–795
  diagnosis of, 794
  drug-induced, 790–793, 792t
  fever with, 96
  hypermagnesemia in, 595
  hypovolemic hyponatremia in, 565
  primary, 565
  secondary, 565
  thyroid storm and, 800
  treatment of, 794–795
Adrenal suppression, in critical illness, 790–793
Advanced Cardiovascular Life Support (ACLS), 373–377, 374f
AEDs. *See* Automatic external defibrillators

Aerosol intolerance, in asthma, 406–407
AFib. *See* Atrial fibrillation
Afterload, cardiac, 176
  cardiogenic shock treatment and, 284
  ECMO and, 290
  noninvasive ventilation and, 437, 437f, 438–441, 439f, 440f
  septic shock and, 299
Agency for Healthcare Research and Quality (AHRQ), 460
Aggrastat. *See* Tirofiban
Agitation
  in alcohol withdrawal, 675t
  definition of, 74
  monitoring, 75, 76t
  PADS algorithm for, 85–87, 86f
  sedation for management of, 74–85
  supportive measures for, 74
AHRQ. *See* Agency for Healthcare Research and Quality
Air embolism, venous, 15–17, 15f
Air hunger, 253
Air-Q, 39t
Air trapping, 401, 402f
Airway, difficult, 23–27, 24f, 25t
Airway care, 456
Airway management, 23–44
  awake fiberoptic intubation for, 38–40, 40t
  endotracheal intubation for, 27–30, 36–38
  in hemorrhagic shock, 264

rapid sequence induction
and intubation for,
31–36
supraglottic airway devices
for, 38, 39t
surgical airway for, 41
in traumatic brain injury, 737t
Airway obstruction, 296, 401,
409
Airway pressure release
ventilation (APRV), 425
Airway pressures, in
mechanical ventilation,
445–446, 446f, 449–451,
449f, 450f
Airway protection, in
extubation, 481
AKA. *See* Alcoholic ketoacidosis
AKI. *See* Acute kidney injury
Alanine aminotransferase
(ALT), 632, 809
Albumin
and anion gap, 513, 513t
and calcium levels/
measurement, 598–600,
599f
for hepatorenal syndrome,
618t
Albumin solutions, 166–168,
168f, 169t, 266t
Albuterol
for acute asthma
exacerbation, 403–405,
406t
for acute COPD exacerbation,
411t
adverse effects of, 405
for anaphylaxis, 307
dosing regimen for, 406t, 411t
for hyperkalemia, 584t, 585
hypokalemia with, 576–577

ipratropium combined with,
405
Alcoholic ketoacidosis (AKA),
530–531
Alcohols, toxic, 831–836
Alcohol use
and acetaminophen toxicity,
808
and hypomagnesemia, 591t
and hyponatremia, 566
and pancreatitis, 96
and thiamine deficiency, 748
Alcohol withdrawal, 671–678
assessment scale for, 672,
674t–675t
clinical features of, 672–673,
673t
management of, 676
symptom-triggered approach
to, 676, 677f
Alcohol withdrawal delirium,
672, 673, 676
Aldosterone, 317–318, 576
Alkaline phosphatase, 632
Alkali therapy, for lactic
acidosis, 523–525
Alkalosis, 505–509. *See also*
Metabolic alkalosis;
Respiratory alkalosis
diagnosis of, 510–511
hypocalcemia in, 600, 600t
hypokalemia in, 577, 578f
hypophosphatemia in, 605t
responses to, 505t, 506–509,
507f, 508t, 509t
strong ion difference in, 516
Alloimmunization, 221
Alteplase, 357t, 395
Altered consciousness, 667–668,
667t, 668t
Alveolar collapse, 444–445

Alveolar consolidation, 459t
Alveolar dead space, 444
Alveolar pressure (Palv), 449–451, 449f, 450f
Alveolar recruitment, 445
Alveolar ventilation (VA), 443–444
Amantadine, 95
American College of Chest Physicians (ACCP), 482
American College of Gastroenterology, 646
American College of Surgeons (ACS), 162, 261, 262t, 265, 729, 730t–731t
American Diabetes Association, 527, 528t
American Heart Association, 281, 392, 393t
American Society for Parenteral and Enteral Nutrition (ASPEN), 741, 781–782, 787
American Society of Health-System Pharmacists, 49
American Society of Regional Anesthesia and Pain Medicine, 59, 60t
American Thoracic Society (ATS), 427, 462, 482
Amiloride, hyperkalemia with, 581t
Amino acids
  in enteral nutrition, 761t, 762t, 764
  in parenteral nutrition, 777–778, 778t
Amino acid solutions, 777–778
Aminocaproic acid. *See* Epsilon-aminocaproic acid
Aminoglycosides, hypomagnesemia with, 591t
Aminophylline, 345
Amiodarone, 334t, 335, 341f, 343, 373
Ammonia, in hepatic encephalopathy, 619–622
Amphotericin B, for candiduria, 661–662
Amylase, 102, 631
Amyl nitrite inhalant, 830t, 831
Analgesia, 64–74
  neuraxial, VTE prophylaxis and, 59, 60t
  non-opioid, 71–74, 71t
  opioid, 65–70
  patient-controlled, 69, 69t
  for traumatic brain injury, 730t
Anaphylactic shock, 304–307
  clinical features of, 304, 304t
  laryngeal edema in, 296
  management of, 305–307
  refractory hypotension in, 306
Anaphylaxis, 304
Anatomic dead space, 444
Andexanet alfa, 271, 718t, 719t
Anemia, 186–209
  cardiac output in, 189–190, 190f
  contributing factors to, ICU-associated, 188–189
  definitions of, 186–188
  hemolytic, in HUS, 219–220
  inflammatory, 188–189
  oxygen extraction in, 190–191, 191f
  phlebotomy and, 189

physiological effects of, 189–192
rates, in ICU, 186
tolerance to, 192
transfusion products for, 193–196, 194t
transfusion triggers in, 192–193
Anemia of chronic disease, 188
Angiographic embolization, 265, 267f
Angiography
in brain death, 686
coronary, 356
in delayed cerebral ischemia, 723
pulmonary, 390, 391f, 392
Angiotensin, in heart failure, 317–318
Angiotensin II, for septic shock, 302t
Anidulafungin, 103, 652, 661
Anion gap (AG), 512–513, 513t, 514t
in alcoholic ketoacidosis, 530–531
in diabetic ketoacidosis, 528t
in lactic acidosis, 520
Antacids, 47
Antibiotics
for acalculous cholecystitis, 642
for acute asthma exacerbation, 409
for acute COPD exacerbation, 411–412
for asymptomatic bacteriuria, 655
for catheter-associated UTIs, 660–661
for *C. difficile* infection, 644–646, 645t
C. difficile infection associated with, 642
for complicated intra-abdominal infections, 650–652
drug fever with, 93t
for fever, 103
for pancreatic infections, 637–638
for selective decontamination, 456
for septic shock, 300t, 303
for sinusitis, 100
for spontaneous bacterial peritonitis, 618–619
for surgical site infections, 99
for traumatic brain injury patients, 738t
for ventilator-associated pneumonia, 465–466, 466t, 467t
Anticholinergic aerosols, 405, 406t
Anticoagulants. *See also specific agents*
for acute coronary syndromes, 361, 362t
alternative, in heparin-induced thrombocytopenia, 214, 215t
for atrial fibrillation, 335–337, 336t, 337t
bleeding with, 270–272
calcium measurement affected by, 600
catheter insertion/removal with use of, 59, 60t

Anticoagulants (*Continued*)
  for pulmonary embolism, 392–393, 394f
  reversal of (*See* Anticoagulation reversal)
  spontaneous intracerebral hemorrhage with, 716–719
  for traumatic brain injury, 737t
  for VTE prophylaxis, 53–56, 54t, 59t
Anticoagulation reversal, 270–271
  algorithm for, 239f
  fresh frozen plasma for, 225, 238t
  prothrombin complex concentrate for, 225, 236–238, 237f, 239f, 270–271, 271t
  rapid warfarin, protocols for, 238t
  for spontaneous intracerebral hemorrhage, 718–719, 718t, 719t
Anticonvulsants. *See* Antiseizure medications
Antidiuretic hormone (ADH)
  for cardiac arrest, 377
  in diabetes insipidus, 560–561
  in heart failure, 317–318, 325
  inappropriate secretion of, syndrome of, 565
  for septic shock, 300t, 302t
Antiepileptics. *See* Antiseizure medications
Antifibrinolytic agents, 234t, 240–241

Antifreeze. *See* Ethylene glycol intoxication
Antifungal agents
  for candiduria, 661–663
  for complicated intra-abdominal infections, 651–652
  empiric, for fever, 103
Antihistamines, for anaphylaxis, 306
Antihypertensive agents
  for acute aortic dissection, 364–367, 366t
  for stroke (ischemic stroke), 710t, 711, 711t
Antimicrobial-coated catheters, 7, 655
Antimicrobial therapy. *See also* Antibiotics; Antifungal agents
  for catheter-associated UTIs, 660–663
  for fever, 103
  for pancreatic infections, 638
  for spontaneous bacterial peritonitis, 618–619
  for ventilator-associated pneumonia, 465–466, 466t, 467t
Antimotility agents, for *C. difficile* infection, 646
Antiplatelet agents
  for acute coronary syndromes, 360, 360t
  for ischemic stroke, 710t
  reversal of, 718t, 719
Antipsychotic agents
  neuroleptic malignant syndrome with, 84, 94, 95, 95t
  for sedation, 83–85

Antipyretic therapy, 103–104
Antiseizure medications
(ASMs)
drug fever with, 93t
for neuropathic pain, 74
for poststroke seizures, 716
for status epilepticus, 692t,
693
for traumatic brain injury,
731t, 738t
Anxiety
in alcohol withdrawal, 674t
definition of, 74
sedation for relief of, 74–85
in spontaneous breathing
trials, 477–478
supportive measures for, 74
Anxiolytic agents, for
spontaneous breathing
trials, 478
Aortic dissection, acute,
361–367
antihypertensive therapy for,
364–367, 366t
clinical presentation of, 363
diagnostic imaging of,
363–364, 364f
management of, 364–367, 365f
pathophysiology of, 361–363
Type A, 363, 367
Type B, 363
Aortography, 363
AP. *See* Acute pancreatitis
Apathetic thyrotoxicosis, 797
Apheresis platelets, 221
Apixaban (Eliquis)
for atrial fibrillation, 336, 337t
bleeding with, 270–271
reversal of, 237f, 239f,
270–271, 718–719, 718t,
719t

Apneal testing, for brain death,
683–686
APRV. *See* Airway pressure
release ventilation
APTEM assay, 233
ARDS. *See* Acute respiratory
distress syndrome
ARDS Clinical Network
(ARDSNet), 423
Argatroban, 215
Arginine, in enteral nutrition,
761t, 762t, 764
Arixtra. *See* Fondaparinux
Arousal, and consciousness,
667, 667t
Arrhythmias. *See*
Dysrhythmias
Arterial blood gases (ABGs)
in acute asthma exacerbation,
409
in acute pancreatitis, 632
in mechanical ventilation,
448
in shock, 254t, 256–257
Arterial injury, venous access
and, 14
Arterial line, in hemorrhagic
shock, 263
Arterial oxygenation (SaO_2),
measurement of, 127
ASB. *See* Asymptomatic
bacteriuria
ASMs. *See* Antiseizure
medications
Aspartate aminotransferase
(AST), 632, 809
ASPEN. *See* American Society
for Parenteral and
Enteral Nutrition
Aspirates, endotracheal,
461–462, 463t, 467t

Aspiration
  bag-valve mask and risk of, 31
  in endotracheal intubation, prevention of, 36–37
  in enteral nutrition, 770
  myasthenia gravis and, 698
Aspiration pneumonitis, 92
Aspirin
  for acute coronary syndromes, 360t
  contraindicated, in thyrotoxicosis, 800
  for fever, 104
  overdoses of, 819–821
  reversal of, 718t, 719
Assist control (A/C), in mechanical ventilation, 452t
Asterixis, 619–620
Asthma
  acute exacerbation of, 400–409
    aerosol intolerance in, 406–407
    antibiotics for, 409
    anticholinergic aerosols for, 405, 406t
    arterial blood gases in, 409
    corticosteroids for, 407, 408t
    drug (dosing) regimens for, 406t
    epinephrine for, 406
    helium-oxygen mixture (Heliox) for, 408–409
    inhaled bronchodilators for, 403–407
    ketamine for, 408
    lactic acidosis in, 523
    leukotriene receptor antagonists for, 408
    magnesium for, 407
    management of, 402–405
    mechanical ventilation for, 412–415
    NAEP protocol for, 402, 404f
    noninvasive ventilation for, 409
    respiratory failure and mortality risk in, 400
    short-acting β_2 agonists for, 403–405, 406t
    terbutaline for, 406
  airway obstruction and air trapping in, 401, 402f
  bronchospasm in, 400–401, 401f
  dynamic hyperinflation in, 401–402
  flow-time ventilator graphics in, 400–402, 401f, 402f, 414–415
  mucous plugging in, 402
  pathophysiology of, 400–402
  volume-pressure loop in, 402, 403f, 413–414, 413f
Asymptomatic bacteriuria (ASB), 655
Asystole, 377
Atelectasis, postoperative, 97–98, 97t
Atelectrauma, mechanical ventilation and, 422–423
Atherosclerosis, 352, 353f, 361, 709
Ativan. *See* Lorazepam
Atlanta classification, of acute pancreatitis, 629, 630t
Atorvastatin, 361

Atrial fibrillation (AFib), 328–330, 330f, 332–337
  adverse consequences of, 333
  anticoagulants for, 335–337, 337t
  arterial pressure tracing in, 333f
  cardioversion for, 335, 337
  CHA_2DS_2-VASc score in, 335, 336t, 848
  heart rate control in, 333–335, 334t
  prevalence and incidence of, 332
  stroke prevention in, 335–337
  stroke risk with, 333, 848
  transition from intravenous to oral therapy for, 335
  treatment of, 333–337
  Wolff-Parkinson-White syndrome and, 336–337
Atrial flutter, 328
Atrioventricular block, 344
Atrioventricular nodal reentrant tachycardia (AVNRT), 328, 330f, 339–340
Atropine, 345, 839t
Atypical antipsychotics
  neuroleptic malignant syndrome with, 84, 94, 95, 95t
  receptor binding profiles of, 84–85, 85t
  for sedation, 83, 84–85
Aura, in seizures, 690
Autoimmune thyroiditis, 800
Automatic external defibrillators (AEDs), 375
Automatisms, 690

Auto-PEEP, 401
AVNRT. *See* Atrioventricular nodal reentrant tachycardia
Awake fiberoptic intubation, 38–40, 40t
Awareness, and consciousness, 667, 667t
Axillary vein thrombosis, PICCs and, 17
Azithromycin, for gastroparesis, 770–771, 771t

B

Bacterial peritonitis, spontaneous, 618–619
Bacteriuria, asymptomatic. *See* Asymptomatic bacteriuria
Bag-valve mask (BVM), 29t, 31, 32
BAL. *See* Bronchoalveolar lavage
Balanced crystalloid solutions, 157–159
Balloon flotation principle, 137–138
Barbiturates, in traumatic brain injury, 730t
Base deficit (BD), 256–257
Basic Life Support (BLS), 371–373, 372t
Basic metabolic panel, in acute pancreatitis, 632
Basilic vein, cannulation of, 12
BD. *See* Base deficit
Bedside echocardiography, 109–123. *See also* Echocardiography
Beer potomania, 566
Behavioral Pain Scale, 64, 65t

Benralizumab, 408
Benzodiazepines, 75–79, 77t
   for alcohol withdrawal, 673, 676, 677f
   delirium with, 669
   overdoses of, 813–814
   for status epilepticus, 692–693, 692t, 693t
   for traumatic brain injury, 731t
β_2 Agonists
   for anaphylaxis, 307
   for hyperkalemia, 584t, 585
   hypokalemia with, 576–577
   short-acting, for asthma, 403–405, 406t
β-Blockers
   for acute aortic dissection, 366t, 367
   for acute coronary syndromes, 359t, 360, 361
   for atrial fibrillation, 333–335, 334t
   bradycardia with, 344, 345, 814–816
   hyperkalemia with, 581t
   for ischemic stroke, 711t
   for multifocal atrial tachycardia, 338
   overdoses of, 345, 814–817
   for ventricular tachycardia, 343
β-Hydroxybutyrate, 525–526, 526f
Bezlotoxumab, for *C. difficile* infection, 644, 645t
Bicarbonate (HCO_3). *See also* Sodium bicarbonate
   in acid-base disorders, 505–509, 505f, 507f, 508t, 509t
   in anion gap, 512–513
   in delta gap, 513–515
   in diabetic ketoacidosis, 530
   for lactic acidosis, 523–525
   reference ranges for, 510
Bilevel positive airway pressure (BiPAP), 431–432, 432f
   face masks for, 433–434, 433f
   postextubation, 483
   prior to endotracheal intubation, 29t
BiPAP. *See* Bilevel positive airway pressure
Biphasic shocks, in defibrillation, 375
Bisphosphonates, for hypercalcemia, 604t
Bivalirudin, 215t, 362t
Blankets
   cooling, 104
   warming, 268, 268f
Bleeding. *See* Hemorrhage/bleeding
Blood, oxygen content of, 186–188, 249–250
Blood bank, 196–198
Blood clot. *See also* Coagulopathy; Thromboembolism
   formation of, stages of, 231
   viscoelastic monitoring for, 231–236
Blood filters, 198
Blood groups, 197
Blood pressure. *See also* Hypertension; Hypotension
   dexmedetomidine and, 82
   heart failure and, 319–322, 320t

opioids and, 70
shock and, 254–255
traumatic brain injury and, 731t
Blood purification, 551
Blood transfusion. *See also specific types*
benefit *vs.* risk of, 206
for hemorrhagic shock
massive, protocol for, 269–270
products for, 265, 266t
hyperkalemia in, 582
hypocalcemia in, 600t, 601
plasma, 224–227
platelet, 221–224
red blood cell, 192–206
risks and adverse events associated with, 198–206, 199t
triggers for, 192–193
type, screen, and cross for, 196
universal donors for, 197
Blood type, 196–197
Blood volume, 187, 188f
BLS. *See* Basic Life Support
BNP. *See* Brain-type natriuretic peptide
Bradyarrhythmias, 344–348
definition and causes of, 344–345
management of, 345–348
temporary pacing for, 347t, 348
Bradycardia
benzodiazepine overdose and, 813
β-blocker toxicity and, 344, 345, 814–816

drug-induced, 345–348
flow chart for management of, 346f
hypermagnesemia and, 595t
shock and, 253, 285
sinus, 344
temporary pacemaker for, 347t, 348
treatment of, 345–348
Brain death, 683–686, 684t–685t
Brain herniation, impending, 733–735, 735t
Brain injury
cardiac arrest and, 380
coma in, 678, 679
seizures in, 689t
traumatic, 727–740 (*See also* Traumatic brain injury)
Brain tissue oxygen tension monitoring ($PbtO_2$), 735, 736t
Brain Trauma Foundation, 729, 730t
Brain-type natriuretic peptide (BNP), 315–317, 388, 479
Breathing trial. *See* Spontaneous breathing trial
Bridion. *See* Sugammadex
Brilinta. *See* Ticagrelor
British Thoracic Society, 462
Bronchoalveolar lavage (BAL), 462–464, 463t
Bronchodilators
for acute asthma exacerbation, 403–407
for anaphylaxis, 307
for COPD, 410
hypokalemia with, 576–577
intolerance of aerosols, 406–407

Bronchoscopy, in ventilator-associated pneumonia, 462–464
Bronchospasm
  in anaphylaxis, 307
  in asthma, 400–401, 401f
Bronchus, feeding tube in, 767, 768f
Brugada criteria, 332
Bubble test, 713, 713f
Bumetanide, 321t
Bundle branch blocks, 344–345

C

CABG. *See* Coronary artery bypass grafting
Calcitonin, 598, 604t
Calcium, 598–603. *See also* Hypercalcemia; Hypocalcemia
  blood samples for measuring, 600
  distribution of, 598
  for drug-induced bradycardia, 345–348
  for hemorrhagic shock, 269
  for hyperkalemia, 584–585, 584t
  hypermagnesemia and, 595
  hypoalbuminemia and, 598–599, 599f
  in lactated Ringer's, 157–158
  normal ranges for, 599t
  in parenteral nutrition, 780t
  physiological functions of, 598
  plasma, 598–600, 599f
  total *vs.* ionized, 598–599, 599f
Calcium acetate, 609

Calcium channel blockers
  for atrial fibrillation, 333–335, 334t
  bradycardia with, 344, 345–348
  for ischemic stroke, 711t
  for multifocal atrial tachycardia, 338
  overdoses of, 816
  for paroxysmal supraventricular tachycardia, 339–340
  for subarachnoid hemorrhage, 722t, 723
  toxicity, treatment of, 345–348
Calcium chloride, 602, 602t
Calcium gluconate, 596, 602, 602t
Calcium oxalate crystals, in ethylene glycol intoxication, 833, 833f
Calcium replacement therapy, 602, 602t
Calculators, clinical, 846–850
Calories
  in enteral nutrition, 759–760, 761t, 762t, 764–765, 766t
  requirements for, 743–745
  restriction of, 745, 746t
Calorimetry, indirect, 744–745
CAM-ICU. *See* Confusion Assessment Method for the ICU
Campylobacter jejuni, 698
Candida albicans, 100, 651–652, 661
Candida auris, 101
Candida glabrata, 101, 661, 662
Candida krusei, 662

Candidal infection/candidiasis
    complicated intra-abdominal, 651–652
    invasive, 101
Candiduria, 661–663
Cannulation sites, 8–12. *See also specific sites*
Capnography, 129, 131–133, 132f
Carbamate poisoning, 836–838
    clinical features of, 836–838, 838t
    diagnosis of, 838
    management of, 838, 839t–840t
    pathogenesis of, 836, 837f
Carbamazepine, for neuropathic pain, 74
Carbohydrates
    endogenous stores of, 747, 747t
    in enteral formulations, 761t, 762
    nutritional requirements for, 747
    in parenteral nutrition, 776–777, 777t
Carbon dioxide (CO_2)
    end-tidal, 129, 131–133, 132f, 263, 377–378, 378f
    removal, in venovenous ECMO, 489
Carbon dioxide (CO_2) colorimetry, 129–131, 130f
Carbon dioxide (CO_2) production (VCO_2), 743–745
Carbon monoxide (CO) oximetry, 126–127, 828

Carbon monoxide poisoning, 825–828
    clinical features of, 826–827, 827t
    CO-oximetry in, 126–127, 828
    cyanide poisoning *vs.*, 830
    diagnosis of, 827–828
    management of, 828
    pathogenesis of, 825, 826f
Carboxyhemoglobin (COHb), 126–127, 825–828, 826f, 827t
Cardiac arrest, 371–385
    advanced life support for, 373–377, 374f
    basic life support for, 371–373, 372t
    defibrillation for, 373, 375–376
    extracorporeal CPR in, 376, 376t, 501–502
    hyperkalemia and, 582
    hypermagnesemia and, 595t
    neurologic outcomes of, 382, 382t
    post-cardiac arrest syndrome after, 380
    post-resuscitation period in, 379–382, 381t
    pregnancy and, 277
    resuscitation monitoring in, 377–379, 378f
    return of spontaneous circulation in, 377–379, 378f
    reversible causes of ("H's" and "T's"), 374, 375t
    sudden, 344–345
    temperature control in, 380, 381t, 382
    time dependence in, 371
    ultrasound in, 379, 379f

Cardiac dysrhythmia. *See* Dysrhythmias
Cardiac filling pressures
  cardiogenic shock and, 278–282, 279f
  PA-catheter measurement of, 144–145, 144t, 280–281
  positive-pressure ventilation and, 438–439, 439f
Cardiac index (CI)
  cardiogenic shock and, 277, 278–279, 279f
  echocardiographic measurement of, 119–120, 120t
  PA-catheter measurement of, 144t, 146
  septic shock and, 301
Cardiac output
  anemia and, 189–190, 190f
  capnographic monitoring of, 131–133, 132f
  cardiogenic shock and, 277, 278–282, 279f
  determinants of, 176
  diuretics and, 319–321
  echocardiographic measurement of, 119–120, 119f, 120t
  errors in measuring, sources of, 143
  fluid resuscitation and, 176–177
  heart failure and, 319
  hemorrhage and, 260, 260f
  hyperchloremia and, 570
  hypocalcemia and, 602
  Impella catheters and, 289
  noninvasive ventilation and, 437, 437f, 440–441
  oxygen delivery in, 249, 250
  positive end-expiratory pressure and, 446, 447f
  preload and, 176–177, 177f
  septic shock and, 299
  thermodilution method of measuring, PA catheter for, 143, 146
Cardiac pump failure, 275, 278–279, 279f. *See also* Cardiogenic shock
Cardiac support, mechanical. *See* Mechanical cardiac support
Cardiac troponin, 354–356
Cardiogenic pulmonary edema
  ARDS *vs.*, 419
  CPAP for, 431, 436–437, 437f, 441
  noninvasive ventilation for, 436–437, 437f, 441
Cardiogenic shock, 275–294
  acute myocardial infarction and, 275, 276f, 279, 285
  addressing underlying causes of, 285
  cardiac surgery and, 277
  cardiac workload in, 284
  dynamic outflow obstruction and, 275–277
  etiologies of, 275–277, 276t
  filling pressures in, 278–282, 279f
  heart failure *vs.*, 278
  hemodynamic changes in, 278–279, 279f
  initial approach to, 254t
  inotropic therapy for, 282–284, 283t
  management of, 280–291, 280t
  mechanical cardiac support for, 285–291

mixed, with septic shock, 285
monitoring and measures in, 280–281
pregnancy and, 277
systemic inflammation in, 279
vasopressors for, 282
venoarterial ECMO for, 289–290, 492–495
venous air embolism and, 16
Cardiomyopathy
hypertrophic, shock in, 275–277
pregnancy and, 277
sepsis-induced, 296
Takotsubo (stress), 296, 297f
thiamine deficiency and, 748–749
Cardiopulmonary resuscitation (CPR), 133, 371–382
advanced life support with, 373–377
basic life support with, 371–373, 372t
chest compressions in, 371–372
extracorporeal, 376, 376t, 501–502, 502t
immediate goal of, 379
lung inflations in, 371, 372–373
post-resuscitation period after, 379–382, 381t
resuscitation monitoring after, 377–379, 378f
time dependence of, 371
Cardiorenal syndrome, 319, 539
Cardiorespiratory monitoring, 1
Cardiovascular parameters. *See also specific measurements*
in PA-catheter monitoring, 143–147, 144t

Cardioversion
for atrial fibrillation, 335, 337
for paroxysmal supraventricular tachycardia, 340
for torsades de pointes, 343
for ventricular tachycardia, 341f, 342
Carotid artery puncture, 14
Caspofungin, 103, 652, 661
Catheter(s). *See also specific types and uses*
anticoagulant use and, 59, 60t
antimicrobial coating of, 7, 655
central venous, 5–7, 5f, 6f
flow rates through, 2, 2f, 3t
infection prevention measures for, 17t, 18
infections related to, 17–18, 99, 656–661, 785
introducer sheaths for, 6–7, 6f, 138
malposition of, 18
midline, 4–5, 4f
peripheral intravenous, 1–2, 2f, 3f, 3t
peripherally inserted central, 7–8, 7f
Poiseuille's Law and, 2, 2f
proper placement of, 18–19, 18f
pulmonary artery, 136–151 (*See also* Pulmonary artery [PA] catheter)
rapid infusion, 2, 3t
removal of, 17t
size of, 1, 3t
temperature measured via, 91
thrombosis related to, 14, 17

Catheter-associated urinary tract infections (CAUTIs), 656–661
  diagnostic criteria for, 660, 660t
  etiology of, 656
  microbiology of, 656–657, 656t
  prevention of, 657–658
  treatment of, 660–661
Catheter-directed therapies (CDT), for pulmonary embolism, 395
Cathflo® Activase®, 785
Cation exchange resins, for hyperkalemia, 584t, 586
CAUTIs. *See* Catheter-associated urinary tract infections
CBC. *See* Complete blood count
CDI. *See Clostridium difficile* infection
CDT. *See* Catheter-directed therapies
Cefepime, 638
Cefotaxime, 619
Ceftazidime/avibactam, 651
Ceftriaxone, 651, 738t
Cellular respiration. *See* Oxidative metabolism
Centers for Disease Control and Prevention (CDC), 455–456
Central diabetes insipidus, 560, 561
Central line-associated bloodstream infection (CLABSI), 17–18, 99, 785
Central line bundle, 17t
Central pontine myelinolysis, 568

Central venous access, 5–12
  antimicrobial coating of, 7
  cannulation sites for, 8–12
  complications of, 13–20
  femoral vein, 11
  flow rate in, 3t
  for hemodialysis, 548–550, 550f
  in hemorrhagic shock, 263
  infection prevention in, 17t, 18
  internal jugular vein, 8–10
  in parenteral nutrition, 784–785
  peripherally inserted central catheters for, 7–8, 7f, 12
  purposes of, 1
  subclavian vein, 10–11
Central venous catheters (CVCs), 5–8
  introducer sheaths for, 6–7, 6f
  malpositioned, 18
  proper placement of, 18–20, 18f, 19f
  right atrial placement of, 20
  triple lumen, 5, 5f
Central venous oxygen saturation ($ScvO_2$), 127–128, 193, 248t, 251–252, 252t, 300
Central venous pressure (CVP)
  in cardiorenal syndrome, 539
  fluid resuscitation and, 178–179
  PA-catheter measurement of, 144–145, 144t
  in right heart failure, 313–314
  venous return affected by, 178–179, 179f
Cephalic vein, cannulation of, 12

Cerebral artery aneurysms, 718–721, 720f
Cerebral blood flow, in traumatic brain injury, 728, 728f, 729
Cerebral edema, 715, 716t
Cerebral ischemia, delayed, 720–721, 722t, 723
Cerebral microdialysis, 736t
Cerebral perfusion pressure (CPP), 729–733, 731t, 735t, 736t
Cerebral salt wasting, 565
Cerebrospinal fluid, draining, in traumatic brain injury, 729–733, 730t, 732f
Cetylpyridinium chloride, 456
CHA$_2$DS$_2$-VASc score, 335, 336t, 848
Charcoal, activated, 615, 820–821, 840t
Chatter, in venovenous ECMO, 490
Chest compressions, 17, 371–373, 372t. *See also* Cardiopulmonary resuscitation
Chest radiography
 of acute respiratory distress syndrome, 419–420, 421f
 for catheter confirmation, 18, 139, 140f
 for endotracheal intubation confirmation, 448, 448f
 for feeding tube confirmation, 766–767, 767f, 768f
 for fever assessment, 102
 of heart failure, 318f
 in myasthenia gravis, 698
 of pneumoperitoneum, 650, 651f
 of pulmonary embolism, 389
 for shock assessment, 254t
 of transfusion-related acute lung injury, 203, 204f
 of ventilator-associated pneumonia, 458–459, 459t
Chlordiazepoxide, for alcohol withdrawal, 676
Chlorhexidine, for oral hygiene, 456
Chlorhexidine-coated catheters, 7
Chloride, 569–572. *See also* Hyperchloremia; Hypochloremia
Chloride/acetate, in parenteral nutrition, 780, 780t
Chlorpromazine, neuroleptic malignant syndrome with, 95
Cholecystitis, acalculous. *See* Acalculous cholecystitis
Cholecystostomy, percutaneous, 93, 642
Choledocholithiasis, pancreatitis with, 634, 635f
Cholestasis, parenteral nutrition and, 786–787
Chromium, 750t, 782
Chronic disease, anemia of, 188
Chronic kidney disease (CKD), 537–538, 538t
Chronic obstructive pulmonary disease (COPD)
 acute exacerbation of, 400, 409–412
 antibiotics for, 411–412

Chronic obstructive pulmonary disease (COPD) (*Continued*)
- bronchodilator therapy for, 410
- corticosteroids for, 408t, 410
- drug (dosing) regimens for, 411t
- mechanical ventilation for, 412–415
- noninvasive ventilation for, 412, 435–436, 435f
- oxygen therapy for, 412
- respiratory failure and mortality risk in, 400
- dynamic hyperinflation in, 413–414, 413f
- hypophosphatemia and, 607
- pathophysiology of, 409
- volume-pressure loop in, 413–414, 413f

Chvostek's sign, 601–602
CI. *See* Cardiac index
CIM. *See* Critical illness myopathy
CIP. *See* Critical illness polyneuropathy
CIRCI. *See* Critical illness-related corticosteroid insufficiency
Circulatory overload, transfusion-related, 202–203, 205t, 223t, 226t
Cirrhosis
- hepatorenal syndrome in, 616
- hyponatremia in, 566
- parenteral nutrition and, 786–787
- serum ammonia levels in, 621

Cisatracurium, 702t, 703
CIWA-AR. *See* Clinical Institute Withdrawal Assessment of Alcohol Scale, Revised
CKD. *See* Chronic kidney disease
CLABSI. *See* Central line-associated bloodstream infection
Clean-contaminated wound, 649t
Clean wound, 649t
Clevidipine, for ischemic stroke, 711t
Clinical calculators, 846–850
Clinical Institute Withdrawal Assessment of Alcohol Scale, Revised (CIWA-AR), 672, 674t–675t, 676, 677f
Clonic seizures, 690
Clopidogrel (Plavix), 48, 360t, 718t, 719
Clostridium difficile infection (CDI), 642–647
- antibiotic-associated, 642
- clinical features of, 643
- colonization rates in, 642, 643t
- colonoscopy in, 644
- diagnosis evaluation of, 643–644
- enteral nutrition and, 772
- fecal microbiota transplantation for, 645t, 647
- fever in, 100
- medical treatment of, 644–646, 645t
- pathogenesis of, 642–643
- preventing spread of, 647, 648f

probiotics and prebiotics for, 646
recolonization for, 646–647
short-chain fatty acids and, 763
surgical treatment of, 646
Clostridium infections, wound/surgical site, 99
Clostridium perfringens, 99
Coagulopathy, 231–245. *See also specific types*
anticoagulation reversal in, 231
consumptive, 217
in hemorrhagic shock, 262, 268–269
hemostatic adjuncts for, 235t, 236–242
in inflammation, 297
stress ulcer risk with, 46, 46t
viscoelastic monitoring for, 231–236, 232f, 233f, 235f
visual patterns associated with, 235f
Cockroft-Gault formula, 537f
Colitis, fulminant *C. difficile*, 643
Colloid fluids, 165–172
albumin solutions, 166–168
comparison of, 169t
crystalloid fluids *vs.*, 170–171
hydroxyethyl starch, 169, 169t
indications for, 171
volume effects of, 166, 166f
Colloid osmotic pressure (COP), 165, 167, 169, 170, 281–282
Colonoscopy, in *C. difficile* infection, 644
Coma, 678–683
bedside evaluation of, 678–683
etiologies of, 678

Glasgow scale for, 681–683, 682t
hypercalcemia and, 603
hypermagnesemia and, 595t
motor responses in, 678
myxedema, 800–801, 801t
ocular motility and reflexes in, 679–681, 681f
pain responses in, 679
pupillary responses in, 679, 680t
Common bile duct (CBD), in acute pancreatitis, 634, 635f
Community-acquired pneumonia (CAP), noninvasive ventilation for, 435f
Compartment syndrome, abdominal, 541, 638
Compatibility, red blood cell, 197
Compensated shock, 253
Complete blood count (CBC), 102, 632
Complex partial seizures, 690
Complicated intra-abdominal infections, 647–652
candidal coverage in, 651–652
definition of, 647
diagnostic evaluation of, 648–650
history and physical in, 648–650
management of, 650–652
postoperative, 647–648, 649t
radiologic imaging of, 650, 651f
source control in, 652
Compression stockings, 57

Computed tomographic angiography (CTA), 390, 391f, 723
Computed tomography (CT)
  of acute aortic dissection, 363–364, 364f
  of acute pancreatitis, 633–634, 634f
  of acute respiratory distress syndrome, 420, 421f
  in complicated intra-abdominal infections, 648–650
  in fever assessment, 102
  of intracerebral hemorrhage, 714f
  of pancreatic infections, 637
  in shock assessment, 254t
Condom catheters (male), 658
Conduction system, cardiac, disturbances in, 344–345
Confusion Assessment Method for the ICU (CAM-ICU), 670, 670t
Consciousness. *See also* Alcohol withdrawal; Brain death; Coma; Delirium
  altered states of, 667–668, 667t, 668f
  definition of, 667
  disorders of, 667–688
  predisposing conditions and, 668, 668f
Constipation, opioids and, 70
Consumptive coagulopathy, 217
Contaminated wound, 649t
Continuous positive airway pressure (CPAP), 431, 432f
  for acute respiratory distress syndrome, 425
  for cardiogenic pulmonary edema, 431, 436–437, 437f, 441
  face masks for, 433
  postextubation, 483
Continuous renal replacement therapy (CRRT), 551–552, 617, 622
Continuous venovenous hemofiltration (CVVH), 551
Contrast agents, acute kidney injury from, 541–543
Convection, in hemofiltration, 551
Cooling blankets, 104
CO-oximetry, 126–127, 828
COP. *See* Colloid osmotic pressure
COPD. *See* Chronic obstructive pulmonary disease
Copper, 750t
Coronary angiography, 356
Coronary artery bypass grafting (CABG), 356, 358
Coronary syndromes, acute. *See* Acute coronary syndromes
Coronary thrombosis, 352–353, 353f
Corticosteroid insufficiency, in critical illness, 790–795
Corticosteroid therapy
  for acute asthma exacerbation, 407, 408t
  for acute COPD exacerbation, 408t, 410
  for acute respiratory distress syndrome, 426–427, 426t
  for anaphylaxis, 307
  for cardiac arrest, 377

contraindicated, in traumatic brain injury, 730t
for critical illness-related corticosteroid insufficiency, 794–795
for extubation, 482
for hypercalcemia, 604t
for hypothyroidism, 802
for myasthenia gravis, 694
for postextubation stridor, 483
for septic shock, 300t, 301
for thyrotoxicosis and thyroid storm, 799t, 800
for TTP, 219
Coumadin. *See* Warfarin
Countercurrent exchange, 550–551
COVID, 297, 435f, 698
CPAP. *See* Continuous positive airway pressure
CPP. *See* Cerebral perfusion pressure
CPR. *See* Cardiopulmonary resuscitation
Craniectomy/craniotomy, decompressive, 735, 735t
C-reactive protein, 102, 254t, 632
Creatinine, serum, 257, 536
Cricoid pressure, in endotracheal intubation, 36–37
Cricothyrotomy, 41
Critical illness myopathy (CIM), 700–701
Critical illness neuromyopathy, 480–481, 700–701
Critical illness polyneuropathy (CIP), 700–701

Critical illness-related corticosteroid insufficiency (CIRCI), 790–795
clinical manifestations of, 793, 793t
diagnosis of, 794
drug-induced, 790–793, 792t
incidence in ICU, 790
pathophysiology of, 790, 791f
treatment of, 794–795
CRRT. *See* Continuous renal replacement therapy
Cryoprecipitate, 226–227
for hemorrhagic shock, 266t, 270
for intracerebral hemorrhage, 715
TEG- or ROTEM-based thresholds for, 234t
treatment algorithm for, 242f
Crystalloid fluids, 153–162. *See also specific types*
for acute pancreatitis, 636
albumin solution *vs.*, 167–168
balanced solutions, 157–159
colloid fluids *vs.*, 170–171
comparison with plasma, 155, 156t
equilibration of, 153, 155f
fluid challenge with, 180
for hemorrhagic shock, 264–265, 266t
for hypochloremia, 572
increased intra-abdominal pressure with, 541
indications for, 171
normal pH fluids, 157, 159–160
osmolarity and osmolality of, 154, 156t

Crystalloid fluids (*Continued*)
  principal effect of, 153
  for septic shock, 300t, 301
  for subarachnoid hemorrhage, 721
  volume distribution and, 153–154
Crystalluria, in ethylene glycol intoxication, 833, 833f
Cstat. *See* Static compliance
CT. *See* Computed tomography
Cuff-leak test, 482–483
Curling's ulcer, 45
Cushing's triad, 733–735
Cushing's ulcer, 45
CVCs. *See* Central venous catheters
CVP. *See* Central venous pressure
CVVH. *See* Continuous venovenous hemofiltration
Cyanide antidote kits, 831
Cyanide poisoning, 247, 523, 828–831
  carbon monoxide poisoning *vs.*, 830
  clinical features of, 829–830
  management of, 830–831, 830t
  nitroprusside and, 320t, 366t, 828
  oxygen delivery and shock in, 247
  pathogenesis of, 828–829, 829f
Cytochrome oxidase, 828–829, 829f
Cytopathic hypoxia, in septic shock, 300
Cytoprotection, for stress ulcer prophylaxis, 47t, 48–49

Cytotoxic edema, 715
Cytotoxic shock, 296–297

D

Dabigatran (Pradaxa)
  for atrial fibrillation, 336, 337t
  bleeding with, 270–271
  reversal of, 237f, 239f, 270–271, 719
Dalteparin (Fragmin), 54t, 56
Dantrolene sodium, 94
ddAVP. *See* Desmopressin
D-dimer, 254t, 387–388
Dead space, 443–444
Death, brain, 683–686, 684t–685t
Death by neurologic criteria (DNC), 683–686, 684t
Decontamination, selective, 456
Decubitus (pressure) ulcers, 101
Deep venous thrombosis (DVT), 52–63
  anticoagulant prophylaxis for, 53–56, 54t, 59t
  catheter-related, 17
  fever with, 92
  heparin-induced thrombocytopenia and, 212
  mechanical aids for, 57–58, 57f
  pulmonary embolism with, 387, 389
  risk factors for, 52–53
  venous duplex ultrasonography of, 389, 390f
Defibrillation, 371, 373, 375–376
Delayed cerebral ischemia (DCI), 720–721, 722t, 723
Delirium, 668–671
  alcohol withdrawal, 672, 673, 676

benzodiazepines and, 75, 77–78
clinical features of, 668–669, 669f
definition of, 74
dementia *vs.*, 671
diagnosis of, 670–671, 670t
gabapentin withdrawal, 678
hyperactive, 669f, 673
hypermagnesemia and, 595t
hypoactive, 668, 669f
management of, 671
PADS algorithm for, 85–87, 86f
predisposing conditions for, 668–669
prevention of, 671
psychosis *vs.*, 671
sedation for management of, 74–85
severe, drugs for, 672t
supportive measures for, 74

Delirium tremens, 673, 673t
Delta gap, 513–515
Dementia, delirium *vs.*, 671
Denervation hypersensitivity, 582
Denitrogenation, 28, 29t
Depression, in thyrotoxicosis, 797
De-resuscitation, 172, 184
Desmopressin (ddAVP), 238–240
for diabetes insipidus, 561
dosing of, 240
indications for, 238–240
mechanism of action, 238
for overcorrection of hyponatremia, 568, 568t
for spontaneous intracerebral hemorrhage, 718t
TEG- or ROTEM-based thresholds for, 234t

Dexamethasone, 426t, 482, 483
Dexmedetomidine, 79t, 82–83, 672t
Dextrans, 169–170
comparison with other colloid fluids, 169t
disadvantages of, 170
features of, 170
for hemorrhagic shock, 266t
preparations of, 169–170

5% Dextrose solutions, 162–165
adverse effects of, 164–165
for hypovolemic hypernatremia, 559–560
in parenteral nutrition, 776, 777t
protein-sparing effects of, 162–163
volume effects of, 163, 164f

10% Dextrose solutions, 776, 777t
50% Dextrose solutions, 776–777, 777t
70% Dextrose solutions, 777, 777t

Diabetes insipidus (DI), 560–561
Diabetes mellitus
enteral nutrition in, 760t
hypomagnesemia in, 591t

Diabetic ketoacidosis (DKA), 527–530
clinical features of, 527, 528t
delta gap in, 514–515
hypophosphatemia in, 530, 605t
insulin for, 527–529, 529t
management of, 527–530, 529t
potassium for, 529–530, 530t

Diabetic ketoacidosis (DKA) (*Continued*)
  predisposing factors for, 527
  volume resuscitation for, 527, 529t
Dialysis. *See* Hemodialysis
Dialysis disequilibrium syndrome, 551
Diarrhea
  C. difficile infection and, 100, 642–647
  enteral nutrition and, 772
  fiber for, 763
  hypokalemia with, 577, 578f
  hypomagnesemia with, 591t
  sodium concentration in, 559t
Diastolic dysfunction, 311–312
Diastolic pressure, pulmonary artery catheter and, 138–139
Diazepam (Valium), 75, 676, 677f, 839t
DIC. *See* Disseminated intravascular coagulation
Difficult airway, 23–27, 24f, 25t
Diffusion, in hemodialysis, 550
Digitalis, 581t, 585, 591t, 592
Digoxin, 333–335, 334t
Dilaudid. *See* Hydromorphone
Diltiazem, 333–335, 334t, 339–340
Diphenhydramine, for anaphylaxis, 306
Diprivan. *See* Propofol
Direct-acting oral anticoagulants (DOACs). *See also specific agents*
  for atrial fibrillation, 336
  hemorrhage associated with, 270–271
  for heparin-induced thrombocytopenia, 214
  reversal of, 236–238, 237f, 239f, 270–271
Dirty or infected wound, 649t
Disseminated intravascular coagulation (DIC), 216–217
  HELLP syndrome *vs.*, 220
  laboratory profile in, 216t, 217
  scoring criteria for, 217, 218t
  TTP *vs.*, 218
Distributive shock, 254t
Diuretics
  for acute kidney injury, 547
  concerns/precautions with, 319–321
  for heart failure, 319–322, 321t, 323f
  for hypercalcemia, 603
  for hypermagnesemia, 596
  for hypervolemic hypernatremia, 561–562
  hypokalemia with, 577, 578f
  hypomagnesemia with, 591, 591t
  hypovolemic hyponatremia with, 564
  potassium-sparing, 576
  for rhabdomyolysis, 544–545
  thiamine deficiency with, 748
DKA. *See* Diabetic ketoacidosis
DNC. *See* Death by neurologic criteria
DO_2. *See* Oxygen delivery
DOACs. *See* Direct-acting oral anticoagulants
Dobhoff feeding tube, 767, 767f
Dobutamine, 282–283, 283t, 303t, 324

Dopamine
  for bradycardia, 345
  low-dose, for acute kidney injury, 547
  for right heart failure, 325
  for septic shock, 302t
Dopaminergic agents, neuroleptic malignant syndrome with, 95
Double defibrillation, 375–376
Double sequential external defibrillation (DSED), 375–376
Droperidol, neuroleptic malignant syndrome with, 95
Drug fever, 93–94, 93t
Drug-induced lactic acidosis, 522–523
Drug-induced pancreatitis, 96
Drug-induced paralysis, 701–704
Drug overdoses. *See* Pharmaceutical drug overdoses
Drug-related hyperthermia, 94–96
DSED. *See* Double sequential external defibrillation
Dual circulation, in venoarterial ECMO, 497
Dual oximetry, 128
Ducanto technique, 37–38
Duodenum, feeding tube in, 766–767, 767f
DVT. *See* Deep venous thrombosis
Dynamic hyperinflation
  adverse consequences of, 414
  in asthma, 401–402, 413–415, 413f
  in COPD, 413–415, 413f
Dynamic outflow obstruction, 275–277, 282
Dysrhythmias, 328–351. *See also specific types*
  central venous access and, 13
  haloperidol and, 84
  hyperkalemia and, 582, 583f
  hypokalemia and, 577–578
  hypomagnesemia and, 591t, 592

E

EACA. *See* Epsilon-aminocaproic acid
ECG. *See* Electrocardiography
Echinocandins, 103, 652, 661
Echocardiography
  of acute aortic dissection, 363
  bedside, 109–123, 389
  in cardiogenic shock, 280
  of hemodynamics, 119–120, 119f, 120t
  of hypovolemia and hypervolemia, 116–119
  in ischemic stroke, 712–713, 713f
  of left ventricular function, 109–113, 111t, 112f
  of pericardium, 115–116, 115t, 116t
  physiological assessments with, 116–120
  of pulmonary embolism, 389
  of right heart failure, 313–314, 315f
  of right ventricular function, 113–115, 114f, 114t
  transesophageal, 121, 121f, 363, 712–713, 713f
  transthoracic, 109–120, 313

ECMO. *See* Extracorporeal membrane oxygenation
ECPR. *See* Extracorporeal cardiopulmonary resuscitation
Eculizumab, 220
Edema, 295–296. *See also specific types and locations*
Edoxaban (Lixiana)
   for atrial fibrillation, 336, 337t
   bleeding with, 270–271
   reversal of, 237f, 239f, 270–271
EDV. *See* End-diastolic volume
EEG. *See* Electroencephalogram
Effient. *See* Prasugrel
Ejection fraction
   atrial fibrillation and, 333–334
   echocardiographic measurement of, 111t, 112–113
   heart failure classification based on, 311–312, 312t
Electrocardiography (ECG)
   in acute aortic dissection, 363
   in acute coronary syndromes, 352–353, 354, 355t
   in atrial fibrillation, 328–330, 330f
   in AV nodal reentrant tachycardia, 328, 330f
   in basic life support, 371
   in carbon monoxide poisoning, 827
   in hemorrhagic shock, 263
   hypercalcemia and, 603
   hyperkalemia and, 582, 583f, 584
   hypokalemia and, 577–578
   in multifocal atrial tachycardia, 329–330, 330f, 338
   in narrow complex tachycardias, 328–330, 330f
   in paroxysmal supraventricular tachycardia, 339
   in supraventricular tachycardia, 331, 331f
   in tachyarrhythmias, 328–343
   in torsades de pointes, 342–343, 342f
   in unstable angina, 354
   in ventricular tachycardia, 331–332, 331f, 340–341
   in wide complex tachycardias, 331–332, 331f
   in Wolff-Parkinson-White syndrome, 336–337
Electroencephalogram (EEG)
   contraindicated, in brain death, 686
   in status epilepticus, 691
Electrolyte(s)
   in parenteral nutrition, 779–780, 780t
   in traumatic brain injury, 737t
Electrolyte disorders, 558–572. *See also specific types*
Electromyography (EMG), 701
Eliquis. *See* Apixaban
ELISA. *See* Enzyme-linked immunosorbent assay
Embolectomy, surgical, for pulmonary embolism, 395, 396f
Embolic stroke, 709, 712

Embolization, angiographic, 265, 267f
EMG. *See* Electromyography
Encephalitis, seizures in, 689t
Encephalopathy
  coma in, 678
  delirium in, 668–669
  hepatic, 614, 619–622, 809
  hypernatremic, 559
  hyponatremic, 566–568
  Wernicke, 591, 676–678, 748–749
End-diastolic volume (EDV), 311–312
Endogenous pyrogens, 91, 104
Endothelial injury, 53
Endotracheal aspirates, 461–462, 463t, 467t
Endotracheal intubation
  adverse events in, minimizing risk of, 27–28
  care in, and prevention of ventilator-associated pneumonia, 455–458
  chest radiograph confirming, 448, 448f
  CO_2 colorimetry for, 129, 130f
  cricoid pressure in, 36–37
  equipment for, 30, 31t
  in hemorrhagic shock, 264
  initial ventilator settings after, 447–448, 447t
  neuromuscular weakness and need for, 695, 696t
  patient positioning for, 28–30, 28f, 30f
  potentially difficult, assessment for, 23–27, 25t
  preoxygenation for, 28, 29t
  preparation for, 27–30
  removal of (extubation), 481–483
  suction-assisted laryngoscopy (Ducanto technique) in, 37–38
  video laryngoscopy in, 37
Endotracheal suctioning, 456–457, 457f
End-tidal carbon dioxide ($ETCO_2$), 129, 131–133, 132f, 263, 377–378, 378f
End-tidal carbon dioxide ($ETCO_2$)–$PaCO_2$ difference, 133, 133t
Energy expenditure, 743–745
Energy yield, of nutrient fuels, 744, 744t
Enoxaparin (Lovenox)
  for pulmonary embolism, 393, 394f
  reversal of, 718t, 719
  thrombocytopenia risk with, 212
  for VTE prophylaxis, 54t, 56
Enteral nutrition, 757–775
  contraindications to, 758, 759t
  creating feeding regimen for, 764–765, 766t
  diarrhea with, 772
  early, benefits of, 757, 757t
  feeding formulas for, 759–762
    calories in, 759–760, 761t, 764–765, 766t
    carbohydrate content of, 761t, 762
    immune-modulating, 760t, 763, 764
    nonprotein calories of, 760
    osmolality of, 760, 761t

Enteral nutrition (*Continued*)
  protein content of, 760–761, 761t, 764–765, 766t
  types and examples of, 760t, 761t
  feeding tube occlusion in, 769
  feeding tube placement for, 766–767, 767f, 768f
  gastroparesis and, 770–772
  general considerations in, 757–759
  implementing feeding regimens for, 768–769
  indications for, 758
  infusion rate for, 765, 766t, 768
  initiation of, 757, 766–769
  modular supplements for, 759, 762–764, 762t
  problems and complications of, 769–772
  regurgitation/aspiration in, 770
  and stress ulcer prophylaxis, 49
  supplemental parenteral nutrition with, 787
  translocation in, 758
  trophic effects of, 757–758
  trophic *vs.* full feedings in, 759
Enterobacter, 455t
Enterococcus, 637, 656t, 657
Entresto. *See* Sacubitril/valsartan
Enzyme-linked immunosorbent assay (ELISA), 213–214, 643
Epidural catheters, VTE prophylaxis and, 59, 60t

Epinephrine
  for acute asthma exacerbation, 406, 839t
  for advanced life support, 373
  aerosolized, for postextubation stridor, 483
  for anaphylaxis, 305, 305t
  avoidance, for acute pancreatitis, 637
  for bradycardia, 345
  for cardiac arrest, 377
  lactic acidosis with, 522
  for septic shock, 300t, 301, 302t
E-point septal separation (EPSS), 111t, 112, 112f
EPS. *See* Extrapyramidal syndrome
Epsilon-aminocaproic acid (EACA), 234t, 240–241
EPSS. *See* E-point septal separation
Eptifibatide (Integrilin), 360t
Erythrocytes. *See* Red blood cell(s)
Erythrocyte transketolase assay, 749
Erythromycin, for gastroparesis, 770–771, 771t
ESBLs. *See* Extended-spectrum beta-lactamases
Escherichia coli infections, 219, 455t, 656t, 657
Esmolol, 334t, 366t, 367, 799t
Esomeprazole, 47t, 48
Esophageal varices. *See* Variceal hemorrhage
Essential trace elements, 750–753
  daily allowances for, 750t
  definition of, 750

in parenteral nutrition, 781–782, 782t
ETCO$_2$. *See* End-tidal carbon dioxide
Ethylene glycol intoxication, 831–834
    clinical features of, 832–833
    crystalluria in, 833, 833f
    management of, 834, 834t
    pathogenesis of, 831–832, 832f
Etomidate, 34t, 793
European Society of Cardiology, 392, 393t
Euthyroid sick syndrome, 796, 797
EVD. *See* External ventricular drain
EXTEM assay, 232
Extended-spectrum beta-lactamases (ESBLs), 651
External ventricular drain (EVD), 729–733, 732f
Extracorporeal cardiopulmonary resuscitation (ECPR), 376, 376t, 486–504, 502t
Extracorporeal Life Support Organization, 486
Extracorporeal membrane oxygenation (ECMO), 486–504
    availability and use of, 486
    comparison of techniques, 502
    for propofol-related infusion syndrome, 81–82
    for pulmonary embolism management, 396
    venoarterial, 486, 492–502
        for cardiogenic shock, 289–290, 492–495
        comparison with other ECMO techniques, 502t
        complications of, 290, 497–500, 501t
        contraindications to, 495t
        differential hypoxemia in, 497–499, 500f
        in extracorporeal cardiopulmonary resuscitation, 376, 376t, 501–502
        general management considerations in, 498t–499t
        indications for, 492–495, 495t
        initial settings for, 496
        lower extremity ischemia in, 499–500
        outcomes of, 290
        physiology in, 495–497, 496f
        retrograde flow in, consequences of, 496–497
        tools for predicting survival in, 495
        troubleshooting in, 497–500
        weaning from, 501
    venovenous, 486–492
        for acute respiratory distress syndrome, 427
        calculators predicting survival with, 486
        carbon dioxide removal in, 489
        chatter and suck-down in, 490–492
        comparison with other ECMO techniques, 502t

Extracorporeal membrane oxygenation (ECMO) (*Continued*)
  contraindications to, 487t
  general management considerations in, 491t–492t
  hemodynamics in, 490
  indications for, 486, 487t
  oxygenation in, 489
  physiology in, 486–487, 488f
  refractory hypoxemia in, 492, 493t
  troubleshooting in, 490–492
  weaning from, 492, 494t
Extrapyramidal syndrome (EPS), 84
Extubation, 481–483
Eye movements, in coma, 679–681, 681f

F

FAC. *See* Fractional area of change
Face masks
  for noninvasive ventilation, 433–434, 433f
  problems with, 27, 27t, 434
Factitious hyperkalemia, 580–581
Factor Eight Inhibitor Bypassing Activity (FEIBA), 236
Famotidine, 47, 47t
Fatty acids
  dietary, 747–748
  in enteral nutrition, 761t, 762–763
  in ketogenesis, 525–526, 526f
  polyunsaturated, 763
  short-chain, 646, 762–763

FCDC. *See* Fulminant *C. difficile* colitis
Febrile nonhemolytic reaction
  to platelet transfusion, 223–224
  to red blood cell transfusion, 93, 195, 200–201
Febrile nonhemolytic reactions, 200–201
Fecal microbiota transplantation (FMT), 645t, 647
Feeding formulas, enteral, 759–762
  calories in, 759–760, 761t, 764–765, 766t
  carbohydrate content of, 761t, 762
  immune-modulating, 760t, 763, 764
  nonprotein calories of, 760
  osmolality of, 760, 761t
  protein content of, 760–761, 761t, 764–765, 766t
  types and examples of, 760t, 761t
Feeding tube. *See also* Enteral nutrition
  occlusion of, 769
  placement of, 766–767, 767f, 768f
FEIBA. *See* Factor Eight Inhibitor Bypassing Activity
Femoral triangle, 11, 12f
Femoral vein
  anatomy and location of, 11, 12f
  cannulation of, 11
Femorofemoral ECMO, 495–497, 496f
Fentanyl, 36, 66t, 67–68, 69t

Fermentable fiber, 762–763
Ferritin, 751
Fever, 91–107
  antipyretic therapy for, 103–104
  assessment of, 101–102
  in cardiac arrest, prevention of, 380, 381t
  definition, in ICU, 91
  drugs as cause of (drug fever), 93–94, 93t
  empiric antimicrobial therapy for, 103
  external cooling for, 104
  iatrogenic, 98
  imaging studies in, 102
  infectious causes of, 98–101
  inflammation vs. infection and, 91–92
  inflammatory (noninfectious) etiologies of, 92–93, 92t
  laboratory tests in, 102
  moderate, and decreased mortality, 103
  patient's medical history and, 101–102
  postoperative, early, 97–98, 97t
  in shock, 255
  in stroke, 710t
  in subarachnoid hemorrhage, 721
  in ventilator-associated pneumonia, 458, 459t
FFP. *See* Fresh frozen plasma
Fiber, in enteral nutrition, 762–763
Fiberoptic intubation, awake, 38–40, 40t
Fibrinogen, 226–227, 233

Fibrinogen concentrate, 241, 242f, 266t, 270, 715
Fibrinolysis
  inhibition of (*See* Antifibrinolytic agents)
  intrapleural, 469
FIBTEM assay, 233
Fick equation, 148
Fidaxomicin, for *C. difficile* infection, 644, 645t
Filters
  blood, 198
  vena cava, 58–59, 59f, 396–397, 737t
Filtration gradient, 540
Fingertip probe, for pulse oximetry, 124–126, 125f
FiO_2. *See* Fraction of inspired oxygen
Five "W's," of postoperative fever, 97–98, 97t
"Flash" pulmonary edema, 321
Fleischner's sign, 389
Flow rates, through catheters, 2, 2f, 3t
Flow-time graphics
  in asthma, 400–402, 401f, 402f, 414–415
  in COPD, 414–415
Fluconazole, 661–663
Fludrocortisone, 795
Fluid challenge, 116–119, 180, 181f, 547
Fluid compartments, body, 153, 154f, 556–557, 556f
Fluid management, 176–185
  in acute kidney injury, 547
  in acute respiratory distress syndrome, 425
  in cerebral edema, 715
  in hyperchloremia, 571

Fluid management (*Continued*)
  in hypernatremia, 559–562
  in hypochloremia, 572
  in hyponatremia, 566–569
  in parenteral nutrition, 784, 784t
  in right heart failure, 322–323
  in subarachnoid hemorrhage, 723
  in venoarterial ECMO, 499t
  in venovenous ECMO, 492t
Fluid resuscitation, 153–175
  for acute pancreatitis, 636
  adrenal insufficiency and, 793
  albumin solutions for, 166–168
  for alcoholic ketoacidosis, 531
  for anaphylactic shock, 306
  central venous pressure in, 178–179
  colloid–crystalloid debate in, 170–171
  colloid fluids for, 165–172
  crystalloid fluids for, 153–162
  de-resuscitation in, 172, 184
  5% dextrose solutions for, 162–165
  for diabetic ketoacidosis, 527, 529t
  equilibration in, 153, 155f
  excess, adverse effects of, 183, 183t
  first-line fluids for, 153
  fluid responsiveness in, 179–182
  for hemorrhagic shock, 264–265, 266t
  hydroxyethyl starch for, 169
  hypertonic saline for, 160–162
  inferior vena cava diameter and, 182
  for ischemic stroke, 712
  isotonic saline for, 154–157
  keys to, 183
  lactated Ringer's for, 157–159
  normal pH fluids for, 157, 159–160
  osmolarity and osmolality in, 154, 156f
  physiology of, 176–182
  preload in, 153, 176–177, 177f
  for rhabdomyolysis, 544
  for shock, 253, 254t, 300t, 301
  stroke volume variation in, 180–181, 182f
  TEG- or ROTEM-based thresholds for, 234, 234t
  for thyroid storm, 800
  venous return in, 177–179
  volume distribution and, 153–154, 154f, 155f, 166, 166f
Flumazenil (Romazicon), 813–814
Focal seizures, 690
Folinic acid, for methanol intoxication, 836
Fomepizole, 834, 834t
Fondaparinux (Arixtra), 54t, 215t, 362t
Formic acid, 832f, 835
Fosphenytoin, 692t, 693
Four-factor prothrombin complex concentrate, 236–238, 238t, 270–271, 271t, 718–719, 718t
4Ts score, 213, 213t
Fractional area of change (FAC), 111t, 114t

Fractional excretion of sodium, 545t, 546
Fractional excretion of urea, 545t, 546
Fractional shortening (FS), 111t
Fraction of inspired oxygen (FiO$_2$), 444, 447t
Fragmin. *See* Dalteparin
Frank-Starling law, 176–177, 177f, 183
FRC. *See* Functional residual capacity
Freezing point depression method, 557
French size, of catheters and needles, 1, 3t
Fresh frozen plasma (FFP), 224–226, 265, 266t
 adverse effects of, 225–226, 226t
 anticoagulation reversal with, 225, 238t
 TEG- or ROTEM-based thresholds for, 234t
FS. *See* Fractional shortening
Fulminant *C. difficile* colitis (FCDC), 643
Functional residual capacity (FRC), 445
Furosemide
 for acute kidney injury, 547
 continuous infusion of, 322, 323f
 for heart failure, 319, 321t, 322, 323f
 for hypercalcemia, 603
 for hypermagnesemia, 596
 for hypervolemic hypernatremia, 561–562
 hypomagnesemia with, 591, 591t
 for rhabdomyolysis, 544
 thiamine deficiency with, 748
Fusion beats, 332, 332f

G

Gabapentin (Neurontin), 74, 699–700
Gabapentin withdrawal, 678
Gag reflex, induced, 339
Gallbladder
 inflammation of (*See* Acalculous cholecystitis)
 parenteral nutrition and, 786–787
Gallstone pancreatitis, 96, 634, 635, 635f
γ-Aminobutyric acid (GABA), in alcohol withdrawal, 671–672
Gastric decompression, 32
Gastric mucosa, stress-related erosion of, 45–51. *See also* Stress ulcer
Gastric secretions, sodium concentration in, 559t
Gastric ultrasound, in RSII preparation, 32, 33f
Gastric varices. *See* Variceal hemorrhage
Gastroparesis, 770–772
Gauge size, of catheters and needles, 1, 3t
GCS. *See* Glasgow Coma Scale
Generalized seizures, 690
Geodon. *See* Ziprasidone
GFR. *See* Glomerular filtration rate
Glasgow Coma Scale (GCS), 681–683, 682t, 727

Glomerular filtration pressure, 540, 540f
Glomerular filtration rate (GFR), 536, 537f
  in chronic kidney disease, 537–538, 538t
  in hypotension, 540, 540f
Glucagon
  for anaphylactic shock, 306
  for β-blockers toxicity, 345, 815–816
  for calcium channel blocker toxicity, 816
Glucocorticoids
  adrenal insufficiency induced by, 792, 792t
  deficiency of, 565
  for hypercalcemia, 604t
Gluconate, in normal pH fluids, 159
Glucose, energy yield from, 744t
Glucose levels
  5% dextrose solutions and, 164–165
  enteral nutrition and, 760t
  parenteral nutrition and, 776–777, 777t, 785
  in post-cardiac arrest patients, 381t
  short-acting $β_2$ agonists and, 405
  sodium and, 562–563
  stroke and, 710t
  subarachnoid hemorrhage and, 721
Glucose loading, hypophosphatemia with, 605t
Glutamine, 762t, 764, 778
Glutathione peroxidase, 752f, 753, 782
Glutathione redox reactions, 752f, 753
Glycogen, endogenous stores of, 747, 747t
Glycopyrrolate, 704
Graded compression stockings (GCS), 57
Gram stain, in ventilator-associated pneumonia, 460–461
Guillain-Barré syndrome, 698–700, 699t

H

Haemophilus influenzae infection, in COPD, 411
Hagen–Poiseuille equation, 189–190, 190f
Haloperidol (Haldol), 83–84, 83t, 95, 672t, 677f
Halothane, malignant hyperthermia with, 94, 94t
Hampton's hump, 389
Hand hygiene, 17t, 647
Harlequin syndrome, 497
Hartmann, Alexis, 157
Hartmann's solution, 157. *See also* Lactated Ringer's
HCO_3. *See* Bicarbonate
Heart block
  β-blocker overdose and, 814
  hyperkalemia and, 582, 583f
  hypermagnesemia and, 595t
Heart dysrhythmias. *See* Dysrhythmias
Heart failure (HF)
  acute, 311–327
  acute kidney injury with, 319, 539
  cardiogenic shock *vs.*, 278

cardiovascular consequences
of, 315–319
diastolic dysfunction in,
311–312
diuretics for, 319–322, 321t,
323f
hyponatremia in, 566
left ventricular ejection
fraction in, 311–312, 312t
management strategies for,
319–325
mortality in, 311
neurohumoral responses in,
315–317
positive-pressure ventilation
and, 441
in post-cardiac arrest
syndrome, 380
prevalence of, 311
renin-angiotensin-
aldosterone system in,
317–318
right, 312–314, 313t, 315f,
322–325, 324f
stages and classes of, 315,
316t
sympathetic nervous system
in, 317
systolic dysfunction in, 311
types of, 311–314
vasodilators for, 319, 320t
venous air embolism and, 15
venous congestion in, 318,
318f
Heart failure with mildly
reduced ejection
fraction (HFmrEF), 312t
Heart failure with preserved
ejection fraction
(HFpEF), 311–312, 312t,
321
Heart failure with reduced
ejection fraction
(HFrEF), 312t, 335
Helium-oxygen mixture
(Heliox), 408–409
HELLP syndrome, 216, 220–221
Helmet, for ventilation, 434
Hematocrit, 186–188
in acute pancreatitis, 632
blood viscosity and, 190
definition of, 187
oxygen extraction and,
190–191
reference ranges for, 186t
tolerance to low levels of, 192
as unreliable marker, in
critically ill patients,
187–188
Hematoma(s)
anticoagulant use and, 59, 60t
venous access and, 13–14
Hemodialysis
for acetaminophen toxicity,
812
for acute kidney injury,
547–551
advantages and
disadvantages of, 551
countercurrent exchange in,
550–551
diffusion in, 550
for ethylene glycol
intoxication, 834
for hemolytic uremic
syndrome, 220
for hyperkalemia, 586
for hypermagnesemia, 596
intravenous access for,
548–550, 550f
mechanism of fluid and
solute removal in, 549f

Hemodialysis (*Continued*)
   for methanol intoxication, 836
   for propofol-related infusion syndrome, 81–82
   for salicylate intoxication, 821
Hemodynamics. *See also specific parameters*
   cardiogenic shock and, 278–279, 279f
   echocardiographic assessment of, 119–120, 119f, 120t
   positive end-expiratory pressure and, 446, 447f
   pulmonary catheter for monitoring, 136–151
   septic shock and, 299
   traumatic brain injury and, 737t
   venoarterial ECMO and, 496–497
   venovenous ECMO and, 490
Hemofiltration
   for acute kidney injury, 547–548, 551–552
   advantages of, 551
   continuous performance of, 551
   convection in, 551
   disadvantages of, 551–552
   mechanism of fluid and solute removal in, 549f
Hemoglobin, 186–188, 249–250
   carbon monoxide poisoning and, 825, 826f
   definition and function of, 187
   iron bound to, 751
   loss, in hemorrhage, 260, 260f
   oximetry of, 124–128
   reference ranges for, 186t
   shock and, 257
   tolerance to low levels of, 192
   as transfusion trigger, 192–193
   as unreliable marker, in critically ill patients, 187–188
Hemolysis, elevated liver function tests, and low platelets (HELLP) syndrome, 216, 220–221
Hemolysis, massive, hypermagnesemia in, 595
Hemolytic reaction, acute, 198–200
Hemolytic uremic syndrome (HUS), 216t, 219–220
Hemorrhage/bleeding, 260–261. *See also specific types and anatomic locations*
   anticoagulation-associated, 270–272
   classification system for, 261, 262t
   control of, 265, 267f
   NSAIDs and, 73
   oxygen delivery in, 260, 260f
   stress ulcers and, 45
   thrombolytic therapy and, 356–357
   unfractionated heparin and, 55
   venous access and, 13–14
Hemorrhagic shock, 260–274
   acidosis in, 262, 267
   airway and breathing in, 264
   class III hemorrhage and onset of, 261, 262t

class IV hemorrhage and
progression of, 261, 262t
clinical evaluation of, 262
coagulopathy in, 262,
268–269
concomitant responses
required in, 262–263,
265
diagnosis of, 265
hypothermia in, 262, 267–268
initial approach to, 254t
lactate levels in, 519, 519f
lethal triad in, 262, 267–269
massive transfusion protocol
for, 269–270
resuscitation for, 262–270
basic adjuncts for, 263–264
goals of, 272, 272f
thromboelastography in, 269,
269t
treatment for hemorrhage in,
265, 267f
Hemostatic adjuncts, 236–242.
See also specific agents
TEG- or ROTEM-based
thresholds for, 234, 234t
topical, 241, 243f
treatment algorithm for,
242f
Hemothorax, venous access
and, 13–14
Heparin. *See also* Low-
molecular-weight
heparin; Unfractionated
heparin
coagulopathy assay with,
233
continuous infusion, 395
for pulmonary embolism,
393–395, 394f
reversal of, 718t, 719

Heparin-induced
thrombocytopenia
(HIT), 212–214
alternative anticoagulant
therapy in, 214, 215t
clinical features of, 212
diagnosis of, 213–214
4Ts score in, 213, 213t
laboratory testing in, 213–214
management of, 214
pathogenesis of, 212
risk factors for, 212
Hepatic encephalopathy, 614,
619–622, 809
clinical features of, 619–620
closure of portosystemic
shunts for, 622, 623f
diagnostic evaluation of,
619–621
grading of, 620t
intracranial pressure in, 622
pathogenesis of, 619
reducing ammonia burden
in, 621–622
serum ammonia levels in,
620–621
Hepatic steatosis, parenteral
nutrition and, 786
Hepatobiliary iminodiacetic
acid (HIDA) scan, 642
Hepatorenal syndrome (HRS),
541, 542t, 616–617, 617t,
618t
Hepcidin, 751
HEPTEM assay, 233
Hetastarch. *See* Hydroxyethyl
starch
HF. *See* Heart failure
HFmrEF. *See* Heart failure with
mildly reduced ejection
fraction

HFNO. *See* High-flow nasal oxygen
HFpEF. *See* Heart failure with preserved ejection fraction
HFrEF. *See* Heart failure with reduced ejection fraction
HIDA scan, 642
High-flow nasal oxygen (HFNO), 438, 483
Histamine H_2 receptor antagonists (H_2RA), 47, 47t
HIT. *See* Heparin-induced thrombocytopenia
HRS. *See* Hepatorenal syndrome
HUS. *See* Hemolytic uremic syndrome
Hydrocortisone
  for critical illness-related corticosteroid insufficiency, 794–795
  for hypercalcemia, 604t
  for hypothyroidism, 802
  for septic shock, 300t, 301
  for thyrotoxicosis and thyroid storm, 799t, 800
Hydrogen peroxide, 751, 752f, 753
Hydrolyzed proteins, 761
Hydromorphone (Dilaudid), 66t, 68, 69t
Hydroxocobalamin, 301, 830t, 831
Hydroxyethyl starch (HES, Hetastarch), 169, 169t, 266t
Hydroxyl radical, 751, 752f
25-Hydroxyvitamin D, 749–750

Hyperactive central nervous system syndrome, 591, 591t
Hyperactive delirium, 669f, 673
Hyperbaric oxygen, for carbon monoxide poisoning, 828
Hypercalcemia, 603, 604t
Hypercapnia, 409, 412, 424, 490
Hypercapnic respiratory failure, noninvasive ventilation for, 435–436, 435f
Hyperchloremia, 569–571, 570t
Hyperchloremic metabolic acidosis, 157
Hypercoagulable state, 52
Hyperglycemia
  5% dextrose solutions and, 164–165
  enteral nutrition in, 760t
  parenteral nutrition and, 785
  short-acting β_2 agonists and, 405
  sodium in, 562–563
  stroke and, 710t
  subarachnoid hemorrhage and, 721
Hyperinflation of lungs, dynamic. *See* Dynamic hyperinflation
Hyperkalemia, 580–586
  atrioventricular block with, 344
  clinical consequences of, 582
  drug-induced, 581–582, 581t
  ECG changes in, 582, 583f, 584
  factitious, 580–581
  mechanisms of, 580–582
  severe
    cardiac stabilization in, 584–585, 584t

Index

definition of, 583
management of, 583–586, 584t
transcellular shift and, 580, 581t
Hyperlactatemia, 518–525
causes of, 520, 521t
in critical care, considerations for, 520–523
in cyanide poisoning, 828–830
drug-induced, 522–523
in ethylene glycol intoxication, 832, 832f, 833
in methanol intoxication, 832f
in shock, 256, 519, 519f, 520
Hypermagnesemia, 595–596
Hypernatremia, 558–562
definition of, 558
extracellular volume in, 558, 558f
hypervolemic, 561–562
hypovolemic, 559–560
normovolemic, 560–561
Hypernociception, 64
Hyperosmolar therapy, for traumatic brain injury, 730t
Hyperparathyroidism, 595, 603
Hyperphosphatemia, 607–609, 608t
Hypersensitivity reactions
to fresh frozen plasma, 226, 226t
to platelet transfusion, 223t, 224
to RBC transfusion, 201–202
Hypertension
in acute aortic dissection, 363, 364–367, 366t
dexmedetomidine and, 82
in heart failure, 319, 320t
portal (*See* Portal hypertension)
spontaneous intracerebral hemorrhage in, 716
in stroke, management of, 710t, 711, 711t
subarachnoid hemorrhage in, 719
Hyperthermia
definition of, 91
drug-related, 94–96
malignant, 94, 94t
Hyperthyroidism. *See* Thyrotoxicosis
Hypertonic fluids, 556–557, 556f
Hypertonic saline, 160–162, 160t
for cerebral edema, 715, 716t
for hyponatremia, 566–567, 566t
for intracranial pressure management, 162, 733
for subarachnoid hemorrhage, 721
for traumatic brain injury, 162
for traumatic shock, 161–162
volume effects of, 160–161, 161f
Hypertriglyceridemia, 564t, 632, 635, 748
Hypertrophic cardiomyopathy, shock in, 275–277
Hypervolemia, echocardiographic assessment of, 116–119
Hypervolemic hypernatremia, 561–562
Hypervolemic hyponatremia, 566, 569

Hypoactive delirium, 668, 669f
Hypoalbuminemia, 513, 598–599, 599f
Hypocalcemia, 600–602
 alkalosis and, 600–601, 600t
 blood transfusion and, 600t, 601
 calcium replacement therapy for, 602, 602t
 clinical manifestations of, 601–602
 hyperphosphatemia and, 608
 hypomagnesemia and, 591t, 592, 600t, 601
 inflammation and, 601
 ionized, 600–602
  causes, in ICU, 600t
  definition of, 600
 predisposing conditions for, 600–601, 600t
 renal failure and, 600t, 601
 torsades de pointes with, 342
Hypochloremia, 571–572, 571t
Hypoglycemia, parenteral nutrition in, 776–777, 777t
Hypokalemia, 576–580
 alkalosis and, 577, 578f
 clinical manifestations of, 577–578
 diabetes insipidus with, 560
 diarrhea and, 577, 578f
 diuretic therapy and, 577, 578f
 ECG changes in, 577–578
 estimated potassium deficits in, 579t
 hypomagnesemia and, 577, 580, 591t, 592
 management of, 578–580
 multifocal atrial tachycardia with, 338

 parenteral nutrition and, 786
 potassium depletion and, 577, 578f
 potassium replacement for, 579–580
 short-acting β_2 agonists and, 405
 torsades de pointes with, 342
 transcellular shift and, 576–577, 578
Hypomagnesemia, 590–594
 clinical manifestations of, 591–592, 591t
 definition of, 590
 diuretics and, 591, 591t
 dysrhythmias with, 591t, 592
 hypocalcemia in, 591t, 592, 600t, 601
 hypokalemia with, 577, 580, 591t
 ICU risks with, 590
 magnesium replacement for, 592–594
 multifocal atrial tachycardia with, 338
 neurological signs of, 591
 predisposing conditions for, 590–591, 591t
 short-acting β_2 agonists and, 405
 thiamine deficiency in, 748
 torsades de pointes with, 342–343, 592
Hyponatremia, 562–569
 diagnostic approach to, 563f
 hypertonic saline for, 566–567, 566t
 hypervolemic, 566, 569
 hypomagnesemia and, 591t
 hypovolemic, 564–565, 569
 management of, 566–569

normovolemic, 565–566, 569
overcorrection of, 568, 568t
pseudohyponatremia vs., 562–563, 564t
subarachnoid hemorrhage and, 721
Hyponatremic encephalopathy, 566–568
Hypo-oncotic fluids, 167
Hypoparathyroidism, hyperphosphatemia in, 607
Hypophosphatemia, 604–607
clinically silent, 606
clinical manifestations of, 606–607
in diabetic ketoacidosis, 530, 605t
hypomagnesemia and, 591t
management of, 607, 607t
mechanisms of, 605t
muscle disorders with, 607
oxidative metabolism in, 606, 606f
in parenteral nutrition, 785–786
predisposing conditions for, 604–605, 605t
short-acting β_2 agonists and, 405
Hypotension
acute kidney injury in, 540, 540f
adrenal insufficiency and, 793
anaphylactic shock and, 304–307
benzodiazepine overdose and, 813
β-blocker overdose and, 814–816

cardiogenic shock and, 277
hypercalcemia and, 603
hypocalcemia and, 602
hypovolemic hypernatremia and, 559–560, 569
ischemic stroke and, 712
morphine and, 67
opioids and, 70
post-resuscitation period and, 382
propofol and, 80
rapid ultrasound for, 109, 110t
traumatic brain injury and, 731t, 737t
venous air embolism and, 16
Hypothermia
cardiac arrest and, 381t, 382
hypokalemia with, 577
shock and, 255, 262, 267–268
Hypothyroidism, 796–797, 800–802
diagnosis of, 801
etiologies of, 800
hyponatremia in, 566
identifying inciting event in, 802
myxedema coma in, 800–801, 801t
treatment of, 802
Hypotonic fluids, 556–557, 556f
Hypoventilation
capnography of, 131
obesity syndrome of, 436
Hypovolemia
acute pancreatitis and, 636
echocardiographic assessment of, 116–119, 117f
fluid resuscitation for (See Fluid resuscitation)
hemorrhage and, 260–261

Hypovolemia (*Continued*)
hypercalcemia and, 603
venous access in patients with, 2
VExUS score in, 117f, 119
Hypovolemic hypernatremia, 559–560, 569
Hypovolemic hyponatremia, 564–565
Hypoxemia
opioids and, 70
pulmonary embolism and, 387, 388t
in venoarterial ECMO, 497–499, 500f
in venovenous ECMO, 490, 492, 493t
Hypoxia
in acute respiratory distress syndrome, 418
in cyanide poisoning, 828–829
cytopathic, in septic shock, 300
measures of, 248, 248t
oxygen measures in, 248t
in shock, 247, 253
in traumatic brain injury, 728, 728f
Hypoxic respiratory failure, noninvasive ventilation for, 436

I
IABP. *See* Intra-aortic balloon pump
IAP. *See* Intra-abdominal pressure
Ibutilide, 337
IC. *See* Intermittent catheterization
ICH. *See* Intracerebral hemorrhage
ICP. *See* Intracranial pressure
Idarucizumab (Praxbind), 271, 718t, 719
IDSA. *See* Infectious Diseases Society of America
i-gel, 39t
IJV. *See* Internal jugular vein
Immune-modulating enteral formulations, 760t, 763, 764
Immunosuppressants, for TTP, 219
Immunotherapy, for myasthenia gravis, 697
Impella heart (catheter) pumps, 288–289, 288f
Impulse generation, cardiac disorder of, 344
Impulse propagation, cardiac disorders of, 344
IMV. *See* Intermittent mandatory ventilation
Indirect calorimetry, 744–745
Indomethacin, 561
Induction agents, for RSII, 34t, 35
Indwelling urinary catheter (IUC)
alternatives to, 658, 659f
appropriate indications for, 657–658, 657t
duration of use, 657
in hemorrhagic shock, 264
infection risk with, 656 (*See also* Catheter-associated urinary tract infections)
prevalence of use, 656

Infection(s). *See also specific infections*
  abdominal, 641–654
  central line-associated, 17–18, 99, 785
  ICU (nosocomial), 98–101
  inflammation *vs.*, and fever, 91–92
  postoperative wound, 99, 647–648, 649t
  transfusions and, 223t, 224, 226t
Infectious Diseases Society of America (IDSA), 91, 103, 644, 655, 661–663
Inferior vena cava
  diameter, and fluid responsiveness, 182
  filter, 58–59, 59f, 396–397, 737t
Inflammation
  acute, consequences of, 295–297
  acute kidney injury in, 538–539, 539t
  anemia of, 188–189
  cardiogenic shock and, 279
  clinical syndromes in, 298–303
  fever as indication of, 91–92
  fever caused by, 92–93, 92t
  hypocalcemia in, 601
  hypophosphatemia in, 605t
  post-cardiac arrest syndrome and, 380
  severe or persistent, 295
Inflammatory mediators, 295
Inflammatory shock, 295–310. *See also* Anaphylactic shock; Septic shock
Inflation of lungs, in mechanical ventilation, 448–451

Influenza, hemolytic uremic syndrome in, 219
Inotropic agents
  for cardiogenic shock, 282–284, 283t
  for right heart failure, 324
  for septic shock, 301, 303t
Insecticides, poisoning from, 836–838
Institute for Healthcare Improvement, 457–458
Insulin
  for diabetic ketoacidosis, 527–529, 529t
  hypokalemia with, 577
Insulin-dextrose, for hyperkalemia, 584t, 585
Integrilin. *See* Eptifibatide
INTEM assay, 232
Intermittent catheterization (IC), 658
Intermittent mandatory ventilation (IMV), 452t
Intermittent pneumatic compression (IPC), 57–58, 57f
Internal jugular vein (IJV)
  anatomy and location of, 8–9, 9f
  approaches to, 9, 9f
  cannulation of, 8–10, 9f, 10f
  carotid artery puncture with catheterization of, 14
  pneumothorax with catheterization of, 13
  venous air embolism with entry to, 16
International Society of Thrombosis and Haemostasis, 217, 218t
Interstitial edema, 156–157, 172

Interstitial edematous pancreatitis, 629
Interstitial nephritis, drugs implicated in, 543t
Intra-abdominal pressure (IAP)
  abdominal compartment syndrome and, 541, 638
  acute pancreatitis and, 638
  crystalloid resuscitation and, 541
Intra-aortic balloon pump (IABP), 285–288, 287f
Intracardiac shunts, cardiac output measurement errors with, 143
Intracerebral hemorrhage (ICH)
  management of, 715
  seizures with, 689t
  spontaneous, 716–719
  stroke management and, 714–715, 714f
Intracranial pressure (ICP)
  elevated, impending brain herniation with, 733–735, 735t
  elevated, management of, 733–735, 734f
  hepatic encephalopathy and, 622
  hypertonic saline and, 162, 733
  monitoring of, 729–733, 732f, 732t
  stroke and, 715
  traumatic brain injury and, 729–735
  treatment threshold of, 731t
Intrapleural fibrinolysis, 469
Intrathoracic pressure
  and noninvasive ventilation, 438–441
  and pulmonary artery catheter, 145
Intravenous immunoglobulin (IVIG), 697, 699
Intraventricular conduction disturbances, 344–345
Introducer sheaths, for catheters, 6–7, 6f, 138
Intubation
  endotracheal (*See* Endotracheal intubation)
  fiberoptic (*See* Awake fiberoptic intubation)
  rapid sequence (*See* Rapid sequence induction and intubation)
Invasive ventilation. *See* Mechanical ventilation
Iodine, 750t, 799t
IPC. *See* Intermittent pneumatic compression
Ipratropium, 405, 406t, 410, 411t, 839t
Iron
  free *vs.* bound, 751
  nutritional requirements for, 750t, 751–752
  and oxidant injury, 751–752, 752f
Iron supplementation, 752
Ischemic stroke, 709–716
  antihypertensive therapy for, 710t, 711, 711t
  antiplatelet therapy for, 710t
  cerebral edema with, 715
  complications of, 714–716
  echocardiography in, 712–713, 713f
  fever in, 710t
  general support measures for, 710t

hyperglycemia in, 710t
hypotension in, 712
intracerebral hemorrhage with, 714–715, 714f
management of, 709–713
mechanical ventilation in, 710
respiratory support/oxygen for, 709, 710t
seizures in, 715–716
thromboprophylaxis for, 710t
Isolation precautions, for *C. difficile* infection, 647, 648f
Isoproterenol, for bradycardia, 345
Isotonic fluids, 556, 556f
Isotonic saline, 154–157
adverse effects of, 156–157
comparison with lactated Ringer's, 157–158
comparison with plasma, 155, 156t
excessive, hypervolemic hypernatremia with, 561–562
features of, 155
for hemorrhagic shock, 266t
for hypercalcemia, 604t
and hyperchloremia, 571
for hypotension, 559–560, 569
for ischemic stroke, 712
normal pH fluids *vs.*, 160
volume effects of, 155–156
IUC. *See* Indwelling urinary catheter

J

Jugular vein, internal. *See* Internal jugular vein
Jugular venous oximetry (SjVO$_2$), 731t, 735, 736t

K

Kayexalate. *See* Sodium polystyrene sulfonate
Keppra. *See* Levetiracetam
Ketamine, 34t, 71t, 73, 408
Ketoacids, 525–526, 526f. *See also* Alcoholic ketoacidosis; Diabetic ketoacidosis
Ketorolac, 71t, 72–73
Kidney Disease Improving Global Outcomes (KDIGO) group, 535
Kidney failure. *See* Acute kidney injury
Kidney function/dysfunction. *See also specific disorders*
in acid-base disorders, 508–509
acute kidney injury criteria and, 535–538, 535t
biomarkers of, 537
chronic kidney disease and, 537–538
in heart failure, 319
hyperchloremia with, 570, 570t
magnesium replacement for, 594
nephrotoxins and, 541–543, 543t
in shock, 256, 257
urinary indices of, 545–546, 545t
King LTS-D, 39t
Klebsiella, 455t, 656t
Knuckle sign, 389

L

Labetalol, 366t, 711t
Lactate, 518–525
acute pancreatitis and, 632

Lactate (*Continued*)
  cyanide poisoning and,
    828–830
  5% dextrose solutions and,
    164
  ethylene glycol intoxication
    and, 832, 832f, 833
  hypoxic measures of, 248t
  lactated Ringer's and,
    158–159
  measurement of, 520
  methanol intoxication and,
    832f
  misconceptions about, 518
  normal measures of, 248t, 519
  prognostic value of, 519–520
  shock and, 256, 519, 519f
Lactated Ringer's, 157–159
  for acute pancreatitis, 636
  adverse effects of, 158–159
  comparison with plasma, 156t
  contraindication to, 158, 592
  for diabetic ketoacidosis, 527
  features of, 157–158
  for hemorrhagic shock, 264,
    266t
  normal pH fluids *vs.*, 159–160
  for shock, 256
Lactic acidosis, 518–525
  alkali therapy for, 523–525
  in critical care, considerations
    for, 520–523
  ICU drugs associated with,
    522–523
  in propofol-related infusion
    syndrome, 81–82
  in septic shock, 520
  in thiamine deficiency,
    520–522, 522f
  thiamine deficiency and,
    748–749

Lactulose, 621
Lansoprazole, for stress ulcer
  prophylaxis, 47t
Laryngeal edema, 296, 481
Laryngeal mask airway (LMA),
  39t
Laryngoscopy
  potentially difficult,
    assessment for, 23–27,
    25t
  suction-assisted, 37–38
  video, 37
Leaky-capillary pulmonary
  edema, 15
Left atrial function, wedge
  pressure and, 141–142
Left ventricular assist devices
  (LVADs), 288–289, 288f
Left ventricular ejection fraction
  (LVEF)
  atrial fibrillation and,
    333–334
  echocardiographic
    measurement of, 111t,
    112–113
  heart failure classification
    based on, 311–312, 312t
Left ventricular end-diastolic
  pressure (LVEDP), 145
Left ventricular function
  EPSS measurement of, 111t,
    112, 112f
  MAPSE measurement of, 112
  noninvasive ventilation and,
    440f
  positive-pressure ventilation
    and, 438–439, 439f
  pulmonary artery wedge
    pressure and, 142, 145
  quantitative assessment of,
    111t, 112–113

Simpson's method for, 112–113
transthoracic echocardiography of, 109–113, 111t, 112f
Left ventricular outflow obstruction, dynamic, 275–277, 282
Left ventricular outflow tract (LVOT), 119–120, 119f
Leg raising, passive, 180, 181f
Lethal triad, in hemorrhagic shock, 262, 267–269
Leucovorin, for methanol intoxication, 836
Leukocyte-reduced red blood cells, 194t, 195
Leukocytes, as percentage in blood volume, 188f
Leukoreduction, 222
Leukotriene receptor antagonists, 408
Levalbuterol, 403, 406t, 411t
Levetiracetam (Keppra), 692t, 693, 731t, 738t
Levodopa, 95
Levosimendan, 283t, 284, 303t
Levothyroxine, 802
Lidocaine, 36, 373
Life support
advanced, 373–377, 374f
basic, 371–373, 372t
extracorporeal, 486 (*See also* Extracorporeal membrane oxygenation)
Limb ischemia
Impella catheter and, 289
intra-aortic balloon pump and, 286–287
venoarterial ECMO and, 499–500

Linezolid, lactic acidosis with, 523
Linoleic acid, 747
Lipase, 102, 631
Lipid(s)
endogenous stores of, 747, 747t
energy yield from, 744t, 747
in enteral nutrition, 763
nutritional requirements for, 747–748
in parenteral nutrition, 779, 786
Lipid emulsions, 779, 786
Liquid feeding. *See* Enteral nutrition
Lithium intoxication, 595
Liver failure, 613–628
acetaminophen toxicity and, 613, 615–616, 807–812
acute (fulminant), 613–614
acute-on-chronic, 613–614, 614t
amino acid dosing in, 778
clinical features of, 614
delirium in, 668–669
enteral nutrition in, 760t
hepatic encephalopathy in, 614, 619–622
hepatorenal syndrome and, 541, 542t, 616–617, 617t, 618t
parenteral nutrition and, 786–787
variceal hemorrhage in, 614, 623–624, 625f
Liver function tests
in acetaminophen toxicity, 809
in acute pancreatitis, 632
in fever assessment, 102
in HELLP syndrome, 220–221

Liver (hepatic) steatosis, in parenteral nutrition, 786
Liver transplantation, 617, 622
Lixiana. *See* Edoxaban
LMA. *See* Laryngeal mask airway
LMWH. *See* Low-molecular-weight heparin
Lockout interval, for patient-controlled analgesia, 69
Lokelma. *See* Sodium zirconium cyclosilicate
Lorazepam (Ativan), 75–79, 77t
  for alcohol withdrawal, 673, 676, 677f
  for status epilepticus, 692–693, 692t
  for traumatic brain injury, 731t
Lovenox. *See* Enoxaparin
Low-molecular-weight heparin (LMWH)
  actions of, 55
  for acute coronary syndromes, 362t
  advantages and disadvantages of, 56
  dosing of, 56
  neuraxial catheters and, 59, 60t
  for pulmonary embolism, 392–393, 394f
  thrombocytopenia risk with, 212
  for VTE prophylaxis, 54t, 55–56
Lung(s)
  dynamic hyperinflation of
    adverse consequences of, 414
    in asthma, 401–402, 413–415, 413f
    in COPD, 413–415, 413f
    monitoring of, 414–415
  feeding tube in, 767
  inflation of
    in basic life support, 371, 372–373
    in mechanical ventilation, 448–451
Lung biopsy, in ventilator-associated pneumonia, 462, 465t, 467t
Lung injury
  transfusion-related acute, 203–205, 204f, 205t, 223t, 224, 226t
  ventilator-induced, 422–423
Lung protective ventilation, 415, 423–425, 423t
"Lung rest," 486–487, 488f
LVADs. *See* Left ventricular assist devices
LVEDP. *See* Left ventricular end-diastolic pressure
LVEF. *See* Left ventricular ejection fraction
LVOT. *See* Left ventricular outflow tract

M

Macronutrient solutions, 776–779, 783t
Magnesium, 589–597. *See also* Hypermagnesemia; Hypomagnesemia
  for acute asthma exacerbation, 407
  as calcium blocker, 595
  depletion of, 577
  function and distribution of, 589–590
  for hypokalemia, 580

ionized (active) form of, 589
for multifocal atrial
tachycardia, 338
in normal pH fluids, 159
in parenteral nutrition, 780t
serum, reference ranges for,
589t
for torsades de pointes, 343
urinary, 589–590, 590f
Magnesium replacement,
592–594, 593t
Magnesium retention test, 594,
594t
Magnetic resonance
angiography (MRA), of
pulmonary embolism,
392
Magnetic resonance cholangiopancreatography
(MRCP), 634, 635f
Magnetic resonance imaging
(MRI)
of acute aortic dissection,
363–364
in fever assessment, 102
Malignant hyperthermia (MH),
94, 94t
Mallampati classification, 26f
Malnutrition, acetaminophen
toxicity in, 808
Malpositioned catheters, 18
Mandibular protrusion test, 24f
Manganese, nutritional intake
of, 750t
Mannitol, 544–545, 715, 735t,
737t
MAOI. *See* Monoamine oxidase
inhibitors, serotonin
syndrome with
MAPSE. *See* Mitral annular
plane systolic excursion

Marfan's syndrome, 361
Mask intolerance, 434
Mask ventilation
complications of, 434
difficult or impossible,
factors associated with,
27, 27t
face masks for, 433–434,
433f
Massive blood loss, 261. *See
also* Hemorrhage;
Hemorrhagic shock
Massive hemolysis,
hypermagnesemia in,
595
Massive transfusion protocol,
269–270
MAT. *See* Multifocal atrial
tachycardia
Maximum inspiratory pressure,
in spontaneous
breathing trial, 475t, 481
McConnell's sign, 389
MCS. *See* Mechanical cardiac
support
MDIs. *See* Metered dose
inhalers
Mean cell volume, 186t
Mean systemic pressure (Pms),
178–179
Mechanical cardiac support
(MCS), 285–291
Mechanical ventilation. *See also
specific methods, settings,
and applications*
for acute respiratory distress
syndrome, 418, 422–427
airway pressures in, 445–446,
446f, 449–451, 449f, 450f
alveolar collapse in, 444–445
alveolar recruitment in, 445

Mechanical ventilation (*Continued*)
　arterial blood gases in, 448
　for asthma exacerbation, acute, 412–415
　asthma flow-time graphics in, 400–402, 401f, 402f
　conventional, 443–453
　for COPD exacerbation, acute, 412–415
　core settings in, 443–446
　fraction of inspired oxygen in, 444, 447t
　for hemorrhagic shock, 264
　hypophosphatemia and, 607
　initial settings in, 447–448, 447t
　liberation (weaning) from, 474–485
　　cardiac assessment in, 479
　　cardiac dysfunction in, 478–479
　　extubation in, 481–483
　　readiness evaluation for, 474, 474t
　　respiratory muscle weakness and, 479–481
　　spontaneous breathing trial for, 475–478, 475t, 476f
　　spontaneous breathing trial failure and, 478–481, 480f
　lung inflation methods in, 448–451
　lung injury in, 422–423
　lung protective protocol for, 415, 423–425, 423t
　monitoring of, 131, 414–415
　patient-controlled analgesia with, 69
　positive end-expiratory pressure in, 444–446, 447t
　preferred/commonly used modes of, 451, 452t
　pressure control, 445–446, 446f, 448–449, 449f
　prone positioning for, 427
　respiratory rate in, 443–444, 447t
　sedation during, 79
　static compliance in, 451
　stress ulcer risk with, 46, 46t
　for stroke patients, 710
　stroke volume variation in, 180–181
　tidal volume in, 443, 447t
　for traumatic brain injury, 737t
　volume control, 448–449, 449f, 450f
Mediastinal hematomas, 13–14
Megacolon, toxic, 643
Mepolizumab, 408
Meropenem, 638, 651
Mestinon. *See* Pyridostigmine
Metabolic acidosis, 505t
　anion and delta gaps in, 515
　diagnosis of, 510–511
　in ethylene glycol intoxication, 833
　gaps in, 511–515
　hyperchloremic, isotonic saline and, 157
　hyperkalemia with, 581, 586
　in methanol intoxication, 835
　mixed, 514
　in propofol-related infusion syndrome, 81–82, 81t
　responses to, 505t, 506–507, 507f, 508t
　salicylate toxicity and, 819

Metabolic alkalosis, 505t
  anion and delta gaps in, 515
  diagnosis of, 510–511
  hypochloremia in, 571t
  hypokalemia with, 577
  responses to, 505t, 507–508, 507f, 508t
"Metabolic carts," 745
Metered dose inhalers (MDIs), 405
Methadone, 66t
Methanol intoxication, 831, 832f, 835–836
Methemoglobin, 126–127, 831
Methicillin-resistant *Staphylococcus aureus*, 455t, 460–461, 467t
Methimazole, 799t
Methylene blue, for septic shock, 301
Methylprednisolone, 377, 426t, 482, 730t, 794–795
Metoclopramide, 95, 770–772, 771t, 772
Metolazone, 321t
Metoprolol, 334t, 338, 359t, 366t, 799t
Metronidazole, 638, 644, 645t, 651
MG. *See* Myasthenia gravis
Micafungin, 103, 652, 661
Microcirculatory dysfunction, 279, 281
Microdialysis, cerebral, 736t
Micronutrients. *See also specific micronutrients*
  in parenteral nutrition, 779–782, 783t
Microvascular shunting, 296
Microvascular thrombosis, 297
Midazolam (Versed), 75–79, 77t
  for alcohol withdrawal, 676
  for RSII, 34t, 36
  for status epilepticus, 692–693, 692t, 693t
  for traumatic brain injury, 731t
Midline catheters, 4–5, 4f
Miller Fisher syndrome, 698
Mill wheel murmur, 16
Milrinone, 283–284, 283t, 303t, 324, 816–817
Mineralocorticoid deficiency, 565
Mini-bronchoalveolar lavage, 464
Minnesota tube, 623–624
Minocycline-coated catheters, 7
Minute ventilation, 443, 506–508
Mitochondria
  cyanide poisoning and, 828–829
  function of, 296
  inflammation and, 296–297
  septic shock and, 300
Mitral annular plane systolic excursion (MAPSE), 112
Mixed acid-based disorders, 510
Mixed cardiogenic-septic shock, 285
Mixed metabolic acidoses, 514
Mixed venous oxygen saturation (SvO_2), 127–128, 248t, 251, 252t, 281, 300
Modular supplements, enteral, 759, 762–764, 762t
Monoamine oxidase inhibitors (MAOI), serotonin syndrome with, 96
Montelukast, 408

Morphine, 66t, 67
  for acute coronary syndromes, 359, 359t
  fentanyl *vs.*, 67–68
  patient-controlled analgesia with, 69t
Mortality prediction, SOFA score-based, 847
Movement disorders, 689–708. *See also* Seizure(s); *specific types*
MRCP. *See* Magnetic resonance cholangiopancreatography
MRI. *See* Magnetic resonance imaging
Mucosal injury, stress-related, 45–51. *See also* Stress ulcer
Mucous plugging, in asthma, 402
Multifocal atrial tachycardia (MAT), 329–330, 330f, 338
Muscle weakness
  hypermagnesemia and, 595t
  hypokalemia and, 577
  respiratory, 479–481, 607
Myasthenia gravis (MG), 694–698
  clinical features of, 695
  diagnosis of, 695
  drugs exacerbating, 694, 694t
  etiologies of, 694
  Guillain-Barré syndrome *vs.*, 698, 699t
  management of, 697–698
  pathophysiology of, 694
  prognosis of, 698
  respiratory failure prediction in, 695, 696t
Myasthenic crisis, 695
Myocardial infarction
  acute, cardiogenic shock with, 275, 276f, 279, 285
  heparin-induced thrombocytopenia and, 212
  hypomagnesemia in, 591t
  non-ST-elevation, 352
    ECG findings in, 354, 355t
    management of, 358
  ST-elevation, 352
    ECG findings in, 354, 355t
    management of, 357–358
Myocardial stunning, 321, 380
Myoclonic seizures, 690
Myoclonus, coma and, 678
Myopathy, critical illness, 700–701
Myxedema coma, 800–801, 801t

N
N-acetylcysteine (NAC), 614, 615–616, 615t, 811–812, 812t
NaCl. *See* Sodium chloride
Naloxone (Narcan), 817–819
Narcan. *See* Naloxone
Narcotic, 65. *See also* Opioid(s)
Narrow complex tachycardias, 328–330, 330f
Nasal cannula, 29t, 32
Nasal oxygen, high-flow, 438, 483
Nasogastric tube (NGT)
  CO_2 colorimetry for placement of, 129–131, 130f
  in hemorrhagic shock, 263
National Asthma Education Program, 402, 404f

National Heart, Lung, and
Blood Institute
(NHLBI), 423
National Institutes of Health
(NIH), 423
Natriuretic peptides, 315–317,
317t, 388, 479
Necrotizing pancreatitis, 629,
636, 637–638
Necrotizing wound infections,
99
Negative pressure "Wick"
systems, 658, 659f
Neostigmine, 703–704
Nephrogenic diabetes
insipidus, 560, 561
Nephrotoxins, 541–543, 543t
Nerve conduction studies, 701
Neuraxial analgesia, VTE
prophylaxis with, 59, 60t
Neurocritical care, 729–737,
730t–731t
Neuroleptic malignant
syndrome (NMS), 84,
94, 95, 95t
Neuromuscular blocking
(NMB) agents, 701–704
awake fiberoptic intubation
vs. use of, 38
commonly used, 702t
indications for, 701
malignant hyperthermia
with, 94
for mechanical ventilation in
ARDS, 426
monitoring with, 703
for organophosphate/
carbamate poisoning,
839t
reversal of, 35, 703–704
for RSII, 35

Neuromuscular weakness
syndromes, 694–704
Neuromyopathy, critical illness,
480–481, 700–701
Neurontin. *See* Gabapentin
Neuropathic pain
drugs for, 74
Guillain-Barré syndrome
and, 699–700
New York Heart Association
Classification, 315,
316t
NGT. *See* Nasogastric tube
NHLBI. *See* National Heart,
Lung, and Blood
Institute
Nicardipine, 366t, 711t
Nimodipine, 722t, 723
Nitrogen, preoxygenation to
remove, 28, 29t
Nitrogen balance, 746
Nitroglycerin, 320t, 324, 358,
359t
Nitroprusside, 320t, 324, 366t,
828
NIV. *See* Noninvasive
ventilation
NMB agents. *See*
Neuromuscular
blocking (NMB) agents
NMS. *See* Neuroleptic
malignant syndrome
Nonfermentable fiber, 762–763
Noninvasive ventilation (NIV),
431–442
for acute asthma
exacerbation, 409
for acute COPD exacerbation,
412, 435–436, 435f
cardiac performance during,
438–441, 439f, 440f

Noninvasive ventilation (NIV) (*Continued*)
- for cardiogenic pulmonary edema, 436–437, 437f, 441
- checklist for, 434t
- evaluating response in, 436
- face masks for, 433–434, 433f
- helmet for, 434
- high-flow nasal oxygen as alternative to, 438
- for hypercapnic respiratory failure, 435–436, 435f
- for hypoxic respiratory failure, 436
- indications and contraindications, 410t
- methods of, 431–434
- for obesity hypoventilation syndrome, 436
- patient selection for, 434–435
- postextubation, 483
- prior to endotracheal intubation, 29t

Non-opioid analgesia, 71–74, 71t

Nonpharmaceutical poisonings, 825–842

Non-ST-elevation myocardial infarction (NSTEMI), 352
- ECG findings in, 354, 355t
- management of, 358

Nonsteroidal anti-inflammatory drugs (NSAIDs). *See also specific drugs*
- actions of, 72
- adverse effects and risks of, 72–73
- for fever, 104
- hyperkalemia with, 581t
- for nephrogenic diabetes insipidus, 561

Norepinephrine
- for acute pancreatitis, 636–637
- for cardiogenic shock, 282
- for delayed cerebral ischemia, 723
- for hepatorenal syndrome, 617, 618t
- for ischemic stroke, 712
- for right heart failure, 325
- for septic shock, 300t, 301, 302t

Normal saline. *See* Isotonic saline

Normosol-R, 156t, 157, 159–160, 266t

Normovolemic hypernatremia, 560–561

Normovolemic hyponatremia, 565–566, 569

North-south syndrome, 497

Nosocomial infections, 98–101. *See also specific infections*
- C. difficile, 647
- RBC transfusions and, 205
- urinary tract infections, 98, 655
- ventilator-associated pneumonia as, 454–473

NRS. *See* Numeric Ranking Scale; Nutritional Risk Screening

NSTEMI. *See* Non-ST-elevation myocardial infarction

Numeric Ranking Scale (NRS), 64

NUTRIC. *See* Nutrition Risk in Critically Ill

Nutrient fuels
- energy yield from, 744, 744t
- oxidation of, 743–744

Nutritional assessment, initial, 741–743
Nutritional requirements, 741–756
  caloric, 743–745
  carbohydrate, 747
  essential trace element, 750–753
  lipid, 747–748
  protein, 746
  substrate, 746–748
  vitamin, 748–750
Nutritional Risk Screening (NRS), 741, 742f
Nutritional support
  in acute pancreatitis, 637
  calorie restriction in, 745, 746t
  enteral nutrition for, 757–775 (*See also* Enteral nutrition)
  goal of, 741
  parenteral nutrition for, 776–789 (*See also* Parenteral nutrition)
  propofol and, 748
  requirements in, 741–756
Nutrition Risk in Critically Ill (NUTRIC), 741–743, 743f

O

O_2ER. *See* Oxygen extraction ratio
Obese patients
  anticoagulant prophylaxis in, 54t, 55
  calorie restriction in, 745, 746t
  endotracheal intubation of, 30
Obesity hypoventilation syndrome, 436
Obstructive shock, 253, 254t, 285
Obstructive sleep apnea, CPAP for, 431
Occult shock, 253, 256
Octreotide, 618t
Oculocephalic reflex, in coma, 679, 681f
Oculovestibular reflex, in coma, 679–681, 681f
Olanzapine (Zyprexa), 83, 84–85, 85t, 95
Oleic acid infusions, 786
Omega-3 fatty acids, 763
Omeprazole, 47t
Opiate, 65
Opioid(s)
  acetaminophen toxicity with, 809
  adrenal insufficiency induced by, 792t, 793
  adverse effects of, 70
  analgesia with, 65–70
  cardiovascular effects of, 70
  definition and terminology, 65–66
  dosing of, 66–67, 66t
  gastrointestinal effects of, 70
  ketorolac co-administered with, 72
  metabolism of, 67
  most frequently used in ICU, 67–68
  overdoses of, 817–819
  patient-controlled analgesia with, 69t
  for spontaneous breathing trials, 478
Opioid conversion, 66–67

Oral hygiene, 455–456, 456f
Organ failure assessment, sequential (SOFA), 846–847
Organophosphate poisoning, 836–838
  clinical features of, 836–838, 838t
  diagnosis of, 838
  management of, 838, 839t–840t
  pathogenesis of, 836, 837f
Osmolality
  feeding (enteral) formula, 760, 761t
  plasma, 557–558
  resuscitation fluid, 154–156, 156t, 158, 163
  urine, 545t, 561
Osmolar gap, 515
Osmolarity, 557
Osmotic activity, 556–558, 556f
  effective, 556
  in fluid distribution/resuscitation, 154–156
  tonicity and, 556–557, 556f
  units of, 557 (*See also* Osmolality)
Osmotic demyelination syndrome, 568
Osmotic nephropathy, drugs implicated in, 543t
Osmotic pressure, 556
Osmotic pressure, colloid, 165, 167, 169, 170, 281–282
Overdoses. *See* Pharmaceutical drug overdoses
Oxalic acid, 832, 832f
Oxidative metabolism
  energy (caloric) requirements for, 743–745
  hypophosphatemia and, 606, 606f
  iron and, 751–752, 752f
  selenium and, 753
  shock and, 247
Oximetry, 124–128
  CO-oximetry, 126–127, 828
  dual, 128
  jugular venous, 731t, 735, 736t
  pulse, 124–126, 125f, 126t, 263
Oxycodone, 66t
Oxygen balance, systemic, 127–128, 248, 248t, 252
Oxygen-carrying capacity, 186–188
Oxygen content, of blood, 187, 249–250
Oxygen delivery (DO_2), 248–250, 249f
  anemia and, 190–191, 191f
  balance with oxygen extraction, 252
  cardiac output and, 249, 250
  cardiogenic shock and, 281
  hemorrhage and, 260, 260f
  normal and hypoxic measures of, 248, 248t
  PA-catheter measurement of, 144t, 148
  shock and, 247, 260, 301
  venovenous ECMO and, 486–489, 488f
Oxygen extraction (O_2EXT), 248, 249f, 251
  anemia and, 190–191, 191f, 193
  balance with oxygen delivery, 252
  definition and calculation of, 190, 251

normal and hypoxic
measures of, 248t
as transfusion trigger, 193
Oxygen extraction ratio (O_2ER),
144t, 149, 248t, 251
Oxygen saturation, 127–128
cardiogenic shock and, 281
central venous, 127–128, 193,
248t, 251–252, 252t, 300
interpretation of measures,
252t
in mechanical ventilation,
444
mixed venous, 127–128, 251,
252t, 281, 300
monitoring of, 1, 124–128,
125f, 126t
septic shock and, 300
in spontaneous breathing
trial failure, 479
Oxygen therapy
for acute COPD exacerbation,
412
for acute coronary
syndromes, 358, 359t
for carbon monoxide
poisoning, 828
high-flow nasal, 438, 483
for post-cardiac arrest
patients, 381t
for stroke, 709, 710t
Oxygen transport, 248–252
normal and hypoxic
measures of, 248t
PA-catheter parameters for,
143–144, 144t, 147–149
Oxygen uptake or consumption
(VO_2), 248–251, 249f,
743–745
cardiogenic shock and, 281
control of, 127–128, 252

normal and hypoxic
measures of, 248t
oxygen delivery and,
248–250, 249f
oxygen extraction and, 248,
249f, 251
PA-catheter measurement of,
144t, 148–149

P

PA catheter. *See* Pulmonary
artery (PA) catheter
Pacemakers, temporary, 347t,
348
Packed red blood cells, 194t,
195, 265, 266t
PADS. *See* Pain, agitation,
delirium, and sedation
(PADS) algorithm
Pain
assessment of, 64, 65t
coma and responses to, 679
neuropathic
drugs for, 74
Guillain-Barré syndrome
and, 699–700
as stressor in ICU, 64
Pain, agitation, delirium,
and sedation (PADS)
algorithm, 85–87, 86f
Pain management, 64–74. *See
also* Analgesia
non-opioid, 71–74
opioid, 65–70
PADS algorithm for, 85–87, 86f
Palv. *See* Alveolar pressure
2-PAM, for organophosphate/
carbamate poisoning,
839t
Pancreatic enzymes, in acute
pancreatitis, 631–632

Pancreatic infections, 637–638
Pancreatitis
  acute, 629–640 (*See also* Acute pancreatitis)
  drug-induced, 96
  fever with, 96
  gallstone, 96, 634, 635, 635f
  hypertriglyceridemic, 632, 635
  hypocalcemia in, 600t
  interstitial edematous, 629
  necrotizing, 629, 636
  severe, 636
Pancuronium, 704
Pantoprazole, for stress ulcer prophylaxis, 47t, 48
Papaver somniferum, 65
Paracetamol. *See* Acetaminophen (paracetamol)
Paralysis
  in critical illness neuromyopathy, 700–701
  drug-induced, 701–704
Parapneumonic effusions, 467–469, 468t
Parathyroid hormone (PTH), 598
Parenteral nutrition (PN), 776–789
  amino acid solutions in, 777–778
  catheter problems in, 784–785
  cholestasis in, 786–787
  complications of, 784–787
  components of, 783t
  creating regimen for, 782–784
  dextrose solutions in, 776–777, 777t
  electrolytes in, 779–780, 780t
  hepatic steatosis in, 786
  hyperglycemia in, 785
  hypertriglyceridemia in, 786
  hypokalemia in, 786
  hypophosphatemia in, 785–786
  indications for, 776
  initiation of, 782
  lipid emulsions in, 779, 786
  macronutrient solutions for, 776–779, 783t
  micronutrients in, 779–782, 783t
  peripheral, 787
  recommended laboratory monitoring in, 781t
  trace elements in, 781–782, 782t
  vitamins in, 780
  volume considerations for, 784, 784t
Paroxysmal supraventricular tachycardia (PSVT), 339–340, 340t
Partial pressure of carbon dioxide (PCO_2)
  in acid-base disorders, 505–510, 505t, 507f, 508t, 509t
  arterial, relationship with $ETCO_2$, 133, 133t
  in cardiac arrest, 377–378, 378f
  in cardiogenic shock, 281
  reference ranges for, 510
  renal response to changes in, 508–509
Partial pressure of carbon dioxide (PCO_2) gap, 281
Passive leg raising (PLR), 180, 181f

Patent foramen ovale (PFO), 713, 713f
Patient-controlled analgesia (PCA), 69, 69t
Patient positioning
 for endotracheal intubation, 28–30, 28f, 30f
 for mechanical ventilation, 427
 for venous air embolism, 16
PAV. *See* Proportional assist ventilation
Paw. *See* Peak airway pressure
PAWP. *See* Pulmonary artery wedge pressure
PbtO$_2$. *See* Brain tissue oxygen tension monitoring
PBW. *See* Predicted body weight
PCA. *See* Patient-controlled analgesia
PCC. *See* Prothrombin complex concentrate
PCI. *See* Percutaneous coronary intervention
PCO$_2$. *See* Partial pressure of carbon dioxide
PCP. *See* Phencyclidine
PCV. *See* Pressure control ventilation
PE. *See* Pulmonary embolism
PEA. *See* Pulseless electrical activity
Peak airway pressure (Paw), 449–451, 449f, 450f
PEEP. *See* Positive end-expiratory pressure
Penicillins, for surgical site infections, 99
Pentobarbital, 693t
Peptamen, 761
Peptide-based enteral formulations, 760t

Percutaneous coronary intervention (PCI), 356, 357–358
Pericardial effusion, transthoracic echocardiography of, 115, 115t
Pericardial tamponade, 115–116, 116t, 285, 363, 379
Pericardium, transthoracic echocardiography of, 115–116, 115t, 116t
Peripheral intravenous access (PIV), 1–5, 3f, 3t
 flow rate in, 2, 2f, 3t
 midline catheters for, 4–5, 4f
Peripherally inserted central catheter (PICC), 7–8, 7f
 benefits of, 12
 infection with, 17–18
 insertion sites for, 12
 malpositioned, 18
 for parenteral nutrition, 784–785
 proper placement of, 18–19, 18f
 thrombosis with, 17
Peripheral neuropathy, thiamine deficiency and, 748–749
Peripheral parenteral nutrition (PPN), 787
Peritonitis, 647–652
 candidal, 651–652
 management of, 650–652
 spontaneous bacterial, 618–619
 surgical exploration in, 650
Permissive hypercapnia, in acute respiratory distress syndrome, 424

PFO. *See* Patent foramen ovale
pH, 505
   in acid-base disorders, 505–509 (*See also* Acid-base disorders)
   gastric, in stress ulcer prophylaxis, 46–50
   reference ranges for, 510
Pharmaceutical drug overdoses, 807–824
   acetaminophen, 807–813
   benzodiazepine, 813–814
   β-blocker, 814–817
   calcium channel blocker, 816
   opioid, 817–819
   salicylate, 819–821
Phencyclidine (PCP), 73
Phenylephrine, 282, 302t, 712
Phenytoin, 731t, 738t
Phlebotomy, blood loss/anemia in, 189
Phosphate binders, 605t, 608–609
Phosphate replacement, 530, 607, 607t
Phosphodiesterase inhibitors
   for β-blocker toxicity, 816–817
   for cardiogenic shock, 283–284, 283t
   for right heart failure, 324
   for septic shock, 303t
Phosphorus, 604–609. *See also* Hyperphosphatemia; Hypophosphatemia
   in enteral formulations, 761t
   normal ranges for, 599t
   in parenteral nutrition, 780t
   physiological functions of, 598, 604
Physiologic dead space, 443–444
PICC. *See* Peripherally inserted central catheter
Piperacillin/tazobactam, 638, 651, 660
PIV. *See* Peripheral intravenous access
Plasma
   calcium in, 598–600, 599f
   comparison of crystalloid fluids with, 155, 156t
   fresh frozen, 224–226, 238t
   hypertonic, in diabetes insipidus, 561
   osmolality of, 557–558
   oxygen dissolved in, 249, 250
Plasma exchange, 219, 220
Plasma fluid volume, 153, 155f, 166, 166f
Plasma-Lyte, 156t, 157, 159–160, 264, 266t, 527, 636
Plasmapheresis, 697, 699
Plasma products/transfusion, 224–227
   for disseminated intravascular coagulation, 217
   for hemorrhagic shock, 265, 266t
Plasma volume, 187, 188f
Plateau pressure (P_{plat}), 424, 450–451
Platelet(s)
   apheresis, 221
   as percentage in blood volume, 188f
   pooled, 221
Platelet count
   in fever assessment, 102
   low, 210 (*See also* Thrombocytopenia)
Platelet mapping, 231
Platelet refractoriness, 223

Platelet transfusions, 221–224
  acute lung injury with, 223t, 224
  adverse effects of, 223–224, 223t
  bacterial and viral transmission via, 223t, 224
  for disseminated intravascular coagulation, 217
  for hemorrhagic shock, 265, 266t
  hypersensitivity reactions to, 223t, 224
  indications for, 221, 222t
  leukoreduction for, 222
  nonhemolytic fever with, 223–224, 223t
  products for, 221–222
  response to, 222–223
  TEG- or ROTEM-based thresholds for, 234t
Plavix. *See* Clopidogrel
Pleural effusion
  drainage of, 469
  in heart failure, 318
  intrapleural fibrinolysis for, 469
  in pulmonary embolism, 388t
  in ventilator-associated pneumonia, 467–469
PLR. *See* Passive leg raising
Pms. *See* Mean systemic pressure
PN. *See* Parenteral nutrition
Pneumatic compression, intermittent, 57–58, 57f
Pneumonia
  community-acquired, noninvasive ventilation for, 435f
  ventilator-associated, 98, 454–473 (*See also* Ventilator-associated pneumonia)
Pneumonitis, aspiration, 92
Pneumoperitoneum, 650, 651f
Pneumothorax, 13, 14f, 253, 285, 379
POCUS. *See* Point-of-care ultrasound
Point-of-care ultrasound (POCUS), 109
  echocardiography, 109–123
  renal, 545
Poiseuille's Law, 2, 2f
Poisoning
  nonpharmaceutical, 825–842
  pharmaceutical drug overdose, 807–824
Polydipsia, primary, 566
Polyethylene glycol, 621
Polymerase chain reaction (PCR), 461, 643
Polymeric formulas, 761
Polyneuropathy
  acute immune-mediated, 698–700
  critical illness, 700–701
Polyunsaturated fatty acids (PUFAs), 763
Pooled platelets, 221
Portal hypertension, 614, 616, 623–624
Portosystemic shunts, 622, 623, 623f
Positioning. *See* Patient positioning
Positive end-expiratory pressure (PEEP), 444–446
  in acute respiratory distress syndrome, 424

Positive end-expiratory pressure (PEEP) (*Continued*)
  airway pressures in, 445–446, 446f
  alveolar collapse prevention in, 444–445
  alveolar recruitment in, 445
  in asthma and COPD, 413–414
  in BiPAP, 432, 432f
  hemodynamic effects of, 446, 447f
  initial setting for, 447t
Positive-pressure ventilation
  for asthma exacerbation, acute, 412–415
  cardiac performance during, 438–441, 439f
  for COPD exacerbation, acute, 412–415
  venous air embolism prevention with, 16
Post-cardiac arrest syndrome, 380
Postcardiotomy shock, 277
Postextubation laryngeal edema, 481
Postoperative fever, 97–98, 97t
Postoperative wound infections, 99, 647–648, 649t
Potassium, 575–588. *See also* Hyperkalemia; Hypokalemia
  depletion of, 577, 578f
  for diabetic ketoacidosis, 529–530, 530t
  distribution of, 575–576, 576f
  in enteral formulations, 761t
  excretion of, 576, 581–582, 581t
  for hypochloremia, 572
  in lactated Ringer's, 157–158
  in parenteral nutrition, 780t
  physiology of, 575–576
  transcellular shift of, 576–577, 578, 580, 581t
Potassium chloride, 579
Potassium phosphate, 607t
Potassium replacement, 579–580
Potassium-sparing diuretics, 576
PPIs. *See* Proton pump inhibitors
PPN. *See* Peripheral parenteral nutrition
Pradaxa. *See* Dabigatran
Prasugrel (Effient), 360t
Praxbind. *See* Idarucizumab
Prebiotics, for *C. difficile* infection, 646
Predicted body weight (PBW)
  for females, 845
  for males, 844
Prednisone, 410, 604t
Pregabalin, 74
Pregnancy
  cardiogenic shock in, 277
  HELLP syndrome in, 220–221
  imaging during, 391
Preload, cardiac, 153, 176–177, 177f
  hemorrhage and, 260
  positive-pressure ventilation and, 438, 439f, 440–441
  septic shock and, 299, 301
Preoxygenation
  for endotracheal intubation, 28, 29t
  for rapid sequence induction and intubation, 32

Pressure control inverse ratio ventilation, 425
Pressure control ventilation (PCV), 445–446, 446f, 448–449, 449f, 452t
Pressure reactivity index (PRx), 735, 736t
Pressure regulated volume control (PRVC), 452t
Pressure support ventilation (PSV), 433, 452t
Pressure support ventilation trial, 477
Pressure ulcers, 101
PRIS. *See* Propofol-related infusion syndrome
Probiotics, for *C. difficile* infection, 646
Procainamide, 337
Procalcitonin, 102, 632
Prokinetic agents, for gastroparesis, 770–771, 771t
Promethazine, 95
Propofol (Diprivan), 79–83, 79t
  actions of, 79–80
  adverse effects of, 80–82
  calories/lipids from, 748
  dosing of, 79t, 80
  emergence from, factors influencing, 80, 80t
  pharmacokinetics of, 79t
  for refractory status epilepticus, 693t
  for RSII, 34t
  for traumatic brain injury, 730t
Propofol-related infusion syndrome (PRIS), 81–82, 81t

Proportional assist ventilation (PAV), 433
Propranolol, 799t
Propylene glycol toxicity, 78, 523
Propylthiouracil (PTU), 799t
Prostaglandin E, in febrile response, 104
Protamine sulfate, 718t, 719
Protected specimen brush (PSB), 464, 465f, 467t
Protein(s)
  energy yield from, 744t
  in enteral nutrition, 760–762, 761t, 762t, 764–765, 766t
  intact *vs.* hydrolyzed, 761
  nutritional requirements for, 746
  in parenteral nutrition, 777–778
Prothrombin complex concentrate (PCC), 236–238
  anticoagulation reversal with, 225, 236–238, 237f, 238t, 239f, 270, 271t, 718–719, 718t
  indications for and administration of, 236–238
  preparations of, 236
  TEG- or ROTEM-based thresholds for, 234t
Proton pump inhibitors (PPIs), 47t, 48, 591t
PRVC. *See* Pressure regulated volume control
PRx. *See* Pressure reactivity index
PSB. *See* Protected specimen brush

Pseudohyperkalemia, 580–581
Pseudohyponatremia, 562–563, 564t
Pseudomonas aeruginosa infections, 411–412, 455t, 656t
Pseudothrombocytopenia, 210
PSV. *See* Pressure support ventilation
PSVT. *See* Paroxysmal supraventricular tachycardia
Psychosis, delirium *vs.*, 671
Pulmonary angiography, 392
Pulmonary artery (PA) catheter, 1, 136–151
  balloon flotation principle and, 137–138
  basics of, 136–139, 137f
  cardiac output measurement by, 143, 146
  in cardiogenic shock, 280–281
  cardiovascular measurements by, 143–147, 144t
  indications for, 136, 136t
  inflatable balloon of, 137, 137f, 138–139
  insertion and placement of, 137–139
  internal channels of, 136–137
  length and diameter of, 136
  monitoring revolutionized by, 136
  optical module connector of, 137, 137f
  oxygen transport measurements by, 143–144, 144t, 147–149
  pressure waveform from, 138–139, 139f, 140f
  radiographic confirmation of, 139, 140f
  respiratory fluctuations and, 145
  in spontaneous breathing trial failure, 479
  temperature measured via, 91
  thermistor/thermal filament of, 137, 137f, 143
  wedge pressure measurement by, 139, 140f, 141–142, 141f, 144t, 145
Pulmonary artery wedge pressure (PAWP)
  in acute respiratory distress syndrome, 420–422
  in cardiogenic shock, 281–282
  PA-catheter measurement of, 139, 140f, 141–142, 144t, 145
  principle of, 141–142, 141f
  pulmonary capillary pressure *vs.*, 142
  in right heart failure, 313–314
  variability in, 145
Pulmonary capillary pressure, 142, 277
Pulmonary edema
  cardiogenic
    ARDS *vs.*, 419
    CPAP for, 431, 436–437, 437f, 441
    noninvasive ventilation for, 436–437, 437f, 441
  diuretics for, 319–322
  "flash," 321
  in heart failure, 318, 318f, 319–322
  in inflammation, 295–296

venous air embolism and, 15
weaning-induced, 478
Pulmonary embolism (PE), 52–63, 387–399
- anticoagulation for, 53–56, 54t, 59t, 392–393, 394f
- bedside echocardiography for, 389
- catheter-directed therapies for, 395
- chest x-ray of, 389
- clinical presentation of, 387
- computed tomographic angiography of, 390, 391f
- diagnostic studies for, 387–392
- ECMO as bridge/supportive therapy in, 396
- fever with, 92
- heparin-induced thrombocytopenia and, 212
- laboratory testing in, 387–389
- magnetic resonance angiography of, 392
- management of, 392–397
- mechanical aids for, 57–58, 57f
- obstructive shock with, 285
- predictive value of clinical findings for, 388t
- pulmonary angiography of, 392
- risk factors for, 52–53
- scoring systems/risk stratification for, 392, 393t
- surgical embolectomy for, 395, 396f
- thrombolytic therapy for, 394–395
- vena cava filters for, 58–59, 58f, 396–397
- venous duplex ultrasonography for, 389
- ventilation-perfusion lung scan for, 390–391

Pulmonary infiltrate, pulmonary embolism and, 388t

Pulmonary vascular resistance, PA-catheter measurement of, 144t, 146–147

Pulmonary vascular resistance index (PVRI), 144t, 147

Pulseless electrical activity (PEA), 377

Pulseless ventricular tachycardia, 376

Pulse oximetry, 124–126, 125f, 126t, 263

Pupillary responses, 679, 680t

PureWick Urine Collection system, 658, 659f

Purpura fulminans, 217

Purulent secretions, in ventilator-associated pneumonia, 458, 459t

Pyelonephritis, candiduria and, 662

Pyridostigmine (Mestinon), for myasthenia gravis, 697

Pyridoxine, for ethylene glycol intoxication, 834

Pyrogens, endogenous, 91, 104

Q

QRS complex
- duration of, 328
- narrow, 328–330, 330f
- wide, 331–332, 331f

QT interval
  haloperidol and, 84
  hypercalcemia and, 603
  hypokalemia and, 577–578
  measurement of, 343
  in torsades de pointes, 342–343
Qualitative cultures, in ventilator-associated pneumonia, 461, 463t
Quantitative cultures, in ventilator-associated pneumonia, 461–462, 463t, 464, 465t
Quetiapine (Seroquel), 83, 84–85, 85t, 95

R

Radiocontrast dye, acute kidney injury from, 541–543
Radionuclide cerebral perfusion scintigraphy, 686
Ramp position, 30, 30f
Ranitidine, 306
Rapid arousal agents, 79–83, 79t
Rapid breathing, in spontaneous breathing trial, 477–478
Rapid infusion catheter (RIC), 2, 3t
Rapid sequence induction and intubation (RSII), 31–36
  gastric decompression for, 32
  gastric ultrasound for, 32, 33f
  induction agents for, 34t, 35
  neuromuscular blockade for, 35
  pharmacological adjuncts in, 36
  preoxygenation for, 32
  preparation for, 32

Rapid thromboelastography (r-TEG), 231
Rapid Ultrasound for Shock and Hypotension (RUSH), 109, 110t
RASS. *See* Richmond Agitation-Sedation Scale
RBCs. *See* Red blood cell(s)
Recruitment maneuvers, in acute respiratory distress syndrome, 427
Red blood cell(s) (RBCs)
  leukocyte-reduced, 194t, 195
  oxygen-carrying capacity of, 186–188
  packed, 194t, 195, 265, 266t
  as percentage in blood volume, 188f
  washed, 194t, 196, 202
Red blood cell (RBC) count, 186t
Red blood cell storage lesions, 196
Red blood cell (RBC) transfusions, 192–206
  acute hemolytic reactions to, 198–200
  acute lung injury related to, 203–205, 204f, 205t
  benefit *vs.* risk of, 206
  circulatory overload in, 202–203, 205t
  compatibility in, 197
  febrile nonhemolytic reaction to, 93, 195, 200–201
  filters for, 198
  for hemolytic uremic syndrome, 220
  for hemorrhagic shock, 265, 266t
  hypersensitivity reactions to, 201–202

lactated Ringer's contraindicated with, 158
nosocomial infections associated with, 205
physiologic effects of, 198
products for, 193–196, 194t
risks and adverse events associated with, 198–206, 199t
triggers for, 192–193
type, screen, and cross for, 196
universal donors for, 197
Red cell mass, 186, 186t
REE. *See* Resting energy expenditure
Refractory status epilepticus, 78, 690–691, 693–694, 693t
Regurgitation, in enteral nutrition, 770
Remifentanil, 34t, 36, 66t, 68
Remimazolam, 79
Renal replacement therapy (RRT), 547–552. *See also* Hemodialysis
continuous, 551–552, 617, 622
for hepatic encephalopathy, 622
for hepatorenal syndrome, 617
for hyperchloremia, 571
indications for, 547, 548f
mechanism of fluid and solute removal in, 549f
techniques of, 547, 548f
Renin, in heart failure, 317–318
Renin-angiotensin-aldosterone system
in heart failure, 317–318
inhibitors of, 361, 582

Reperfusion, in acute coronary syndromes, 356–358
Respiratory acidosis, 505t
diagnosis of, 510–511
hyperkalemia with, 581
responses to, 505t, 507f, 509, 509t
Respiratory alkalosis, 505t
diagnosis of, 510–511
hypokalemia with, 577
hypophosphatemia in, 605t
responses to, 505t, 507f, 509, 509t
salicylate toxicity and, 819
Respiratory depression
in benzodiazepine overdose, 813
opioids and, 70, 817
propofol and, 80
Respiratory distress, hypermagnesemia and, 595t
Respiratory distress syndrome. *See* Acute respiratory distress syndrome
Respiratory failure
acute asthma and, 400
COPD and, 400
Guillain-Barré syndrome and, 698
hypercapnic, noninvasive ventilation for, 435–436, 435f
hypoxic, noninvasive ventilation for, 436
lipid emulsions and, 786
myasthenia gravis and, 695, 696t
venovenous ECMO for, 486–492

Respiratory fluctuations, and pulmonary artery catheter, 145
Respiratory muscle weakness
  hypophosphatemia and, 607
  mechanical ventilation/ weaning and, 479–481
  monitoring for, 481
  predisposing conditions for, 480–481
Respiratory quotient, 743
Respiratory rate (RR)
  in mechanical ventilation, 443–444, 447t
  in metabolic acidosis, 506
  in metabolic alkalosis, 507–508
  shock and, 253
  in spontaneous breathing trial, 475t, 478
Resting energy expenditure (REE), 743–745
Resuscitation, cardiopulmonary. *See* Cardiopulmonary resuscitation
Resuscitation fluids, 153–175. *See also* Fluid resuscitation
Reteplase, for acute coronary syndromes, 357t
Reticulocyte count, 186t
Retroperitoneal hematomas, 13–14
Return of spontaneous circulation (ROSC), 377–379, 378f
Reversal of anticoagulation, 225, 270–271
  algorithm for, 239f
  fresh frozen plasma for, 225, 238t
  prothrombin complex concentrate for, 225, 236–238, 237f, 239f, 270–271, 271t
  rapid warfarin, protocols for, 238t
  for spontaneous intracerebral hemorrhage, 718–719, 718t, 719t
Reversal of neuromuscular blockade, 35, 703–704
Rewarming, in hemorrhagic shock, 268, 268f
Rhabdomyolysis
  acute kidney injury in, 543–545
  diagnostic criteria for, 544t
  hypocalcemia in, 600t
  hypophosphatemia and, 607
  malignant hyperthermia and, 94
  management of, 544–545
  propofol-related infusion syndrome and, 81t
  surgical site infections and, 99
Rheumatologic diseases, fever with, 96
RHF. *See* Right heart failure
Rh immunoglobulin, 197
RIC. *See* Rapid infusion catheter
Richmond Agitation-Sedation Scale (RASS), 75, 76t, 676, 677f
Rifampin-coated catheters, 7
Rifaximin, 621–622, 644
RIFLE score, 535
Right atrium, catheter tip in, 20
Right heart failure (RHF), 312–314
  causes of, 312, 313t

echocardiography of, 313–314, 315f
management of, 322–325, 324f
vasoactive agents for, 324–325
volume management in, 322–323
Right ventricle, normal and abnormal anatomy of, 314f
Right-ventricular assist devices (RVADs), 288
Right ventricular dysfunction, 312
Right ventricular function, 113–115, 114f, 114t
Ringer, Sydney, 157
Ringer's solution. *See* Lactated Ringer's
Risk, Injury, Failure, Loss of kidney function, and End-stage kidney disease (RIFLE) score, 535
Risperidone (Risperdal), 83, 84–85, 85t, 95
Rivaroxaban (Xarelto), 718–719, 718t
for atrial fibrillation, 336, 337t
bleeding with, 270–271
reversal of, 237f, 239f, 270–271
Rocuronium, 701–704, 702t
for organophosphate/carbamate poisoning, 839f
reversal of, 35, 703–704
for RSII, 35
Romazicon. *See* Flumazenil
R on T phenomenon, 342
ROSC. *See* Return of spontaneous circulation
Rotational thromboelastometry (ROTEM), 231, 232–236, 232f, 234t, 235f
RR. *See* Respiratory rate
RR intervals
in narrow complex tachycardias, 328–330
uniformity of, 328
RSII. *See* Rapid sequence induction and intubation
RUSH. *See* Rapid Ultrasound for Shock and Hypotension
RVADs. *See* Right-ventricular assist devices

S

SABAs. *See* Short-acting β_2 agonists
Sacubitril/valsartan (Entresto), 361
SAH. *See* Subarachnoid hemorrhage
SALAD. *See* Suction-assisted laryngoscopic and airway decontamination
Salicylate intoxication, 819–821
Saline
albumin solution *vs.*, 167–168
for diabetic ketoacidosis, 527
excess administration, hyperchloremia with, 570t
for hemorrhagic shock, 264, 266t
for hypercalcemia, 603, 604t
hypertonic, 160–162, 160t (*See also* Hypertonic saline)
isotonic, 154–157, 559 (*See also* Isotonic saline)

Saline *versus* Albumin Fluid Evaluation (SAFE) Study, 167–168
Salt wasting, cerebral, 565
SaO_2. *See* Arterial oxygenation
SAPS (Simplified Acute Physiology Score) II, 849–850
SAVE Score, 495
SBP. *See* Spontaneous bacterial peritonitis
SBT. *See* Spontaneous breathing trial
SBTube, 623–624, 625f
SCD. *See* Sequential compression devices
SCV. *See* Subclavian vein
$ScvO_2$. *See* Central venous oxygen saturation
$SCVO_2$, normal and hypoxic measures of, 248t
SE. *See* Status epilepticus
Sedation, 74–85
  antipsychotic agents for, 83–85
  benzodiazepines for, 75–79
  dexmedetomidine for, 79t, 82–83
  in hemorrhagic shock, 264
  monitoring, 75, 76t
  PADS algorithm for, 85–87, 86f
  procedural, capnography for, 131
  propofol for, 79–83, 79t
  rapid arousal agents for, 79–83, 79t
Sedation "holidays," 77–78
Sedative-hypnotic drugs
  delirium with, 668–669
  sinus bradycardia with, 344
  in traumatic brain injury, 730t

Seizure(s), 689–694
  abnormal movements in, 690
  alcohol withdrawal and, 673, 673t
  β-blocker overdose and, 814
  complex partial, 690
  continuous and recurrent (*See* Status epilepticus)
  generalized *vs.* focal, 690
  hypocalcemia and, 601
  lactic acidosis in, 523
  new-onset, conditions causing, 689t
  stroke and, 689t, 715–716
  traumatic brain injury and, 731t, 738t
  types of, 689–690
Seldinger technique, 8–9, 13
Selective decontamination, 456
Selective serotonin reuptake inhibitors (SSRIs), serotonin syndrome with, 96
Selenium, 750t, 753, 782
Sellick maneuver, 36–37
Semi-elemental formulas, 761
Sengstaken-Blakemore tube (SBTube), 623–624, 625f
Sepsis
  acute kidney injury in, 538–539
  definition of, 299
  delirium in, 668–669
  hypocalcemia in, 600t, 601
  selenium in, 753
  thrombocytopenia in, 211
Sepsis-induced cardiomyopathy (SICM), 296
Septic shock, 299–303
  antimicrobial therapy for, 300t, 303

corticosteroid therapy for, 300t, 301
cytopathic hypoxia in, 300
hemodynamics in, 299
initial management of, 300–303, 300t
inotropic agents for, 301, 303t
lactate levels in, 519, 520
mitochondrial dysfunction in, 300
mixed, with cardiogenic shock, 285
off-label therapy for, 301
vasopressor therapy for, 300t, 301, 302t
volume infusion for, 300t, 301
Sequential compression devices (SCD), 58
Sequential organ failure assessment (SOFA), 846–847
Seroquel. *See* Quetiapine
Serotonin release assay, 214
Serotonin syndrome, 95–96, 96t
Sevelamer, 608, 608t
Sevoflurane, 94, 94t
SGA devices. *See* Supraglottic airway (SGA) devices
Shock, 247–259. *See also specific types*
blood pressure in, 254–255
cardiogenic, 254t, 275–294
coinciding and evolving states of, 247
compensated, 253
cytotoxic, 296–297
definition of, 247
distributive, 254t
fever and hypothermia in, 255
general features of, 253–257

hemorrhagic, 260–274
hypertonic saline for, 161–162
inflammatory, 295–310
initial approach to, 253, 254t
laboratory markers of, 254t, 256–257
lactate levels in, 256, 519, 519f
liver failure and, 614
mixed cardiogenic-septic, 285
neurological signs in, 255
obstructive, 253, 254t, 285
occult, 253, 256
oxygen transport in, 248–252
rapid ultrasound for, 109, 110t
renal function in, 256, 257
septic, 299–303
signs and symptoms of, 253–256
skin assessment in, 255
undifferentiated, 253, 254t
venous air embolism and, 16
vital signs in, 253–255
Short-acting β_2 agonists (SABAs), 403–405, 406t
Short-chain fatty acids (SCFAs), 646, 762–763
SI. *See* Stroke index
SIADH. *See* Syndrome of inappropriate ADH secretion
SICM. *See* Sepsis-induced cardiomyopathy
SID. *See* Strong ion difference
"Silent chest," 400
Silver sulfadiazine-coated catheters, 7
Simplified Acute Physiology Score (SAPS) II, 849–850
Simpson's method, for left ventricular function, 112–113

Sinus bradycardia, 344
Sinusitis, 100
Sinus tachycardia, 328
SjVO$_2$. *See* Jugular venous oximetry
Skin antisepsis, for central line, 17t
Skin signs, in shock, 255
Smoke inhalation, 825. *See also* Carbon monoxide poisoning
Sniffing position, 28f, 30
Society for Healthcare Epidemiology of America (SHEA), 644
Society of Cardiovascular Angiography and Interventions (SCAI), 278t
Society of Critical Care Medicine (SCCM), 49, 91, 103, 426–427, 741, 787
Society of Interventional Radiology, 59, 59t
Sodium, 558–569. *See also* Hypernatremia; Hyponatremia
 aldosterone and retention of, 576
 average concentration, in select fluids, 559t
 fractional excretion of, 545t, 546
 hyperglycemia and, 562–563
 importance in fluid distribution, 558
 in parenteral nutrition, 780t
 pseudohyponatremia and, 562–563, 564t
 spot urine, 545–546, 545t, 564
 in traumatic brain injury, 735t, 737t
Sodium bicarbonate
 as buffer, ineffectiveness of, 523, 524f
 dosing of, 525
 for hyperkalemia, 585
 hypocalcemia with, 600
 for lactic acidosis, 523–525
Sodium chloride (NaCl)
 in crystalloid fluids, 153
 in hypertonic saline, 160–162, 160t
 in isotonic saline, 154–157
 in lactated Ringer's, 157–158
 23.4 %, precautions with, 162, 163f
Sodium intake, and hyperchloremia, 570t
Sodium phosphate, 607t
Sodium polystyrene sulfonate (SPS, Kayexalate), for hyperkalemia, 586
Sodium thiosulfate, for cyanide poisoning, 830t, 831
Sodium zirconium cyclosilicate (SZC, Lokelma), for hyperkalemia, 584t, 586
SOFA. *See* Sequential organ failure assessment
Spironolactone, 576, 581t
SPN. *See* Supplemental parenteral nutrition
SpO$_2$. *See* Oxygen saturation
Spontaneous bacterial peritonitis (SBP), 618–619
Spontaneous breathing trial (SBT), 475–481
 acute cardiac dysfunction in, 478–479

failure of, 478–481, 480f
measurements to predict outcome of, 475t
pressure support, 477
rapid breathing in, 477–478
respiratory muscle weakness and, 479–481
success *vs.* failure in, 477–478
tidal volumes in, 475t, 478
T-piece, 476, 476f
Spontaneous intracerebral hemorrhage, 716–719
anticoagulation reversal for, 718–719, 718t, 719t
etiologies of, 716
general supportive measures for, 717t
management of, 716–719
Spot urine potassium, 577, 578f, 580
Spot urine sodium, 545–546, 545t, 564
SPS. *See* Sodium polystyrene sulfonate
SSRIs. *See* Selective serotonin reuptake inhibitors
"Stacking breaths," 401
Staphylococcal infections
catheter-associated UTI, 656t, 657
pancreatic, 637
sinusitis, 100
ventilator-associated pneumonia, 454, 455t, 460–461, 467t
wound/surgical site, 99
Staphylococcus aureus
in catheter-associated UTIs, 656t
in pancreatic infections, 637
in sinusitis, 100
in ventilator-associated pneumonia, 454, 455t, 460–461, 467t
Staphylococcus epidermidis, 99, 100
Static compliance (Cstat), 451
Statins, for acute coronary syndromes, 361
Status epilepticus (SE), 690–694
coma in, 678
definition of, 690
nonconvulsive, 691–694, 691t
prognosis of, 694
refractory, 78, 690–691, 693–694, 693t
super-refractory, 691
treatment of, 691–694, 692t, 693t
ST-elevation myocardial infarction (STEMI), 352
ECG findings in, 354, 355t
management of, 357–358
Steroids. *See* Corticosteroid therapy
Stewart approach, to acid-base analysis, 515–516
Stomach, feeding tube in, 766–767
Stool, potassium in, 576
Streptococcal infections
in COPD, 411
in hemolytic uremic syndrome, 219
wound/surgical site, 99
Streptococcus pneumoniae, 219, 411
Stress, physiological
hyponatremia in, 566
hypophosphatemia in, 605t
Stress (Takotsubo) cardiomyopathy, 296, 297f

Stress ulcer, 45–51
    bleeding and mortality with, 45
    clinically silent, 45
    pathophysiology of, 45
    risk factors for, 46, 46t
Stress ulcer prophylaxis (SUP), 46–50
    antacids for, 47
    C. difficile infection with, 642
    cytoprotection for, 47t, 48–49
    discontinuation of, 50
    enteral feedings and, 49
    histamine H_2 receptor antagonists for, 47, 47t
    proton pump inhibitors for, 47t, 48
Stridor, postextubation, 482–483
Stroke
    acute, in ICU, 709–726
    antihypertensive therapy for, 710t, 711, 711t
    antiplatelet therapy for, 710t
    atrial fibrillation and prevention of, 335–337
    atrial fibrillation and risk of, 333, 848
    cerebral edema with, 715
    coma in, 678
    complications of, 714–716
    echocardiography in, 712–713, 713f
    embolic, 709, 712
    fever in, 710t
    general support measures for, 710t
    heparin-induced thrombocytopenia and, 212
    hyperglycemia in, 710t
    hypotension in, 712
    intracerebral hemorrhage with, 714–715, 714f
    ischemic, 709–716
    management of, 709–713
    mechanical ventilation in, 710
    respiratory support/oxygen in, 709, 710t
    seizures in, 689t, 715–716
    spontaneous intracerebral hemorrhage and, 716–719
    subarachnoid hemorrhage and, 719–723
    thromboprophylaxis for, 710t
    venous air embolism and, 15
Stroke index (SI), 146
Stroke volume
    echocardiographic measurement of, 116–120, 117f, 119f, 120t
    noninvasive ventilation and, 437, 437f
    PA-catheter measurement of, 144t, 146
    preload and, 176–177, 177f
Stroke volume variation (SVV), 180–181, 182f
Strong ion difference (SID), 515–516
Subarachnoid hemorrhage (SAH), 719–723
    aneurysm management in, 721
    delayed cerebral ischemia in, 720–721, 722t, 723
    epidemiology of, 719
    etiologies of, 719

general supportive measures for, 722t
management of, 721–723
pathophysiology of, 720–721, 720f
seizure with, 689t
Subclavian vein (SCV)
anatomy and location of, 9f, 10
cannulation of, 10–11
pneumothorax with catheterization of, 13
proper catheter placement in, 18–19
surface landmarks for, 11
thrombosis, PICCs and, 17
venous air embolism with entry to, 16
Subglottic secretions, clearing, 457, 457f
Substrates, nutritional, 746–748
Succinylcholine, 701–704, 702t
contraindications to, 35
hyperkalemia with, 581–582
malignant hyperthermia with, 94, 94t
reversal of, 703–704
for RSII, 35
Suck-down, in venovenous ECMO, 490–492
Sucralfate, 47t, 48–49, 49t
Suction-assisted laryngoscopic and airway decontamination (SALAD), 37–38
Suction swabs and toothbrushes, 456, 456f
Sudden cardiac arrest, 344–345
Sugammadex (Bridion), 35, 704

SUP. *See* Stress ulcer prophylaxis
Superior vena cava, oxygen saturation in. *See* Central venous oxygen saturation
Superoxide radical, 751, 752f
Super-refractory status epilepticus, 691
Supplemental parenteral nutrition (SPN), 787
Supraglottic airway (SGA) devices, 38, 39t
Supraventricular tachycardia (SVT), 331, 331f
Supraventricular tachycardia, paroxysmal, 339–340
Surgical airway, 41
Surgical site infections (SSI), 99, 647–648, 649t
SvO_2. *See* Mixed venous oxygen saturation
SVR. *See* Systemic vascular resistance
SVRI. *See* Systemic vascular resistance index
SVT. *See* Supraventricular tachycardia
SVV. *See* Stroke volume variation
Swabs, suction, 456, 456f
Sweat, 559t, 576
Sympathetic nervous system, in heart failure, 317
Syndrome of inappropriate ADH secretion (SIADH), 565
Systemic inflammatory response syndrome (SIRS), 298, 298t

Systemic vascular resistance (SVR)
  cardiogenic shock and, 278–281
  echocardiographic measurement of, 120t
  PA-catheter measurement of, 144t, 146–147, 280–281
  propofol and, 80
Systemic vascular resistance index (SVRI), 120t, 144t, 147
Systolic dysfunction, 311
SZC. *See* Sodium zirconium cyclosilicate

T

Tachyarrhythmias, 328–343. *See also specific types*
  flow diagram for evaluation of, 329f
  narrow complex, 328–330
  wide complex, 331–332, 331f
Tachycardia(s)
  AV nodal reentrant, 328, 330f, 339–340
  flow diagram for evaluation of, 329f
  hypomagnesemia and, 342–343, 592
  multifocal atrial, 329–330, 330f, 338
  narrow complex, 328–330, 330f
  pulmonary embolism and, 387, 388t
  short-acting β_2 agonists and, 405
  supraventricular, 331, 331f
  supraventricular paroxysmal, 339–340
  ventricular, 331–332, 331f, 340–343
  wide complex, 331–332, 331f
TACO. *See* Transfusion-associated circulatory overload
Takotsubo cardiomyopathy, 296, 297f
TAPSE. *See* Tricuspid annular plane systolic excursion
TBI. *See* Traumatic brain injury
TEE. *See* Transesophageal echocardiography
TEG. *See* Thromboelastography
Teichholz method, 111t
Temperature, body. *See also* Fever; Hypothermia
  cardiac arrest and, 380, 381t, 382
  measurement of, 91
  traumatic brain injury and, 737t
Temporary pacemakers, 347t, 348
Tenecteplase, 356, 357t
Tension pneumothorax, 253, 285, 379
Terbutaline, 406
Terlipressin, 617, 618t
Tetany, hypocalcemia and, 601
THAM. *See* Tris-hydroxymethyl aminomethane
Thermal diffusion flowmetry, 736t
Thermistor-equipped catheters, 91, 137, 137f, 143, 264
Thermodilution cardiac output, 143, 146
Thiamine
  deficiency of, 748–749
    lactic acidosis in, 520–522, 522f

Wernicke encephalopathy in, 591, 676–678, 748–749
for ethylene glycol intoxication, 834
magnesium and, 591, 748
physiological function of, 748
reference range of, 749
Thiamine pyrophosphate (TTP), 749
Thiazide diuretics, hypovolemic hyponatremia with, 564
Thiosulfate, for cyanide poisoning, 830t, 831
Thoracostomy, tube, 469
Thoracotomy, in ventilator-associated pneumonia, 469
Thorazine, neuroleptic malignant syndrome with, 95
Three-factor prothrombin complex concentrate, 236, 238t
Thrombocytopenia, 210–230
causes in critically ill patients, 211, 211t
definition of, 210
disseminated intravascular coagulation and, 216–217, 216t
HELLP syndrome and, 216, 220–221
hemolytic uremic syndrome and, 216t, 219–220
heparin-induced, 212–214
pseudothrombocytopenia vs., 210
thrombotic microangiopathies and, 214–221
thrombotic thrombocytopenic purpura and, 216t, 217–219
Thromboelastography (TEG), 231, 232f, 233f, 234–236, 234t, 235f, 269, 269t
Thromboelastometry, rotational, 231, 232–236, 232f, 234t, 235f
Thromboembolism
atrial fibrillation and, 333, 335–337
heparin-induced thrombocytopenia and, 212
venous (*See* Venous thromboembolism)
Thrombolytic therapy
for acute coronary syndromes, 356–357, 357t
bleeding attributed to, 356–357
contraindications to, 395
intracerebral hemorrhage with, 714–715, 714f
for pulmonary embolism, 394–395
Thromboprophylaxis, for ischemic stroke, 710t
Thrombosis
catheter-related, 14, 17
coronary, 352–353, 353f
intra-aortic balloon pump and, 286–287
microvascular, 297
prevention, in acute coronary syndromes, 360–361, 360t, 362t

Thrombotic microangiopathies, 214–221
  cardinal features of, 214
  laboratory profiles in, 216t
  types of, 216 (*See also specific types*)
Thrombotic thrombocytopenic purpura (TTP), 216t, 217–219
Thymoma, myasthenia gravis and, 698
Thyroid function/dysfunction, 795–802
  evaluation of, 795–797
  test findings of, 796–797, 796t
Thyroiditis, autoimmune, 800
Thyroid-stimulating hormone (TSH), 796, 796t, 798, 801
Thyroid storm, 96, 797–800, 799t
Thyromental distance, 26f
Thyrotoxicosis, 797–800
  apathetic, 797
  clinical manifestations of, 797, 798t
  diagnosis of, 797–798
  fever with, 96
  treatment of, 799–800, 799t
Thyroxine, 795, 796t, 797–798, 801
Ticagrelor (Brilinta), 360t
Tidal volume (V_t)
  in mechanical ventilation, 443, 447t
  in metabolic acidosis, 506
  in spontaneous breathing trial, 475t, 478
Tidal volume charts
  for females, 845
  for males, 844
Tigecycline, 651
TIPS. *See* Transjugular intrahepatic portosystemic shunt
Tirofiban (Aggrastat), 360t
Tissue factor, 216–217, 231–236
Tissue perfusion, in cardiogenic shock, 281
Tissue plasminogen activator
  for acute coronary syndromes, 356–357, 357t
  for catheter occlusion, in parenteral nutrition, 785
  intracerebral hemorrhage with, 714–715, 714f
  for intrapleural fibrinolysis, 469
  for pulmonary embolism, 395
TOF. *See* Train-of-four monitoring
Tonicity, 556–557, 556f
Tonic seizures, 690
Toothbrushes, suction, 456, 456f
Topical hemostatic agents, 241, 243f
Topicalization method, of intubation, 38–40, 40t
Torsades de pointes, 342–343
  drugs causing, 84, 343, 343t
  ECG findings of, 342–343, 342f
  hypomagnesemia and, 342–343, 592
  treatment of, 343
Torsemide, 321t
Toxic alcohols, 831–836
Toxicity (poisoning)
  nonpharmaceutical, 825–842
  pharmaceutical drug overdose, 807–824
Toxic megacolon, 643

Toxidromes, lactic acidosis with, 523
T-piece trial, 476, 476f
Trace elements
  daily allowances for, 750t
  essential, 750–753
  in parenteral nutrition, 781–782, 782t
Trachea, feeding tube in, 767
Tracheostomy, 41
Train-of-four monitoring (TOF), 703
Tralement trace elements injection, 781–782, 782t
TRALI. *See* Transfusion-related acute lung injury
Tranexamic acid (TXA), 234t, 240–241, 270
Transesophageal echocardiography (TEE), 121, 121f
  of acute aortic dissection, 363
  in ischemic stroke, 712–713, 713f
Transferrin, 751
Transfusion. *See* Blood transfusion
Transfusion-associated circulatory overload (TACO), 202–203, 205t, 223t, 226t
Transfusion-related acute lung injury (TRALI), 203–205, 204f, 205t, 223t, 224, 226t
Transjugular intrahepatic portosystemic shunt (TIPS), 622, 623, 623f
Transketolase enzyme, 749
Translocation, in enteral feedings, 758

Transthoracic echocardiography (TTE), 109–120
  of hypovolemia and hypervolemia, 116–119
  of left ventricular function, 109–113, 111t, 112f
  of pericardium, 115–116, 115t, 116t
  physiological assessments with, 116–120
  of right heart failure, 313–314, 315f
  of right ventricular function, 113–115, 114f, 114t
  transesophageal *vs.*, 121, 121f
  types of exams in, 109
Traumatic brain injury (TBI), 727–740
  advanced neuromonitoring in, 735, 736t
  cerebrospinal fluid drainage in, 729–733, 730t, 732f
  definition of, 727
  diffuse, 727t
  focal, 727t
  general ICU management of, 737, 737t–738t
  hyperosmolar therapy for, 730t
  hypertonic saline for, 162
  impending brain herniation in, 733–735, 735t
  intracranial pressure management in, 733–735, 734f
  intracranial pressure monitoring in, 729–733, 732f, 732t
  moderate, 727
  mortality and morbidity in, 727

Traumatic brain injury (TBI) (*Continued*)
  neurocritical care management in, 729–737, 730t–731t
  pathophysiology of, 727–728, 728f
  severe, 727
  structural, types of, 727t
  treatment thresholds in, 731t
Traumatic shock, hypertonic saline for, 161–162
Tremors, in alcohol withdrawal, 675t
Tricuspid annular plane systolic excursion (TAPSE), 113–115, 114f
Tricuspid regurgitation, 143
Triglycerides
  acute pancreatitis and, 632, 635
  dietary, 747–748
  in ketogenesis, 525–526
  in parenteral nutrition, 779, 786
  propofol and, 748
  pseudohyponatremia and, 564t
Triiodothyronine, 795, 797–798, 801
Trimethoprim-sulfamethoxazole (TMP-SMX), 581t, 582
Triple-lumen central venous catheter, 5, 5f
Tris-hydroxymethyl aminomethane (THAM), 525
Trophic feedings, 759
Troponin(s)
  in acute coronary syndromes, 354–356
  in pulmonary embolism, 388–389
Trousseau's sign, 602
TSH. *See* Thyroid-stimulating hormone
4Ts score, 213, 213t
TTE. *See* Transthoracic echocardiography
TTP. *See* Thiamine pyrophosphate; Thrombotic thrombocytopenic purpura
Tube feedings. *See* Enteral nutrition
Tube thoracostomy, 469
Tumor lysis syndrome, 581, 600t, 607
23.4% sodium chloride, 162, 163f
TXA. *See* Tranexamic acid
Tylenol. *See* Acetaminophen (paracetamol)
Type and cross, 196
Type and hold, 196
Type and screen, 196

U

UA. *See* Unstable angina
Ulcer(s)
  pressure, 101
  stress, 45–51 (*See also* Stress ulcer)
Ultrasound
  of acalculous cholecystitis, 93, 641–642
  of acute kidney injury, 545
  of airway, 27
  of biliary-related acute pancreatitis, 634
  in cardiac arrest, 379, 379f

in ECMO-related limb
    ischemia, 499–500
of femoral vein, 11
in fever assessment, 102
gastric, in RSII preparation,
    32, 33f
of heart (*See*
    Echocardiography)
of internal jugular vein, 8–10,
    10f
of pneumothorax, 13
point-of-care, 109, 545
rapid, for shock and
    hypotension, 109,
    110t
transcranial, in brain death,
    686
of venous air embolism, 16
venous duplex, of DVT/
    pulmonary embolism,
    389, 390f
of ventilator-associated
    pneumonia, 459t, 467
in viscoelastic monitoring,
    236
Ultrasound guidance, for
    thoracentesis, 468
Undifferentiated shock, 253
Unfractionated heparin
actions of, 54
for acute coronary
    syndromes, 362t
complications with, 55
dosing of, 55
low-dose, 55
neuraxial catheters and, 59,
    60t
for pulmonary embolism,
    393, 394f
reversal of, 718t, 719
thrombocytopenia risk with,
    212

for VTE prophylaxis, 53–55,
    54t
Uniform Determination of
    Death Act, 683
Units and conversions, 843
Universal donor red blood cells,
    197
Unstable angina (UA), 352–353
ECG findings in, 354
management of, 358
Urea, fractional excretion of,
    545t, 546
Uremia, delirium in, 668–669
Urinary catheter. *See* Indwelling
    urinary catheter
Urinary crystals, in ethylene
    glycol intoxication, 833,
    833f
Urinary indices, for acute
    kidney injury, 545–546,
    545t
Urinary magnesium test, 594,
    594t
Urinary tract infections (UTIs),
    655–665
asymptomatic bacteriuria
    vs., 655
candidal, 661–663
catheter-associated, 656–661
ICU (nosocomial), 98, 655
Urine
hypotonic, in diabetes
    insipidus, 561
magnesium in, 589–590, 590f
potassium in, 576, 577, 578f,
    580
sodium concentration in,
    545–546, 545t, 559t, 564
Urine alkalinization, 821, 821t
Urine osmolality
in diabetes insipidus, 545t,
    561

Urine osmolality (*Continued*)
  in hyponatremia, 543t, 562–566
  in syndrome of inappropriate ADH secretion, 565
Urticaria, transfusion-related, 201–202, 224, 226, 226t
UTIs. *See* Urinary tract infections

V

V_t. *See* Tidal volume
VA. *See* Alveolar ventilation
VA ECMO. *See* Venoarterial ECMO
Vagal maneuvers, 339
Valium. *See* Diazepam
Valproic acid, 692t, 693
Valsalva maneuver, 339
Vancomycin, 644, 645t
VAP. *See* Ventilator-associated pneumonia
Variceal hemorrhage, 614, 623–624
  management of, 623–624, 624t
  Minnesota tube for, 623–624
  portosystemic shunt for, 623, 623f
  SBTube for, 623–624, 625f
Vascular resistance. *See also* Pulmonary vascular resistance; Systemic vascular resistance
  PA-catheter measurement of, 144t, 146–147
Vasoconstriction
  in heart failure, 317–318
  in shock, 255
Vasoconstrictors, for cardiogenic shock, 282

Vasodilators, for heart failure, 319, 320t, 324–325
Vasogenic edema, 715
Vasoplegia, 296, 299, 301
Vasopressin. *See* Antidiuretic hormone
Vasopressors
  acidosis/bicarbonate and, 524–525
  for acute pancreatitis, 636–637
  for cardiogenic shock, 282
  for delayed cerebral ischemia, 723
  for ischemic stroke, 712
  for post-cardiac arrest patients, 381t, 382
  for right heart failure, 325
  for septic shock, 300t, 301, 302t
  for venovenous ECMO support, 490
VATS. *See* Video-assisted thoracoscopic surgery
VCO_2. *See* Carbon dioxide (CO_2) production
VCV. *See* Volume control ventilation
VDUS. *See* Venous duplex ultrasonography
Vecuronium, 704
Velocity-time interval (VTI), 119, 119f, 280
Vena cava filters, 58–59, 58f, 396–397, 737t
Venoarterial ECMO (VA ECMO), 486, 492–502
  for cardiogenic shock, 289–290, 492–495
  comparison with other ECMO techniques, 502t

complications of, 290, 497–500, 501t
contraindications to, 495t
differential hypoxemia in, 497–499, 500f
in extracorporeal cardiopulmonary resuscitation, 376, 376t, 501–502
general management considerations in, 498t–499t
indications for, 492–495, 495t
initial settings for, 496
lower extremity ischemia in, 499–500
outcomes of, 290
physiology in, 495–497, 496f
retrograde flow in, consequences of, 496–497
tools for predicting survival in, 495
troubleshooting in, 497–500
weaning from, 501
Venous access, 1–22
cannulation sites for, 8–12
catheter location and placement for, 18–20, 18f, 19f
central, 5–12 (*See also* Central venous access)
complications of, 13–20
femoral vein, 11
for hemodialysis, 548–550, 550f
in hemorrhagic shock, 263
infection prevention in, 17t, 18
internal jugular vein, 8–10
in parenteral nutrition, 784–785
peripheral, 1–5 (*See also* Peripheral intravenous access)
purposes of, 1
subclavian vein, 10–11
Venous air embolism, 15–17, 15f
Venous capacitance, 178
Venous congestion, 117f, 318–322, 318f, 539
Venous duplex ultrasonography (VDUS), 389, 390f
Venous oxygen saturation, 127–128
cardiogenic shock and, 281
central, 127–128, 193, 248t, 251–252, 252t, 300
interpretation of measures, 252t
mixed, 127–128, 248t, 251, 252t, 281, 300
normal and hypoxic measures of, 248t
septic shock and, 300
Venous return
central venous pressure and, 178–179, 179f
determinants of, 177–178
fluid resuscitation and, 177–179
passive leg raising and, 180
Venous stasis, 53
Venous thromboembolism (VTE), 52–63. See *also* Deep venous thrombosis; Pulmonary embolism
anticoagulant prophylaxis for, 53–56, 54t, 59t
catheter-related, 14, 17
epidemiology of, 52
fever with, 92

Venous thromboembolism (VTE) (*Continued*)
- mechanical aids for, 56–57, 56f
- myasthenia gravis and, 697
- percutaneous interventional procedures for, 59
- risk factors for, 52–53
- subarachnoid hemorrhage and, 721
- traumatic brain injury and, 737t
- vena cava filters for, 58–59, 58f

Venovenous ECMO (VV ECMO), 486–492
- for acute respiratory distress syndrome, 427
- calculators predicting survival with, 486
- carbon dioxide removal in, 489
- chatter and suck-down in, 490–492
- comparison with other ECMO techniques, 502t
- contraindications to, 487t
- general management considerations in, 491t–492t
- hemodynamics in, 490
- indications for, 486, 487t
- oxygenation in, 489
- physiology in, 486–487, 488f
- refractory hypoxemia in, 492, 493t
- troubleshooting in, 490–492
- weaning from, 492, 494t

Ventilation
- mechanical (*See* Mechanical ventilation)
- minute, 443, 506–508
- noninvasive (*See* Noninvasive ventilation)

Ventilation-perfusion (V/Q) lung scan, 390–391

Ventilator-associated pneumonia (VAP), 98, 454–473
- antimicrobial therapy for, 465–466, 466t, 467t
- blood cultures in, 460
- bronchoalveolar lavage in, 462–464, 467t
- chest radiography of, 458–459, 459t
- clinical manifestations of, 458–460, 459t
- common isolates in, 454, 455t
- community-acquired pneumonia *vs.*, 454
- culture thresholds for diagnosis of, 467t
- definition of, 454
- endotracheal aspirates in, 461–462, 463t, 467t
- general information on, 454
- Gram stain in, 460–461
- incidence of, 454
- intrapleural fibrinolysis in, 469
- invasive specimen sampling in, 462
- lung biopsy in, 462, 465t, 467t
- microbiological evaluation of, 460–464
- mortality rate in, 454, 466
- MRSA polymerase chain reaction in, 461
- parapneumonic effusions in, 467–469, 468t

prevention of, 455–458, 738t
  clearing subglottic secretions for, 457, 457f
  routine airway care for, 456
  routine oral hygiene for, 455–456, 456f
  selective decontamination for, 456
  ventilator bundles for, 457–458, 458t
protected brush specimen in, 464, 465f, 467t
qualitative cultures in, 461, 463t
quantitative cultures in, 461–462, 463t, 464, 465t
signs and symptoms of, 458, 459t
simple take-home for diagnosis of, 460
surgical drainage in, 469
thoracentesis in, 468–469
Ventilator bundles, 457–458, 458t
Ventricular dysrhythmia, central venous access and, 13
Ventricular fibrillation, 376
Ventricular filling (preload), 153, 176–177, 177f
Ventricular tachycardia (VT), 331–332, 331f, 340–343
  cardioversion for, 341f, 342
  diagnosis of, 340–341
  ECG findings of, 331–332, 331f, 340–341
  hypomagnesemia and, 342–343, 592
  management of, 341–342, 341f, 343
  pulseless, 376

Verapamil, 333–335, 338
Versed. *See* Midazolam
VExUS score, 117f, 119
Video-assisted thoracoscopic surgery (VATS), 469
Video laryngoscopy, 37
Virchow, Rudolf, 52
Virchow's triad, 52, 52t
Viscoelastic monitoring, 231–236, 232f, 233f, 234t, 235f
Vital signs, in shock, 253–255
Vitamin(s)
  in parenteral nutrition, 780
  requirements for, 748–750
Vitamin B1. *See* Thiamine
Vitamin D
  in calcium metabolism, 598
  deficiency of, 749–750
  recommended daily intake of, 750
Vitamin deficiencies, 748–750
Vitamin K, 225, 270
Vitamin K antagonist (VKA)-associated hemorrhage, 270
Vivonex, 761
VO_2. *See* Oxygen uptake
Volatile anesthetics, malignant hyperthermia with, 94, 94t
Volume control ventilation (VCV), 448–449, 449f, 450f
Volume distribution, 153–154, 154f
  colloid fluids and, 166, 166f
  crystalloid fluids and, 153–154, 155f
  osmotic activity and, 154, 556–558

Volume-pressure loop
  in asthma, 402, 403f, 413–414, 413f
  in COPD, 413–414, 413f
Volume support ventilation (VSV), 452t
Volutrauma, 422, 451
Vomiting, opioids and, 70
von Willebrand factor, 226–227, 238
VSV. *See* Volume support ventilation
VT. *See* Ventricular tachycardia
VTE. *See* Venous thromboembolism
VTI. *See* Velocity-time interval
VV ECMO. *See* Venovenous ECMO

W

"W's," of postoperative fever, 97–98, 97t
Warfarin (Coumadin)
  for atrial fibrillation, 336, 337t
  for heparin-induced thrombocytopenia, 214
  reversal of, 225, 237–238, 238t, 718–719, 718t
Warming blankets, 268, 268f
Washed red blood cells, 194t, 196, 202
Weaning, from external ventricular drain, 733
Weaning, from mechanical ventilation, 474–485
  cardiac assessment in, 479
  cardiac dysfunction in, 478–479
  extubation in, 481–483
  readiness evaluation for, 474, 474t
  respiratory muscle weakness and, 479–481
  spontaneous breathing trial for, 475–478, 475t, 476f
  spontaneous breathing trial failure and, 478–481, 480f
Weaning, from venoarterial ECMO, 501
Weaning, from venovenous ECMO, 492, 494t
Weaning-induced pulmonary edema (WIPO), 478
Wedge pressure. *See* Pulmonary artery wedge pressure
Weight, predicted body
  for females, 845
  for males, 844
Wernicke encephalopathy, 591, 676–678, 748–749
Westermark sign, 389
West Haven System, 620t
Wet beriberi, 748–749
White blood cell count (WBC), in fever assessment, 102
Whole blood
  for hemorrhagic shock, 265, 266t
  platelets separated from, 221
  transfusion of, 194–195, 194t
"Wick" systems, 658, 659f
Wide complex tachycardias, 331–332, 331f
WIPO. *See* Weaning-induced pulmonary edema
Withdrawal
  alcohol, 671–678
  gabapentin, 678

Wolff-Parkinson-White (WPW) syndrome, 336–337
Wood alcohol. *See* Methanol intoxication
Wound classification, 649t
Wound infections
　necrotizing, 99
　surgical site (postoperative), 99, 647–648, 649t

X
Xarelto. *See* Rivaroxaban

Z
Zika virus, 698
Zinc, 750t
Ziprasidone (Geodon), 83, 84–85, 85t, 672t
Zyprexa. *See* Olanzapine

NOTES

NOTES

NOTES

NOTES

NOTES

NOTES